VOLUME NINETY FOUR

ADVANCES IN PHARMACOLOGY

New Targets for the Treatment of Hypertension and Associated Diseases

VOLUME NINETY FOUR

ADVANCES IN PHARMACOLOGY

New Targets for the Treatment of Hypertension and Associated Diseases

Edited by

WILLIAM B. CAMPBELL

Department of Pharmacology and Toxicology,
Medical College of Wisconsin,
Milwaukee, WI, United States

JOHN D. IMIG

Drug Discovery Center,
Medical College of Wisconsin,
Milwaukee, WI, United States

ELSEVIER

ACADEMIC PRESS
An imprint of Elsevier

Academic Press is an imprint of Elsevier
50 Hampshire Street, 5th Floor, Cambridge, MA 02139, United States
525 B Street, Suite 1650, San Diego, CA 92101, United States
The Boulevard, Langford Lane, Kidlington, Oxford OX5 1GB, United Kingdom
125 London Wall, London, EC2Y 5AS, United Kingdom

First edition 2022

ISBN: 978-0-323-91087-3
ISSN: 1054-3589

Publisher: Zoe Kruze
Developmental Editor: Jhon Michael Peñano
Production Project Manager:
Vijayaraj Purushothaman
Cover Designer: Matthew Limbert

Typeset by STRAIVE, India

Contents

Contributors

Heather Alcala
Western University of Health Sciences, Pomona, CA, United States

Bradley T. Andresen
Western University of Health Sciences, Pomona, CA, United States

Dominique Brown
Western University of Health Sciences, Pomona, CA, United States

Massimiliano Camilli
Department of Cardiovascular Medicine, Fondazione Policlinico Universitario A. Gemelli IRCCS, Rome

Prasad Chunduri
School of Biomedical Sciences, The University of Queensland, Brisbane, QLD, Australia

A.H. Jan Danser
Department of Internal Medicine, Division of Vascular Disease and Pharmacology, Erasmus Medical Center, Erasmus University, Rotterdam, The Netherlands

Ghezal Froogh
Department of Pharmacology, New York Medical College School of Medicine, Valhalla, NY, United States

Victor Garcia
Department of Pharmacology, New York Medical College School of Medicine, Valhalla, NY, United States

Valentin K. Gribkoff
Section on Endocrinology, Department of Internal Medicine, Yale University School of Medicine, New Haven, CT; TheraStat LLC, Weston, MA, United States

John D. Imig
Drug Discovery Center, Medical College of Wisconsin, Milwaukee, WI, United States

Annika A. Jüttner
Department of Internal Medicine, Division of Vascular Disease and Pharmacology, Erasmus Medical Center, Erasmus University, Rotterdam, The Netherlands

Raouf A. Khalil
Vascular Surgery Research Laboratories, Division of Vascular and Endovascular Surgery, Brigham and Women's Hospital, Harvard Medical School, Boston, MA, United States

Michal Laniado Schwartzman
Department of Pharmacology, New York Medical College School of Medicine, Valhalla, NY, United States

Roberto Levi
Department of Pharmacology, Weill Cornell Medicine, New York, NY, United States

Scott P. Levick
Physiology and Pharmacology, West Virginia University, Morgantown, WV, United States

Pierantonio Menna
Department of Health Sciences, Campus Bio-Medico University and Fondazione Policlinico, Rome, Italy

Giorgio Minotti
Department of Medicine, Campus Bio-Medico University and Fondazione Policlinico, Rome, Italy

Peter Oelschlaeger
Western University of Health Sciences, Pomona, CA, United States

Shrey A. Patel
School of Biomedical Sciences, The University of Queensland, Brisbane, QLD, Australia

Anton J.M. Roks
Department of Internal Medicine, Division of Vascular Disease and Pharmacology, Erasmus Medical Center, Erasmus University, Rotterdam, The Netherlands

Salvatore Salomone
Department of Biomedical and Biotechnological Science, University of Catania, Catania, Italy

Emanuela Salvatorelli
Department of Medicine, Campus Bio-Medico University and Fondazione Policlinico, Rome, Italy

Maria Angela Sortino
Department of Biomedical and Biotechnological Science, University of Catania, Catania, Italy

Simona Federica Spampinato
Department of Biomedical and Biotechnological Science, University of Catania, Catania, Italy

Raymond J. Winquist
Alkermes Pharmaceuticals Inc., Waltham, MA, United States

HaiFeng Yang
Vascular Surgery Research Laboratories, Division of Vascular and Endovascular Surgery, Brigham and Women's Hospital, Harvard Medical School, Boston, MA, United States

CHAPTER ONE

The CYP/20-HETE/GPR75 axis in hypertension

Ghezal Froogh, Victor Garcia, and Michal Laniado Schwartzman*
Department of Pharmacology, New York Medical College School of Medicine, Valhalla, NY, United States
*Corresponding author: e-mail address: michal_schwartzman@nymc.edu

Contents

Abstract

20-Hydroxyeicosatetraenoic acid (20-HETE) is a bioactive lipid generated from the ω-hydroxylation of arachidonic acid (AA) by enzymes of the cytochrome P450 (CYP) family, primarily the CYP4A and CYP4F subfamilies. 20-HETE is most notably identified as a modulator of vascular tone, regulator of renal function, and a contributor to the onset and development of hypertension and cardiovascular disease. 20-HETE-mediated signaling promotes hypertension by sensitizing the vasculature to constrictor stimuli, inducing endothelial dysfunction, and potentiating vascular inflammation. These bioactions are driven by the activation of the G-protein coupled receptor 75 (GPR75), a 20-HETE receptor (20HR). Given the capacity of 20-HETE signaling to drive pro-hypertensive mechanisms, the CYP/20-HETE/GPR75 axis has the potential to be a significant therapeutic target for the treatment of hypertension and cardiovascular diseases associated with increases in blood pressure. In this chapter, we review 20-HETE-mediated cellular mechanisms that promote hypertension, highlight important data in humans such as genetic variants in the CYP genes that potentiate 20-HETE production and describe recent findings in humans with 20HR/GPR75

Advances in Pharmacology, Volume 94
ISSN 1054-3589
https://doi.org/10.1016/bs.apha.2022.02.003

mutations. Special emphasis is given to the 20HR and respective receptor blockers that have the potential to pave a path to translational and clinical studies for the treatment of 20-HETE-driven hypertension, and obesity/metabolic syndrome.

Abbreviations

17-ODYA	17-octadecynoic acid
1-ABT	1-aminobenzotriazole
20-HEDE	20-hydroxyeicosa-6(*Z*),15(*Z*)-dienoic acid
20-HEDGE	*N*-[20-hydroxyeicosa-6(*Z*),15(*Z*)-dienoyl]glycine
20-HETE	20-hydroxyeicosatetraenoic acid
20HR	20-HETE receptor
20HRBs	20-HETE receptor blockers
20-SOLA	[2,5,8,11,14,17-hexaoxanonadecan-19-yl 20-hydroxyicosa-6(Z),15(Z)-dienoate]
AA	arachidonic acid
AAA	*N*-disodium succinate-20-hydroxyeicosa-6(Z),15(Z)-diencarboxamide
ACE	angiotensin converting enzyme
Ang II	angiotensin II
AR	androgen receptors
ARB	angiotensin receptor blocker
AT1R	angiotensin type II receptor
BKca	Ca^{2+} activated K^{+} channels
CSA	cross sectional area
c-Src	Src-type tyrosine kinase
CYP	cytochrome P450
DDMS	dibromo-dodecenyl-methylsulfimide
DHT	dihydrotestosterone
DOCA	deoxycoricosterone
EETs	epoxyeicosatrienoic acids
EGFR	epidermal growth factor receptor
eNOS	endothelial nitric oxide synthase
FFAR-1	free fatty acid receptor 1
GPR40	G-protein coupled receptor 40
GPR75	G-protein coupled receptor 75
GSIS	glucose stimulated insulin secretion
HET-0016	N-hydroxy-N′-(4-butyl-2-methylphenyl)-formamidine
HIF-1α	hypoxia-inducible factor-1α
HSP90	heatschock protein 90
ICAM-1	intercellular cell adhesion molecule-1
IKK	inhibitor of kappa B kinase
MAPK	mitogen activated protein kinase
NE	norepinephrine
NFκB	nuclear factor kappa B
NHE3	sodium-hydrogen exchanger 3
NKCC2	Na-K-CL cotransporter 2
NO	nitric oxide

PKC	protein kinase C
pLOF	predicted loss of function
PPARs	peroxisome proliferator activated receptors
PT	proximal tubule
ROS	reactive oxygen species
SD	Sprague-Dawley
SNPs	single nucleotide polymorphisms
SPR	surface plasmon resonance
TALH	thick ascending limb of Henle
TGF-β	transforming growth factor β
TRPC6	transient receptor potential cation channel 6
VEGF	vascular endothelial growth factor
VEGFR2	vascular endothelial growth factor receptor 2
VSMCs	vascular smooth muscle cells

1. Introduction

The role of 20-hydroxyeicosatetraenoic acid (20-HETE) as a regulator of blood pressure first surfaced in 1981 with findings in three separate studies that arachidonic acid (AA) could be metabolized by cytochrome P450 (CYP) enzymes to generate a yet to be identified vasoactive lipid (Capdevila et al., 1981; Morrison & Pascoe, 1981; Oliw, Lawson, Brash, & Oates, 1981). Following this initial discovery, researchers identified several CYP enzymes that are differentially expressed in the kidneys of hypertensive rats, which correspond to the generation of, and promote elevations in, 20-HETE levels (Iwai & Inagami, 1991; Sacerdoti, Abraham, McGiff, & Schwartzman, 1988). The first study to link 20-HETE to blood pressure regulation was conducted by Sacerdoti et al. (Sacerdoti et al., 1989), demonstrating that depletion of CYP-derived AA metabolites reduced blood pressure in the spontaneously hypertensive rats. Since then, various studies have identified 20-HETE to mediate pro-hypertensive and pro-inflammatory signals. The mechanisms that drive these conditions include the activation of the renin-angiotensin system (RAS) through the induction and activation of angiotensin converting enzyme (ACE), the uncoupling of endothelial nitric oxide synthase (eNOS) and the promotion of pro-inflammatory mediators including reactive oxygen species (ROS), adhesion molecules and cytokines. With the discovery of the 20-HETE receptor

(20HR), G-protein coupled receptor 75 (GPR75), pharmacological targeting of 20-HETE signaling can be fine-tuned for the treatment of hypertension and cardiovascular disease.

2. 20-HETE biosynthesis, regulation, and metabolism

20-HETE is produced by the CYP4 family of enzymes, primarily by enzymes of the CYP4A and CYP4F subfamilies (Hardwick, 2008), all of which catalyze the hydroxylation of fatty acids including AA at the terminal carbons (ω/ω-1). The primary producers of 20-HETE in human tissues are the CYP4A11 and CYP4F2 isoforms (Hardwick, 2008; Lasker et al., 2000), while in rats the major isoforms are CYP4A1 and CYP4A2/4A3 (Helvig, Dishman, & Capdevila, 1998; Nguyen, Wang, Reddy, Falck, & Schwartzman, 1999; Xu, Falck, Ortiz de Montellano, & Kroetz, 2004), and CYP4a12 in mice (Holla et al., 2001; Muller et al., 2007). Expression of CYP4 enzymes are tightly regulated and influenced by transcriptional activators such as the peroxisome proliferator activated receptors (PPARs) and androgen receptor (AR), and undergo post-translational regulation by microRNAs (Hardwick, Osei-Hyiaman, Wiland, Abdelmegeed, & Song, 2009; Hiratsuka, Matsuura, Watanabe, Sato, & Suzuki, 1996; Rocic & Schwartzman, 2018; Wu, Gupta, Garcia, Ding, & Schwartzman, 2014). Moreover, both the transcription and translation of CYPs are influenced by diet and environmental factors (Gilani et al., 2018; Hardwick, 2008; Hardwick et al., 2013).

Known as an eicosanoid of the microcirculation, 20-HETE is synthesized across the vessel wall of resistant arteries, predominantly by vascular smooth muscle cells (VSMCs) (Gebremedhin et al., 1998; Harder et al., 1994; Marji, Wang, & Laniado-Schwartzman, 2002; Miyata & Roman, 2005) (Fig. 1). 20-HETE is also synthesized in other tissues including liver, brain, lung, heart, kidney, small intestine, pancreas, and conductive vessels (Capdevila, Falck, & Estabrook, 1992; Edson & Rettie, 2013; Macica, Balazy, Falck, Mioskowski, & Carroll, 1993; Schwartzman et al., 1990; Tunaru et al., 2018; Yousif, Benter, & Roman, 2009; Zhu, Zhang, Medhora, & Jacobs, 2002). Interestingly, the vascular endothelium except for the pulmonary endothelium (Zhu et al., 2002) does not generate 20-HETE under homeostasis, but activates the cellular machinery to synthesize 20-HETE under hypoxic conditions (Chen et al., 2016; Joseph et al., 2017). Peripheral blood myeloid and bone marrow cells (such as neutrophils, platelets, and endothelial progenitor cells) can also generate 20-HETE and

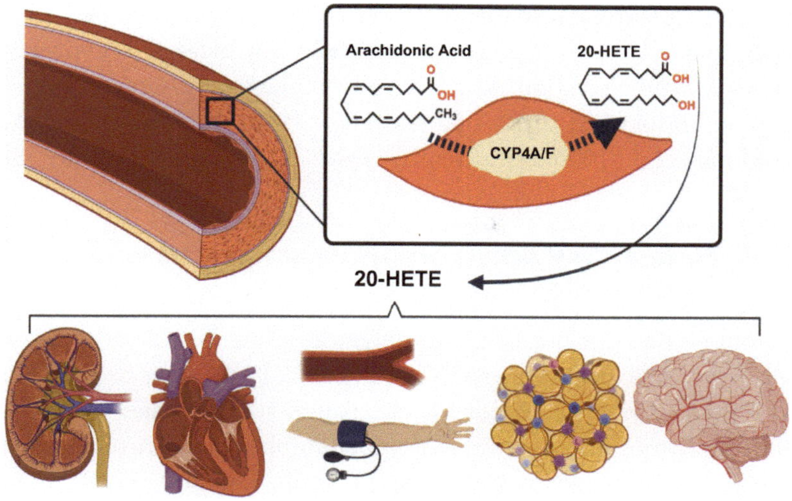

Fig. 1 20-HETE Synthesis and Target Organs. 20-HETE producing CYP isoforms CYP4A and CYP4F reside across the vasculature in vascular smooth muscle cells (VSMCs). 20-HETE elicits its bioactions across various target organs/tissues including the kidney, heart, brain and adipose. Elevation in 20-HETE is associated with the onset and development of hypertension, obesity, stroke and myocardial infarction.

contribute to its circulatory levels (Chen et al., 2014; Hill & Murphy, 1992; Rosolowsky, Falck, & Campbell, 1996; Tsai, Croft, Puddey, Beilin, & Barden, 2011).

The production of 20-HETE is stimulated by autocoids such as angiotensin II (Ang II), endothelin, and norepinephrine (NE) (Carroll et al., 1997; Croft, McGiff, Sanchez-Mendoza, & Carroll, 2000; Hercule & Oyekan, 2000; Lima, Yanes, Davis, & Reckelhoff, 2013; Ljuca & Drevensek, 2010; Speed, George, Arany, Cockrell, & Granger, 2011; Tsai et al., 2011; Uddin, Muthalif, Karzoun, Benter, & Malik, 1998). In addition, androgens are potent stimulators of 20-HETE production, a mechanism that involves transcriptional activation of CYP gene expression, as mentioned, via the AR (Wu & Schwartzman, 2011). Androgen-driven increases in 20-HETE synthesis through the use of dihydrotestosterone (DHT) is commonly utilized to study 20-HETE-dependent actions in vivo (Ding et al., 2013; Holla et al., 2001; Liu, Wu, Liu, Lai, & Zhao, 2012; Singh et al., 2007).

By contrast, nitric oxide (NO), superoxide, and carbon monoxide serve to inhibit 20-HETE production (Alonso-Galicia, Hudetz, Shen, Harder, & Roman, 1999; Minamiyama et al., 1997; Oyekan, Youseff, Fulton, Quilley, & McGiff, 1999; Sun et al., 1998; Wang et al., 2003).

Moreover, 20-HETE can be metabolized by cyclooxygenases, lipoxygenases, and CYP monooxygenases, as well as by alcohol dehydrogenase via a β-oxidation reaction to various metabolites with largely unknown bioactivity (Hill, Fitzpatrick, & Murphy, 1992; Kaduce et al., 2004; Rosolowsky et al., 1996; Schwartzman, Falck, Yadagiri, & Escalante, 1989).

3. Human CYP polymorphisms associated with hypertension

Numerous single nucleotide polymorphisms (SNPs) of the human 20-HETE producing enzymes, CYP4F2 and CYPA11, have been identified to correlate with hypertension in population-based studies. Among the CYP4F2 polymorphisms, the V433M polymorphism is positively associated with blood pressure and urinary 20-HETE levels (Fava et al., 2008; Hu et al., 2011; Munshi et al., 2012; Ward et al., 2008). The V433M isoform results from a guanine to adenosine missense mutation at nucleotide 1347 resulting in a valine to methionine substitution at amino acid 433 (Stec, Roman, Flasch, & Rieder, 2007). This polymorphism renders CYP4F2 inactive, thereby blunting CYP4F2-dependent 20-HETE production (Stec, Roman, et al., 2007). The hypothesis behind why the V433M polymorphism is associated with hypertension even though it results in a decrease in CYP4F2 activity may be due to a shift in 20-HETE production to alternate 20-HETE producing pathways. This is observed in Cyp4a14 knockout mice, which have elevated 20-HETE levels resulting from elevations in Cyp4a12 (Holla et al., 2001). Furthermore, male carriers of the V433M-allele present with higher diastolic blood pressure compared to females, indicating a sex-dependent characteristic in this allele (Fava, Ricci, Melander, & Minuz, 2012).

With regard to CYP4A11 polymorphisms, one of the major genetic variants is T8590C. T8590C results from a thymidine to cytosine substitution at nucleotide 8590, resulting in a phenylalanine to serine substitution at amino acid 434, the functional consequence of which is a reduction in the catalytic activity of the CYP4A11 enzyme (Gainer et al., 2005). T8590C has been correlated with hypertension, but the evidence is inconclusive due to contradictory reports. For example, multiple studies have reported T8590C to be associated with an increased risk of hypertension in certain ethnic groups but not others (Gainer et al., 2005, 2008; Lino Cardenas et al., 2012; Mayer et al., 2005). One study, in particular, did not report any differences in systolic or diastolic blood pressure among carriers of the T8590C variant (Ward et al., 2008), highlighting the need for additional research on the contribution of T8590C to the development of hypertension.

4. The 20-HETE receptors

Decades of research exploring the cellular mechanisms driven by 20-HETE across endothelial cells and VSMCs have identified several key signaling pathways to be at the forefront of the pro-inflammatory and pro-hypertensive actions of 20-HETE. In endothelial cells, 20-HETE-dependent uncoupling of eNOS, reduction in NO bioavailability, induction of endothelial ACE expression and increases in circulating Ang II levels are all mediated via an epidermal growth factor receptor (EGFR)-mitogen activated protein kinase (MAPK)-inhibitor of κB kinase (IKKβ)-nuclear factor (NF) κB-dependent pathway (Fig. 2) (Cheng et al., 2012, 2008, 2010; Garcia, Shkolnik, Milhau, Falck, & Schwartzman, 2016). In VSMCs, 20-HETE sensitization of the contractile apparatus is mediated via inhibition of the BKca channel and activation of the L-type Ca channel (Miyata & Roman, 2005; Randriamboavonjy, Busse, & Fleming, 2003; Zou et al., 1996). These extensively studied signaling pathways hinted at the presence of a G-protein coupled receptor, which was identified by Garcia and colleagues to be GPR75, a member of the Gq-coupled Rhodopsin subfamily of receptors (Tarttelin et al., 1999). GPR75 is a high affinity 20HR essential for the binding of 20-HETE and activation of these downstream signals (Garcia et al., 2017; Pascale et al., 2021). GPR75 is expressed in various tissues including the vasculature, liver, eye, kidney, lung, brain and beyond (Garcia et al., 2017). In a mouse model of 20-HETE-dependent hypertension, the increase in blood pressure is prevented and reversed by knocking down GPR75, further strengthening the notion that 20-HETE binding to its receptor is necessary for eliciting its action (Garcia et al., 2017).

Interestingly, studies examining glucose stimulated insulin secretion (GSIS) in pancreatic islets in mice have observed the emerging role of a new receptor that binds 20-HETE. G-protein coupled receptor 40 (GPR40), known as a free fatty acid receptor (FFAR-1) has been shown to bind 20-HETE, with low affinity, that serves to amplify GSIS responses (Tunaru et al., 2018). This lipid-receptor is not exclusive to 20-HETE as it also binds various fatty acids including epoxyeicosatrienoic acids (EETs)

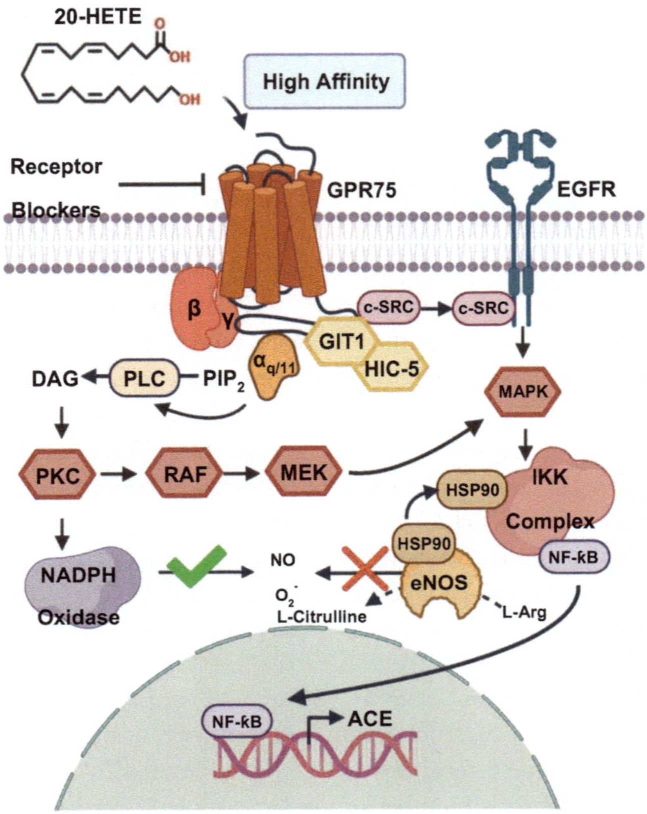

Fig. 2 20-HETE Receptor (GPR75) Signaling in Endothelial Cells. The binding to and activation of the 20-HETE receptor (GPR75) via 20-HETE leads to Gαq/11 driven signaling and the transactivation of the epidermal growth factor receptor (EGFR) via a GIT1 –/ c-SRC-dependent pathway that stimulates the activation of MAPK and the IKK complex. Activated IKK initiates two events; firstly, IKK triggers the translocation of NF-KB to the nucleus where it binds the promotor region of the angiotensin converting enzyme (ACE) gene leading to the increased transcription of ACE. Secondly, IKK activation promotes the endothelial nitric oxide synthase (eNOS) uncoupling through recruitment of the chaperone protein HSP90 away from eNOS resulting in decreased nitric oxide (NO) bioavailability. Moreover, 20-HETE receptor signaling promotes the activation protein kinase C (PKC) driven mechanisms including increases in NADPH oxidase-derived ROS generation. Taken together, these signaling events promote endothelial dysfunction and initiate pro-inflammatory signaling pathways that promote the development of hypertension and inflammation.

with a similar low affinity (Grundmann, Bender, Schamberger, & Eitner, 2021; Park et al., 2018; Tunaru et al., 2018). Thus far, there has not been a role for the 20-HETE/GPR40 pairing in the context of vascular function or hypertension.

5. 20-HETE and the kidney in hypertension

In the kidney, 20-HETE plays an important role in the regulation of the pressure natriuretic response (Ito et al., 2006; Williams et al., 2007). This normal physiological response, which results in the increase in renal sodium excretion in response to rising arterial pressure to the kidneys, is significantly impaired with inhibitors of 20-HETE synthesis (Ito et al., 2006; Williams, Sarkis, et al., 2007). Within the kidney, 20-HETE is synthesized in the proximal tubule (PT), medullary thick ascending limb of Henle (TALH), the glomerulus and the vasculature (Imig et al., 1996; Ito & Roman, 1999; Lin, Abraham, & Schwartzman, 1994; Omata, Abraham, & Schwartzman, 1992; Schwartzman, Ferreri, Carroll, Songu-Mize, & McGiff, 1985). 20-HETE inhibits Na-K-ATPase activity and the internalization of the sodium-hydrogen exchanger 3 (NHE3) in the PT (Nowicki et al., 1997; Ribeiro, Dubay, Falck, & Mandel, 1994) and prevents K efflux and Na uptake via the Na-K-Cl cotransporter 2 (NKCC2) in the medullary TALH (Escalante, Erlij, Falck, & McGiff, 1994; Wang & Lu, 1995). In the glomerulus, 20-HETE is essential for the maintenance of a glomerular filtration barrier to albumin by preventing transforming growth factor (TGF-β)-mediated glomerular injury in hypertension (Dahly-Vernon et al., 2005; Luo et al., 2009; Williams, Sharma, Anjaiahh, Falck, & Roman, 2007). 20-HETE increases constriction of the afferent arteriole in response to elevations in perfusion pressure. Blockade of 20-HETE formation diminishes the vasoconstrictor response to both elevations in transmural pressure and is believed to be a mediator of tubulo-glomerular feedback responses (Zhao, Inscho, Bondlela, Falck, & Imig, 2001; Zou et al., 1994).

Importantly, in Lewis rats inhibition of 20-HETE synthesis elevates blood pressure and sodium reabsorption through mechanisms that involve the medullary thick ascending limbs and outer medullary regions (Stec, Mattson, & Roman, 1997; Zou, Drummond, & Roman, 1996). In the Dahl salt-sensitive, deoxycorticosterone acetate (DOCA)-salt and high-fat-induced hypertensive rats stimulation of renal 20-HETE production lowers blood pressure (Honeck et al., 2000; Wilson, Alonso-Galicia, & Roman, 1998; Zhou et al., 2006). Interestingly, polymorphisms in the CYP4A11 gene associated with a significant reduction in its catalytic activity are correlated with decreases in urinary excretion of 20-HETE and the development of salt-sensitive hypertension in humans (Laffer et al., 2008; Williams, Hopkins, Jeunemaitre, & Brown, 2011). Taken together these findings are evidence of the reno-protective actions of 20-HETE that are disrupted with inhibition of 20-HETE in the tubular regions of the kidney.

In contrast, mice expressing the human CYP4A11 under the control of its native promoter are hypertensive (Savas et al., 2016); these studies have identified CYP4A11 and 20-HETE as potential risk factors for salt-sensitive human hypertension by perturbation of the renal renin-angiotensin axis. Likewise, overexpressing the dominant 20-HETE synthase in mice (Cyp4a12) across the proximal tubule increases 20-HETE synthesis in this region and promotes salt-sensitive hypertension (Gilani et al., 2020). Interestingly, in two-kidney one clip Goldblatt hypertensive rats and in Ren-2 transgenic rats, where the resultant hypertension is due to the continuous activation of the RAS and is Ang II-dependent, urinary excretion of 20-HETE is significantly increased and inhibition of 20-HETE synthesis attenuates the development of hypertension (Certikova Chabova et al., 2010; Walkowska et al., 2010). Thus, the inhibition of 20-HETE production in the kidney can lead to hypertension due to disruption of the pressure natriuretic mechanism, while 20-HETE overproduction in the kidney can promote hypertension due to exacerbation of its pro-hypertensive effects across the vasculature.

6. 20-HETE, vascular smooth muscle cells (VSMCs) and hypertension

As previously mentioned, VSMCs are one of the primary sites for 20-HETE synthesis. The autocrine bioactions of 20-HETE are multifaceted and influence the sensitization of the vasculature to vasoconstrictors such as Ang II, NE, and endothelin (Hercule & Oyekan, 2000; Imig et al., 1996; Kohagura et al., 2001; Zhang et al., 2001). The sensitization to vasoconstrictor stimuli by 20-HETE is mediated by multiple mechanisms; firstly, 20-HETE signaling facilitates phosphorylation, and therefore inhibition, of the Ca^{2+} activated K^{+} channels (BKca) by protein kinase C (PKC), MAPK, and Src-type tyrosine kinases (c-Src), leading to VSMC depolarization (Garcia & Schwartzman, 2017; Miyata & Roman, 2005). This process has been shown to require the presence and activation of the 20HR/GPR75 (Garcia et al., 2017). Consequently, the fall in membrane potential also increases calcium efflux via voltage-gated L type Ca^{2+} channels and transient receptor potential cation channel 6 (TRPC6), a non-voltage-gated Ca^{2+} entry/depolarization channel, leading to vasoconstriction and contributing to myogenic tone (Inoue et al., 2009). 20-HETE can further promote VSMC contraction by increasing Rho-kinase activity and promoting the phosphorylated state of myosin light chain, thereby enhancing the sensitivity of the contractile apparatus (Randriamboavonjy et al., 2003). In addition to sensitizing the VSMC to constrictor stimuli, thus enhancing vascular reactivity and blood pressure, 20-HETE signaling increases mitochondrial superoxide/ROS (Lakhkar et al., 2016), as well as promotes VSMC migration and proliferation (Muthalif et al., 2001; Stec, Gannon, Beaird, & Drummond, 2007), actions that can significantly contribute to vascular remodeling in hypertension (Ding et al., 2013; Garcia et al., 2015; Yaghini et al., 2005). There is also evidence that 20-HETE of smooth muscle origin can affect endothelial function. Study by Jiang et al. (Jiang et al., 2004) demonstrated that smooth muscle-specific CYP4A2 overexpression promotes capillary growth by stimulating endothelial cell proliferation.

7. 20-HETE, endothelial cell dysfunction and activation

While the vascular endothelium is not a common source of 20-HETE synthesis, it is a major cellular target for 20-HETE's bioactions. 20-HETE promotes endothelial dysfunction through the uncoupling eNOS from its chaperone protein, heat shock protein 90 (HSP90), which in turn reduces NO bioavailability. This results in impaired endothelial-dependent vasorelaxation and potentiates the generation of pro-hypertensive and pro-fibrotic signals driven by reductions in both eNOS activity and NO (Cheng et al., 2012, 2008). 20-HETE also stimulates superoxide formation in endothelial cells and elicits increases in vascular endothelial growth factor (VEGF) synthesis (Guo et al., 2007; Medhora et al., 2008). Additionally, elevations in 20-HETE are closely associated with endothelial cell activation, indicated by increases in endothelial expression of adhesion molecules including intracellular cell adhesion molecule 1 (ICAM-1) and the synthesis of inflammatory cytokines IL-6, IL-8 and TNFα (Hoopes, Garcia, Edin, Schwartzman, & Zeldin, 2015; Ishizuka et al., 2008). Interestingly, hypoxia drives endothelial cell CYP expression and subsequent 20-HETE levels, a process that is vital for ischemia-induced angiogenesis. This process requires the synthesis and presence of 20-HETE which drives changes in hypoxia-inducible factor-1 α (HIF-1α), VEGF and VEGF receptor 2 (VEGFR2) in ischemic tissues (Chen, Ackerman, & Guo, 2012; Chen et al., 2014, 2016; Guo et al., 2009).

8. 20-HETE and the renin angiotensin system (RAS)

The RAS is a key regulator of blood pressure and vascular function that is tightly regulated by various enzymes across several effector tissues. Studies by Inoue et al. (Inoue et al., 2009) demonstrates that long-term endothelial CYP4A overexpression in Sprague-Dawley (SD) rats augments 20-HETE levels, resulting in endothelial dysfunction, hypertension, and renal injury. Follow-up studies by Sodhi et al. (Sodhi et al., 2010) found that the elevation in blood pressure was attenuated by administration of an ACE inhibitor (Lisinopril) or an angiotensin type II receptor (AT1R) blocker (losartan). Interestingly, blood pressure rebounds once treatment ends, indicating a 20-HETE-dependent activation of RAS. Indeed, endothelial-specific overexpression of CYP4A increased expression of ACE and AT1R, as well as plasma and tissue Ang II levels (Sodhi et al., 2010). These outcomes were counteracted by treatment with HET-0016, a non-specific inhibitor of 20-HETE synthesis. This is in agreement with studies demonstrating that 20-HETE activates both the transcription and activity of ACE in endothelial cells (Cheng et al., 2012; Garcia et al., 2016). As mentioned previously, the increase in ACE expression by 20-HETE is mediated through transactivation of the EGFR that promotes downstream signals, culminating in the translocation of the transcription factor NF-κB into the nucleus (Akbulut et al., 2009; Garcia et al., 2016). The translocation of NF-κB then elicits the activation of the ACE promoter region, thus driving gene expression, which sets the stage for elevations in Ang II and blood pressure in a feed forward mechanism.

9. 20-HETE and vascular remodeling

Persistent elevations in blood pressure promote a host of cardiovascular changes across the vasculature including dynamic changes to the vascular wall in the form of vascular remodeling. Vascular remodeling is characterized by increases in media thickness, media: lumen and cross sectional area (CSA). Increases in vascular remodeling have been observed in multiple rodent studies that utilized several models of 20-HETE-dependent hypertension (Ding et al., 2013; Garcia et al., 2017, 2015). Interestingly, while the prevention and normalization of 20-HETE-driven increases in blood pressure can be achieved by targeting the RAS, such as with lisinopril or losartan, these drugs fail to prevent 20-HETE-dependent changes in media thickness, media: lumen and CSA. In these studies, 20-HETE antagonism and the knockdown of the 20HR/GPR75 in vivo prevented any changes in blood pressure and vascular remodeling (Ding et al., 2013; Garcia et al., 2017, 2015). Therefore, 20-HETE-dependent vascular remodeling can occur in the presence of normalized blood pressure, suggesting that patients presently prescribed an ACE inhibitor or AT1 receptor blocker (ARB) may have persistent increases in vascular remodeling without any intervention targeting the 20-HETE-GPR75 axis.

10. 20-HETE and cardio-metabolic disease

In addition to its potent role in the regulation of blood pressure, 20-HETE impairs insulin signaling, and consequently can contribute to obesity and obesity-driven hypertension. In studies by Gilani et al. (Gilani et al., 2021, 2018) high-fat diet fed mice overexpressing the dominant 20-HETE producing enzyme, cyp4a12, exhibited greater rate of weight gain, were hyperglycemic and had impaired glucose metabolism compared to control animals. Moreover, *Gpr75* null mice are protected from high-fat diet-driven adiposity and insulin resistance (Akbari et al., 2021). Interestingly in humans, several predicted loss of function (pLOF) GPR75 variants are associated with leanness and protection from obesity (Akbari et al., 2021). These studies highlight the significance of GPR75 in the regulation of blood pressure, as well as provides evidence for the importance of GPR75-dependent signaling in cardio-metabolic disease, a research niche that is ripe for in-depth scientific exploration.

11. 20-HETE synthesis inhibitors and 20-HETE receptor blockers (20HRBs)

The potent actions of 20-HETE have continuously prompted researchers to develop pharmacological agents that target either the synthesis of 20-HETE via CYP inhibitors/inducers or the actions of 20-HETE via receptor blockers/antagonists. The first wave of agents seeking to target 20-HETE synthesis were ketoconazole, and miconazole. These compounds, however, are non-specific and inhibit the production of other eicosanoids and numerous CYP enzymes (Roman & Fan, 2018). Similar results are observed with 1-Aminobenzotriazole (1-ABT) and 17-octadecynoic acid (17-ODYA), which also block the formation of EETs along with 20-HETE (Ortiz de Montellano & Reich, 1984). Subsequent strides went on to develop the formamide derivative N-hydroxy-N′-(4-butyl-2-methylphenyl)-formamidine (HET-0016). HET-0016's mechanism of action is through a non-competitive, irreversible inhibition of CYP4As, thus preventing omega hydroxylation (Miyata et al., 2001). Recently, TS-011, a more potent analog of HET0016 has been developed, but is currently not widely used across rodent studies (Marumo, Eto, Wake, Omura, & Nabekura, 2010). Thus far, the most selective 20-HETE synthesis inhibitor is dibromo-dodecenyl-methylsulfimide (DDMS) with a 10-fold selectivity for CYP4A11, which minimally influences the synthesis of EETs (Chen et al., 2019; Wang et al., 1998).

In addition to the 20-HETE synthesis inhibitors, there is an ever-growing list of 20-HETE receptor blockers (20HRBs), previously referred to as 20-HETE antagonists, that are undergoing characterization across various small animal models. The first generation of 20-HETE antagonists include 20-hydroxyeicosa-6(*Z*),15(*Z*)-dienoic acid (20-HEDE) and *N*-[20-hydroxyeicosa-6(*Z*),15(*Z*)-dienoyl]glycine (20-HEDGE) (Alonso-Galicia, Falck, Reddy, & Roman, 1999; Regner et al., 2009). Like 20-HETE, 20-HEDE and 20-HEDGE are lipid derived analogues that maintain many of the same hydrophobic properties of 20-HETE and therefore are not water soluble. Next, two water soluble compounds [2,5,8,11,14,17-hexaoxanonadecan-19-yl 20-hydroxyicosa-6(Z),15(Z)-dienoate] (20-SOLA) and N-disodium succinate-20-hydroxyeicosa-6(Z),15(Z)-diencarboxamide (AAA) were developed that can block 20-HETE binding and activity in vitro (Cardenas et al., 2019; Pascale et al., 2021) and in vivo (Gilani et al., 2021, 2018; Pandey et al., 2017; Savas et al., 2016). Evidence for the efficacy of AAA to bind directly to the 20HR has been confirmed in surface plasmon resonance (SPR) binding studies (Pascale et al., 2021), setting the stage for the characterization and development of future 20HRBs.

12. Conclusion

Hypertension is a multifaceted disease driven by a complex etiology. A mix of environmental and genetic factors contribute to the onset and progression of hypertension, of which the molecular mechanisms have yet to be fully elucidated. Extensive studies in our lab and others have identified 20-HETE as one of the key mechanistic contributors to the development of hypertension, and related cardiovascular diseases (Fig. 3). The recent discovery of GPR75 as the 20HR provides researchers with a key and specific

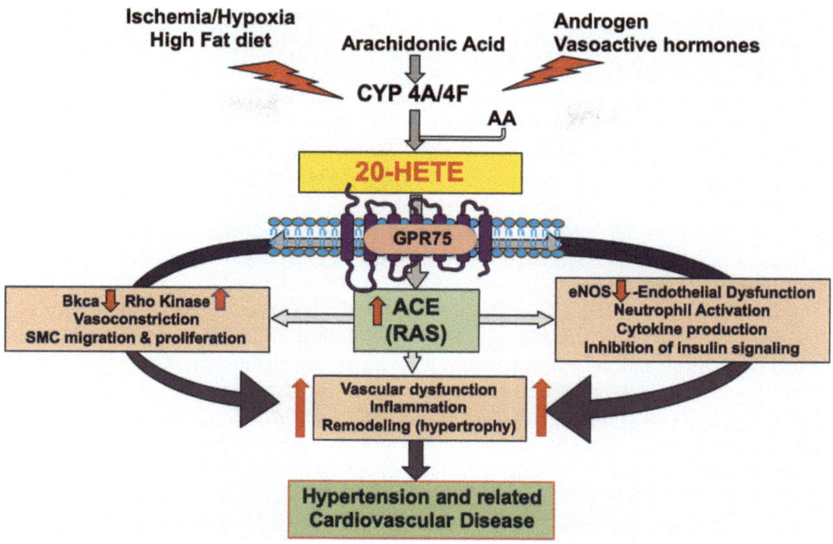

Fig. 3 The postulated outcomes of 20-HETE-GPR75 pairing in the vasculature and its contribution to hypertension and related cardiovascular diseases.

therapeutic target for drug development to treat hypertension and its associated vascular and cardiac complications.

Conflict of interest statement

The authors have no conflicts of interest to declare.

References

Akbari, P., Gilani, A., Sosina, O., Kosmicki, J. A., Khrimian, L., Fang, Y. Y., et al. (2021). Sequencing of 640,000 exomes identifies GPR75 variants associated with protection from obesity. *Science*, *373*(6550). https://doi.org/10.1126/science.abf8683.

Akbulut, T., Regner, K. R., Roman, R. J., Avner, E. D., Falck, J. R., & Park, F. (2009). 20-HETE activates the Raf/MEK/ERK pathway in renal epithelial cells through an EGFR- and c-Src-dependent mechanism. *American Journal of Physiology. Renal Physiology*, *297*(3), F662–F670. https://doi.org/10.1152/ajprenal.00146.2009.

Alonso-Galicia, M., Falck, J. R., Reddy, K. M., & Roman, R. J. (1999). 20-HETE agonists and antagonists in the renal circulation. *The American Journal of Physiology*, *277*(5 Pt 2), F790–F796.

Alonso-Galicia, M., Hudetz, A. G., Shen, H., Harder, D. R., & Roman, R. J. (1999). Contribution of 20-HETE to vasodilator actions of nitric oxide in the cerebral microcirculation. *Stroke*, *30*(12), 2727–2734, discussion 2734.

Capdevila, J. H., Falck, J. R., & Estabrook, R. W. (1992). Cytochrome P450 and the arachidonate cascade. *The FASEB Journal*, *6*(2), 731–736. https://doi.org/10.1096/fasebj.6.2.1537463.

Capdevila, J., Parkhill, L., Chacos, N., Okita, R., Masters, B. S. S., & Estabrook, R. W. (1981). The oxidative metabolism of arachidonic acid by purified cytochrome P-450. *Biochemical and Biophysical Research Communications, 101*, 1357–1363.

Cardenas, S., Colombero, C., Panelo, L., Dakarapu, R., Falck John, R., Costas Monica, A., et al. (2019). GPR75 receptor mediates 20-HETE-signaling and metastatic features of androgen-insensitive prostate cancer cells. *Biochimica et Biophysica Acta - Molecular and Cell Biology of Lipids, 1865*, 158573–158580. https://doi.org/10.1016/j.bbalip.2019.158573.

Carroll, M. A., Balazy, M., Huang, D. D., Rybalova, S., Falck, J. R., & McGiff, J. C. (1997). Cytochrome P450-derived renal HETEs: Storage and release. *Kidney International, 51*(6), 1696–1702. https://doi.org/10.1038/ki.1997.234.

Certikova Chabova, V., Walkowska, A., Kompanowska-Jezierska, E., Sadowski, J., Kujal, P., Vernerova, Z., et al. (2010). Combined inhibition of 20-hydroxy-eicosatetraenoic acid formation and of epoxyeicosatrienoic acids degradation attenuates hypertension and hypertension-induced end-organ damage in ren-2 transgenic rats. *Clinical Science (London, England), 118*(10), 617–632. https://doi.org/10.1042/cs20090459.

Chen, L., Ackerman, R., & Guo, A. M. (2012). 20-HETE in neovascularization. *Prostaglandins & Other Lipid Mediators, 98*(3–4), 63–68. https://doi.org/10.1016/j.prostaglandins.2011.12.005.

Chen, L., Ackerman, R., Saleh, M., Gotlinger, K. H., Kessler, M., Mendelowitz, L. G., et al. (2014). 20-HETE regulates the angiogenic functions of human endothelial progenitor cells and contributes to angiogenesis in vivo. *The Journal of Pharmacology and Experimental Therapeutics, 348*(3), 442–451. https://doi.org/10.1124/jpet.113.210120.

Chen, L., Joseph, G., Zhang, F. F., Nguyen, H., Jiang, H., Gotlinger, K. H., et al. (2016). 20-HETE contributes to ischemia-induced angiogenesis. *Vascular Pharmacology, 83*, 57–65. https://doi.org/10.1016/j.vph.2016.04.002.

Chen, L., Tang, S., Zhang, F. F., Garcia, V., Falck, J. R., Schwartzman, M. L., et al. (2019). CYP4A/20-HETE regulates ischemia-induced neovascularization via its actions on endothelial progenitor and preexisting endothelial cells. *American Journal of Physiology. Heart and Circulatory Physiology, 316*(6), H1468–h1479. https://doi.org/10.1152/ajpheart.00690.2018.

Cheng, J., Garcia, V., Ding, Y., Wu, C. C., Thakar, K., Falck, J. R., et al. (2012). Induction of angiotensin-converting enzyme and activation of the renin-angiotensin system contribute to 20-Hydroxyeicosatetraenoic acid-mediated endothelial dysfunction. *Arteriosclerosis, Thrombosis, and Vascular Biology, 32*(8), 1917–1924. https://doi.org/10.1161/atvbaha.112.248344.

Cheng, J., Ou, J. S., Singh, H., Falck, J. R., Narsimhaswamy, D., Pritchard, K. A., Jr., et al. (2008). 20-Hydroxyeicosatetraenoic acid causes endothelial dysfunction via eNOS uncoupling. *American Journal of Physiology. Heart and Circulatory Physiology, 294*(2), H1018–H1026.

Cheng, J., Wu, C. C., Gotlinger, K. H., Zhang, F., Falck, J. R., Narsimhaswamy, D., et al. (2010). 20-hydroxy-5,8,11,14-eicosatetraenoic acid mediates endothelial dysfunction via IkappaB kinase-dependent endothelial nitric-oxide synthase uncoupling. *The Journal of Pharmacology and Experimental Therapeutics, 332*(1), 57–65. https://doi.org/10.1124/jpet.109.159863.

Croft, K. D., McGiff, J. C., Sanchez-Mendoza, A., & Carroll, M. A. (2000). Angiotensin II releases 20-HETE from rat renal microvessels. *American Journal of Physiology. Renal Physiology, 279*(3), F544–F551. https://doi.org/10.1152/ajprenal.2000.279.3.F544.

Dahly-Vernon, A. J., Sharma, M., McCarthy, E. T., Savin, V. J., Ledbetter, S. R., & Roman, R. J. (2005). Transforming growth factor-beta, 20-HETE interaction, and glomerular injury in dahl salt-sensitive rats. *Hypertension, 45*(4), 643–648. https://doi.org/10.1161/01.hyp.0000153791.89776.43.

Ding, Y., Wu, C. C., Garcia, V., Dimitrova, I., Weidenhammer, A., Joseph, G., et al. (2013). 20-HETE induces remodeling of renal resistance arteries independent of blood pressure elevation in hypertension. *American Journal of Physiology. Renal Physiology, 305*(5), F753–F763. https://doi.org/10.1152/ajprenal.00292.2013.

Edson, K. Z., & Rettie, A. E. (2013). CYP4 enzymes as potential drug targets: Focus on enzyme multiplicity, inducers and inhibitors, and therapeutic modulation of 20-hydroxyeicosatetraenoic acid (20-HETE) synthase and fatty acid omega-hydroxylase activities. *Current Topics in Medicinal Chemistry, 13*(12), 1429–1440. (Retrieved from http://www.ncbi.nlm.nih.gov/pmc/articles/PMC4245146/pdf/nihms643755.pdf).

Escalante, B., Erlij, D., Falck, J. R., & McGiff, J. C. (1994). Cytochrome P-450 arachidonate metabolites affect ion fluxes in rabbit medullary thick ascending limb. *The American Journal of Physiology, 266*(6 Pt 1), C1775–C1782.

Fava, C., Montagnana, M., Almgren, P., Rosberg, L., Lippi, G., Hedblad, B., et al. (2008). The V433M variant of the CYP4F2 is associated with ischemic stroke in male swedes beyond its effect on blood pressure. *Hypertension, 52*(2), 373–380. https://doi.org/10.1161/hypertensionaha.108.114199.

Fava, C., Ricci, M., Melander, O., & Minuz, P. (2012). Hypertension, cardiovascular risk and polymorphisms in genes controlling the cytochrome P450 pathway of arachidonic acid: A sex-specific relation? *Prostaglandins & Other Lipid Mediators, 98*(3–4), 75–85. https://doi.org/10.1016/j.prostaglandins.2011.11.007.

Gainer, J. V., Bellamine, A., Dawson, E. P., Womble, K. E., Grant, S. W., Wang, Y., et al. (2005). Functional variant of CYP4A11 20-hydroxyeicosatetraenoic acid synthase is associated with essential hypertension. *Circulation, 111*(1), 63–69. https://doi.org/10.1161/01.cir.0000151309.82473.59.

Gainer, J. V., Lipkowitz, M. S., Yu, C., Waterman, M. R., Dawson, E. P., Capdevila, J. H., et al. (2008). Association of a CYP4A11 variant and blood pressure in black men. *The Journal of the American Society of Nephrology, 19*(8), 1606–1612. https://doi.org/10.1681/ASN.2008010063.

Garcia, V., Gilani, A., Shkolnik, B., Pandey, V., Zhang, F. F., Dakarapu, R., et al. (2017). 20-HETE signals through G-protein-coupled receptor GPR75 (Gq) to affect vascular function and trigger hypertension. *Circulation Research, 120*(11), 1776–1788. https://doi.org/10.1161/circresaha.116.310525.

Garcia, V., Joseph, G., Shkolnik, B., Ding, Y., Zhang, F. F., Gotlinger, K., et al. (2015). Angiotensin II receptor blockade or deletion of vascular endothelial ACE does not prevent vascular dysfunction and remodeling in 20-HETE-dependent hypertension. *American Journal of Physiology. Regulatory, Integrative and Comparative Physiology, 309*(1), R71–R78. https://doi.org/10.1152/ajpregu.00039.2015.

Garcia, V., & Schwartzman, M. L. (2017). Recent developments on the vascular effects of 20-hydroxyeicosatetraenoic acid. *Current Opinion in Nephrology and Hypertension, 26*(2), 74–82. https://doi.org/10.1097/mnh.0000000000000302.

Garcia, V., Shkolnik, B., Milhau, L., Falck, J. R., & Schwartzman, M. L. (2016). 20-HETE activates the transcription of angiotensin-converting enzyme via nuclear factor-kappaB translocation and promoter binding. *The Journal of Pharmacology and Experimental Therapeutics, 356*(3), 525–533. https://doi.org/10.1124/jpet.115.229377.

Gebremedhin, D., Lange, A. R., Narayanan, J., Aebly, M. R., Jacobs, E. R., & Harder, D. R. (1998). Cat cerebral arterial smooth muscle cells express cytochrome P450 4A2 enzyme and produce the vasoconstrictor 20-HETE which enhances L-type Ca2+ current. *The Journal of Physiology, 507*(Pt 3), 771–781.

Gilani, A., Agostinucci, K., Hossain, S., Pascale, J. V., Garcia, V., Adebesin, A. M., et al. (2021). 20-HETE interferes with insulin signaling and contributes to obesity-driven insulin resistance. *Prostaglandins & Other Lipid Mediators, 152*, 106485. https://doi.org/10.1016/j.prostaglandins.2020.106485.

Gilani, A., Agostinucci, K., Pascale, J. V., Hossain, S., Kandhi, S., Pandey, V., et al. (2020). Proximal tubular-targeted overexpression of the Cyp4a12-20-HETE synthase promotes salt-sensitive hypertension in male mice. *American Journal of Physiology. Regulatory, Integrative and Comparative Physiology*. https://doi.org/10.1152/ajpregu.00089.2020.

Gilani, A., Pandey, V., Garcia, V., Agostinucci, K., Singh, S. P., Schragenheim, J., et al. (2018). High-fat diet-induced obesity and insulin resistance in CYP4a14(−/−) mice is mediated by 20-HETE. *American Journal of Physiology. Regulatory, Integrative and Comparative Physiology*, *315*(5), R934–r944. https://doi.org/10.1152/ajpregu.00125.2018.

Grundmann, M., Bender, E., Schamberger, J., & Eitner, F. (2021). Pharmacology of free fatty acid receptors and their allosteric modulators. *International Journal of Molecular Sciences*, *22*(4). https://doi.org/10.3390/ijms22041763.

Guo, A. M., Arbab, A. S., Falck, J. R., Chen, P., Edwards, P. A., Roman, R. J., et al. (2007). Activation of vascular endothelial growth factor through reactive oxygen species mediates 20-hydroxyeicosatetraenoic acid-induced endothelial cell proliferation. *The Journal of Pharmacology and Experimental Therapeutics*, *321*(1), 18–27. https://doi.org/10.1124/jpet.106.115360.

Guo, A. M., Scicli, G., Sheng, J., Falck, J. C., Edwards, P. A., & Scicli, A. G. (2009). 20-HETE can act as a nonhypoxic regulator of HIF-1alpha in human microvascular endothelial cells. *American Journal of Physiology. Heart and Circulatory Physiology*, *297*(2), H602–H613. https://doi.org/10.1152/ajpheart.00874.2008.

Harder, D. R., Gebremedhin, D., Narayanan, J., Jefcoat, C., Falck, J. R., Campbell, W. B., et al. (1994). Formation and action of a P-450 4A metabolite of arachidonic acid in cat cerebral microvessels. *The American Journal of Physiology*, *266*(5 Pt 2), H2098–H2107.

Hardwick, J. P. (2008). Cytochrome P450 omega hydroxylase (CYP4) function in fatty acid metabolism and metabolic diseases. *Biochemical Pharmacology*, *75*(12), 2263–2275.

Hardwick, J. P., Eckman, K., Lee, Y. K., Abdelmegeed, M. A., Esterle, A., Chilian, W. M., et al. (2013). Eicosanoids in metabolic syndrome. *Advances in Pharmacology*, *66*, 157–266. https://doi.org/10.1016/b978-0-12-404717-4.00005-6.

Hardwick, J. P., Osei-Hyiaman, D., Wiland, H., Abdelmegeed, M. A., & Song, B. J. (2009). PPAR/RXR regulation of fatty acid metabolism and fatty acid omega-hydroxylase (CYP4) isozymes: Implications for prevention of lipotoxicity in fatty liver disease. *PPAR Research*, *2009*, 952734. https://doi.org/10.1155/2009/952734.

Helvig, C., Dishman, E., & Capdevila, J. H. (1998). Molecular, enzymatic and regulatory characterization of rat kidney cytochromes P450 4A2 and 4A3. *The Biochemist*, *37*, 12546–12558.

Hercule, H. C., & Oyekan, A. O. (2000). Cytochrome P450 omega/omega-1 hydroxylase-derived eicosanoids contribute to endothelin(a) and endothelin(B) receptor-mediated vasoconstriction to endothelin-1 in the rat preglomerular arteriole. *The Journal of Pharmacology and Experimental Therapeutics*, *292*(3), 1153–1160.

Hill, E., Fitzpatrick, F., & Murphy, R. C. (1992). Biological activity and metabolism of 20-hydroxyeicosatetraenoic acid in the human platelet. *British Journal of Pharmacology*, *106*(2), 267–274.

Hill, E., & Murphy, R. C. (1992). Quantitation of 20-hydroxy-5,8,11,14-eicosatetraenoic acid (20-HETE) produced by human polymorphonuclear leukocytes using electron capture ionization gas chromatography/mass spectrometry. *Biological Mass Spectrometry*, *21*(5), 249–253. https://doi.org/10.1002/bms.1200210505.

Hiratsuka, M., Matsuura, T., Watanabe, E., Sato, M., & Suzuki, Y. (1996). Sex and strain differences in constitutive expression of fatty acid omega-hydroxylase (CYP4A-related proteins) in mice. *Journal of Biochemistry*, *119*(2), 340–345.

Holla, V. R., Adas, F., Imig, J. D., Zhao, X., Price, E., Jr., Olsen, N., et al. (2001). Alterations in the regulation of androgen-sensitive Cyp 4a monooxygenases cause hypertension. *Proceedings of the National Academy of Sciences of the United States of America*, *98*(9), 5211–5216. https://doi.org/10.1073/pnas.081627898.

Honeck, H., Gross, V., Erdmann, B., Kargel, E., Neunaber, R., Milia, A. F., et al. (2000). Cytochrome P450-dependent renal arachidonic acid metabolism in desoxycorticosterone acetate-salt hypertensive mice. *Hypertension, 36*(4), 610–616.

Hoopes, S. L., Garcia, V., Edin, M. L., Schwartzman, M. L., & Zeldin, D. C. (2015). Vascular actions of 20-HETE. *Prostaglandins & Other Lipid Mediators, 120*, 9–16. https://doi.org/10.1016/j.prostaglandins.2015.03.002.

Hu, B. C., Li, Y., Li, F. H., Zhang, Y., Sheng, C. S., Fan, H. Q., et al. (2011). Peripheral and central augmentation indexes in relation to the CYP4F2 polymorphisms in Chinese. *Journal of Hypertension, 29*(3), 501–508. https://doi.org/10.1097/HJH.0b013e328342673c.

Imig, J. D., Zou, A. P., Stec, D. E., Harder, D. R., Falck, J. R., & Roman, R. J. (1996). Formation and actions of 20-hydroxyeicosatetraenoic acid in rat renal arterioles. *The American Journal of Physiology, 270*(1 Pt 2), R217–R227.

Inoue, R., Jensen, L. J., Jian, Z., Shi, J., Hai, L., Lurie, A. I., et al. (2009). Synergistic activation of vascular TRPC6 channel by receptor and mechanical stimulation via phospholipase C/diacylglycerol and phospholipase A2/omega-hydroxylase/20-HETE pathways. *Circulation Research, 104*(12), 1399–1409. https://doi.org/10.1161/circresaha.108.193227.

Inoue, K., Sodhi, K., Puri, N., Gotlinger, K. H., Cao, J., Rezzani, R., et al. (2009). Endothelial-specific CYP4A2 overexpression leads to renal injury and hypertension via increased production of 20-HETE. *American Journal of Physiology. Renal Physiology, 297*(4), F875–F884. https://doi.org/10.1152/ajprenal.00364.2009.

Ishizuka, T., Cheng, J., Singh, H., Vitto, M. D., Manthati, V. L., Falck, J. R., et al. (2008). 20-Hydroxyeicosatetraenoic acid stimulates nuclear factor-kappaB activation and the production of inflammatory cytokines in human endothelial cells. *The Journal of Pharmacology and Experimental Therapeutics, 324*(1), 103–110. https://doi.org/10.1124/jpet.107.130336.

Ito, O., Nakamura, Y., Tan, L., Ishizuka, T., Sasaki, Y., Minami, N., et al. (2006). Expression of cytochrome P-450 4 enzymes in the kidney and liver: Regulation by PPAR and species-difference between rat and human. *Molecular and Cellular Biochemistry, 284*(1–2), 141–148. https://doi.org/10.1007/s11010-005-9038-x.

Ito, O., & Roman, R. J. (1999). Regulation of P-450 4A activity in the glomerulus of the rat. *The American Journal of Physiology, 276*(6), R1749–R1757. https://doi.org/10.1152/ajpregu.1999.276.6.R1749.

Iwai, N., & Inagami, T. (1991). Isolation of preferentially expressed genes in the kidneys of hypertensive rats. *Hypertension, 17*(2), 161–169. https://doi.org/10.1161/01.hyp.17.2.161.

Jiang, M., Mezentsev, A., Kemp, R., Byun, K., Falck, J. R., Miano, J. M., et al. (2004). Smooth muscle—Specific expression of CYP4A1 induces endothelial sprouting in renal arterial microvessels. *Circulation Research, 94*(2), 167–174. https://doi.org/10.1161/01.res.0000111523.12842.fc.

Joseph, G., Soler, A., Hutcheson, R., Hunter, I., Bradford, C., Hutcheson, B., et al. (2017). Elevated 20-HETE impairs coronary collateral growth in metabolic syndrome via endothelial dysfunction. *American Journal of Physiology. Heart and Circulatory Physiology, 312*(3), H528–H540. https://doi.org/10.1152/ajpheart.00561.2016.

Kaduce, T. L., Fang, X., Harmon, S. D., Oltman, C. L., Dellsperger, K. C., Teesch, L. M., et al. (2004). 20-hydroxyeicosatetraenoic acid (20-HETE) metabolism in coronary endothelial cells. *The Journal of Biological Chemistry, 279*(4), 2648–2656. https://doi.org/10.1074/jbc.M306849200.

Kohagura, K., Arima, S., Endo, Y., Chiba, Y., Ito, O., Abe, M., et al. (2001). Involvement of cytochrome P450 metabolites in the vascular action of angiotensin II on the afferent arterioles. *Hypertension Research, 24*(5), 551–557. https://doi.org/10.1291/hypres.24.551.

Laffer, C. L., Gainer, J. V., Waterman, M. R., Capdevila, J. H., Laniado-Schwartzman, M., Nasjletti, A., et al. (2008). The T8590C polymorphism of CYP4A11 and 20-hydroxyeicosatetraenoic acid in essential hypertension. *Hypertension, 51*(3), 767–772. https://doi.org/10.1161/hypertensionaha.107.102921.

Lakhkar, A., Dhagia, V., Joshi, S. R., Gotlinger, K., Patel, D., Sun, D., et al. (2016). 20-HETE-induced mitochondrial superoxide production and inflammatory phenotype in vascular smooth muscle is prevented by glucose-6-phosphate dehydrogenase inhibition. *American Journal of Physiology. Heart and Circulatory Physiology, 310*(9), H1107–H1117. https://doi.org/10.1152/ajpheart.00961.2015.

Lasker, J. M., Chen, W. B., Wolf, I., Bloswick, B. P., Wilson, P. D., & Powell, P. K. (2000). Formation of 20-hydroxyeicosatetraenoic acid, a vasoactive and natriuretic eicosanoid, in human kidney. Role of Cyp4F2 and Cyp4A11. *The Journal of Biological Chemistry, 275*(6), 4118–4126.

Lima, R., Yanes, L. L., Davis, D. D., & Reckelhoff, J. F. (2013). Roles played by 20-HETE, angiotensin II and endothelin in mediating the hypertension in aging female spontaneously hypertensive rats. *American Journal of Physiology. Regulatory, Integrative and Comparative Physiology, 304*(3), R248–R251. https://doi.org/10.1152/ajpregu.00380.2012.

Lin, F., Abraham, N. G., & Schwartzman, M. L. (1994). Cytochrome P450 arachidonic acid omega-hydroxylation in the proximal tubule of the rat kidney. *Annals of the New York Academy of Sciences, 744*, 11–24.

Lino Cardenas, C. L., Devos, A., Toure, A., Cardenas Garcia, J., Kenani, A., Migot-Nabias, F., et al. (2012). Arachidonic acid omega-hydroxylase CYP4A11: Inter-ethnic variations in the 8590T>C loss-of-function variant. *Molecular Biology Reports, 39*(2), 1503–1508. https://doi.org/10.1007/s11033-011-0888-x.

Liu, X., Wu, J., Liu, H., Lai, G., & Zhao, Y. (2012). Disturbed ratio of renal 20-HETE/EETs is involved in androgen-induced hypertension in cytochrome P450 4F2 transgenic mice. *Gene, 505*(2), 352–359. https://doi.org/10.1016/j.gene.2012.02.029.

Ljuca, F., & Drevensek, G. (2010). Endothelin-1 induced vascular smooth muscle cell proliferation is mediated by cytochrome p-450 arachidonic acid metabolites. *Bosnian Journal of Basic Medical Sciences, 10*(3), 223–226.

Luo, P., Zhou, Y., Chang, H. H., Zhang, J., Seki, T., Wang, C. Y., et al. (2009). Glomerular 20-HETE, EETs, and TGF-beta1 in diabetic nephropathy. *American Journal of Physiology. Renal Physiology, 296*(3), F556–F563. https://doi.org/10.1152/ajprenal.90613.2008.

Macica, C., Balazy, M., Falck, J. R., Mioskowski, C., & Carroll, M. A. (1993). Characterization of cytochrome P-450-dependent arachidonic acid metabolism in rabbit intestine. *The American Journal of Physiology, 265*(4 Pt 1), G735–G741.

Marji, J. S., Wang, M. H., & Laniado-Schwartzman, M. (2002). Cytochrome P-450 4A isoform expression and 20-HETE synthesis in renal preglomerular arteries. *American Journal of Physiology. Renal Physiology, 283*(1), F60–F67. https://doi.org/10.1152/ajprenal.00265.2001.

Marumo, T., Eto, K., Wake, H., Omura, T., & Nabekura, J. (2010). The inhibitor of 20-HETE synthesis, TS-011, improves cerebral microcirculatory autoregulation impaired by middle cerebral artery occlusion in mice. *British Journal of Pharmacology, 161*(6), 1391–1402. https://doi.org/10.1111/j.1476-5381.2010.00973.x.

Mayer, B., Lieb, W., Gotz, A., Konig, I. R., Aherrahrou, Z., Thiemig, A., et al. (2005). Association of the T8590C polymorphism of CYP4A11 with hypertension in the MONICA Augsburg echocardiographic substudy. *Hypertension, 46*(4), 766–771. https://doi.org/10.1161/01.HYP.0000182658.04299.15.

Medhora, M., Chen, Y., Gruenloh, S., Harland, D., Bodiga, S., Zielonka, J., et al. (2008). 20-HETE increases superoxide production and activates NAPDH oxidase in pulmonary artery endothelial cells. *American Journal of Physiology. Lung Cellular and Molecular Physiology, 294*(5), L902–L911. https://doi.org/10.1152/ajplung.00278.2007.

Minamiyama, Y., Takemura, S., Imaoka, S., Funae, Y., Tanimoto, Y., & Inoue, M. (1997). Irreversible inhibition of cytochrome P450 by nitric oxide. *The Journal of Pharmacology and Experimental Therapeutics*, *283*(3), 1479–1485. (Retrieved from https://www.ncbi.nlm.nih.gov/pubmed/9400024).

Miyata, N., & Roman, R. J. (2005). Role of 20-hydroxyeicosatetraenoic acid (20-HETE) in vascular system. *Journal of Smooth Muscle Research*, *41*(4), 175–193. (Retrieved from https://www.jstage.jst.go.jp/article/jsmr/41/4/41_4_175/_pdf).

Miyata, N., Taniguchi, K., Seki, T., Ishimoto, T., Sato-Watanabe, M., Yasuda, Y., et al. (2001). HET0016, a potent and selective inhibitor of 20-HETE synthesizing enzyme. *British Journal of Pharmacology*, *133*(3), 325–329. https://doi.org/10.1038/sj.bjp.0704101.

Morrison, A. R., & Pascoe, N. (1981). Metabolism of arachidonate through NADPH-dependent oxygenase of renal cortex. *Proceedings of the National Academy of Sciences of the United States of America*, *78*, 7375–7378.

Muller, D. N., Schmidt, C., Barbosa-Sicard, E., Wellner, M., Gross, V., Hercule, H., et al. (2007). Mouse Cyp4a isoforms: Enzymatic properties, gender- and strain-specific expression, and role in renal 20-hydroxyeicosatetraenoic acid formation. *The Biochemical Journal*, *403*(1), 109–118. https://doi.org/10.1042/bj20061328.

Munshi, A., Sharma, V., Kaul, S., Al-Hazzani, A., Alshatwi, A. A., Shafi, G., et al. (2012). Association of 1347 G/a cytochrome P450 4F2 (CYP4F2) gene variant with hypertension and stroke. *Molecular Biology Reports*, *39*(2), 1677–1682. https://doi.org/10.1007/s11033-011-0907-y.

Muthalif, M. M., Uddin, M. R., Fatima, S., Parmentier, J. H., Khandekar, Z., & Malik, K. U. (2001). Small GTP binding protein Ras contributes to norepinephrine-induced mitogenesis of vascular smooth muscle cells. *Prostaglandins & Other Lipid Mediators*, *65*(1), 33–43.

Nguyen, X., Wang, M. H., Reddy, K. M., Falck, J. R., & Schwartzman, M. L. (1999). Kinetic profile of the rat CYP4A isoforms: Arachidonic acid metabolism and isoform-specific inhibitors. *The American Journal of Physiology*, *276*(6), R1691–R1700. https://doi.org/10.1152/ajpregu.1999.276.6.R1691.

Nowicki, S., Chen, S. L., Aizman, O., Cheng, X. J., Li, D., Nowicki, C., et al. (1997). 20-Hydroxyeicosa-tetraenoic acid (20 HETE) activates protein kinase C. role in regulation of rat renal Na+,K+-ATPase. *The Journal of Clinical Investigation*, *99*(6), 1224–1230. https://doi.org/10.1172/jci119279.

Oliw, E. H., Lawson, J. A., Brash, A. R., & Oates, J. A. (1981). Arachidonic acid metabolism in rabbit renal cortex. Formation of two novel dihydroxyeicosatrienoic acids. *The Journal of Biological Chemistry*, *256*, 9924–9931.

Omata, K., Abraham, N. G., & Schwartzman, M. L. (1992). Renal cytochrome P-450-arachidonic acid metabolism: Localization and hormonal regulation in SHR. *The American Journal of Physiology*, *262*(4 Pt 2), F591–F599.

Ortiz de Montellano, P. R., & Reich, N. O. (1984). Specific inactivation of hepatic fatty acid hydroxylases by acetylenic fatty acids. *The Journal of Biological Chemistry*, *259*(7), 4136–4141. (Retrieved from https://www.ncbi.nlm.nih.gov/pubmed/6706995).

Oyekan, A. O., Youseff, T., Fulton, D., Quilley, J., & McGiff, J. C. (1999). Renal cytochrome P450 omega-hydroxylase and epoxygenase activity are differentially modified by nitric oxide and sodium chloride. *The Journal of Clinical Investigation*, *104*(8), 1131–1137. https://doi.org/10.1172/jci6786.

Pandey, V., Garcia, V., Gilani, A., Mishra, P., Zhang, F. F., Paudyal, M. P., et al. (2017). The blood pressure-lowering effect of 20-HETE blockade in Cyp4a14(−/−) mice is associated with natriuresis. *The Journal of Pharmacology and Experimental Therapeutics*, *363*(3), 412–418. https://doi.org/10.1124/jpet.117.243618.

Park, S. K., Herrnreiter, A., Pfister, S. L., Gauthier, K. M., Falck, B. A., Falck, J. R., et al. (2018). GPR40 is a low-affinity epoxyeicosatrienoic acid receptor in vascular cells. *The Journal of Biological Chemistry*, *293*(27), 10675–10691. https://doi.org/10.1074/jbc.RA117.001297.

Pascale, J. V., Park, E. J., Adebesin, A. M., Falck, J. R., Schwartzman, M. L., & Garcia, V. (2021). Uncovering the signalling, structure and function of the 20-HETE-GPR75 pairing: Identifying the chemokine CCL5 as a negative regulator of GPR75. *British Journal of Pharmacology*, *178*(18), 3813–3828. https://doi.org/10.1111/bph.15525.

Randriamboavonjy, V., Busse, R., & Fleming, I. (2003). 20-HETE-induced contraction of small coronary arteries depends on the activation of rho-kinase. *Hypertension*, *41*(3 Pt 2), 801–806. https://doi.org/10.1161/01.hyp.0000047240.33861.6b.

Regner, K. R., Zuk, A., Van Why, S. K., Shames, B. D., Ryan, R. P., Falck, J. R., et al. (2009). Protective effect of 20-HETE analogues in experimental renal ischemia reperfusion injury. *Kidney International*, *75*(5), 511–517. https://doi.org/10.1038/ki.2008.600.

Ribeiro, C. M., Dubay, G. R., Falck, J. R., & Mandel, L. J. (1994). Parathyroid hormone inhibits Na(+)-K(+)-ATPase through a cytochrome P-450 pathway. *The American Journal of Physiology*, *266*(3 Pt 2), F497–F505.

Rocic, P., & Schwartzman, M. L. (2018). 20-HETE in the regulation of vascular and cardiac function. *Pharmacology & Therapeutics*, *192*, 74–87. https://doi.org/10.1016/j.pharmthera.2018.07.004.

Roman, R. J., & Fan, F. (2018). 20-HETE: Hypertension and beyond. *Hypertension*, *72*(1), 12–18. https://doi.org/10.1161/HYPERTENSIONAHA.118.10269.

Rosolowsky, M., Falck, J. R., & Campbell, W. B. (1996). Metabolism of arachidonic acid by canine polymorphonuclear leukocytes synthesis of lipoxygenase and omega-oxidized metabolites. *Biochimica et Biophysica Acta*, *1300*(2), 143–150.

Sacerdoti, D., Abraham, N. G., McGiff, J. C., & Schwartzman, M. L. (1988). Renal cytochrome P-450-dependent metabolism of arachidonic acid in spontaneously hypertensive rats. *Biochemical Pharmacology*, *37*(3), 521–527. https://doi.org/10.1016/0006-2952(88)90223-7.

Sacerdoti, D., Escalante, B., Abraham, N. G., McGiff, J. C., Levere, R. D., & Schwartzman, M. L. (1989). Treatment with tin prevents the development of hypertension in spontaneously hypertensive rats. *Science*, *243*(4889), 388–390. https://doi.org/10.1126/science.2492116.

Savas, U., Wei, S., Hsu, M. H., Falck, J. R., Guengerich, F. P., Capdevila, J. H., et al. (2016). 20-Hydroxyeicosatetraenoic acid (HETE)-dependent hypertension in human cytochrome P450 (CYP) 4A11 transgenic mice: Normalization of blood pressure by sodium restriction, hydrochlorothiazide, or blockade of the type 1 angiotensin ii receptor. *The Journal of Biological Chemistry*, *291*(32), 16904–16919. https://doi.org/10.1074/jbc.M116.732297.

Schwartzman, M. L., Falck, J. R., Yadagiri, P., & Escalante, B. (1989). Metabolism of 20-hydroxyeicosatetraenoic acid by cyclooxygenase. Formation and identification of novel endothelium-dependent vasoconstrictor metabolites. *The Journal of Biological Chemistry*, *264*(20), 11658–11662.

Schwartzman, M. L., Ferreri, N. R., Carroll, M. A., Songu-Mize, E., & McGiff, J. C. (1985). Renal cytochrome P450-related arachidonate metabolite inhibits (Na++K+)ATPase. *Nature*, *314*, 620.

Schwartzman, M. L., Martasek, P., Rios, A. R., Levere, R. D., Solangi, K., Goodman, A. I., et al. (1990). Cytochrome P450-dependent arachidonic acid metabolism in human kidney. *Kidney International*, *37*(1), 94–99. https://doi.org/10.1038/ki.1990.13.

Singh, H., Cheng, J., Deng, H., Kemp, R., Ishizuka, T., Nasjletti, A., et al. (2007). Vascular cytochrome P450 4A expression and 20-hydroxyeicosatetraenoic acid synthesis contribute to endothelial dysfunction in androgen-induced hypertension. *Hypertension*, *50*(1), 123–129. https://doi.org/10.1161/hypertensionaha.107.089599.

Sodhi, K., Wu, C. C., Cheng, J., Gotlinger, K., Inoue, K., Goli, M., et al. (2010). CYP4A2-induced hypertension is 20-hydroxyeicosatetraenoic acid- and angiotensin II-dependent. *Hypertension*, *56*(5), 871–878. https://doi.org/10.1161/hypertensionaha.110.154559.

Speed, J. S., George, E. M., Arany, M., Cockrell, K., & Granger, J. P. (2011). Role of 20-hydroxyeicosatetraenoic acid in mediating hypertension in response to chronic renal medullary endothelin type B receptor blockade. *PLoS One*, *6*(10), e26063. https://doi.org/10.1371/journal.pone.0026063.

Stec, D. E., Gannon, K. P., Beaird, J. S., & Drummond, H. A. (2007). 20-Hydroxyeicosatetraenoic acid (20-HETE) stimulates migration of vascular smooth muscle cells. *Cellular Physiology and Biochemistry*, *19*(1–4), 121–128. https://doi.org/10.1159/000099200.

Stec, D. E., Mattson, D. L., & Roman, R. J. (1997). Inhibition of renal outer medullary 20-HETE production produces hypertension in Lewis rats. *Hypertension*, *29*(1 Pt 2), 315–319.

Stec, D. E., Roman, R. J., Flasch, A., & Rieder, M. J. (2007). Functional polymorphism in human CYP4F2 decreases 20-HETE production. *Physiological Genomics*, *30*(1), 74–81. https://doi.org/10.1152/physiolgenomics.00003.2007.

Sun, C. W., Alonso-Galicia, M., Taheri, M. R., Falck, J. R., Harder, D. R., & Roman, R. J. (1998). Nitric oxide-20-hydroxyeicosatetraenoic acid interaction in the regulation of K+ channel activity and vascular tone in renal arterioles. *Circulation Research*, *83*(11), 1069–1079.

Tarttelin, E. E., Kirschner, L. S., Bellingham, J., Baffi, J., Taymans, S. E., Gregory-Evans, K., et al. (1999). Cloning and characterization of a novel orphan G-protein-coupled receptor localized to human chromosome 2p16. *Biochemical and Biophysical Research Communications*, *260*(1), 174–180. https://doi.org/10.1006/bbrc.1999.0753.

Tsai, I. J., Croft, K., Puddey, I. B., Beilin, L. J., & Barden, A. E. (2011). 20-Hydroxyeicosatetraenoic acid synthesis is increased in human neutrophils and platelets by angiotensin ii and Endothelin-1. *American Journal of Physiology. Heart and Circulatory Physiology*, *300*(4), H1194–H1200.

Tunaru, S., Bonnavion, R., Brandenburger, I., Preussner, J., Thomas, D., Scholich, K., et al. (2018). 20-HETE promotes glucose-stimulated insulin secretion in an autocrine manner through FFAR1. *Nature Communications*, *9*(1), 177. https://doi.org/10.1038/s41467-017-02539-4.

Uddin, M. R., Muthalif, M. M., Karzoun, N. A., Benter, I. F., & Malik, K. U. (1998). Cytochrome P-450 metabolites mediate norepinephrine-induced mitogenic signaling. *Hypertension*, *31*(1 Pt 2), 242–247.

Walkowska, A., Skaroupkova, P., Huskova, Z., Vanourkova, Z., Chabova, V. C., Tesar, V., et al. (2010). Intrarenal cytochrome P-450 metabolites of arachidonic acid in the regulation of the nonclipped kidney function in two-kidney, one-clip Goldblatt hypertensive rats. *Journal of Hypertension*, *28*(3), 582–593. https://doi.org/10.1097/HJH.0b013e328334dfd4.

Wang, M. H., Brand-Schieber, E., Zand, B. A., Nguyen, X., Falck, J. R., Balu, N., et al. (1998). Cytochrome P450-derived arachidonic acid metabolism in the rat kidney: Characterization of selective inhibitors. *The Journal of Pharmacology and Experimental Therapeutics*, *284*, 966–973.

Wang, W., & Lu, M. (1995). Effect of arachidonic acid on activity of the apical K+ channel in the thick ascending limb of the rat kidney. *The Journal of General Physiology*, *106*(4), 727–743.

Wang, M. H., Wang, J., Chang, H. H., Zand, B. A., Jiang, M., Nasjletti, A., et al. (2003). Regulation of renal CYP4A expression and 20-HETE synthesis by nitric oxide in pregnant rats. *American Journal of Physiology. Renal Physiology*, *285*(2), F295–F302. https://doi.org/10.1152/ajprenal.00065.2003.

Ward, N. C., Tsai, I. J., Barden, A., van Bockxmeer, F. M., Puddey, I. B., Hodgson, J. M., et al. (2008). A single nucleotide polymorphism in the CYP4F2 but not CYP4A11 gene is associated with increased 20-HETE excretion and blood pressure. *Hypertension*, *51*(5), 1393–1398. https://doi.org/10.1161/hypertensionaha.107.104463.

Williams, J. S., Hopkins, P. N., Jeunemaitre, X., & Brown, N. J. (2011). CYP4A11 T8590C polymorphism, salt-sensitive hypertension, and renal blood flow. *Journal of Hypertension*, *29*(10), 1913–1918. https://doi.org/10.1097/HJH.0b013e32834aa786.

Williams, J. M., Sarkis, A., Lopez, B., Ryan, R. P., Flasch, A. K., & Roman, R. J. (2007). Elevations in renal interstitial hydrostatic pressure and 20-hydroxyeicosatetraenoic acid contribute to pressure natriuresis. *Hypertension*, *49*(3), 687–694. https://doi.org/10.1161/01.hyp.0000255753.89363.47.

Williams, J. M., Sharma, M., Anjaiahh, S., Falck, J. R., & Roman, R. J. (2007). Role of endogenous CYP450 metabolites of arachidonic acid in maintaining the glomerular protein permeability barrier. *American Journal of Physiology. Renal Physiology*, *293*(2), F501–F505. https://doi.org/10.1152/ajprenal.00131.2007.

Wilson, T. W., Alonso-Galicia, M., & Roman, R. J. (1998). Effects of lipid-lowering agents in the dahl salt-sensitive rat. *Hypertension*, *31*(1 Pt 2), 225–231.

Wu, C. C., Gupta, T., Garcia, V., Ding, Y., & Schwartzman, M. L. (2014). 20-HETE and blood pressure regulation: Clinical implications. *Cardiology in Review*, *22*(1), 1–12. https://doi.org/10.1097/CRD.0b013e3182961659.

Wu, C. C., & Schwartzman, M. L. (2011). The role of 20-HETE in androgen-mediated hypertension. *Prostaglandins & Other Lipid Mediators*, *96*(1–4), 45–53. https://doi.org/10.1016/j.prostaglandins.2011.06.006.

Xu, F., Falck, J. R., Ortiz de Montellano, P. R., & Kroetz, D. L. (2004). Catalytic activity and isoform-specific inhibition of rat cytochrome p450 4F enzymes. *The Journal of Pharmacology and Experimental Therapeutics*, *308*(3), 887–895. https://doi.org/10.1124/jpet.103.059626.

Yaghini, F. A., Zhang, C., Parmentier, J. H., Estes, A. M., Jafari, N., Schaefer, S. A., et al. (2005). Contribution of arachidonic acid metabolites derived via cytochrome P4504A to angiotensin II-induced neointimal growth. *Hypertension*, *45*(6), 1182–1187. https://doi.org/10.1161/01.HYP.0000168051.04275.ea.

Yousif, M. H., Benter, I. F., & Roman, R. J. (2009). Cytochrome P450 metabolites of arachidonic acid play a role in the enhanced cardiac dysfunction in diabetic rats following ischaemic reperfusion injury. *Autonomic & Autacoid Pharmacology*, *29*(1–2), 33–41. https://doi.org/10.1111/j.1474-8673.2009.00429.x.

Zhang, F., Wang, M. H., Krishna, U. M., Falck, J. R., Laniado-Schwartzman, M., & Nasjletti, A. (2001). Modulation by 20-HETE of phenylephrine-induced mesenteric artery contraction in spontaneously hypertensive and Wistar-Kyoto rats. *Hypertension*, *38*(6), 1311–1315. (Retrieved from http://hyper.ahajournals.org/content/38/6/1311.full.pdf).

Zhao, X., Inscho, E. W., Bondlela, M., Falck, J. R., & Imig, J. D. (2001). The CYP450 hydroxylase pathway contributes to P2X receptor-mediated afferent arteriolar vasoconstriction. *American Journal of Physiology. Heart and Circulatory Physiology*, *281*(5), H2089–H2096 (Retrieved from http://ajpheart.physiology.org/content/ajpheart/281/5/H2089.full.pdf).

Zhou, Y., Huang, H., Chang, H. H., Du, J., Wu, J. F., Wang, C. Y., et al. (2006). Induction of renal 20-hydroxyeicosatetraenoic acid by clofibrate attenuates high-fat diet-induced hypertension in rats. *The Journal of Pharmacology and Experimental Therapeutics*, *317*(1), 11–18. https://doi.org/10.1124/jpet.105.095356.

Zhu, D., Zhang, C., Medhora, M., & Jacobs, E. R. (2002). CYP4A mRNA, protein, and product in rat lungs: Novel localization in vascular endothelium. *Journal of Applied Physiology (Bethesda, MD: 1985)*, *93*(1), 330–337. https://doi.org/10.1152/japplphysiol.01159.2001.

Zou, A. P., Drummond, H. A., & Roman, R. J. (1996). Role of 20-HETE in elevating loop chloride reabsorption in dahl SS/Jr rats. *Hypertension, 27*(3 Pt 2), 631–635.
Zou, A. P., Fleming, J. T., Falck, J. R., Jacobs, E. R., Gebremedhin, D., Harder, D. R., et al. (1996). 20-HETE is an endogenous inhibitor of the large-conductance ca(2+)-activated K+ channel in renal arterioles. *The American Journal of Physiology, 270*(1 Pt 2), R228–R237.
Zou, A. P., Imig, J. D., Ortiz de Montellano, P. R., Sui, Z., Falck, J. R., & Roman, R. J. (1994). Effect of P-450 omega-hydroxylase metabolites of arachidonic acid on tubuloglomerular feedback. *The American Journal of Physiology, 266*(6 Pt 2), F934–F941.

CHAPTER TWO

Orally active epoxyeicosatrienoic acid analogs in hypertension and renal injury

John D. Imig*
Drug Discovery Center, Medical College of Wisconsin, Milwaukee, WI, United States
*Corresponding author: e-mail address: jdimig@mcw.edu

Contents

Abstract

Epoxyeicosatrienoic acids (EETs) are arachidonic acid metabolites synthesized by cytochrome P450 epoxygenases. Biological activities for EETs include vasodilation, decreasing inflammation, opposing apoptosis, and inhibiting renal sodium reabsorption. These actions are beneficial in lowering blood pressure and slowing kidney disease progression. Furthermore, evidence in human and experimental animal studies have found that decreased EET levels contribute to hypertension and kidney diseases. Consequently, EET mimics/analogs have been developed as a potential therapeutic for hypertension and acute and chronic kidney diseases. Their development has resulted in EET analogs that are orally active with favorable pharmacological profiles. Analogs for 8,9-EET, 11,12-EET, and 14,15-EET have been tested in several hypertension and kidney disease animal models. More recently, kidney targeted EET analogs have been synthesized and tested against drug-induced nephrotoxicity. Experimental evidence has demonstrated compelling therapeutic potential for EET analogs to oppose cardiovascular and kidney diseases. These EET analogs lower blood pressure, decrease kidney inflammation, improve vascular endothelial function, and decrease kidney fibrosis and apoptosis. Overall, these preclinical studies support the likelihood that EET analogs will advance to clinical trials for hypertension and associated comorbidities or acute and chronic kidney diseases.

Advances in Pharmacology, Volume 94
ISSN 1054-3589
https://doi.org/10.1016/bs.apha.2022.02.004

Abbreviations

11,12-ether-EET-8-ZE	11-nonyloxy-undec-8(Z)-enoic acid
11,12-tetra-EET-8-ZE	11,12-transoxidoeicosa-8(Z)-enoic acid
11,12,20-THE8ZE	11,12,20-trihydroxy-eicosa-8(Z)-enoic acid
14,15-EE5ZE	14,15-epoxy-5 (Z)-enoic acid
DHETs	dihydroxyeicosatrienoic acids
EETs	epoxyeicosatrienoic acids
FSPF	focal glomerular sclerosis permeability factor
HETEs	hydroxyeicosatetraenoic acids
NUDSA	11-nonyloxy-undec-8(Z)-enoic acid
sEH	soluble epoxide hydrolase
UUO	unilateral ureter obstruction

1. Introduction

Cardiovascular diseases afflict one in every three adults worldwide with hypertension being the most prevalent (Jeemon et al., 2021; Ogunniyi, Commodore-Mensah, & Ferdinand, 2021). Hypertension is also the leading cause of cardiovascular and renal disease morbidity and mortality (Jeemon et al., 2021). Factors contributing to hypertension include an elevated renin-angiotensin system, inflammation, increased sympathetic activity, and increased vasoconstriction (McMaster, Kirabo, Madhur, & Harrison, 2015). Blood pressure becomes elevated due to decreased sodium excretion, increased peripheral vascular resistance, and increased cardiac output (Titze & Luft, 2017). Anti-hypertensive drugs act to increase sodium excretion, reduce cardiac output, and reduce peripheral vascular resistance (Ojha et al., 2021). Classes of anti-hypertensive drugs include renin-angiotensin system inhibitors, diuretics, vasodilators, and β-blockers (Khan & Imig, 2018; Ojha et al., 2021). These anti-hypertensive drugs are effective in lowering blood pressure to improve health outcomes in subjects with hypertension (Ojha et al., 2021). Although these drugs are effective, uncontrolled and drug resistant hypertension prevalence remains approximately 50% (Egan & Laken, 2011).

A major gap for anti-hypertensive therapies is the lack of drugs that act on multiple mechanisms of blood pressure regulation that can avoid drug resistance with chronic treatment (Egan & Laken, 2011). Diuretics are effective anti-hypertensive drugs that target renal epithelial cell sodium transport. This class of drugs results in an initial increase in sodium excretion to decrease venous return and cardiac output resulting in a lowering of blood pressure. Over time the ability of diuretics to increase sodium excretion wanes while actions to decrease peripheral vascular resistance by ill-defined mechanisms contributes to their ability to lower blood pressure (Khan & Imig, 2018). β-blockers act on the heart to decrease heart rate and lower cardiac output to combat hypertension (Khan & Imig, 2018). Unfortunately, the dependence on cardiac output to control blood pressure decreases with age and β-blockers become less effective in older adults (Joyner, Wallin, & Charkoudian, 2016). Vasodilators such as calcium channel blockers act on the vascular smooth muscle to lower total peripheral resistance and blood pressure (Khan & Imig, 2018). Finally, renin-angiotensin system inhibitors are effective at multiple blood pressure mechanisms. Angiotensin converting enzyme inhibitors and angiotensin type 1 (AT1) receptor blockers increase sodium excretion, decrease inflammation, and decrease peripheral vascular resistance (Khan & Imig, 2018). Unfortunately, all these anti-hypertensive drugs tend to become less effective with chronic administration and treatment of hypertension with 2–4 anti-hypertensive drugs is common (Egan & Laken, 2011). In addition, end organ damage, morbidity, and mortality remain a major healthcare problem with hypertension (Kućmierz, Frąk, Młynarska, Franczyk, & Rysz, 2021; Piskorz, 2020). Research continues to identify factors that act at kidney epithelial cells, endothelial and vascular smooth muscle cells, and inflammatory cells contributing to blood pressure regulation and hypertension.

A promising target for hypertension, kidney diseases, and cardiovascular diseases is epoxyeicosatrienoic acids (EETs). EETs are epoxylipids generated from arachidonic acid by CYP2C and CYP2J epoxygenase enzymes (Capdevila, Falck, & Imig, 2007; Imig, 2012). There are four regioisomeric EETs synthesized from arachidonic acid; 5,6-EET; 8,9-EET; 11,12-EET; and 14,15-EET. CYP2C and CYP2J enzymes generate predominantly 11,12-EET and 14,15-EET with less amounts of 5,6-EET and 8,9-EET (Capdevila et al., 2007). Epoxygenase enzymes are found in renal epithelial cells and endothelial cells with highest expression in liver, kidney, lung, and heart (Imig, 2012; Zeldin, 2011). EETs have also been demonstrated to be generated by inflammatory cells (Bystrom et al., 2011). The kidney and cardiovascular actions of EETs have been extensively investigated.

Physiological actions described for EETs are beneficial in cardiovascular and kidney diseases (Fan & Roman, 2017; Imig, 2012; Roman, 2002). In general, 11,12-EET and 14,15-EET are the most physiologically active EET regioisomers (Imig, 2012). EETs act to inhibit sodium reabsorption through inhibition of epithelial cell sodium channels (ENaC) and actions on epithelial cell potassium channels (Pavlov et al., 2011; Sun et al., 2010; Wang et al., 2020, 2014). EETs released from endothelial cells activate vascular smooth large-conductance calcium-activated (K_{Ca}) channels resulting in membrane hyperpolarization and vasodilation (Archer et al., 2003; Campbell et al., 2002; Campbell, Gebremedhin, Pratt, & Harder, 1996). Anti-inflammatory actions for EETs have been demonstrated in several physiological circumstances (Fleming, 2007; Imig, 2012). EETs have also been demonstrated to oppose apoptosis and organ fibrosis (Imig et al., 2021; Oni-Orisan, Alsaleh, Lee, & Seubert, 2014) (Fig. 1). These multiple physiological actions described for EETs make these epoxy fatty acids an attractive target that effects multiple mechanisms of blood pressure regulation and end organ damage associated with hypertension.

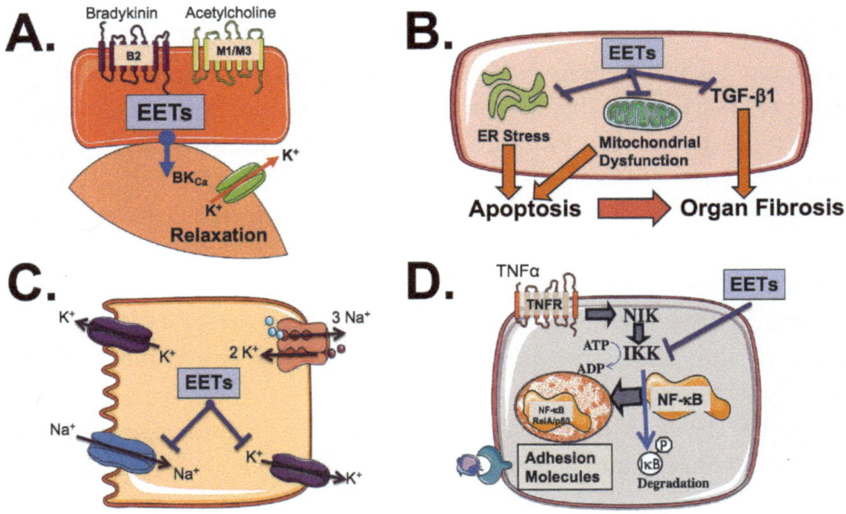

Fig. 1 Epoxyeicosatrienoic acid (EET) biological actions on (A) vascular smooth muscle, (B) renal cortical collecting duct cells, (C) organ apoptosis and fibrosis, and (D) inflammation. *A:* Endothelial-derived EETs activate vascular smooth muscle cell large conductance K^+ channels (BK_{Ca}) resulting in hyperpolarization and vasodilation; *B:* EETs inhibit kiendy cortical collecting duct apical Na^+ channels (ENaC) and basolateral K^+ channels to decrease sodium reabsorption; *C:* EETs decrease endoplasmic reticulum (ER) stress, combat mitochondrial dysfunction, and inhibit transforming growth factor β1 (TGF-β1) to reduce apoptosis and decrease organ fibrosis; *D:* Tumor necrosis factor α (TNFα) activates a sequence of cell signaling events resulting in nuclear factor-κB (NF-κB) translocation to the nucleus to increase adhesion molecule levels to cause inflammatory cell infiltration. EETs act to prevent IKK phosphorylation and activation of NF-κB to decrease inflammation. Remodeling.

There have been attempts to develop drugs that increase EETs to treat hypertension. These past efforts to develop an anti-hypertensive drug that manipulated EET levels focused on inhibition of the enzyme soluble epoxide hydrolase (sEH) that degraded EETs to their less active or inactive diols (Imig & Hammock, 2009). Indeed, sEH inhibitors were demonstrated to increase EET levels and be anti-hypertensive in several hypertension animal models (Imig & Hammock, 2009). However, clinical trials with sEH inhibitors failed to move past Phase II clinical trials (Imig, 2018). EET mimics (analogs) drugs have been another avenue being pursued to treat hypertension, cardiovascular diseases, and kidney diseases (Campbell, Imig, Schmitz, & Falck, 2017). This article will focus on EET analog drugs to combat hypertension and kidney diseases.

2. CYP Epoxygenase, sEH, and EET regulation in human hypertension

A major impetus for developing EET analogs for hypertension and kidney diseases is the evidence from human studies that decreased EET generation by CYP epoxygenase enzymes or increased sEH activity to decrease EET levels associate with cardiovascular and kidney diseases (Bellien & Joannides, 2013) (Fig. 2). Human *CYP2C8* and *CYP2C9* gene variants result in decreased epoxygenase activity (Bellien & Joannides, 2013; Morisseau & Hammock, 2013). Likewise, *CYP2C* and *CYP2J* polymorphisms have been investigated in various ethnic groups including Asian, African Americans, Europeans, and Arabs with confounding results on associations with hypertension (Bellien & Joannides, 2013; Dreisbach et al., 2005; Morisseau & Hammock, 2013). Essential hypertension in a cohort of Russians associates with the *CYP2J2* genetic variant (Polonikov et al., 2008). A lower frequency of the *CYP2C9*3* genetic variant was found to associate with hypertension in Asian females (Yu et al., 2004). A more recent study in a Russian cohort determined that polymorphisms in *CYP2C8* associated with increased risk for essential hypertension (Polonikov et al., 2017). Combinations of *CYP2C8* and *CYP2C19* variants were also found to associate with essential hypertension in this Russian cohort (Polonikov et al., 2017). On the other hand, several of the gene variants with decreased epoxygenation rates failed to demonstrate an association with hypertension. The *CYP2J2*7* genetic variant results in reduced *CYP2J2* transcription and lower plasma EET levels failed to associate with human hypertension (King et al., 2005). *CYP2C* human genetic variants in Caucasian and African American cohorts were also found

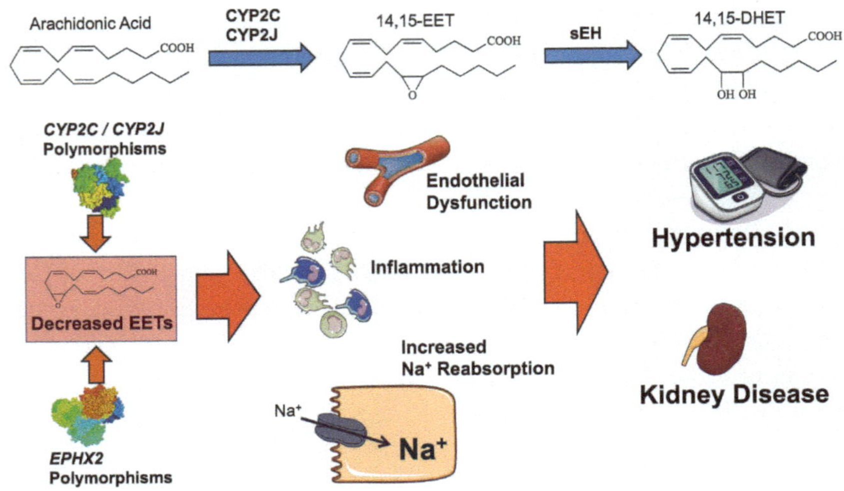

Fig. 2 Diagram depicting pathways of cytochrome P450 (CYP) arachidonic metabolism (Top) and changes in pathway that contribute to hypertension and kidney disease (Bottom). *TOP:* CYP2C and CYP2J enzymes generate epoxyeicosatrienoic acid (EETs). Soluble epoxide hydrolase (sEH) can hydrate EETs to form dihydroxyeicosatrienoic acids (DHETEs). *BOTTOM: CYP2C, CYP2J,* and *EPHX2* polymorphisms result in decreased EET levels. Decreased EET levels result in endothelial dysfunction, inflammation, increased sodium reabsorption that contribute to hypertension and kidney disease.

to not associate with hypertension (Dreisbach et al., 2005; Spiecker et al., 2004). Regarding sEH, a genetic variant in the gene responsible for sEH, *EPHX2*, which results in reduced sEH activity and decreased EET degradation associated with a lower hypertension incidence in a Chinese cohort (Bellien & Joannides, 2013). Overall, these genetic association studies provide varied evidence that decreased EET generation could contribute to human hypertension.

Although an association between hypertension and EET levels is varied, there is overwhelming evidence that increased sEH activity or reduced epoxygenase activity is associated with cardiovascular disease and endothelial dysfunction in humans (Bellien et al., 2006; Bellien, Iacob, et al., 2012; Bellien, Remy-Jouet, et al., 2012; Lee et al., 2011) (Fig. 2). A *CYP2J2* genetic variant that results in decreased plasma EET levels associates with increased risk for coronary artery disease (Spiecker et al., 2004). The *EPHX2* Arg55 polymorphism that increases sEH activity also associates with a greater risk for coronary artery disease (Lee et al., 2011). This *EPHX2* genetic variant results in impaired endothelial function as determined by decreased human forearm blood flow responses to bradykinin (Lee et al., 2011).

In humans with renovascular disease there is a decrease in plasma EET levels which supports a contribution of EETs to vascular and kidney disease (Bellien & Joannides, 2013; Elijovich, Milne, Brown, Laniado-Schwartzman, & Laffer, 2018). Chronic obstructive pulmonary disease patients have decreased plasma EET levels and endothelial dysfunction as assessed by forearm blood flow responses to bradykinin (Yang et al., 2017). Another study found an inability to induce EET release during flow mediated dilation that contributed to endothelial dysfunction in human hypertension (Bellien, Iacob, et al., 2012; Bellien, Remy-Jouet, et al., 2012). Conversely, the *EPHX2* Gln287 genetic variant that decreases sEH activity enhances human forearm blood flow responses to bradykinin (Lee et al., 2011). Intriguingly, plasma EET levels have been found to be elevated in coronary artery disease patients and following an ischemic stroke event in patients (Wang et al., 2010; Ward et al., 2011). Decreased *EPHX2* expression was also found in heart biopsies of heart failure patients (Monti et al., 2008). These findings suggest that decreased sEH activity and increased EETs could be a compensatory mechanism in cardiovascular disease and that genetic variants that reduce EET levels can contribute to cardiovascular diseases.

More recent studies have demonstrated that EET levels can importantly contribute to salt-sensitive hypertension (Capdevila et al., 2014; Elijovich et al., 2018; Imig, Jankiewicz, & Khan, 2020) (Fig. 2). One human study determined urine and plasma EET levels in salt-resistant and salt-sensitive normotensive subjects (Elijovich et al., 2018). Findings of this study found that urine EET levels represent kidney generation and correlate with inhibition of ENaC and sodium excretion. On the other hand, plasma EET levels did not correlate with aldosterone and salt regulation (Elijovich et al., 2018). Thus, plasma EET levels appear to be more reflective of systemic EET regulation that could contribute to cardiovascular diseases. Evaluation of EET levels in primary aldosteronism provide additional evidence for a contribution to salt regulation and blood pressure control. Primary aldosteronism leads to elevated aldosterone levels that act on renal epithelial cells to cause the body to retain more sodium and lose potassium resulting in hypertension. EET levels were determined in patients with primary aldosteronism before and after surgical resection of an aldosterone-secreting adenoma or medical treatment with a mineralocorticoid antagonist (Luther et al., 2021). Circulating plasma EET concentrations were found to increase following treatment of primary aldosteronism (Luther et al., 2021). These findings suggest that aldosterone actions could be mediated in part by decreasing the vasodilatory and natriuretic EETs. Taken together, these studies provide evidence for EET regulation of renal epithelial sodium transport and blood pressure in humans.

3. EET contribution to experimental hypertension and kidney disease

Extensive evaluation of animal disease models has demonstrated the contribution for increased sEH activity and decreased EET levels to hypertension and kidney diseases (Imig, 2018; Imig et al., 2020). These animal studies have determined CYP2C, CYP2J, and sEH protein expression, as well as, plasma, kidney, vascular, heart, and urine EET and dihydroxyeicosatrienoic acid (DHET) levels (Imig et al., 2020). Hypertension and kidney disease models have been evaluated under conditions of pharmacological and genetic manipulation of EET levels (Imig et al., 2020). Overall, these experimental animal studies have found that decreased EET levels contribute to vascular and renal epithelial dysfunction resulting in elevated blood pressure and kidney damage (Imig, 2018; Imig et al., 2020) (Fig. 2).

The exact contribution of increased sEH activity and decreased EET levels to elevate blood pressure have been extensively studied in rodent models of hypertension (Imig et al., 2020). Angiotensin II hypertension results in an increase in renal microvascular sEH protein expression resulting in a decrease in EET levels (Zhao, Pollock, Inscho, Zeldin, & Imig, 2003; Zhao et al., 2004). Overexpression human renin and angiotensinogen genes in rats (dTGR) results in decreased kidney CYP2C11 and CYP2C23 protein expression (Kaergel et al., 2002). Likewise, renin (*Ren*)-2 transgenic rats have decreased renal EET levels after 5/6 renal mass reduction to induce chronic kidney disease (Čertíková Chábová et al., 2019). Taken together, decreased kidney EET levels in angiotensin II dependent hypertension contribute to increased renal vascular resistance, renal inflammation, and decreased sodium excretion.

The importance of EETs to respond to dietary salt and increase sodium excretion to maintain water and electrolyte homeostasis has been demonstrated. Rats and mice increase kidney EET levels in response to a high salt diet (Capdevila et al., 2014; Imig et al., 2020; Makita et al., 1994; Zhao et al., 2003). Importantly, salt-sensitive hypertension occurs when there is an inability for kidney EET levels to increase in response high dietary salt levels (Capdevila et al., 2014; Zhao et al., 2003). Dahl salt-resistance rats increase EET levels in response to a high salt diet whereas Dahl salt-sensitive rats fail to increase renal protein expression of either CYP2C23 or CYP2C11

(Liclican, McGiff, Falck, & Carroll, 2008). Likewise, kidney and vascular CYP2C11 and CYP2C23 protein expression fail to increase in rats infused with angiotensin II and fed a high salt diet (Zhao et al., 2003). Decreased CYP2C levels also results in an inability to respond to a high salt diet (Capdevila et al., 2014; Zhao et al., 2003). Mice deficient in *CYP2C44* have decreased renal EET levels, elevated ENaC activity, and develop salt-sensitive hypertension (Capdevila et al., 2014). Salt-sensitive hypertension also occurs with genetic deletion of *CYP4A10* that results in suppression of *CYP2C44* and decreased kidney EET levels (Nakagawa et al., 2006). These findings demonstrate that an increase in renal EET levels is essential to handle an increase in dietary salt to maintain electrolyte and water homeostasis and blood pressure regulation.

Genetic manipulations in mice to increase EET levels have provided evidence for the potential therapeutic value for this pathway in hypertension (Imig & Hammock, 2009; Imig et al., 2020). *EPHX2* gene deficient mice have a lower resting blood pressure (Luria et al., 2007; Manhiani et al., 2009; Sinal et al., 2000). These *EPHX2* knockout mice also had lower blood pressure in deoxycorticosterone (DOCA)-salt hypertension (Manhiani et al., 2009). Increased EET levels, improved renal vascular function, and decreased renal inflammation in *EPHX2* knockout mice were responsible for the lower blood pressure in DOCA-salt hypertension (Manhiani et al., 2009). Transgenic mice expressing human endothelial *CYP2J2* or *CYP2C8* to increase vascular EETs had anti-hypertensive actions (Lee et al., 2010). These endothelial *CYP2J2* and *CYP2C8* transgenic mice had an attenuated renal microvascular endothelin-1 constrictor response and enhanced acetylcholine dilator response. Angiotensin II hypertension and L-NAME hypertension were attenuated in the transgenic mice expressing endothelial *CYP2J2* and *CYP2C8*. In addition to lowering blood pressure, these genetic mice studies found that increasing endothelial EET decreased inflammation and could combat kidney injury in hypertension (Lee et al., 2010). These findings in genetic animals clearly demonstrate that increasing EETs can combat hypertension, improve endothelial function, and decrease organ damage.

In addition to hypertension, there has been extensive evaluation of EETs in kidney diseases (Fan & Roman, 2017; Imig, 2018). Kidney diseases are associated with endothelial dysfunction, inflammation, and epithelial cell apoptosis. Decreased EET levels and increased sEH activity can contribute to kidney disease through vascular dysfunction, inflammation, and fibrosis (Fan & Roman, 2017; Imig, 2018). Increased renal epithelial cell sEH expression correlates with proteinuria and kidney inflammation in IgA nephropathy (Wang et al., 2013; Wang et al., 2014). Intriguingly, a metabolic analysis of urine identified EETs as predictive markers in acute and chronic experimental glomerulonephritis (Han et al., 2020). This study also found activated sEH and decreased *CYP2C23* gene expression in chronic glomerulonephritis (Han et al., 2020). Increased kidney sEH expression was also identified in nephrotoxicity caused by the anti-cancer multikinase inhibitor, sorafenib (Jankiewicz et al., 2021). Likewise, chemotherapy associated cisplatin nephrotoxicity had lower EET levels that contributed to epithelial cell endoplasmic reticulum stress and apoptosis (Khan et al., 2013). Unilateral ureter obstruction (UUO) in mice with progressive renal fibrosis that mimics chronic kidney disease have increased sEH protein expression and a decrease in the kidney EET to DHET ratio (Kim et al., 2015; Kim, Imig, Yang, Hammock, & Padanilam, 2014). Radiation-induced nephrotoxicity was also found to be associated with reduced renal mRNA and protein expressions of CYP2C11 and decreased urinary EET levels (Hye Khan et al., 2016; Imig et al., 2016). Decreased EET levels contributed to renal microvascular endothelial dysfunction in radiation-induced nephrotoxicity (Imig et al., 2016). Similarly, a decrease in EET levels during acute ischemic kidney injury contributes to endothelial dysfunction and epithelial cell apoptosis (Lee et al., 2012; Zhu et al., 2016). Infiltration of inflammatory cells into the vascular smooth muscle cell also occurs with decreased endothelial cell EET generation (Behmoaras et al., 2015). Interestingly, reduced EET generation by macrophages results in a profibrotic macrophage transcriptome (Behmoaras et al., 2015). Consequently, several studies in animal models have consistently found increased sEH expression or decreased EET levels that contributes to progression of kidney diseases.

Overall, there have been compelling experimental findings in humans and animal models to demonstrate that increased sEH activity or decreased EET levels contribute to hypertension and kidney diseases (Bellien & Joannides, 2013; Imig, 2018). These findings have led to the postulate that pharmacological manipulation to inhibit sEH activity or increase EET levels could be anti-hypertensive and oppose kidney diseases. The development of sEH inhibitors have advanced to clinical trials for hypertension, diabetes, and chronic obstructive pulmonary disease (GlaxoSmithKline, 2013; Imig & Hammock, 2009; Lazaar et al., 2016). However, there are drawbacks associated with sEH inhibitors as a therapeutic approach. The use of sEH inhibitors results in an indirect increase in EETs and other epoxy fatty acids, requires a functioning CYP2C or CYP2J epoxygenase to generate EETs, and results in an increase in EETs that are metabolically labile (Campbell et al., 2017; Imig & Hammock, 2009). Development of EET mimics can circumvent these drawbacks of sEH inhibitors by directly providing an active EET that is metabolically stable and independent of CYP2C or CYP2J activity (Campbell et al., 2017). EET mimics have progressed significantly and demonstrated promise in animal disease models (Campbell et al., 2017; Imig, 2018). Therefore, the development of EET mimics as a pharmacological treatment for hypertension and kidney disease will be focus of subsequent sections.

4. Therapeutic development of EET mimics/analogs

Therapeutic development of EET mimics has been ongoing for 25 years. The initial development of EET mimics focused on improving stability to allow determination of biological actions in *in vitro* and *ex vivo* experimental settings (Pfister, Gauthier, & Campbell, 2010; Sudhahar, Shaw, & Imig, 2010). A primary problem with EETs is the need to store at −80 °C and under nitrogen or argon gas. Even under these conditions, EETs must be checked for degradation and purity (Pfister et al., 2010; Sudhahar et al., 2010). This greatly limited early investigations to determine EET biological actions. A first step in the development of 11,12-EET and 14,15-EET mimics was to prevent degradation by β-oxidation and esterification into phospholipids (Gauthier, Falck, Reddy, & Campbell, 2004; Imig, Inscho, Deichmann, Reddy, & Falck, 1999). Modifications were made to the carboxylic acid by synthesizing methyl esters (Me) and sulfonamides (SI) for 11,12-EET and 14,15-EET (Falck et al., 2003; Gauthier et al., 2004; Imig et al., 1999). This series was extensively tested for vascular actions (Pfister et al., 2010; Sudhahar et al., 2010). 11,12-EET-SI, 11,12-EET-Me, 14,15-EET-Me, and 14,15-EET-SI resulted in vasodilation of coronary arteries and renal arterioles (Gauthier et al., 2004; Imig et al., 1999). These EET mimics were also determined to activate vascular smooth muscle cell K_{Ca} channels to cause hyperpolarization and relaxation (Gauthier et al., 2004; Imig et al., 1999). These initial successful findings with EET mimics provided the impetus to move toward developing EET analog drugs.

Another issue with testing EET for biological actions was their limited solubility that required the use of solvents such as ethanol and dimethylsulfoxide (DMSO) (Campbell et al., 2017; Pfister et al., 2010). In addition, EET metabolism by sEH to the biologically less active or inactive DHETs limited their evaluation in experimental settings (Campbell et al., 2017; Imig et al., 2020). Thus, next steps for EET mimic development included the elimination of carbon double bonds to improve solubility and substitutions to the oxygen of the epoxide to resist metabolism by sEH (Campbell et al., 2017; Falck et al., 2009; Pfister et al., 2010). The initial replacements for the 11,12- and 14,15- epoxide oxygen included sulfur and ether moieties (Campbell et al., 2017; Pfister et al., 2010; Sudhahar et al., 2010). These changes resulted in EET mimics with improved solubility that could resist metabolism by sEH (Campbell et al., 2017). Several 11,12-EET and 14,15-EET mimics were tested for biological activity and compared to the native EETs (Campbell et al., 2017; Falck et al., 2014). A series of 11,12-EET mimics included 11,12-EET-SI, 11-nonyloxy-undec-8(Z)-enoic acid (11,12-ether-EET-8-ZE), and 11,12-transoxidoeicosa-8(Z)-enoic acid (11,12-tetra-EET-8-ZE) that were found to have biological actions comparable to 11,12-EET (Imig et al., 2010; Imig, Dimitropoulou, Reddy, White, & Falck, 2008). These 11,12-EET analogs provided evidence that 11,12-EET utilizes cyclic adenosine monophosphate (cAMP) and protein phosphatase 2A (PP2A) dependent pathways to activate K_{Ca} channels in mesenteric and renal arterioles (Imig et al., 2008). Although several of the EET mimics had comparable biological activities, there were structural changes to EETs that had reduced activity (Falck et al., 2014; Imig et al., 2008). Interestingly, the elimination of carbon double bonds resulted in the discovery of EET antagonists like 14,15-epoxy-5(Z)-enoic acid (14,15-EE5ZE) and 11,12,20-trihydroxy-eicosa-8(Z)-enoic acid (11,12,20-THE8ZE) (Bukhari et al., 2012; Gauthier et al., 2002; Gauthier, Jagadeesh, Falck, & Campbell, 2003). Carbon chain length for EET mimics was also modified and tested for biological activity (Campbell et al., 2017; Imig et al., 2010). What emerged was a structure activity relationship for 11,12-EET and 14,15-EET. Structural requirements for 11,12-EET and 14,15-EET vasorelaxation are: (1) a carboxylic acid or acidic proton at C(1); (2) *cis*-8,9-olefin; (3) *cis*-epoxide; (4) 20-carbon chain (Campbell et al., 2017; Falck et al., 2014) (Fig. 3).

A key step in the development of EET analogs was further modifications and testing in *in vivo* experimental settings. 11,12-EET analogs based on the 11-nonyloxy-undec-8-(Z)-enoic acid structure with better solubility and resistance to β-oxidation were synthesized (Imig et al., 2010). Substitution of the epoxide with an acyclic ether led to a series of 11,12-EET analogs that included the aspartic amide of 11-nonyloxy-undec-8(Z)-enoic acid, NUDSA (Imig et al., 2010; Sodhi et al., 2009). NUDSA when administered by intraperitoneal injection lowered blood pressure and improved vascular function in

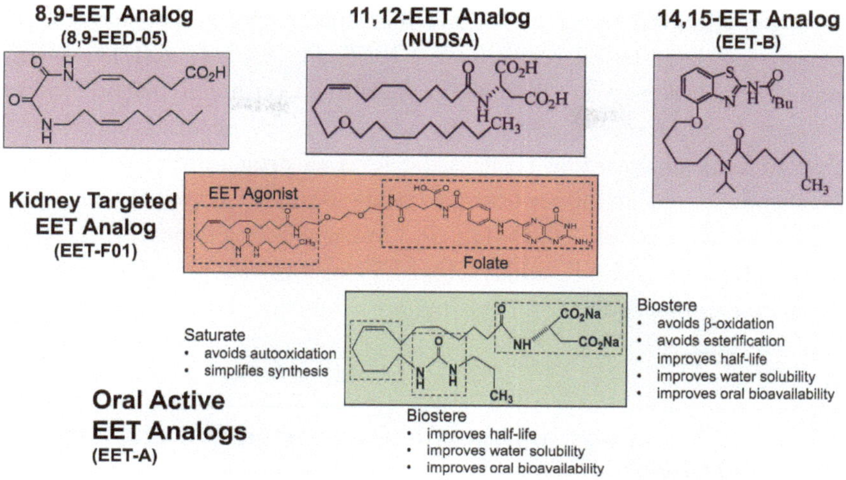

Fig. 3 Development of epoxyeicosatrienoic acid (EET) analogs. *TOP:* Regioisomeric EET analogs for 8,9-EET, 11,12-EET, and 14,15-EET. *MIDDLE:* Folate conjugation of EET analogs results in kidney targeted EET analogs. *BOTTOM:* Modifications in EET analogs that result in orally active EET analogs.

hypertension and obesity (Sodhi et al., 2009). This finding provided the incentive to develop EET analogs that could be administered orally over long periods of time. The development of orally active EET analogs focused on a third generation of 14,15-EET analogs (Falck et al., 2014) (Fig. 3). A major objective was to synthesize 14,15-EET analogs that minimized or prevented β-oxidation and esterification while improving water solubility, obtaining oral bioavailability, and extending the *in vivo* half-life (Campbell et al., 2017; Falck et al., 2014). Changes were made to the epoxide and significant changes to the carboxylic acid including tetrazoles and oxathiadiazole-2-oxides (Falck et al., 2014). As a result, >30 analogs were generated and provided several 14,15-EET analogs with good water solubility that were orally bioavailable with a reasonable half-life for chronic administration in preclinical hypertension and kidney disease animal models (Falck et al., 2014; Khan, Liu, et al., 2013; Khan, Manthati, et al., 2013).

The development of orally bioavailable 8,9-EET, 11,12-EET, and 14,15-EET analogs has led to extensive testing in cardiovascular and renal diseases (Campbell et al., 2017; Imig, 2018). Administration of 11,12-EET and 14,15-EET have been extensively tested in cardiovascular diseases, acute kidney injury, and chronic kidney disease with positive results (Campbell et al., 2017; Imig, 2018). Intriguingly, 8,9-EET analogs are effective for glomerular diseases whereas 11,12-EET or 14,15-EET analogs do not act at the glomerulus to combat increases in glomerular permeability (Sharma et al., 2009). Excitingly, 8,9-EET, 11,12-EET, and 14,15-EET analogs could each act as a therapeutic for distinct cardiovascular and kidney diseases. A more recent development has been the generation of kidney targeted EET analogs that reduces the level of drug needed to achieve a therapeutic effect in kidney diseases while avoiding potential side effects (Imig, Hye Khan, et al., 2021) (Fig. 3). On the whole, phenotypic screening of 8,9-EET, 11,12-EET, and 14,15-EET analogs has provided clear and convincing evidence that EET analogs are drug candidates (Campbell et al., 2017; Imig, 2018).

5. EET analogs in preclinical hypertension and kidney disease

EET analogs were first tested *in vivo* on cardiovascular disease in 2009 with intraperitoneal injection of the 11,12-EET analog, NUDSA, to mice with metabolic syndrome (Sodhi et al., 2009). This opened the door for several studies that administered 11,12-EET and 14,15-EET analogs chronically to preclinical hypertension, heart disease, and kidney disease animal models. A breakthrough came in 2013 with the development of 14,15-EET analogs such as EET-A that could be synthesized in gram quantities and administered orally to rodents (Khan, Liu, et al., 2013). In the subsequent 8 years there was an explosion of publications finding that EET analogs have therapeutic potential to combat cardiovascular and kidney diseases.

Hypertension is a cardiovascular disease where EET analogs have been extensively evaluated for their ability to lower blood pressure, improve endothelial function, and prevent end organ damage (Imig, 2018; Imig et al., 2020) (Fig. 4). NUDSA administration by injection for 5 days to heme-oxygenase 2 knockout mice with metabolic syndrome resulted in decreased blood pressure and improved endothelial-dependent vasodilation (Sodhi et al., 2009). Experimental studies in angiotensin hypertension demonstrated the ability for NUDSA and other 11,12-EET analogs to lower blood pressure following a single injection. Notably, EET analogs that failed to cause vasodilation also failed to lower blood pressure (Imig et al., 2010). Initial studies administering EET analogs orally to spontaneously hypertensive rats (SHR) found that EET analogs required 3 days to lower blood pressure which returned to hypertensive levels after withdrawing EET analog treatment (Hye Khan et al., 2014). On the other hand, findings in

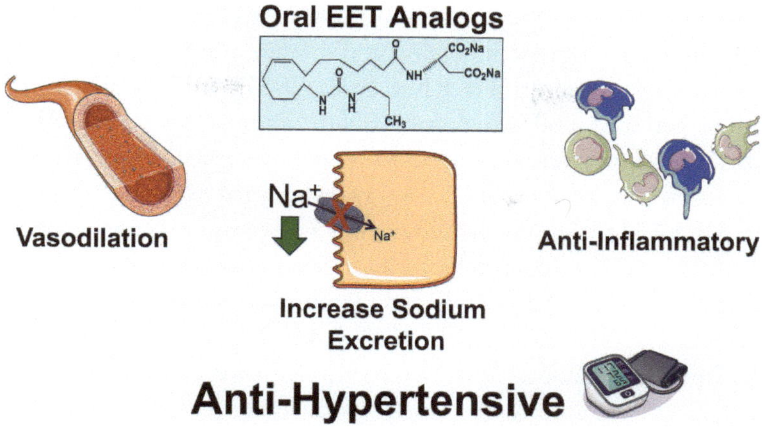

Fig. 4 Diagram depicting epoxyeicosatrienoic acid (EET) analog actions that result in lowering blood pressure to combat hypertension. EET analogs act on vascular smooth muscle cells to cause vasodilation (left), inhibit epithelial sodium channels (ENaC) to increase sodium excretion (middle), and decrease activation of inflammatory cells (right).

SHR and WKY rats demonstrate that EET analogs given centrally have an opposite action on blood pressure regulation (Sellers et al., 2005). Intracerebroventricular injection of an sEH inhibitor to SHR and WKY rats or an EET analog, 11-NODA to WKY rats resulted in an increase in heart rate and blood pressure (Sellers et al., 2005). This finding provides evidence that the central actions for EET analogs could be opposite peripheral actions and suggest that the peripheral actions of EET analogs predominate or EET analogs do not cross the blood–brain barrier. In accordance with peripheral actions of EET analogs predominating, SHR administered an intravenous infusion of EET-A demonstrate an increase in renal blood flow and cortical blood flow that precedes a decrease in blood pressure (Walkowska et al., 2021). These data support the notion that decreased renal vascular resistance contributes to the blood pressure lowering actions for EET analogs. A longer 2-week oral treatment with EET-A was demonstrated to have anti-hypertensive actions in Cyp1a1-*Ren*-2 transgenic rats with malignant angiotensin-dependent hypertension (Jíchová et al., 2016). Likewise, chronic treatment with EET-A and EET-B was determined in SHR and angiotensin hypertension (Hye Khan et al., 2014). Findings in these studies determined that EET-A and EET-B lowered blood pressure through peripheral actions on resistance arteries to cause vasodilation and on renal tubular cells to inhibit ENaC and promote sodium excretion.

Additional studies in *Cyp2c44* knockout mice provided strong evidence that EET analogs acting peripherally on resistance arteries and kidney ENaC to lower blood pressure (Hye Khan et al., 2014). EET-A dilated afferent arterioles, reduced collecting duct ENaC expression and activity, and lowered blood pressure in *Cyp2c44* knockout mice with salt-sensitive hypertension (Capdevila et al., 2014; Hye Khan et al., 2014). Another major action for EET analogs in hypertension is decreasing systemic and renal inflammation. EET analogs decrease monocyte chemoattractant-1 (MCP-1) levels and reduce renal macrophage inflammation in several rodent models of hypertension (Hye Khan et al., 2014; Khan, Manthati, et al., 2013). The anti-inflammatory actions described for EET analogs also likely contribute to their blood pressure lowering effects in hypertension. Taken together these studies demonstrate that EET analogs act on resistance arteries, renal epithelial sodium channels, and inflammatory cells to lower blood pressure in hypertension (Fig. 4).

Vascular, heart, and kidney organ protective actions for EET analogs were also demonstrated in hypertension (Imig, 2018; Imig, Hye Khan, et al., 2021). A consistent finding has been that endothelial dysfunction in hypertension is reduced by chronic EET analog treatment (Imig et al., 2020). As mentioned previously, the 11,12-EET analog, NUDSA improved the aortic dilator responses to acetylcholine in metabolic syndrome mice (Sodhi et al., 2009). Likewise, the 14,15-EET analog, EET-A improved endothelial-dependent dilation of mesenteric resistance arteries in angiotensin hypertension (Hye Khan et al., 2014). Kidney afferent arteriolar endothelial-dependent dilation improved, and blood pressure decreased with EET-A treatment in radiation-induced nephropathy and hypertension (Hye Khan et al., 2016). EET analogs have also been demonstrated to protect the heart from injury in hypertension (Khan, Manthati, et al., 2013; Neckář et al., 2019). SHR with myocardial infarction and administered EET-B for 7 weeks demonstrated decreased heart failure that was associated with reduced myocardial inflammation and fibrosis (Neckář et al., 2019). EET-B has also been demonstrated to decrease cardiac fibrosis in Dahl salt-sensitive hypertension (Khan, Manthati, et al., 2013). Similarly, EET-A treatment reduces ischemic arrhythmias and cardiac hypertrophy in angiotensin-dependent hypertension (Neckář et al., 2012). Lastly, kidney injury in hypertension is reduced by EET analog treatment. Several studies have demonstrated that EET-A and EET-B decrease renal injury in hypertension. These studies have found decreased kidney inflammation, fibrosis, and glomerular injury with EET analog treatment in hypertension

(Imig et al., 2020). It is difficult to determine the contribution of the anti-hypertensive actions vs direct EET analog actions on decreasing progressive kidney injury in hypertension. However, EET-B treatment to Dahl salt-sensitive hypertension did not lower blood pressure while decreasing renal fibrosis and glomerular injury (Khan, Manthati, et al., 2013). This finding demonstrated that EET analogs in addition to lowering blood pressure could have direct actions on the kidney to arrest the progression of chronic kidney disease in hypertension.

The beneficial effects of EET analogs to treat chronic kidney diseases of various etiologies has been consistently demonstrated (Imig, 2018; Imig et al., 2020) (Fig. 5). EET analogs were first tested in drug-induced and radiation-induced nephrotoxicity (Hye Khan et al., 2016; Khan, Liu, et al., 2013). Kidney injury induced by the chemotherapeutic drug cisplatin was prevented by oral administration of EET analogs. EET analogs, EET-A or EET-B reduced blood urea nitrogen (BUN), albuminuria, and kidney injury molecule-1 (KIM-1) levels in cisplatin-induced nephrotoxicity in rats. EET analogs also decreased cisplatin mediated renal injury by reducing oxidative stress, endoplasmic reticulum stress, and apoptosis. Further kidney analysis revealed that EET analogs reduced B-cell lymphoma 2 (Bcl2)-proapoptotic signaling and caspase 3 activity (Khan, Liu, et al., 2013).

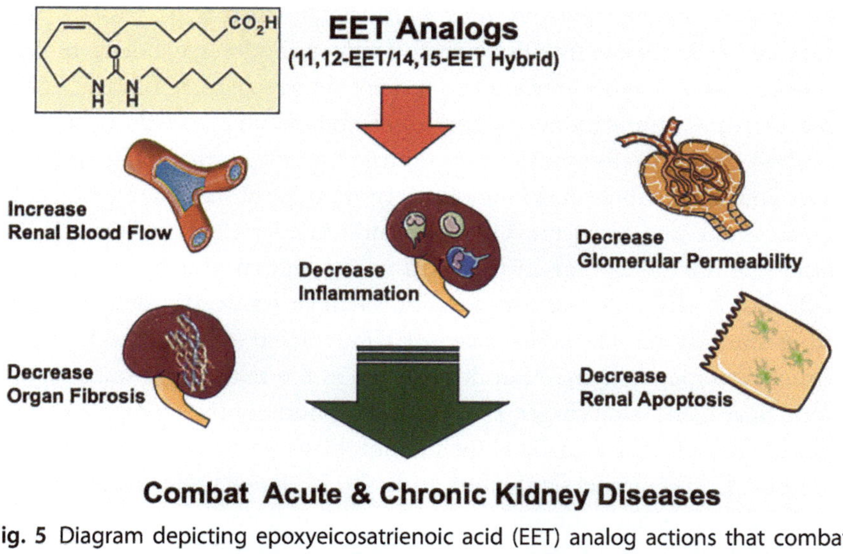

Fig. 5 Diagram depicting epoxyeicosatrienoic acid (EET) analog actions that combat acute and chronic kidney diseases. EET analogs increase renal blood flow, decrease inflammation, and decrease glomerular permeability that decrease kidney fibrosis and apoptosis to slow or arrest the progression of acute and chronic kidney diseases.

Likewise, experimental studies in radiation nephropathy provided evidence for kidney anti-apoptotic actions for EET analogs (Hye Khan et al., 2016). EET-A given 2 days following radiation exposure reduced kidney injury as determined by BUN and histopathological changes that were associated with actions on the p53/Fas/FasL (Fas ligand) apoptotic pathway (Hye Khan et al., 2016). The ability for EET analogs to oppose the renal injury that occurs with the calcineurin inhibitor, cyclosporine has also been determined. EET-B administered for 1 month decreased renal injury caused by cyclosporine (Yeboah et al., 2016). Cyclosporine mediated kidney oxidative stress, inflammation, fibrosis, and apoptosis were reduced in rats treated with EET-B. Additionally, EET-B reduced apoptosis in cultured renal epithelial cells exposed to cyclosporine *via* decreases in endoplasmic reticulum stress and glucose-regulated protein 78 (GRP78) levels (Yeboah et al., 2016). Taken together, these studies demonstrate that EET analogs have anti-inflammatory, anti-oxidative stress, and anti-apoptotic to protect the kidney from radiation- and drug-induced nephrotoxicity (Fig. 5).

Chronic kidney disease studies have demonstrated the ability for EET analogs to slow or arrest progression to end stage renal disease (Imig, 2018). As described, initial studies in hypertension provided evidence that EET analogs could directly act at the kidney to slow the progression of chronic kidney disease (Imig et al., 2020). EET analogs decrease inflammation and fibrosis and improve renal hemodynamics in hypertension (Imig et al., 2020). Evidence in kidney disease animal models have demonstrated decreased EET levels contribute to kidney disease (Fan & Roman, 2017; Imig, 2018). Chronic kidney disease UUO mice have markedly lower renal *Cyp2c44* and *Cyp2j5* expression supporting the notion that decreased EET levels could contribute to kidney damage (Kim et al., 2014). Importantly, experimental studies in the UUO chronic kidney disease mouse model found that 14,15-EET or EET-A had strong anti-fibrotic actions (Skibba et al., 2017). EET-A treatment to UUO mice reduced kidney collagen and α-smooth muscle actin levels. EET-A acted to prevent increased epithelial to mesenchymal transducers such as the zinc-finger transcription factor Snail1 and zinc finger *E*-box binding homeobox 1 (ZEB-1) while reducing myofibroblast markers such as fibroblast-specific protein 1 (FSP-1), E-cadherin, and fibronectin (Skibba et al., 2017). These findings demonstrate that EET analogs have anti-inflammatory and anti-fibrotic actions to decrease progression of chronic kidney disease (Fig. 5).

The ability for EET analogs to reduce glomerular injury has been demonstrated in hypertension and chronic kidney disease (Imig, 2018;

Imig et al., 2020). In addition, EET analogs have been evaluated in glomerular kidney diseases including focal segmental glomerulosclerosis and lupus nephritis (Imig, 2018). Glomerular injury was assessed in 20-week-old female NZBWF1 systemic lupus nephritis mice treated with EET-A (Hye Khan, Stavniichuk, Sattar, Falck, & Imig, 2019). EET-A treatment for 3 months in NZBWF1 systemic lupus nephritis decreased glomerular injury but did not lower plasma levels of anti-dsDNA antibodies. Glomerular infiltration of CD43 positive immune B cells and F4/80 positive macrophages in lupus nephritis mice were decreased by EET-A treatment. Kidney inflammation levels of CXC (chemokine C-X-C motif) chemokines and receptors, tumor necrosis factor-α (TNF-α), interleukin-6 (IL-6), and interleukin-1β (IL-1β) were reduced by EET-A in lupus nephritis mice (Hye Khan et al., 2019). Interestingly, 8,9-EET analogs but not 11,12-EET or 14,15-EET analogs can combat focal segmental glomerular sclerosis (Sharma et al., 2009). Unlike the kidney cortex which produces predominantly 11,12-EET and 14,15-EET, glomeruli production of 8,9-EET accounts for approximately 40% of the total EET production (Katoh et al., 1991). Experimental studies evaluated regioisomeric EET actions to prevent focal glomerular sclerosis permeability factor (FSPF) increase in glomerular permeability (Sharma et al., 2009). FSPF-induced permeability increases in isolated rat glomeruli were reduced by 8,9-EET but not 5,6-EET, 11,12-EET, 14,15-EET, or DHETs. In addition, a synthetic 8,9-EET analogs containing two double bonds (8,9-EED) inhibited the effect of FSPF on the glomerular filtration barrier (Sharma et al., 2009). Taken together, these finding suggests that 11,12-EET and 14,15-EET analogs can combat glomerular inflammation while 8,9-EET analogs appear to directly protect the glomerular barrier from factors that increase permeability (Fig. 5).

EET analogs are also effective in combating acute kidney injury. Renal ischemia reperfusion injury is reduced by renal artery administration of an 11,12-EET/14,15-EET hybrid analog where the epoxide mimic is located in between the two positions (Hoff et al., 2019). EET analog treatment decreased serum creatinine, BUN, and kidney infiltration of CD68 positive macrophages. Renal medullary and cortical oxygenation determined by high temporal resolution parametric magnetic resonance imaging (MRI) was improved by EET analog administration into the renal artery following renal ischemia reperfusion. EET analog treatment decreased renal epithelial cell apoptosis *via* improved phosphoinositide 3-kinase (PI3K)- and mammalian target of rapamycin complex 2 (mTORC2)-dependent rephosphorylation of protein kinase B (Akt) and inactivation of glycogen synthase kinase β

(GSK3β) (Hoff et al., 2019). The beneficial actions for EET analogs in renal ischemia reperfusion injury are consistent with increased susceptibility in acute kidney injury patients with increased sEH activity and a decreased epoxide to diol ratio (Shuey et al., 2017).

Kidney targeted EET analogs is a recent development that allows for EET analogs to achieve a therapeutic effect in kidney diseases at lower doses while reducing side effects. Folate-conjugation of drugs can target the kidney due to the high concentration of folate receptors which permit epithelial cell uptake of the folate-conjugated drug (Kipp et al., 2018; Knight et al., 2012). The concept of folate-conjugated drugs was successfully demonstrated with tempol and rapamycin (Kipp et al., 2018; Knight et al., 2012). More recently, an EET analog backbone connected to folic acid *via* an ethyleneoxydiamine linker, EET-F01, was synthesized and tested in drug-induced nephrotoxicity (Imig, Hye Khan, et al., 2021). EET-F01 was compared to EET-A in cisplatin-induced nephrotoxicity. Initial studies demonstrated that EET-F01, but not EET-A levels were detected in the kidney tissue following 6 h of intravenous administration. Despite an almost 2 ×-greater molecular weight, EET-F01 administered intraperitoneally *via* an osmotic pump effectively decreased cisplatin nephrotoxicity at a 10-fold lower weighted dose than EET-A. EET-F01 reduced levels of kidney injury markers BUN, KIM-1, and NAG (*N*-acetyl-beta-D-glucosaminidase (NAG). Kidney histology also revealed decreased cisplatin-induced tubular damage in rats treated with EET-F01. EET-F01 demonstrated anti-inflammatory actions and reduced kidney IL-6, TNF-α, and interleukin-10 (IL-10) levels in cisplatin nephrotoxicity (Imig, Hye Khan, et al., 2021). These findings demonstrate that a kidney targeted EET analog, EET-F01, demonstrates excellent potential as a therapeutic for kidney diseases.

6. Advances toward clinical trials

The therapeutic potential for EET analogs for hypertension and kidney diseases includes evidence from human studies and preclinical animal model studies (Bellien & Joannides, 2013; Campbell et al., 2017; Imig et al., 2020). Human studies have clearly established genetic polymorphisms in *CYP2C* and *CYP2J* enzymes that decrease EET production or *EPHX2* that increase sEH activity associate with hypertension and kidney diseases (Bellien & Joannides, 2013). Changes in urinary and plasma EET and DHET levels can also be predictive of cardiovascular and kidney diseases

(Bellien & Joannides, 2013). Importantly, vascular endothelial health is diminished in humans with decreased EET levels (Bellien & Joannides, 2013). These human studies provided the impetus for developing therapeutics that increase EET levels.

Although EET analogs have lagged compared to the development of sEH inhibitors, EET analogs are now positioned to advance from preclinical animal studies to human clinical trials. The precise molecular targets for EET regioisomers is still yet to be identified which has required phenotypic screening for EET analogs (Campbell et al., 2017). In addition, a structure–activity relationship for EET analogs needed to be established. A further complexity was that the synthesis process for EET analogs needed to achieve gram quantities. EET analogs have now been developed for 8,9-EET, 11,12-EET, and 14,15-EET which have been tested in experimental hypertension and kidney disease animal models (Campbell et al., 2017; Imig et al., 2020). The findings of these studies have identified 8,9-EET analogs as effective for glomerular diseases whereas 11,12-EET and 14,15-EET analogs are more efficacious in hypertension and chronic kidney diseases.

Other aspects in EET analog development include hybrid 11,12-EET/14,15-EET analogs, EET analogs with sEH inhibitory activity, and kidney targeted EET analogs (Falck et al., 2014; Hoff et al., 2019; Imig, Hye Khan, et al., 2021). Initial studies found that a hybrid 11,12-EET/14,15-EET analog prevented renal ischemia reperfusion injury (Hoff et al., 2019). The overall therapeutic potential in hypertension and kidney disease for the hybrid 11,12-EET/14,15-EET analogs remains to be determined. Several of the EET analogs that have been synthesized also have variable sEH inhibitory activity (Falck et al., 2014). The ability for dual EET analog/sEH inhibitors has not been extensively tested. However, experimental studies have provided evidence that combining sEH inhibitors with EET analogs does not provide additive anti-hypertensive effects (Červenka et al., 2018). This finding supports the notion that sEH inhibitors and EET analogs have overlapping actions and questions the need to further investigate dual EET analog/sEH inhibitors. Finally, a recent breakthrough has been the development of kidney targeted EET analogs. The kidney targeted EET analog, EET-F01 has been demonstrated to prevent drug-induced nephrotoxicity (Imig, Hye Khan, et al., 2021). Therefore, the future for EET analogs as a therapeutic for hypertension and kidney diseases looks promising.

EET analogs have consistently been demonstrated to improve endothelial function, decrease inflammation, decrease endoplasmic reticulum stress, and oppose apoptosis (Campbell et al., 2017; Imig et al., 2020).

These activities suggests that EET analogs could be beneficial in treating several other types of diseases. EET analogs have already been tested in cardiac disease models and have been found to improve heart function (Imig, Hye Khan, et al., 2021; Oni-Orisan et al., 2014). EET analogs could be expanded to non-alcoholic fatty liver disease, diabetes, retinopathies, pre-eclampsia, neuropathies, and organ transplantation. Human studies have previously demonstrated decreased EET levels in insulin resistance and pre-eclampsia (Gangadhariah et al., 2017; Herse et al., 2012; Jiang et al., 2013). Experimental studies in diabetes and pre-eclampsia animal models have not yet tested EET analogs. Supplementing organ transplantation solutions with endogenous EETs demonstrated positive effects on organ preservation (Yang, Zhang, Yim, & He, 2003); however, EET analogs have not been evaluated. Therefore, there are several other diseases where EET analogs need to be tested for therapeutic actions.

7. Conclusion

In conclusion, EET analogs have demonstrated exceptional therapeutic potential to combat hypertension and kidney diseases (Campbell et al., 2017; Imig et al., 2020). Experimental studies have demonstrated oral activity and an excellent pharmacological profile for EET analogs (Campbell et al., 2017; Imig et al., 2020). EET analogs are effective for short-term and long-term administration without significant side effects or toxicities (Campbell et al., 2017; Imig et al., 2020). Defining and identifying the appropriate use for treating humans is the next major hurdle. Human studies could provide valuable information that allows prioritization of clinical indications and patient populations that would best benefit from EET analog treatment. Accordingly, there is a bright future for EET analogs to treat hypertension and acute and chronic kidney diseases.

Acknowledgments

This work was supported by the National Institute of Diabetes and Digestive and Kidney Diseases DK126452. Servier Medical Art was used to generate Figs. 1, 2, 4, and 5 and is licensed by Servier under a Creative Commons Attribution 3.0 Unported License.

Conflict of interest statement

Dr. Imig has patents that cover the composition of matter for EET analogs. There are no other conflicts of interest, financial or otherwise, as declared by the author.

References

Archer, S. L., Gragasin, F. S., Wu, X., Wang, S., McMurtry, S., Kim, D. H., et al. (2003). Endothelium-derived hyperpolarizing factor in human internal mammary artery is 11,12-epoxyeicosatrienoic acid and causes relaxation by activating smooth muscle BK(ca) channels. *Circulation, 107*, 769–776.

Behmoaras, J., Diaz, A. G., Venda, L., Ko, J. H., Srivastava, P., Montoya, A., et al. (2015). Macrophage epoxygenase determines a profibrotic transcriptome signature. *Journal of Immunology, 194*, 4705–4716.

Bellien, J., Iacob, M., Gutierrez, L., Isabelle, M., Lahary, A., Thuillez, C., et al. (2006). Crucial role of NO and endothelium-derived hyperpolarizing factor in human sustained conduit artery flow-mediated dilatation. *Hypertension, 48*, 1088–1094.

Bellien, J., Iacob, M., Remy-Jouet, I., Lucas, D., Monteil, C., Gutierrez, L., et al. (2012). Epoxyeicosatrienoic acids contribute with altered nitric oxide and endothelin-1 pathways to conduit artery endothelial dysfunction in essential hypertension. *Circulation, 125*, 1266–1275.

Bellien, J., & Joannides, R. (2013). Epoxyeicosatrienoic acid pathway in human health and diseases. *Journal of Cardiovascular Pharmacology, 61*, 188–196.

Bellien, J., Remy-Jouet, I., Iacob, M., Blot, E., Mercier, A., Lucas, D., et al. (2012). Impaired role of epoxyeicosatrienoic acids in the regulation of basal conduit artery diameter during essential hypertension. *Hypertension, 60*, 1415–1421.

Bukhari, I. A., Shah, A. J., Gauthier, K. M., Walsh, K. A., Konduru, S. R., Imig, J. D., et al. (2012). 11,12,20-trihydroxy-eicosa-8(Z)-enoic acid: A selective inhibitor of 11,12-EET induced relaxations of bovine coronary and rat mesenteric arteries. *American Journal of Physiology. Heart and Circulatory Physiology, 302*, H1574–H1583.

Bystrom, J., Wray, J. A., Sugden, M. C., Holness, M. J., Swales, K. E., Warner, T. D., et al. (2011). Endogenous epoxygenases are modulators of monocyte/macrophage activity. *PLoS One, 6*, e26591.

Campbell, W. B., Deeter, C., Gauthier, K. M., Ingraham, R. H., Falck, J. R., & Li, P. L. (2002). 14,15-Dihydroxyeicosatrienoic acid relaxes bovine coronary arteries by activation of K(ca) channels. *American Journal of Physiology. Heart and Circulatory Physiology, 282*, H1656–H1664.

Campbell, W. B., Gebremedhin, D., Pratt, P. F., & Harder, D. R. (1996). Identification of epoxyeicosatrienoic acids as endothelium-derived hyperpolarizing factors. *Circulation Research, 78*, 415–423.

Campbell, W. B., Imig, J. D., Schmitz, J. M., & Falck, J. R. (2017). Orally active Epoxyeicosatrienoic acid analogs. *Journal of Cardiovascular Pharmacology, 70*, 211–224.

Capdevila, J. H., Falck, J. R., & Imig, J. D. (2007). Roles of the cytochrome P450 arachidonic acid monooxygenases in the control of systemic blood pressure and experimental hypertension. *Kidney International, 72*, 683–689.

Capdevila, J. H., Pidkovka, N., Mei, S., Gong, Y., Falck, J. R., Imig, J. D., et al. (2014). The Cyp2c44 epoxygenase regulates epithelial sodium channel activity and the blood pressure responses to increased dietary salt. *The Journal of Biological Chemistry, 289*, 4377–4386.

Čertíková Chábová, V., Kujal, P., Vaňourková, Z., Škaroupková, P., Sadowski, J., Kompanowska-Jezierska, E., et al. (2019). Addition of endothelin A-receptor blockade spoils the beneficial effect of combined renin-angiotensin and soluble epoxide hydrolase inhibition: Studies on the course of chronic kidney disease in 5/6 nephrectomized ren-2 transgenic hypertensive rats. *Kidney & Blood Pressure Research, 44*, 1493–1505.

Červenka, L., Husková, Z., Kopkan, L., Kikerlová, S., Sedláková, L., Vaňourková, Z., et al. (2018). Two pharmacological epoxyeicosatrienoic acid-enhancing therapies are effectively antihypertensive and reduce the severity of ischemic arrhythmias in rats with angiotensin II-dependent hypertension. *Journal of Hypertension, 36*, 1326–1341.

Dreisbach, A. W., Japa, S., Sigel, A., Parenti, M. B., Hess, A. E., Srinouanprachanh, S. L., et al. (2005). The prevalence of CYP2C8, 2C9, 2J2, and soluble epoxide hydrolase polymorphisms in African Americans with hypertension. *American Journal of Hypertension, 18*, 1276–1281.

Egan, B. M., & Laken, M. A. (2011). Is blood pressure control to less than 140/less than 90 mmHg in 50% of all hypertensive patients as good as we can do in the USA: Or is this as good as it gets? *Current Opinion in Cardiology, 26*, 300–307.

Elijovich, F., Milne, G. L., Brown, N. J., Laniado-Schwartzman, M., & Laffer, C. L. (2018). Two pools of epoxyeicosatrienoic acids in humans: Alterations in salt-sensitive normotensive subjects. *Hypertension, 71*, 346–355.

Falck, J. R., Kodela, R., Manne, R., Atcha, K. R., Puli, N., Dubasi, N., et al. (2009). 14,15-Epoxyeicosa-5,8,11-trienoic acid (14,15-EET) surrogates containing epoxide bioisosteres: Influence upon vascular relaxation and soluble epoxide hydrolase inhibition. *Journal of Medicinal Chemistry, 52*, 5069–5075.

Falck, J. R., Koduru, S. R., Mohapatra, S., Manne, R., Atcha, R., Manthati, V. L., et al. (2014). 14,15-Epoxyeicosa-5,8,11-trienoic acid (14,15-EET) surrogates: carboxylate modifications. *Journal of Medicinal Chemistry, 57*, 6965–6972.

Falck, J. R., Reddy, L. M., Reddy, Y. K., Bondlela, M., Krishna, U. M., Ji, Y., et al. (2003). 11,12-epoxyeicosatrienoic acid (11,12-EET): Structural determinants for inhibition of TNF-alpha-induced VCAM-1 expression. *Bioorganic & Medicinal Chemistry Letters, 13*, 4011–4014.

Fan, F., & Roman, R. J. (2017). Effect of cytochrome P450 metabolites of arachidonic acid in nephrology. *The Journal of the American Society of Nephrology, 28*, 2845–2855.

Fleming, I. (2007). DiscrEET regulators of homeostasis: Epoxyeicosatrienoic acids, cytochrome P450 epoxygenases and vascular inflammation. *Trends in Pharmacological Sciences, 28*, 448–452.

Gangadhariah, M. H., Dieckmann, B. W., Lantier, L., Kang, L., Wasserman, D. H., Chiusa, M., et al. (2017). Cytochrome P450 epoxygenase-derived epoxyeicosatrienoic acids contribute to insulin sensitivity in mice and in humans. *Diabetologia, 60*, 1066–1075.

Gauthier, K. M., Deeter, C., Krishna, U. M., Reddy, Y. K., Bondlela, M., Falck, J. R., et al. (2002). 14,15-Epoxyeicosa-5(Z)-enoic acid: A selective epoxyeicosatrienoic acid antagonist that inhibits endothelium-dependent hyperpolarization and relaxation in coronary arteries. *Circulation Research, 90*, 1028–1036.

Gauthier, K. M., Falck, J. R., Reddy, L. M., & Campbell, W. B. (2004). 14,15-EET analogs: Characterization of structural requirements for agonist and antagonist activity in bovine coronary arteries. *Pharmacological Research, 49*, 515–524.

Gauthier, K. M., Jagadeesh, S. G., Falck, J. R., & Campbell, W. B. (2003). 14,15-epoxyeicosa-5(Z)-enoic-mSI: A 14,15- and 5,6-EET antagonist in bovine coronary arteries. *Hypertension, 42*, 555–561.

GlaxoSmithKline. (2013). *A study to assess the safety, tolerability, pharmacokinetics and pharmacodynamics of single doses of GSK2256294 in healthy volunteers, and single and repeat doses of GSK2256294 in adult male moderately obese smokers.* http://clinicaltrials.gov/ct2/show/NCT01762774?term=epoxide+hydrolase&rank=2.

Han, K. H., Kim, B., Ji, S. C., Kang, H. G., Cheong, H. I., Cho, J. Y., et al. (2020). Mechanism of chronic kidney disease progression and novel biomarkers: A metabolomic analysis of experimental glomerulonephritis. *Metabolites, 10*, 169.

Herse, F., Lamarca, B., Hubel, C. A., Kaartokallio, T., Lokki, A. I., Ekholm, E., et al. (2012). Cytochrome P450 subfamily 2J polypeptide 2 expression and circulating epoxyeicosatrienoic metabolites in preeclampsia. *Circulation, 126*, 2990–2999.

Hoff, U., Bubalo, G., Fechner, M., Blum, M., Zhu, Y., Pohlmann, A., et al. (2019). A synthetic epoxyeicosatrienoic acid analogue prevents the initiation of ischemic acute kidney injury. *Acta Physiologica (Oxford, England), 227*, e13297.

Hye Khan, M. A., Fish, B., Wahl, G., Sharma, A., Falck, J. R., Paudyal, M. P., et al. (2016). Epoxyeicosatrienoic acid analogue mitigates kidney injury in a rat model of radiation nephropathy. *Clinical Science (London, England)*, *130*, 587–599.

Hye Khan, M. A., Pavlov, T. S., Christain, S. V., Neckář, J., Staruschenko, A., Gauthier, K. M., et al. (2014). Epoxyeicosatrienoic acid analogue lowers blood pressure through vasodilation and sodium channel inhibition. *Clinical Science (London, England)*, *127*, 463–474.

Hye Khan, M. A., Stavniichuk, A., Sattar, M. A., Falck, J. R., & Imig, J. D. (2019). Epoxyeicosatrienoic acid analog EET-A blunts development of lupus nephritis in mice. *Frontiers in Pharmacology*, *10*, 512.

Imig, J. D. (2012). Epoxides and soluble epoxide hydrolase in cardiovascular physiology. *Physiological Reviews*, *92*, 101–130.

Imig, J. D. (2018). Prospective for cytochrome P450 epoxygenase cardiovascular and renal therapeutics. *Pharmacology & Therapeutics*, *192*, 1–19.

Imig, J. D., Dimitropoulou, C., Reddy, D. S., White, R. E., & Falck, J. R. (2008). Afferent arteriolar dilation to 11, 12-EET analogs involves PP2A activity and Ca^{2+}-activated K^+ channels. *Microcirculation*, *15*, 137–150.

Imig, J. D., Elmarakby, A., Nithipatikom, K., Wei, S., Capdevila, J. H., Tuniki, V. R., et al. (2010). Development of epoxyeicosatrienoic acid analogs with in vivo anti-hypertensive actions. *Frontiers in Vascular Physiology*, *1*, 157.

Imig, J. D., & Hammock, B. D. (2009). Soluble epoxide hydrolase as a therapeutic target for cardiovascular diseases. *Nature Reviews. Drug Discovery*, *8*, 794–805.

Imig, J. D., Hye Khan, M. A., Burkhan, A., Chen, G., Adebesin, A. M., & Falck, J. R. (2021). Kidney-targeted epoxyeicosatrienoic acid analog, EET-F01, reduces inflammation, oxidative stress, and cisplatin-induced nephrotoxicity. *International Journal of Molecular Sciences*, *22*, 2793.

Imig, J. D., Hye Khan, M. A., Sharma, A., Fish, B. L., Mandel, N. S., & Cohen, E. P. (2016). Radiation-induced afferent arteriolar endothelial-dependent dysfunction involves decreased epoxygenase metabolites. *American Journal of Physiology. Heart and Circulatory Physiology*, *310*, H1695–H1701.

Imig, J. D., Inscho, E. W., Deichmann, P. C., Reddy, K. M., & Falck, J. R. (1999). Afferent arteriolar vasodilation to the sulfonimide analog of 11, 12-epoxyeicosatrienoic acid involves protein kinase a. *Hypertension*, *33*, 408–413.

Imig, J. D., Jankiewicz, W. K., & Khan, A. H. (2020). Epoxy fatty acids: From salt regulation to kidney and cardiovascular therapeutics: 2019 Lewis K. *Dahl Memorial Lecture. Hypertension*, *76*, 3–15.

Jankiewicz, W. K., Barnett, S. D., Stavniichuk, A., Belayet, J. B., Hwang, S. H., Hammock, B. D., et al. (2021). Dual sEH/COX-2 inhibition using PTUPB – A promising approach to antiangiogenesis-induced nephrotoxicity. *Frontiers in Pharmacology*, *12*, 744776.

Jeemon, P., Séverin, T., Amodeo, C., Balabanova, D., Campbell, N. R. C., Gaita, D., et al. (2021). World heart federation roadmap for hypertension - a 2021 update. *Global Heart*, *16*, 63.

Jiang, H., McGiff, J. C., Fava, C., Amen, G., Nesta, E., Zanconato, G., et al. (2013). Maternal and fetal epoxyeicosatrienoic acids in normotensive and preeclamptic pregnancies. *American Journal of Hypertension*, *26*, 271–278.

Jíchová, Š., Kopkan, L., Husková, Z., Doleželová, Š., Neckář, J., Kujal, P., et al. (2016). Epoxyeicosatrienoic acid analog attenuates the development of malignant hypertension, but does not reverse it once established: A study in Cyp1a1-ren-2 transgenic rats. *Journal of Hypertension*, *34*, 2008–2025.

Joyner, M. J., Wallin, B. G., & Charkoudian, N. (2016). Sex differences and blood pressure regulation in humans. *Experimental Physiology*, *101*, 349–355.

Kaergel, E., Muller, D. N., Honeck, H., Theuer, J., Shagdarsuren, E., Mullally, A., et al. (2002). P450-dependent arachidonic acid metabolism and angiotensin II-induced renal damage. *Hypertension*, *40*, 273–279.

Katoh, T., Takahashi, K., Capdevila, J., Karara, A., Falck, J. R., Jacobson, H. R., et al. (1991). Glomerular stereospecific synthesis and hemodynamic actions of 8,9-epoxyeicosatrienoic acid in rat kidney. *The American Journal of Physiology*, *261*, F578–F586.

Khan, M. A. H., & Imig, J. D. (2018). Antihypertensive drugs. *Reference Module in Biomedical Sciences*. https://doi.org/10.1016/B978-0-12-801238-3.96704-7.

Khan, M. A. H., Liu, J., Kumar, G., Skapek, S. X., Falck, J. R., & Imig, J. D. (2013). Novel orally active epoxyeicosatrienoic acid (EET) analogs attenuate cisplatin nephrotoxicity. *The FASEB Journal*, *27*, 2946–2956.

Khan, M. A. H., Manthati, V., Errabelli, R., Pavlov, T. S., Staruschenko, A., Falck, J. R., et al. (2013). An orally active epoxyeicosatrienoic acid analog attenuates kidney injury in hypertensive dahl salt sensitive rat. *Hypertension*, *62*, 905–913.

Kim, J., Imig, J. D., Yang, J., Hammock, B. D., & Padanilam, B. J. (2014). Inhibition of soluble epoxide hydrolase prevents renal interstitial fibrosis and inflammation. *American Journal of Physiology. Renal Physiology*, *307*, F971–F980.

Kim, J., Yoon, S. P., Toews, M. L., Imig, J. D., Hwang, S. H., Hammock, B. D., et al. (2015). Pharmacological inhibition of soluble epoxide hydrolase prevents renal interstitial fibrogenesis in obstructive nephropathy. *American Journal of Physiology. Renal Physiology*, *308*, F131–F139.

King, L. M., Gainer, J. V., David, G. L., Dai, D., Goldstein, J. A., Brown, N. J., et al. (2005). Single nucleotide polymorphisms in the CYP2J2 and CYP2C8 genes and the risk of hypertension. *Pharmacogenetics and Genomics*, *15*, 7–13.

Kipp, K. R., Kruger, S. L., Schimmel, M. F., Parker, N., Shillingford, J. M., Leamon, C. P., et al. (2018). (2018) comparison of folate-conjugated rapamycin versus unconjugated rapamycin in an orthologous mouse model of polycystic kidney disease. *American Journal of Physiology. Renal Physiology*, *315*, F395–F405.

Knight, S. F., Kundu, K., Joseph, G., Dikalov, S., Weiss, D., Murthy, N., et al. (2012). Folate receptor-targeted antioxidant therapy ameliorates renal ischemia-reperfusion injury. *The Journal of the American Society of Nephrology*, *23*, 793–800.

Kućmierz, J., Frąk, W., Młynarska, E., Franczyk, B., & Rysz, J. (2021). Molecular interactions of arterial hypertension in its target organs. *International Journal of Molecular Sciences*, *22*, 9669.

Lazaar, A. L., Yang, L., Boardley, R. L., Goyal, N. S., Robertson, J., Baldwin, S. J., et al. (2016). Pharmacokinetics, pharmacodynamics and adverse event profile of GSK 2256294, a novel soluble epoxide hydrolase inhibitor. *British Journal of Clinical Pharmacology*, *81*, 971–979.

Lee, C. R., Imig, J. D., Edin, M. L., Foley, J., DeGraff, L. M., Bradbury, J. A., et al. (2010). Endothelial expression of human cytochrome P450 epoxygenases lowers blood pressure and attenuates hypertension-induced renal injury in mice. *The FASEB Journal*, *24*, 3770–3781.

Lee, C. R., Pretorius, M., Schuck, R. N., Burch, L. H., Bartlett, J., Williams, S. M., et al. (2011). Genetic variation in soluble epoxide hydrolase (EPHX2) is associated with forearm vasodilator responses in humans. *Hypertension*, *57*, 116–122.

Lee, J. P., Yang, S. H., Lee, H. Y., Kim, B., Cho, J. Y., Paik, J. H., et al. (2012). Soluble epoxide hydrolase activity determines the severity of ischemia-reperfusion injury in kidney. *PLoS One*, *7*, e37075.

Liclican, E. L., McGiff, J. C., Falck, J. R., & Carroll, M. A. (2008). Failure to upregulate the adenosine2A receptor-epoxyeicosatrienoic acid pathway contributes to the development of hypertension in dahl salt-sensitive rats. *American Journal of Physiology. Renal Physiology*, *295*, F1696–F1704.

Luria, A., Weldon, S. M., Kabcenell, A. K., Ingraham, R. H., Matera, D., Jiang, H., et al. (2007). Compensatory mechanism for homeostatic blood pressure regulation in Ephx2 gene-disrupted mice. *The Journal of Biological Chemistry*, *282*, 2891–2898.

Luther, J. M., Wei, D. S., Ghoshal, K., Peng, D., Adler, G. K., Turcu, A. F., et al. (2021). Treatment of primary aldosteronism increases plasma epoxyeicosatrienoic acids. *Hypertension*, *77*, 1323–1331.

Makita, K., Takahashi, K., Karara, A., Jacobson, H. R., Falck, J. R., & Capdevila, J. H. (1994). Experimental and/or genetically controlled alterations of the renal microsomal cytochrome P450 epoxygenase induce hypertension in rats fed a high salt diet. *The Journal of Clinical Investigation*, *94*, 2414–2420.

Manhiani, M., Quigley, J. E., Knight, S. F., Tasoobshirazi, S., Moore, T., Brands, M. W., et al. (2009). Soluble epoxide hydrolase gene deletion attenuates renal injury and inflammation with DOCA-salt hypertension. *American Journal of Physiology. Renal Physiology*, *297*, F740–F748.

McMaster, W. G., Kirabo, A., Madhur, M. S., & Harrison, D. G. (2015). Inflammation, immunity, and hypertensive end-organ damage. *Circulation Research*, *116*, 1022–1033.

Monti, J., Fischer, J., Paskas, S., Heinig, M., Schulz, H., Gösele, C., et al. (2008). Soluble epoxide hydrolase is a susceptibility factor for heart failure in a rat model of human disease. *Nature Genetics*, *40*, 529–537.

Morisseau, C., & Hammock, B. D. (2013). Impact of soluble epoxide hydrolase and epoxyeicosanoids on human health. *Annual Review of Pharmacology and Toxicology*, *53*, 37–58.

Nakagawa, K., Holla, V. R., Wei, Y., Wang, W. H., Gatica, A., Wei, S., et al. (2006). Salt-sensitive hypertension is associated with dysfunctional Cyp4a10 gene and kidney epithelial sodium channel. *The Journal of Clinical Investigation*, *116*, 1696–1702.

Neckář, J., Hye Khan, M. A., Gross, G. J., Cyprová, M., Hrdlička, J., Kvasilová, A., et al. (2019). Epoxyeicosatrienoic acid analog EET-B attenuates post-myocardial infarction remodeling in spontaneously hypertensive rats. *Clinical Science (London, England)*, *133*, 939–951.

Neckář, J., Kopkan, L., Husková, Z., Kolář, F., Papoušek, F., Kramer, H. J., et al. (2012). Inhibition of soluble epoxide hydrolase by cis-4-[4-(3-adamantan-1-ylureido) cyclohexyl-oxy]benzoic acid exhibits antihypertensive and cardioprotective actions in transgenic rats with angiotensin II-dependent hypertension. *Clinical Science (London, England)*, *122*, 513–525.

Ogunniyi, M. O., Commodore-Mensah, Y., & Ferdinand, K. C. (2021). Race, ethnicity, hypertension, and heart disease: JACC focus seminar 1/9. *Journal of the American College of Cardiology*, *78*, 2460–2470.

Ojha, U., Ruddaraju, S., Sabapathy, N., Ravindran, V., Worapongsatitaya, P., Haq, J., et al. (2021). Current and emerging classes of pharmacological agents for the management of hypertension. *American Journal of Cardiovascular Drugs*, *8*, 1–15.

Oni-Orisan, A., Alsaleh, N., Lee, C. R., & Seubert, J. M. (2014). Epoxyeicosatrienoic acids and cardioprotection: The road to translation. *Journal of Molecular and Cellular Cardiology*, *74*, 199–208.

Pavlov, T. S., Ilatovskaya, D. V., Levchenko, V., Mattson, D. L., Roman, R. J., & Staruschenko, A. (2011). Effects of cytochrome P-450 metabolites of arachidonic acid on the epithelial sodium channel (ENaC). *American Journal of Physiology. Renal Physiology*, *301*, F672–F681.

Pfister, S. L., Gauthier, K. M., & Campbell, W. B. (2010). Vascular pharmacology of epoxyeicosatrienoic acids. *Advances in Pharmacology*, *60*, 27–59. https://doi.org/10.1016/B978-0-12-385061-4.00002-7. PMID: 21081214. PMCID: PMC3373307.

Piskorz, D. (2020). Hypertensive mediated organ damage and hypertension management. How to assess beneficial effects of antihypertensive treatments? *High Blood Pressure & Cardiovascular Prevention*, *27*, 9–17.

Polonikov, A., Bykanova, M., Ponomarenko, I., Sirotina, S., Bocharova, A., Vagaytseva, K., et al. (2017). The contribution of CYP2C gene subfamily involved in epoxygenase pathway of arachidonic acids metabolism to hypertension susceptibility in Russian population. *Clinical and Experimental Hypertension*, *39*, 306–311.

Polonikov, A. V., Ivanov, V. P., Solodilova, M. A., Khoroshaya, I. V., Kozhuhov, M. A., Ivakin, V. E., et al. (2008). A common polymorphism G-50T in cytochrome P450 2J2 gene is associated with increased risk of essential hypertension in a Russian population. *Disease Markers*, *24*, 119–126.

Roman, R. J. (2002). P-450 metabolites of arachidonic acid in the control of cardiovascular function. *Physiological Reviews*, *82*, 131–185.

Sellers, K. W., Sun, C., Diez-Freire, C., Waki, H., Morisseau, C., Falck, J. R., et al. (2005). Novel mechanism of brain soluble epoxide hydrolase-mediated blood pressure regulation in the spontaneously hypertensive rat. *The FASEB Journal*, *19*, 626–628.

Sharma, M., McCarthy, E. T., Reddy, D. S., Patel, P. K., Savin, V. J., Medhora, M., et al. (2009). 8,9-Epoxyeicosatrienoic acid protects the glomerular filtration barrier. *Prostaglandins & Other Lipid Mediators*, *89*, 43–51.

Shuey, M. M., Billings, F. T., 4th, Wei, S., Milne, G. L., Nian, H., Yu, C., et al. (2017). Association of gain-of-function EPHX2 polymorphism Lys55Arg with acute kidney injury following cardiac surgery. *PLoS One*, *12*, e0175292.

Sinal, C. J., Miyata, M., Tohkin, M., Nagata, K., Bend, J. R., & Gonzalez, F. J. (2000). Targeted disruption of soluble epoxide hydrolase reveals a role in blood pressure regulation. *The Journal of Biological Chemistry*, *275*, 40504–40510.

Skibba, M., Hye Khan, M. A., Kolb, L. L., Yeboah, M. M., Falck, J. R., Amaradhi, R., et al. (2017). Epoxyeicosatrienoic acid analog decreases renal fibrosis by reducing epithelial-to-mesenchymal transition. *Frontiers in Pharmacology*, *8*, 406.

Sodhi, K., Inoue, K., Gotlinger, K. H., Canestraro, M., Vanella, L., Kim, D. H., et al. (2009). Epoxyeicosatrienoic acid agonist rescues the metabolic syndrome phenotype of HO-2-null mice. *The Journal of Pharmacology and Experimental Therapeutics*, *331*, 906–916.

Spiecker, M., Darius, H., Hankeln, T., Soufi, M., Sattler, A. M., Schaefer, J. R., et al. (2004). Risk of coronary artery disease associated with polymorphism of the cytochrome P450 epoxygenase CYP2J2. *Circulation*, *110*, 2132–2136.

Sudhahar, V., Shaw, S., & Imig, J. D. (2010). Epoxyeicosatrienoic acid analogs and vascular function. *Current Medicinal Chemistry*, *17*, 1181–1190.

Sun, P., Lin, D. H., Yue, P., Jiang, H., Gotlinger, K. H., Schwartzman, M. L., et al. (2010). High potassium intake enhances the inhibitory effect of 11,12-EET on ENaC. *The Journal of the American Society of Nephrology*, *21*, 1667–1677.

Titze, J., & Luft, F. C. (2017). Speculations on salt and the genesis of arterial hypertension. *Kidney International*, *91*, 1324–1335.

Walkowska, A., Červenka, L., Imig, J. D., Falck, J. R., Sadowski, J., & Kompanowska-Jezierska, E. (2021). Early renal vasodilator and hypotensive action of epoxyeicosatrienoic acid analog (EET-A) and 20-HETE receptor blocker (AAA) in spontaneously hypertensive rats. *Frontiers in Physiology*, *12*, 622882.

Wang, C. P., Hung, W. C., Yu, T. H., Chiu, C. A., Lu, L. F., Chung, F. M., et al. (2010). Genetic variation in the G-50T polymorphism of the cytochrome P450 epoxygenase CYP2J2 gene and the risk of younger onset type 2 diabetes among Chinese population: Potential interaction with body mass index and family history. *Experimental and Clinical Endocrinology & Diabetes*, *118*, 346–352.

Wang, Q., Pang, W., Cui, Z., Shi, J., Liu, Y., Liu, B., et al. (2013). Upregulation of soluble epoxide hydrolase in proximal tubular cells mediated proteinuria-induced renal damage. *American Journal of Physiology. Renal Physiology*, *304*, F168–F176.

Wang, M. X., Wang, L. J., Xiao, Y., Zhang, D. D., Duan, X. P., & Wang, W. H. (2020). Epoxyeicosatrienoic acid metabolites inhibit Kir4.1/Kir5.1 in the distal convoluted tubule. *American Journal of Physiology. Renal Physiology*, *318*, F1369–F1376.

Wang, W. H., Zhang, C., Lin, D. H., Wang, L., Graves, J. P., Zeldin, D. C., et al. (2014). Cyp2c44 epoxygenase in the collecting duct is essential for the high K+ intake-induced antihypertensive effect. *American Journal of Physiology. Renal Physiology*, *307*, F453–F460.

Ward, N. C., Croft, K. D., Blacker, D., Hankey, G. J., Barden, A., Mori, T. A., et al. (2011). Cytochrome P450 metabolites of arachidonic acid are elevated in stroke patients compared with healthy controls. *Clinical Science (London, England)*, *121*, 501–507.

Yang, L., Cheriyan, J., Gutterman, D. D., Mayer, R. J., Ament, Z., Griffin, J. L., et al. (2017). Mechanisms of vascular dysfunction in COPD and effects of a novel soluble epoxide hydrolase inhibitor in smokers. *Chest*, *151*, 555–563.

Yang, Q., Zhang, R. Z., Yim, A. P., & He, G. W. (2003). Effect of 11,12-epoxyeicosatrienoic acid as an additive to St. Thomas' cardioplegia and University of Wisconsin solutions on endothelium-derived hyperpolarizing factor-mediated function in coronary microarteries: Influence of temperature and time. *The Annals of Thoracic Surgery*, *76*, 1623–1630.

Yeboah, M. M., Hye Khan, M. A., Chesnik, M. A., Sharma, A., Paudyal, M. P., Falck, J. R., et al. (2016). The epoxyeicosatrienoic acid analog PVPA ameliorates cyclosporine-induced hypertension and renal injury in rats. *American Journal of Physiology. Renal Physiology*, *311*, F576–F585.

Yu, B. N., Luo, C. H., Wang, D., Wang, A., Li, Z., Zhang, W., et al. (2004). CYP2C9 allele variants in Chinese hypertension patients and healthy controls. *Clinica Chimica Acta*, *348*, 57–61.

Zeldin, D. C. (2011). Epoxygenase pathways of arachidonic acid metabolism. *The Journal of Biological Chemistry*, *276*, 36059–36062.

Zhao, X., Pollock, D. M., Inscho, E. W., Zeldin, D. C., & Imig, J. D. (2003). Decreased renal cytochrome P450 2C enzymes and impaired vasodilation are associated with salt-sensitive hypertension. *Hypertension*, *41*, 709–714.

Zhao, X., Yamamoto, T., Newman, J. W., Kim, I. H., Watanabe, T., Hammock, B. D., et al. (2004). Soluble epoxide hydrolase inhibition protects the kidney from hypertension-induced damage. *The Journal of the American Society of Nephrology*, *15*, 1244–1253.

Zhu, Y., Blum, M., Hoff, U., Wesser, T., Fechner, M., Westphal, C., et al. (2016). Renal ischemia/reperfusion injury in soluble epoxide hydrolase-deficient mice. *PLoS One*, *11*, e0145645.

Further reading

Fu, M., Yu, J., Chen, Z., Tang, Y., Dong, R., Yang, Y., et al. (2021). Epoxyeicosatrienoic acids improve glucose homeostasis by preventing NF-κB-mediated transcription of SGLT2 in renal tubular epithelial cells. *Molecular and Cellular Endocrinology*, *523*, 111149.

Imig, J. D. (2015). Epoxyeicosatrienoic acids, hypertension, and kidney injury. *Hypertension*, *65*, 476–482.

Imig, J. D., Cervenka, L., & Neckar, J. (2021). Epoxylipids and soluble epoxide hydrolase in heart diseases. *Biochemical Pharmacology*, *195*, 114866.

Wang, Q., Liang, Y., Qiao, Y., Zhao, X., Yang, Y., Yang, S., et al. (2018). Expression of soluble epoxide hydrolase in renal tubular epithelial cells regulates macrophage infiltration and polarization in IgA nephropathy. *American Journal of Physiology. Renal Physiology*, *315*, F915–F926.

CHAPTER THREE

Pharmacological developments in antihypertensive treatment through nitric oxide—cGMP modulation

Annika A. Jüttner, A.H. Jan Danser, and Anton J.M. Roks*
Department of Internal Medicine, Division of Vascular Disease and Pharmacology, Erasmus Medical Center, Erasmus University, Rotterdam, The Netherlands
*Corresponding author: e-mail address: a.roks@erasmusmc.nl

Contents

Advances in Pharmacology, Volume 94
ISSN 1054-3589
https://doi.org/10.1016/bs.apha.2022.01.001

Abstract

Treatment of hypertension until now has been directed at inhibition of vasoconstriction, of cardiac contractility and of blood volume regulation. Despite the arsenal of drugs available for this purpose, the control of target blood pressure is still a difficult goal to reach in outpatients. The nitric oxide–cyclic guanosine monophosphate signaling is one of the most important mediators of vasodilation. It might therefore be a potential and most welcome drug target for optimization of the treatment of hypertension. In this chapter we review the problems that can occur in this signaling system, the attempts that have been made to correct these problems, and those that are still under investigation. Recently developed, clinically safe medicines that are currently approved for other applications, such as myocardial infarction, await to be tested for essential systemic hypertension. We conclude that despite many years of research without translation, stimulation of nitric oxide—cyclic guanosine monophosphate is still a viable strategy in the prevention of the health risk posed by chronic hypertension.

Abbreviations

ADMA assymetric dimethylarginine
Ang II angiotensin II
BH4 tetrahydrobiopterin
BP blood pressure
cGMP cyclic guanine monophosphate
CYB5R3 cytochrome b5 reductase isoform 3
DHFR dihydrofolate reductase
DOCA deoxycorticosterone acetate
EDH endothelium-derived hyperpolarization
eNOS endothelial nitric oxide synthase
ETC electron transport chain
GAPDH glyceraldehyde 3-phosphate dehydrogenase
GPER G protein-coupled estrogen receptor
LOX lipoxidase
NADPH nicotinamide-adenine-dinucleotide phosphate
NO nitric oxide
Nox NADPH oxidase
Nrf2 nuclear factor erythroid 2-related factor 2
sGC soluble guanylyl cyclase
PDE phosphodiesterase
PKG protein kinase G
RAAS renin-angiotensin aldosterone system

ROS	reactive oxygen species
SHR(SP)	spontaneously hypertensive rat (stroke prone)
Sirt	sirtuin
SOD2	superoxide dismutase 2
VASP	vasodilator-stimulated phosphoprotein
VSMC	vascular smooth muscle cell
XO	xanthine oxidase

1. Introduction

1.1 Hypertension, a risk factor that is not optimally treated

The treatment of hypertension is of major importance in reducing the risk for cardiovascular disease, but is still not optimal (Collaborators, 2016). According to the latest figures of the National Center for Chronic Disease Prevention and Health Promotion in the United States (www.cdc.gov) only 48% of hypertensive patients reaches the target blood pressure (BP). Currently, treatment of essential hypertension is primarily based on life style adaptation supplemented with pharmacotherapy when necessary. Life style adaptation to reduce cardiovascular risk comprises reduction of sodium intake to lower BP, often accompanied by measures to reduce obesity such as dietary lipid and carbohydrate lowering, and increase of exercise, and by cessation of smoking. When life style adaptation is not effective, essential hypertension can be battled with antihypertensive pharmacotherapy. The standard arsenal of BP lowering medicines consists of β-adrenergic receptor antagonists, which reduce cardiac contractility, calcium channel blockers, which reduce vasoconstriction, diuretics, which reduce blood volume, and renin-angiotensin aldosterone system (RAAS) blockers, which decrease both blood volume and vasoconstriction. Since this range of medicines was found to be insufficient to reach target BP in all patients, the search for other strategies has continued. This chapter will discuss one of the strategies: the improvement of signaling of one of the most important vasodilator mechanisms, the nitric oxide (NO) – cyclic guanosine monophosphate (cGMP) pathway.

In addition to essential hypertension there are the special forms of hypertension such as secondary hypertension and pulmonary hypertension. Secondary hypertension, i.e. hypertension that is caused by other underlying diseases, e.g. diabetes or adrenal tumors, require treatment of the underlying disease, and this will not be further discussed in this book chapter. Pulmonary hypertension is already targeted by NO–cGMP signaling modulation, and will be occasionally mentioned as an example of the efficacy of this class of drugs.

1.2 The NO–cGMP signaling cascade

The NO–cGMP signaling cascade is of the most important vasodilator mechanisms. Furthermore, it has been implicated in vascular remodeling as an anti-fibrotic and anti-hypertrophic messenger system (Ataei Ataabadi et al., 2020). NO–cGMP signaling is also known to regulate BP through other mechanisms such as cardiac and renal effects, but this is out of the scope of the present outline, and we refer to extensive reports on this topic (Mergia & Stegbauer, 2016; Rainer & Kass, 2016). This chapter focusses on vascular NO–cGMP signaling, one of the best-studied cardiovascular signaling systems, and the modes of intervention with this pathway that are relevant for the treatment of hypertension.

An overview of the signaling cascade is provided in Fig. 1. The main source of vascular NO is endothelial NO synthase (eNOS) (Golshiri, Ataei Ataabadi, Portilla Fernandez, Jan Danser, & Roks, 2019). This eNOS is phosphorylation-activated at Ser1177 upon cytosolic Ca^{2+} increase. Forming dimers, NADPH-derived electrons are transferred to the N-terminal catalytic center, prompting the eNOS to release NO from L-arginine, leaving L-citrullin as a by-product (Fig. 1). Tetrahydrobiopterin (BH_4) serves as a co-factor herein (Li, Youn, & Cai, 2015).

NO transfers to soluble guanylyl cyclase (sGC) in vascular smooth muscle cells (VSMCs), and by binding to a ferrous heme group in sGC it strongly increases the enzyme's GTP to cGMP conversion rate. The resulting increase of cGMP activates protein kinase G (PKG), which subsequently phosphorylates vasodilator-stimulated phosphoprotein (VASP) at serine 239. VASP dephosphorylates actin-myosin through activation of myosin light chain phosphatase (Fig. 1), which results in relaxation (Schafer et al., 2003). Furthermore, cGMP- or oxidation-activated PKG decreases Ca^{2+} and RhoA/Rho kinase activation, and hyperpolarizes VSMC by activation of K^+ channels (Fig. 1) (Marinko et al., 2015; Schafer et al., 2003).

The intracellular levels of cGMP are tightly controlled by phosphodiesterases (PDEs; Fig. 1) that act in defined subcellular loci, sometimes as confined as in the immediate proximity of specific receptors or enzymes (Ataei Ataabadi et al., 2020). For BP regulation, PDE1 and PDE5 have been identified as important cGMP-metabolizing subtypes in the vascular system (Ataei Ataabadi et al., 2020).

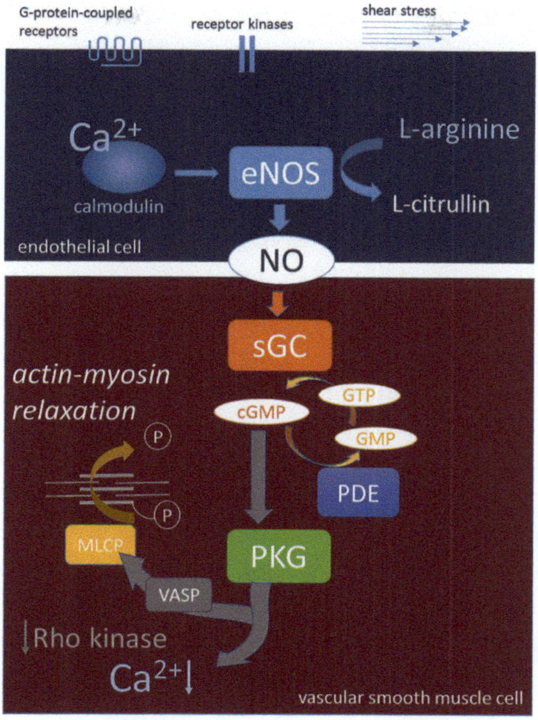

Fig. 1 Overview of the vascular NO–cGMP–PKG signaling cascade. The NO–cGMP signaling axis. The eNOS enzyme can be activated by G protein coupled receptor stimulation that increases intracellular Ca^{2+}. Further inducers are receptor kinases, eg. insulin and vascular endothelial growth factor receptor, and shear stress. The latter is a blood flow-induced mechanosensing response that is transferred intracellularly by various extracellular matrix and membrane components, amongst which the glycocalix and integrins (Baeyens, Bandyopadhyay, Coon, Yun and Schwartz, 2016). An in-depth explanation of the basic cascade is given in the body text.

1.3 Mechanisms that disturb NO–cGMP signaling

NO–cGMP signaling can be reduced as a consequence of decreased NO production due to reduced eNOS transcription and translation, eNOS protein oxidation leading to uncoupling of its co-factor BH_4, reduced cGMP production by sGC, decreased PKG activity, and increased cGMP metabolism by PDEs. Reactive oxygen species (ROS) play an important role in eNOS and sGC inactivation, and involves superoxides ($O\cdot^-$) produced by various sources. Superoxide directly reacts with NO to form peroxynitrite ($OONO^-$), thus decreasing NO bioavailability (Goldstein & Czapski, 1995). In this book chapter we systematically describe what mechanisms decrease

NO–cGMP signaling, how this relates to hypertension, and what can be done in order to restore signaling in blood vessels by targeting these mechanisms.

2. Strategies to improve eNOS activity

2.1 General aspects of eNOS

Several lines of evidence show that decreased NO production is involved in BP increase. Suppression of NO synthesis by administration of the NOS inhibitor L-monomethylarginine or genetic deletion of the eNOS gene leads to hypertension in mice (Huynh et al., 2020). However, in conditions that are associated with increased occurrence of hypertension, eNOS expression levels often do not correspond with BP. For example, aged rats with an increased BP show increased eNOS and the Ca^{2+}-independent inducible NOS (iNOS), but a decreased activation of eNOS (Cernadas et al., 1998). Also, in humans eNOS is increased in diabetes (Hink et al., 2001), while NO vasodilation is decreased. Thus, it is unlikely that in modulation of eNOS transcription and translation would be sufficient to optimally treat hypertension. Therefore, various other approaches have been chosen.

2.2 Uncoupling of eNOS

A factor that limits eNOS activity is uncoupling of BH_4 (Forstermann & Li, 2011). Uncoupling of BH_4 is caused by its oxidation and conversion into dihydrobiopterin (BH_2), or by glutathionylation of cysteins in eNOS (Tejero, Shiva, & Gladwin, 2019). The uncoupled eNOS produces superoxide instead of NO, exacerbating oxidative stress, which was demonstrated in vessels from hypertensive subjects (Landmesser et al., 2003). On the one hand this explains that despite increased eNOS, NO response can be decreased. On the other hand, this mechanism might undermine the effectiveness of increasing NO levels with molecular donors or increasing eNOS expression, and therefore may limit the clinical potential of eNOS-increasing agents. Thus, inhibition of uncoupling may be an important treatment strategy.

Increase of BH_4 is a possible strategy to bypass uncoupling. Under normal physiological conditions BH_2 can be reduced to BH_4 by dihydrofolate reductase (DHFR), but DHFR is downregulated during oxidative stress in endothelial cells. Folic acid supplementation increases DHFR, thereby reducing BP (Gao, Chalupsky, Stefani, & Cai, 2009; Gao et al., 2012). Sepiapterin, a BH_4 precursor, acutely improves endothelium-dependent vasodilation in the SHR aorta (Schuhmacher et al., 2010), and abrogation of its synthesis in mice causes hypertension (Sumi-Ichinose et al., 2017) but does not lower BP in dexamethasone-hypertensive rats (Thida et al., 2010). A possible explanation is suppression of the BH_4 production enzyme sepiapterin reductase by dexamethasone, as demonstrated in deoxycorticosterone acetate (DOCA)-salt hypertension (Youn et al., 2012). However, in angiotensin II-induced hypertension the sepiapterin reductase pathway is intact. Therefore, as a drug target in hypertension the sepiapterin pathway appears to be conditional, complicating its development into a clinical therapy.

AVE compounds, such as AVE 9488, are small molecules, found by high throughput screening, that enhance eNOS transcription, thus augmenting eNOS protein (Forstermann & Li, 2011; Wohlfart et al., 2008). Although these compounds are binding the promotor region of the eNOS gene, little is known about their mechanism of action. In parallel to increasing eNOS protein, these compounds were found to decrease uncoupling (Fig. 2) (Forstermann & Li, 2011). For reasons unknown, attempts to increase eNOS expression with AVE compound have not (yet) found clinical follow up, despite beneficial remodeling effects in rodent models of atherosclerosis and myocardial infarction (Forstermann & Li, 2011).

2.3 Assymetric dimethylarginine

NO production can be disturbed due to assymetric dimethylarginine (ADMA; Fig. 2), an endogenously inhibitor of L-arginine. L-Arginine enters the cell through amino acid channels, for which ADMA competes and thus lowers the intracellular L-arginine. Secondly, ADMA competes with

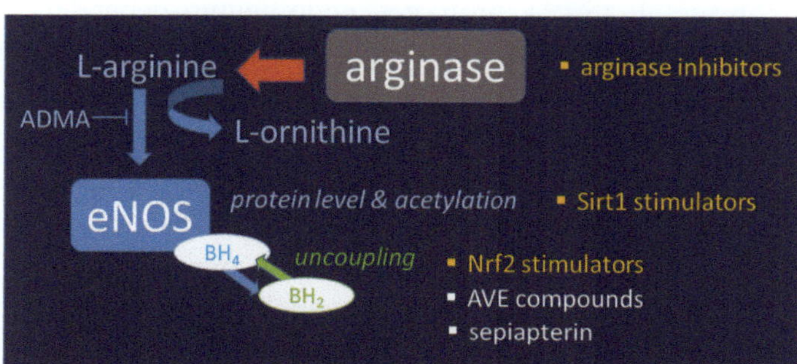

Fig. 2 Potential interventions in endothelial cells. Targeting of eNOS for treatment of hypertension. Bulleted items represent drug classes. Drug class names in white, yellow and green letters are resp. not under clinical development, clinically tested for other indications than hypertension, or in use as antihypertensive medicines.

L-arginine for eNOS binding. ADMA has been shown to contribute to decreased vasodilation in many conditions, and to be decreased by several clinical cardiovascular drugs, but attempts to employ directed interventions, such as L-arginine supply and increased intake of ω3-fatty acids did not reach a clinical effect (Tousoulis et al., 2015). In addition to ADMA L-arginine levels can be lowered by the enzyme L-arginase (Fig. 2), which degrades L-arginine. L-arginase inhibitor Nω-hydroxy-nor-L-arginine has shown antihypertensive effect in animal models and promotes (NO-mediated) vasodilation, among others in the forearm of diabetic patients with coronary artery disease (Bagnost et al., 2010; Kovamees, Shemyakin, & Pernow, 2014). The small-molecule L-arginase inhibitor INCB001158 is under clinical testing for the treatment of solid tumors, in which it has a favorable effect on immune cells. A clinical test in hypertensive patients is therefore feasible.

2.4 Improvement of aging-related eNOS inactivation: Sirtuins and resveratrol

Aging is the single largest risk factor for developing hypertension associated with reduced NO – cGMP signaling originating from eNOS inactivation by oxidative stress (Lakatta & Levy, 2003). Aging essentially reflects a drastic metabolic switch caused by accumulating macromolecular damage, leading to a shift from growth and cell repair to molecular maintenance pathways, which is detrimental to rejuvenation of tissues (Lopez-Otin, Blasco, Partridge, Serrano, & Kroemer, 2013). The family of sirtuins is a group of versatile enzymes, predominantly protein deacetylases, that is involved in this switch by modulation of among others nutrient sensing and DNA repair. However, they also display other roles, some affecting NO–cGMP signaling. Sirtuin 1 (Sirt1) promotes endothelium-dependent vascular relaxation by activating eNOS through deacetylation of lysin residues (Mattagajasingh et al., 2007) (Fig. 2). Conversely, reduction of arterial Sirt1 expression and activity is linked to vascular endothelial dysfunction during aging (Donato et al., 2011). Treatment with the Sirt1 activator SRT1720 reduced local superoxide production and inflammation while also elevating eNOS expression and protein levels (Gano et al., 2014; Li et al., 2016), but BP data are not available. The natural polyphenol resveratrol also acts as Sirt1 activator (Howitz et al., 2003) while additionally activating nuclear factor erythroid 2-related factor 2 (Nrf2), a transcriptional driver of anti-oxidant pathways (Ungvari et al., 2010). This results in increased eNOS activity through deacetylation on one hand (Mattagajasingh et al., 2007) and reduced eNOS uncoupling by decreasing ROS levels and enhancing BH_4 bioavailability on the other hand (Ungvari et al., 2010). Resveratrol was also reported as an inhibitor of asymmetric dimethylarginine, an endogenous inhibitor of eNOS (Scalera, Fulge, Martens-Lobenhoffer, Heimburg, & Bode-Boger, 2009). However, resveratrol administration did not significantly affect systolic or diastolic BP in clinical trials (Fogacci et al., 2019). Resveratrol has shown paradoxical results, both inhibiting and stimulating senescence of endothelial cells, an important determinant of decreased NO–cGMP signaling. The senescence-augmenting effect of resveratrol in ROS-induced senescence in endothelial cells was observed in parallel with a senescence attenuating role of Sirt1 (Botden et al., 2012). It was proposed that resveratrol, as well as other alleged agonists SRT1720, SRT2183, and SRT1460, is not directly stimulating Sirt1, and might therefore not be specific enough (Pacholec et al., 2010). SRT1720, which restores endothelial-dependent NO vasodilation in aged mice, lowered hypertension induced by angiotensin II (Ang II) infusion or by genetic deletion of Klotho, a kidney-derived aging-suppressing protein (Chen, Zhang, Cai, Zhao, & Dai, 2015; Gano et al., 2014; Gao et al., 2016). More direct compounds, such as BF175, have been developed since (Hong et al., 2018), and one clinically applicable, orally deliverable, compound, SRT2104, has shown efficacy in psoriasis (Hoffmann et al., 2013; Krueger et al., 2015), as based on its anti-inflammatory properties. Therefore, Sirt1 stimulation could be explored for hypertension in a clinical setting.

3. (Re)Activation of sGC

3.1 Structure and activation of sGC

The cGMP-generating enzyme sGC is present in various forms, its main active form being a heterodimer between sGCα and heme-containing subunit sGCβ, as meticulously reviewed elsewhere, and, based entirely on this review, summarized here (Stuehr, Misra, Dai, & Ghosh, 2021). Both sGCα and sGCβ are build up in the following N- to C-terminal order: heme binding domain (H-NOX), Per-Arnt-Sim (PAS) domain, coiled-coil (CC) domain, catalytic domain. Only the sGCβ actually binds heme. The subunits start as monomers, which are at all times present in the cytosol. Heme produced by the mitochondria is provided to sGCβ, which in its heme-free form is called apo-sGCβ. The heme group is delivered by glyceraldehyde 3-phosphate dehydrogenase, or GAPDH (Dai, Sweeny, Schlanger, Ghosh, & Stuehr, 2020). The heme donation requires binding of Hsp90 to apo-sGCβ and the ATP-ase activity of this chaperone. Upon incorporation of heme, Hsp90 is released, allowing heme-replete sGCβ to dimerize with sGCα. Thus, sGC becomes active, acting both in the cytosol as well as the cell membrane. NO in low levels stimulates sGC maturation, putatively helping heme incorporation and leading to subsequent heterodimerization. At very low levels or even absence of NO, inadequate sGC maturation might further contribute to hypertension.

3.2 Supplementation of NO to activate sGC

To increase cGMP production by sGC, NO supplementation can be applied by administration of organic and inorganic nitrates as NO donors. Nitrates supply NO or SNO groups that activate sGC mostly by enzymatic denitration, although spontaneous release of NO can occur for some nitrates, as reviewed elsewhere (Abrams, 1991). This could potentially improve pathophysiological conditions with low NO bioavailability, but its use in essential hypertension is limited by nitrate tolerance and induction of endothelial dysfunction when given chronically (Sage et al., 2000; Schulz et al., 2002). This nitrate tolerance is based on various mechanisms including exhaustion of enzymatic denitration, increase of PDE1 and PDE5, and inactivation of sGC by nitrosylation (Abrams, 1991; Beuve, 2017; Chen, Knight, & Yan, 2018). Inorganic nitrate supplementation has been tested in old mice and was found to improve endothelial function, yet without affecting BP (Rossman et al., 2021). Therefore, the use of NO donors is momentarily limited to angina pectoris and acute hypertensive emergencies. In a recent systematic review (Pak et al., 2014) it was found that in almost 14% of all patients admitted to hospital emergency departments acute hypertension (BP $\geq$ 180 mmHg) occurs. About 1% of all patients with chronic hypertension are affected by hypertensive emergency. Hypertensive emergency accounts for 27.5% of all emergency department visits for medical urgencies and emergencies. Apart from administration of nitrates other anti-hypertensive substances can be used, e.g. Ca^{2+} antagonists, α- or β-adrenergic receptor antagonists or α2 agonist clonidin, the loop diuretic furosemide, or RAAS blockers (Pak et al., 2014).

3.3 Activation of sGC with sGC stimulators

To support NO-mediated cGMP production by heme-containing sGC, sGC stimulators can be applied (Fig. 3). This drug class, of which the compounds BAY 41, riociguat (BAY 63; Adempas) and vericiguat (BAY 102; Verquvo) are the typical examples, stimulates heme-containing sGC

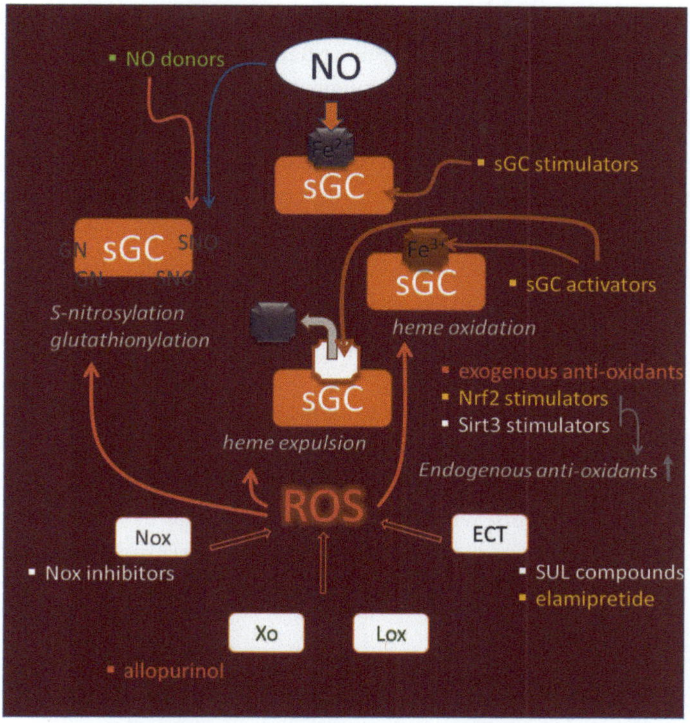

Fig. 3 Potential interventions in smooth muscle cells: sGC and oxidative stress. Stimulation, or prevention and bypassing of deactivation of sGC are an important antihypertensive strategies. The amount of NO and the cell's redox status importantly affect oxidation (Fe^{3+} formation and heme expulsion), S-glutathionylation (GN) and S-nitrosylation (SNO) of sGC, with consequences for BP maintenance. Various drug classes (bulleted items) have potential for clinical application. Drug class names in white, yellow and green letters are resp. not under clinical development, clinically tested for other indications than hypertension, or in use as antihypertensive medicines. Drug classes in red have failed in clinical trials.

to produce cGMP independently of NO (Evgenov et al., 2006). As reviewed recently (Ataei Ataabadi et al., 2020), there is ample evidence of cGMP increase and vasodilation of sGC stimulators and activators in various animal and vascular species, amongst which in coronary arteries. This translates in BP reduction in various animal models, seemingly without the tolerance problem observed for nitrates. In addition, the drugs provide cardiac and renal protection, and recently the VICTORIA trial showed a protective effect in patients with heart failure and reduce ejection fraction (Armstrong et al., 2020). Further trials in heart failure are warranted, as thoroughly discussed elsewhere (Cordwin, Berei, & Pogue, 2021).

With respect to hypertension, Adempas (riociguat) has been clinically registered for the treatment of pulmonary arterial hypertension (PAH) and chronic thromboembolic pulmonary hypertension (CTEPH). An anti-hypertensive effect of the sGC stimulator praliciguat was observed in healthy subjects and hypertensive patients with type 2 diabetes (Hanrahan et al., 2019, 2020). Momentarily, there are, surprisingly, no clinical studies ongoing to further develop sGC stimulator therapy for the treatment of essential hypertension.

3.4 Deactivation of sGC

Deactivation of sGC oxidation is a possible mechanism that inhibits NO–cGMP signaling (Fig. 3). Comprehensive overviews of oxidation-inactivated forms of sGC and the mechanisms of their formation and recuperation can be found elsewhere (Beuve, 2017; Stuehr et al., 2021). Essential knowledge for understanding the difference in sGC stimulators vs. activators and their potential clinical use described in the next paragraph is provided here.

There are two targets of oxidation: the heme group and cysteïns. The heme group normally contains (ferrous) Fe^{2+}, which can be oxidized to (ferric) Fe^{3+} (Fig. 3). If oxidization persists, the sGC heterodimer is inactivated. It is unclear if the heme group is lost, and the low dissociation constant of ferric heme for sGC, although being higher than for ferrous heme, argues against this (Ghosh, Stasch, Papapetropoulos, & Stuehr, 2014; Surmeli & Marletta, 2012). However, Fe^{3+} can be reduced again by cytochrome b5 reductase isoform 3 (CYB5R3), reactivating sGC (Rahaman et al., 2017). The exploration of heme oxidation and its effects has mainly been conducted under in vitro conditions, using isolated sGC. The physiological conditions under which this plays a role in NO–cGMP signaling remain to be identified.

Second to heme oxidation Cys residues of both sGC subunits can be S-glutathionylated (addition of glutathione group to cysteines) or S-nitrosylated by NO (formation of SNO groups: Fig. 3). S-nitrosylation and its consequences for sGC activation has been comprehensively reviewed recently (Beuve, 2017), and is summarized here. The number of Cys residues in sGC is unusually high for the protein's size. S-nitrosylation is associated with sGC inactivation, dissociation of the heterodimer, and renewed binding of Hsp90. Heme oxidation promotes these events, but it is unknown in which order these events occur, leaving open the question of causality (Stuehr et al., 2021). The S-nitrosylation of sGC has been observed in *in vitro* models in which sGC was exposed to high amounts of NO, and in vivo in a mouse asthma model featuring inducible NOS activation (Ghosh et al., 2016). S-nitrosylation can be reversed by thioredoxin-1 and thioreductase, and this mechanism of de- and reactivation of sGC is implicated in the decreased vasodilation observed in a rat model of Ang II–induced hypertension (Choi, Allahdadi, Tostes, & Webb, 2011; Choi, Tostes, & Webb, 2011). From the oxidation and S-nitrosylation events an elegant model of sGC regulation can be designed, in which low amounts of NO stimulate cGMP generation, and high amounts of NO lead to a negative feedback by means of S-nitrosylation (Beuve, 2017), which in turn might be a mechanism explaining the tolerance to nitrates after repeated use (Fig. 3). Dissociation of sGC subunits allow subsequent Hsp90 binding to (apo-)sGCβ, refurbishing with heme, and renewed heterodimerization with eligible sGCα. In the presence of oxidated heme this circulatory mechanism of sGC regulation is accelerated, but ferric-to-ferrous heme reduction by CYB5R3 might serve as an escape route (Stuehr et al., 2021). Yet, many steps, such as expression regulation and the sequence of Hsp90 binding, dimerization and dissociation awaits to be explored or confirmed (Stuehr et al., 2021).

3.5 Reactivation of sGC: sGC activators

NO cannot activate heme-depleted sGC. Similarly, the sGC stimulators, although being NO-independent, are only increasing cGMP production by intact, heme-containing sGC. Stimulators are thought to perform their function by binding outside of the heme pocket sGC (Stuehr et al., 2021). Therefore, nitrates or sGC stimulators are no optimal options if oxidation of sGC has occurred.

To bypass the problem of sGC oxidation, sGC activators have been developed (Evgenov et al., 2006) (Fig. 3). Activators, of which BAY 58-2667 (cinaciguat) and BAY 60-2770 are the typical examples, support sGC maturation without the need of Hsp90, GAPDH nor heme, leading to the formation of activated dimers that produce cGMP at a high rate without the need for NO. It is presumed that sGC activators replace the heme group, and thus keep the sGC in the active conformation to produce cGMP, which again is NO-independent (Stuehr et al., 2021). In addition, given the independency from Hsp90, sGC activators might also support the reactivation of nitrosylated sGC (Stuehr et al., 2021). This still needs to be unraveled.

The sGC activators have only been marginally tested on BP effects. In preclinical studies it was shown that BAY 60-2770 caused vasodilation in the rat monocrotalin model of pulmonary hypertension (Pankey et al., 2011). In the ZSF1 rat model of diabetic nephropathy it was shown that sGC activator BI704704 lowered BP (Boustany-Kari et al., 2016). In human studies cinaciguat provoked BP lowering in acute heart failure, abrogating further studies for this indication, yet supporting clinical potential in hypertension (Ataei Ataabadi et al., 2020). Extensive testing of sGC activators in various forms of clinical hypertension is warranted, but, surprisingly, not currently endeavored.

4. PKG activation as a drug target

4.1 PKG structure and activation by cGMP

There are 2 subtypes of PKG: PKG-I and -II. For vascular and cardiac function, PKG-I is of importance (Ataei Ataabadi et al., 2020). PKG is encoded by the *PRKG1* gene in humans. Alternative splicing produces two isoforms, PKG Iα and Iβ. PKG 1α is known to be the most sensitive subunit to activation by cGMP; about 10x more sensitive than PKG 1β (Francis, Busch, Corbin, & Sibley, 2010). Toward the C-terminus of PKG an auto-inhibiting domain and subsequently by two cGMP-binding promoter regions, A and B, are present. Binding of cGMP abrogates auto-inhibition, thus activating the C-terminal catalytic part of PKG (Francis et al., 2010). The activation of PKG is associated with homodimer formation by either of the two PKG isomers PKG Iα or Iβ, and with translocation from cytosol to cell membrane (Takimoto et al., 2009). To dimerize a leucine zipper (LZ) is present at the N-terminal end of each isomer, and dimerization involves disulfide bridging of Cys-42 (Sheehe et al., 2018).

PKG activation by cGMP leads to lowering of cytosolic Ca^{2+} concentration and of contractile sensitivity to Ca^{2+} through phosphorylation and activation of MLC phosphatase via the myosin phosphatase target subunit 1, as well as through inhibition of the Rho/ Rho kinase contractile pathway (Fig. 1). Lowering of Ca^{2+} and inhibition of Rho kinase can involve the regulator of G-protein signaling 2 (RGS2), a GTP-ase that attenuates Gq/11-coupled receptors (Qiao et al., 2014; Sheehe et al., 2018).

4.2 PKG activation by oxidation: Deviation to hyperpolarization

Next to cGMP binding, PKG can also be activated by oxidation, of which H_2O_2 is a naturally occurring mediator (Sheehe et al., 2018). The oxidation of PKG requires 500 μmol/L H_2O_2 which is at least 100x higher than currently measured cytoplasmic levels. Therefore, H_2O_2 is expected to reach the required levels only in microdomains that contain high amounts of specific enzymes that serve the purpose, but this needs to be confirmed (Sheehe et al., 2018). Oxidation results into constitutive activation of PKG, targeting large conductance calcium-activated potassium channels (Fig. 4) (BK_{Ca}; K_{Ca} 1.1). Phosphorylation-activation of BK_{Ca} leads to hyperpolarization, preventing Ca^{2+}-induced vasoconstriction. In PKG Iα the Cys-117 residue in the promotor region A is responsible for oxidative activation of the catalytic function, whereas Cys-42 serves the dimerization that is required to support this task (Sheehe et al., 2018). Thus, oxidation of PKG on the one hand mimics BK_{Ca} potassium channel-mediated hyperpolarization induced by cGMP, but on the other hand it decreases activation by cGMP, lowering V_{max} of target phosphorylation (Sheehe et al., 2018). At first glance this is confusing in light of the proposition that potassium channels are activated by PKG through phosphorylation (Prysyazhna, Rudyk, & Eaton, 2012). However, cGMP-induced V_{max} and disulfide formation do not appear to be coupled. In contrast to oxidation-mediated vasodilation, NO–cGMP vasodilation is not dependent on dimerization, as demonstrated

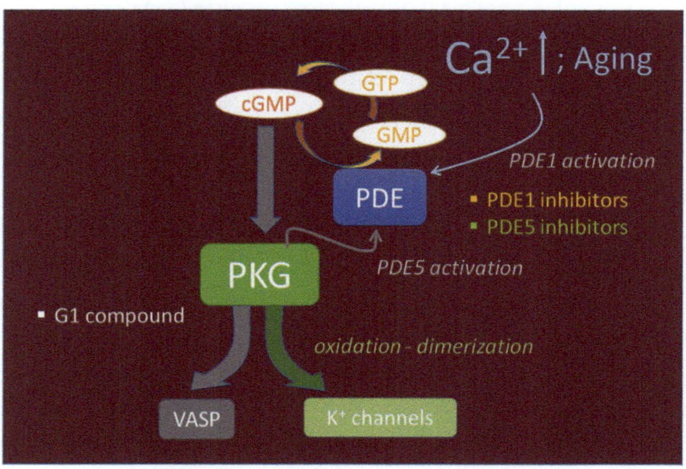

Fig. 4 Possible modulations in smooth muscle cells: PDE and PKG. Drugs targeting PKG or the calcium-dependent enzyme PDE1 could become instrumental in BP management. Apart from NO–cGMP signaling PKG also mediates K+ channel-mediated hyperpolarization as a mechanism of vascular relaxation. PDE5 inhibition is currently used for pulmonary hypertension and erectile dysfunction. PDE1 inhibition is emerging as a clinically applicable drug in heart failure, and might be especially interesting for BP management in aging. Drugs modulating PKG activity, such as G1 compound, are in a very early phase of development.

in C42S knock-in mice (Prysyazhna et al., 2012). Disulfide formation on the other hand determines the affinity for substrate (Burgoyne, Prysyazhna, Rudyk, & Eaton, 2012). Cumulatively, evidence from diverse studies suggest that cGMP initially prevents dimerization, yet after longer stimulation it leads to a prolonged H_2O_2 increase, PKG dimerization and BP lowering (Burgoyne et al., 2012; Feelisch et al., 2020; Rudyk, Prysyazhna, Burgoyne, & Eaton, 2012). This latter mechanism is especially important for resistance vessels that are strongly dependent on EDH /potassium channels.

4.3 PKG oxidation: Relation to nitrate tolerance, PDE5 and reactivation

When PKG is oxidized it cannot be activated by cGMP, potentially explaining the tolerance to repeated nitrite use in hypertension (Rudyk et al., 2012). Interesting to note is the observation that PKG activation by cGMP leads to subsequent activation of PDE5 through phosphorylation of its serine 92 (Thomas, Francis, & Corbin, 1990), which can serve as a negative feedback mechanism. In cardiac myocytes it was shown that Cys-42-dependent dimerization of PKG is needed for this PDE5 activation as it allows PKG to take its required cytosolic co-localization with PDE5 after oxidation (Nakamura et al., 2018). Independently from phosphorylation, PDE5 is activated by cGMP binding at its GAF A region (Rybalkin, Rybalkina, Shimizu-Albergine, Tang, & Beavo, 2003). The collective data cited above suggest that cGMP activation of PKG leads to translocation to the cell membrane, subsequently oxidation leads to dimerization aided by Cys-42, and ultimately reappearance of PKG in the cytosol occurs. Whether this is the end of a cycle that renders PKG sensitive again for modulation by cGMP and PDE5 is unknown. In conclusion, cGMP and oxidation by H_2O_2 collaborate in a fashion to stimulate vasodilation through PKG in temporally orchestrated activation of respectively cGMP-dependent phosphorylation targets, EDH/potassium channels, and PDE5. How this orchestration determines responses to NO–cGMP modulating medicines needs to be further investigated. In a study using a mouse aortic co-arctation model of heart failure it was suggested that PDE5 inhibitor sildenafil is less optimal than sGC activator treatment with BAY602770 due to dependency on PKG dimerization (Nakamura et al., 2018). This was indeed demonstrated by ineffectiveness of sildenafil treatment in mice carrying a dimerization-inhibiting PKG C42S mutation. However, in wild type mice sildenafil was as efficient as BAY 60-2770. Nevertheless, one should remain vigilant to the potential therapy-modulating effect of PKG oxidation.

4.4 PKG as a drug target in hypertension

G1 is a small molecule drug that activates PKGIα (Fig. 4) (Burgoyne, Prysyazhna, Richards, & Eaton, 2017). It relaxed arteries similarly to sGC activator cinaciguat and in angiotensin II-infused mice it temporarily lowered mean arterial pressure. The disappearance of the BP effect suggests a tolerance phenomenon, e.g. activation of oxidized PKGIα by thioredoxin. In a subsequent study, the same investigators reported that resveratrol, normally considered an anti-oxidant, was also capable of inducing PKGIα oxidation (Prysyazhna et al., 2019). Consequently, like G1, it relaxed preconstricted arteries, and lowered BP in angiotensin II-infused mice. Another possibility to activate PKG might be through the recently discovered indoleamine 2,3-dioxygenase 1/*cis*-WOOH pathway (Stanley et al., 2019), but this is in a stage that is too early to sketch any perspective.

5. PDE inhibitors

5.1 General aspects, structure and regulation of activity

PDEs form a large group of 11 distinctive families with a total of over 100 members (Golshiri et al., 2019). Structurally, the PDE's all contain a relatively conserved catalytic domain in the C-terminal halve of the protein., determining their affinity for each of the cyclic nucleotides cAMP or cGMP (Kokkonen & Kass, 2017). In the N-terminal halve, regulatory sequences can be found that determine the activity of the PDE, and these can be modulated by protein kinase A, cGMP or Ca^{2+}/calmodulin (Kokkonen & Kass, 2017). The cGMP-metabolizing PDE1 and 5 are subtypes in VSMC that are candidate targets for the treatment of hypertension (Fig. 4) (Laursen et al., 2017; Tousoulis, Androulakis, Papageorgiou, & Stefanadis, 2012). PDE1 has cGMP-metabolizing activity in its unbound state, and this is strongly increased by binding of Ca^{2+}/calmodulin. PDE5 is activated by binding of cGMP to its GAF domain, as explained above. The relative importance of the Ca^{2+}-dependent dual cGMP- and cAMP-degrading PDE1, and the cGMP-specific PDE5 depends on the (patho)physiologic conditions at play. Cytosolic Ca^{2+} levels and a proliferative state favors a role of PDE1 (Rybalkin, Rybalkina, Beavo, & Bornfeldt, 2002; Yan, 2015). Thus PDE1 and PDE5 represent two distinct drug targets, and their inhibition has been tested in various models.

5.2 Involvement of PDE1 in BP regulation

PDE1A null mice display low BP (Wang et al., 2017). PDE1 selective inhibitors from Lundbeck A/S, Denmark, Lu AF41228 and Lu AF58027, cause NO-dependent relaxation of mesenteric arteries, and when given intravenously lower BP in Wistar rats (Laursen et al., 2017). Lu AF41228 also decreased BP when given orally to conscious animals. The selective PDE1 inhibitor ITI-214 (lenrispodun) restores defective NO-dependent vascular relaxation in mice with an advanced state of non-atherosclerotic vascular aging (Golshiri et al., 2021). This effect of lenrispodun was strongly pronounced in aged arteries as compared to healthy arteries, and was associated with BP lowering, which was not observed in healthy mice. Lenrispodun, which was shown to be safe during Phase 2 clinical studies in patients with heart failure (www.intracellulartherapies.com), therefore has promise as a clinical agent to lower BP and improve organ perfusion in the aged vasculature.

5.3 PDE5 inhibition in blood pressure

PDE5 inhibitors (sildenafil, vardenafil, and tadalafil) are being prescribed clinically for erectile dysfunction and pulmonary hypertension. Extensive reviews of the literature were recently published (Andersson, 2018; Roy, Kloner, Salloum, & Jovin, 2021), of which the highlights are summarized here. PDE5 was found to be abundantly present in vascular smooth muscle of the pulmonary artery and corpus cavernosum. The development of PDE5 inhibitor sildenafil as a treatment for erectile dysfunction resulted in the first clinical report more than 2 decades ago (Goldstein et al., 1998). More recently, the rationale to employ PDE5 inhibition in pulmonary hypertension was exploited. Apart from its abundant presence in pulmonary arteries, PDE5 was found to be increased in pulmonary hypertension (Corbin, Beasley, Blount, & Francis, 2005). The first clinical evidence for improved exercise capacity was reported in 2005 (Galie et al., 2005). PDE5 inhibition has now been accepted as a safe pharmacotherapy to alleviate symptoms of pulmonary arterial hypertension in humans, amongst which in children (Andersson, 2018).

In relation to systemic hypertension, short term PDE5 inhibitor treatment has BP-lowering effect in patients already taking other antihypertensive drugs (Kloner, 2005; Manuel et al., 2017; Tousoulis et al., 2012). Therefore PDE5 inhibition might be interesting for treatment of essential hypertension. More insight in the possibility to use PDE5 inhibition in essential hypertension comes from preclinical studies. Disappointingly, the BP-lowering effect of PDE5 inhibition appears to be short-lived, as shown in spontaneously hypertensive rats (SHR) (Gardiner et al., 2004). Elusively, another study showed long term (4 months) BP-lowering by sildenafil in SHR, but only starting 2 months after initiation of treatment (Yaguas et al., 2010). In mice with progressed non-atherosclerotic vascular aging, 8 weeks of treatment with sildenafil restored NO vasodilation without lowering BP (Golshiri et al., 2020). Opposite to lenrispodun however, sildenafil lowered diastolic BP in healthy mice only, emphasizing the conditionality of both PDE1 and PDE5 inhibition. Whether this might have a relation to the exclusive interaction of PDE5 with sGC or to any counter-regulation by a change of balance in activity of both PDE's during selective inhibition of either one of them needs to be further inspected.

The effect of PDE5 inhibition alone on arterial pressure was found to be minimal in a hemodynamic study in patients with coronary artery disease, which reported a maximal 5 mmHg lowering of mean arterial pressure after a single bolus of 100 mg sildenafil (Herrmann, Chang, Klugherz, & Mahoney, 2000). Altogether, the use of PDE5 inhibition as a chronic treatment for essential hypertension does not yet have substantial ground. However, recently an interest for the use of PDE5 inhibition in cardiac disease has emerged. PDE5 was found to be low in the healthy heart but increased in heart diseases. PDE5 inhibition was found to be effective in various preclinical models of ischemia reperfusion injury, pressure overload and in chemotoxicity (Roy et al., 2021). A recent meta-analysis, accumulating effects in over 1000 treated and 750 control patients with various congenital and non-congenital cardiac problems revealed a potential beneficial effect on remodeling and inotropy (Giannetta et al., 2014).

6. Interventions targeted at reduction of ROS

6.1 General aspects

As has become clear from the preceding sections, ROS play an important role in the decrease of NO–cGMP function. Hence, reduction of excessive ROS production could be an interventional target in hypertension. Superoxide ($O_2^{\cdot -}$), hydrogen peroxide (H_2O_2) and hydroxyl radical ($HO^{\cdot}$) are highly reactive ROS. Main ROS sources in the cardiovascular system are NADPH-oxidase (Nox), xanthine oxidase (XO), lipoxygenase (Lox), uncoupled eNOS and mitochondria (Fig. 3) (Brown & Griendling, 2015). There is an arsenal of possibilities to increase NO–cGMP signaling and reduce BP through modulation of these sources, as summarized below. For a more in-depth analysis we refer to a recent review (Tejero et al., 2019).

6.2 XO and Lox

XO has been suggested to play a role in the pathogenesis of hypertension, since its activity is increased in hearts of hypertensive rats (Janssen, de Jong, Pasini, & Ferrari, 1993). Purine-like XO inhibitors (XOI) like allopurinol and oxypurinol are used in gout and hyperuricemia (Bredemeier et al., 2018) (Fig. 3) (Pacher, Nivorozhkin, & Szabo, 2006). Endothelial function was highly improved by XO inhibition after treating patients with chronic heart failure (Farquharson, Butler, Hill, Belch, & Struthers, 2002; George, Carr, Davies, Belch, & Struthers, 2006) and heavy smokers (Guthikonda, Sinkey, Barenz, & Haynes, 2003). However, a meta-analysis comparing XOI subtypes revealed a significant reduction of hypertension and cardiovascular events by purine-like XOI, whereas non-purine like XOI like febuxostat and topiroxostat had no significant cardiovascular protective effect and BP reduction remained inconsistent (Bredemeier et al., 2018; Yao et al., 2020). The CARES randomized trial in gout patients with a progressed cardiovascular disease showed a similar rate of cardiovascular events in febuxostat- vs allopurinol-treated, but a higher all cause and cardiovascular death rate (White et al., 2018). XOI have multiple serious side effects (Feig, Soletsky, & Johnson, 2008; Gingles et al., 2019). Therefore, further clinical development in hypertension might not be realistic.

Lox catalyzes oxygenation of polyunsaturated fatty acids like arachidonic acid. It was shown that Lox, upregulated in hypertension, consumes NO while forming superoxide as byproduct, thus scavenging NO on the one hand, and producing ROS on the other hand. But Lox is only a limited target because it is also involved in endothelial vasodilator eicosanoid production, as shown for 15-Lox (Coffey et al., 2001; Mashima & Okuyama, 2015).

6.3 Nox inhibition

Nox isoforms 1, 2, 4 and 5 are expressed in cardiovascular cells, residing either in the plasma membrane or also in the mitochondrial membrane in the case of Nox 4 (Zhang, Murugesan, Huang, & Cai, 2020), and are upregulated by Ang II. This upregulation results in ROS accumulation in endothelial cells, and VSMC in cell culture and vessels (Virdis, Neves, Amiri, Touyz, & Schiffrin, 2004). Apart from providing superoxides for chemical modification of NO, Nox might oxidize proteins in the

NO–cGMP pathway. Accordingly, Nox 1 was recently identified as an deactivator of sGC (Neves et al., 2021), but it is unknown whether this is relevant for hypertension. Nox 1 inactivation of sGC can be bypassed by the sGC activator BAY 58, providing clinical potential (Neves et al., 2021). Nevertheless, inhibition of Nox remains of interest as it will reach more oxidation targets than sGC alone. The ideal Nox-inhibitor is highly specific for Nox and isoform selective. Nox-inhibitors can be subdivided into three classes: (1) low specificity, (2) moderate isoform selectivity and improved Nox specificity and (3) Nox-specific and isoform selective (Zhang et al., 2020).

Apocynin inhibits the assembly of Nox-subunits (Johnson et al., 2002), as well as the action of other enzymes that, like Nox, use flavin as a co-factor. Treatment of DOCA)-salt-induced hypertensive mice or Ang II-induced hypertensive mice (Ang II mice) with apocynin reduced superoxide production and BP while also restoring NO bioavailability (Virdis et al., 2004; Youn et al., 2012). Increased ROS generation and impaired ACh-induced vasodilation in aortas of SHR were improved by acute treatment with apocynin, as well as with Nox-inhibitors VAS2870 and VAS3947 (Wind, Beuerlein, Armitage, et al., 2010, Wind, Beuerlein, Eucker, et al., 2010).

GKT137831 (setanaxib) and GKT136901 are more selective towards Nox isoform by targeting Nox1/4. Setanaxib treatment blocks ROS-induced liver fibrosis in WT and superoxide dismutase 1 (SOD1) KO mice by down-regulating markers of oxidative stress, inflammation, and fibrosis (Aoyama et al., 2012). Paradoxically, in SHR GKT137831-therapy increased BP and perivascular macrophage infiltration, resulting in increased perivascular fibrosis, thus exacerbating features of vascular aging. In contrast, the Nox1 inhibitor ML171 treatment modestly reduced BP and perivascular fibrosis in these animals (Nosalski et al., 2020). Nox4 inhibition by GLX351322 counteracts glucose intolerance in high-fat diet-treated mice and is thus a potential type 2 diabetes mellitus treatment (Anvari, Wikström, Walum, & Welsh, 2015). BP data for this model are not available. The Nox2 inhibitor GSK2795039 showed significant inhibition of ROS formation *in vitro* and in a murine model of acute pancreatitis (Hirano et al., 2015). Our results in a smooth muscle specific accelerated aging mouse model also indicate an improvement of ACh-induced vasodilation in aorta after acute treatment with GSK2795039, as well as with apocynin (Ataei Ataabadi et al., 2021). Thus, preclinical results with the few subtype-specific Nox inhibitors that are available are not clearly indicative yet for successful application in hypertension.

Apart from direct inhibition of Nox by allosteric interaction of a drug, Nox can be attenuated through transcriptional targeting. G protein-coupled estrogen receptors (GPER) regulate Nox1 expression, which is upregulated during atherosclerosis, hypertension, fibrosis, and diabetes. Small molecules blocking GPER downregulate Nox1 expression leading to a new class of compounds, Nox1 down-regulators, e.g. G36 (Barton, Meyer, & Prossnitz, 2019). Nox1 expression is significantly increased in Ang II-infused hypertensive mice compared to WT, and normalized by treatment with G36. G36 significantly decreased BP in Ang II mice and also improved ACh-induced vasodilation (Meyer et al., 2016). This new compound class might thus be a potential treatment for hypertension when Nox1 is involved.

6.4 Administration of exogenous and upgrade of endogenous antioxidants

ROS can be decreased by administering exogenous antioxidants. Supplementation of molecular antioxidants such as vitamin E and C decreased oxidative stress in DOCA-induced hypertensive rats (Seifi et al., 2009), while simultaneously impairing coronary endothelial function and myocardial perfusion in normal pigs (Versari et al., 2006). Clinical studies to explore the effects on CVD with such compounds were without success (Myung et al., 2013). Therefore, there are no further endeavors to pursue this strategy for hypertension treatment.

Another possible approach is to increase endogenous antioxidants. Antioxidants, including SOD, glutathione peroxidase, catalase and peroxiredoxin, are part of cellular defense mechanism to prevent oxidant accumulation by degrading ROS to less reactive, harmless oxygen species (Brown & Griendling, 2015). In response to oxidative stress, transcription factor Nrf2 is activated leading to transcription of antioxidant genes (Luo, Aslam, Welch, & Wilcox, 2015). In isolated arteries and VSMC from stroke-prone SHR Nrf2-activation and transcription are downregulated compared to control rats. This is paralleled by decreased SOD activity, increased basal ROS production, and impaired endothelial function. Acute treatment of isolated vessels with the Nrf2-activator L-sulforaphane normalized endothelium-dependent vasodilation to control level (Lopes, Neves, Tostes, Montezano, & Touyz, 2015). Treatment with Nrf2-activator *tert*-butylhydroquinone in Ang II-mice prevented oxidative stress markers and BP increase, whilst normalizing endothelial function (Wang et al., 2018). Hence, Nrf2-activating drugs could potentially be used in hypertension (Fig. 1). Unfortunately, the BEACON trial, which studied the renal effect in patients with type II diabetes with stage 4 renal failure, had to be discontinued after 9 months due to excessive cardiovascular death (de Zeeuw et al., 2013). Nevertheless, clinical trials are ongoing, amongst which in pulmonary hypertension, diabetes and renal diseases (Robledinos-Anton, Fernandez-Gines, Manda, & Cuadrado, 2019). The Nrf2-activator bardoxolone has shown efficacy on glomerular filtration rate in Alport syndrome kidney failure (Chertow et al., 2021).

6.5 Attenuation of mitochondrial ROS

Mitochondria are a source of both ROS and NO. Functions of mitochondria include ATP-production by oxidative phosphorylation, maintenance of cellular redox balance and ROS production. During normal mitochondrial oxidative phosphorylation a small percentage of electron spillover occurs at complex I and III of the electron transport chain (ETC), reducing oxygen to superoxide. Under pathophysiological conditions, such as atherosclerosis, and during aging high levels of superoxide are produced (Lakatta & Levy, 2003). Peroxynitrite produced through interaction with NO can further inhibit complex I, II and III, cytochrome oxidase, ATP synthase, and SOD, leading to further ROS-related derailment of NO–cGMP signaling (Bottani et al., 2020). Multiple inherited mitochondrial diseases are featured by reduced NO–cGMP signaling (Bottani et al., 2020). *Vice versa*, NO reversibly inhibits cytochrome c oxidase in ETC complex IV. Depending on the oxidative state of cytochrome c oxidase, NO can either compete with O_2 to bind to the enzyme's reduced form, resulting in decreased NO metabolism and increased ROS production, or bind to its oxidized form resulting in oxidation of NO to nitrate (Taylor & Moncada, 2010)). Those mechanisms in mitochondria decrease NO bioavailability additionally. Furthermore, NO–cGMP decreases peroxisome proliferator-activated receptor gamma coactivator 1α. This is a transcriptional coactivator that supports increased mitochondrial biogenesis. Thus, mitochondria and NO–cGMP are reciprocally coupled, representing a potential drug target in hypertension.

SOD2 (also known as manganese SOD; mnSOD) is the mitochondrial SOD. *Sod2*$^{+/-}$ mice develop salt-sensitive hypertension (Rodriguez-Iturbe et al., 2007). The human *SOD2* Val16A polymorphism is associated with diabetic nephropathy and CVD (Mollsten, Jorsal, Lajer, Vionnet, & Tarnow, 2009). Decreased SOD2 activity due to hyperacetylation caused by genetic Sirt3 removal in mice leads to an exaggerated BP increase during Ang II infusion (Dikalova et al., 2017). Sirt3 knock out exacerbates cardiac dysfunction and Ang II-induced ROS formation in hypertensive mice (Dikalova et al., 2020; Su, Zeng, Liu, & Chen, 2020). BP as well as senescence markers are increased in Sirt3 KO mice compared to WT. Conversely, Sirt3-overexpression in Ang II- and DOCA-mice significantly reduced BP and superoxide production while also normalizing endothelial NO production and endothelial-dependent relaxation in aorta compared to Ang II mice (Dikalova et al., 2020). MitoTEMPO, a mitochondria-targeting compound, mimics SOD2 when accumulating in mitochondrial membrane. In DOCA- and Ang II-infused hypertensive mice mitoTEMPO treatment reduced superoxide level and Nox activity as well as BP. SOD2 overexpression in those mice led to similar results (Dikalova et al., 2010). Thus, Sirt3/SOD2 is an interesting target mechanism (Fig. 1). Clinically applicable drugs would need to be developed first to make a translational step.

The ubiquinone MitoQ accumulates in mitochondria driven by electrochemical gradient and is then locally converted to its active ubiquinol form preventing lipid peroxidation and mitochondrial damage (James, Cochemé, Smith, & Murphy, 2005; Kelso et al., 2001). In SHRSP, chronic MitoQ treatment significantly reduced BP, as well as superoxide production in aorta compared to vehicle-treated SHRSP (Graham et al., 2009). In a clinical trial, MitoQ acutely and chronically improved vascular endothelial function while also reducing aortic stiffness and markers of oxidative stress. It was well tolerated, although BP was unaffected (Rossman et al., 2018).

6-chromanol derived Sulfateq (Sul) compounds (Fig. 3) preserve mitochondrial membrane potential by activating complex I and IV of the ETC. Thus, mitochondrial ROS production is reduced, ATP production preserved and mitochondrial mass increased (Hajmousa et al., 2017; Lambooy et al., 2017). Mitochondrial ROS also leads to renal damage and endothelial dysfunction and this was ameliorated by Sul-121 treatment in a mouse model of type 2 diabetes (Lambooy et al., 2017). Moreover, anti-inflammatory and antioxidant properties of Sul-121 enable its use for treatment of chronic obstructive pulmonary disease (Han et al., 2016). Finally, Sul-121, more precisely its (*R*)-enantiomer, significantly reduces BP, at least in part due to a pleiotropic antagonism of α_1 adrenergic receptors (Nakladal et al., 2019). Hence, Sul compounds are interesting drugs that allow mitochondrial antioxidant protection and BP lowering (Fig. 1).

Another mitochondrial intervention target is cardiolipin. This peroxisome proliferator-activated receptor gamma coactivator 1α-regulated phospholipid is required for an optimal function of ADP/ATP carrier (Hoffmann, Stöckl, Schlame, Beyer, & Klingenberg, 1994). It binds to complexes I, III, IV and is required for their structural integrity as well as enzymatic activity (Fiedorczuk et al., 2016; Lange, Nett, Trumpower, & Hunte, 2001; Shinzawa-Itoh et al., 2007). Oxidative stress-induced peroxidation of cardiolipin has been implicated in renal and cardiac ischemia-related disease (Vähäheikkilä et al., 2018). Elamipretide (Fig. 3), a protein drug that supports cardiolipin in a still unknown way, is vasoprotective, assisted BP reduction in patients undergoing renal artery stent placement, and restored cardiac eNOS and cGMP in a canine heart failure model (Dai et al., 2011; Eirin et al., 2018; Saad et al., 2017; Sabbah, Gupta, Singh-Gupta, Zhang, & Lanfear, 2018; Yuan et al., 2018). Although ineffective on BP in Ang II-induced and diabetic hypertension (Dai et al., 2011; Eisner, Picard, & Hajnoczky, 2018), elamipretide remains under intensive exploration, and has reached the clinical phase for use in a mitochondrial disease, Barth syndrome, thus remaining an attractive candidate drug to test in hypertension.

7. Conclusion

Antihypertensive treatment based on improvement of NO – cGMP is a viable concept. Whereas strategies to reduce ROS are still in their development phase, drugs to intervene in proteins of the NO – cGMP signaling cascade have already reached a clinical status. Nitrates will in all likelihood be limited to their current use in angina pectoris and acute hypertension. The effectiveness of PDE1 and 5 inhibitors appears to be conditional, with PDE5 inhibition being momentarily limited to pulmonary hypertension, and PDE1 apparently being more effective in the aged vasculature. This needs to be further interrogated, which could already partly take place in the clinic. Activators and stimulators of sGC are of use in pulmonary hypertension, and look promising for application in essential hypertension. Similarly, arginase inhibition is clinically feasible, having shown antihypertensive effectiveness in animal models and applicability in human cancer. An overview of the most important compounds discussed in this book chapter is provided in Table 1.

Whether all these treatment options will reach the clinic depends on a number of factors. Firstly, for intervention in ROS the question arises how excessive ROS can be eliminated without affecting beneficial effects. The contrast between H_2O_2-mediated deactivation of sGC vs activation of PKG is illustrative. Secondly, until now intervention in NO–cGMP signaling is limited to specific condition of hypertension, and for essential

Table 1 overview of clinical and experimental medicines used to improve NO – cGMP signaling, the models they have been tested in, their vascular and BP effects, and implications for clinical use or development.

Name/class	Models	Vascular and BP effect	Opportunities/threads
arginase inhibitors	Various rodent models and humans	Lowers BP in rodents; improves forearm blood flow in humans	Clinical grade compounds developed; currently tested for cancer
L-arginine	Rodents; humans	Lowering in rodents	Not effective in human trial
AVE compounds	Protective in atherosclerosis and cardiac disease models	Not assessed	Development appears to have been stopped
Elamipretide	Various animal models and humans	Vasoprotective, increases vasodilation; inconsistent BP lowering effects (not in Ang II and diabetes models)	Lowered BP in patients receiving stent; in development for clinical mitochondrial disease
Exogenous, molecular anti-oxidants	Animal models; humans	Various vascular protective effects were claimed	Not effective in human cardiovascular disease trials; not pursued in hypertension
G1 compound	Ang II infusion rat model	Vasodilation and BP lowering	Biphasic effect, possibly tolerance
Nox inhibitors	Various rodent models	Vasoprotective, BP effects are inconsistent	No clinical compound available
Nrf2 stimulators	Various animal models and humans	Vascular protective, improved vasodilation and lowered BP in Ang II infusion model	Clinical compounds available; increased cardiovascular events in diabetic patients with renal failure
Nitrates	Various models and humans	Vasodilation and BP lowering	Used in clinical against emergency hypertension; induces tolerance
PDE1 inhibitors	Various rodent models and humans	Vasodilation and BP lowering; more active in aged mice	Clinical compound available and safe in heart failure patients

Table 1 overview of clinical and experimental medicines used to improve NO − cGMP signaling, the models they have been tested in, their vascular and BP effects, and implications for clinical use or development.—cont'd

Name/class	Models	Vascular and BP effect	Opportunities/threads
PDE5 inhibitors	Various rodent models and humans	Vasodilation and BP lowering (biphasic)	Used in clinic for pulmonary hypertension; might be less effective in systemic hypertension, but potentiates other antihypertensive treatments
Sepiapterin	Dexamethasone treated rats	Vasodilation but no BP decrease	Possibly complicated by sepiapterin reductase increase. Still opportunities in other models
sGC stimulators and activators	Various rodent models and humans	Vasodilation and lowers BP	Clinically safe, used in pulmonary hypertension; modest effect on systemic BP in heart failure patients; Trials in hypertension do not seem to be planned
Sirt1 stimulators	Aged mice; Ang II infusion model	Improves NO production and attenuates BP increase by Ang II	Clinical compound available
Sirt3 stimulators/ SOD2 inhibitors	Ang II infusion model	Improves vasodilation and lowers BP	No clinical compound available yet
SUL compounds	Pulmonary hypertension model	Vascular protective, BP lowering	Still in early development

hypertension calcium antagonists, β-adrenergic receptor antagonists, renin-angiotensin-aldosterone system antagonists and diuretics are available. For hypertension related to diabetes combination with glycemic control is available. Some will argue that the currently available medicines are inadequate causing the observed therapy resistance (40–60% of the clinical cases, depending on the definition of hypertension). However, others would argue that patient adherence is a strong confounding factor that needs to be approached first (Feyz et al., 2018). This question might withhold pharmaceutical companies to invest in the development of novel medicine, especially in essential hypertension where the etiology is unknown. In conclusion, antihypertensive intervention in NO–cGMP is certainly not obsolete, and the growth of our pharmacological knowledge might translate in clinical application, which will strongly depend on the incentive of clinical and corporate parties to endorse this development.

Conflict of interest

AJMR has received financial support for preclinical studies from Intracellular Therapies, USA, and Sulfateq BV, The Netherlands.

References

Abrams, J. (1991). Interactions between organic nitrates and thiol groups. *American Journal of Medicine*, *91*(3C), 106S–112S.

Andersson, K. E. (2018). PDE5 inhibitors - pharmacology and clinical applications 20 years after sildenafil discovery. *British Journal of Pharmacology*, *175*(13), 2554–2565.

Anvari, E., Wikström, P., Walum, E., & Welsh, N. (2015). The novel NADPH oxidase 4 inhibitor GLX351322 counteracts glucose intolerance in high-fat diet-treated C57BL/6 mice. *Free Radical Research*, *49*(11), 1308–1318.

Aoyama, T., Paik, Y. H., Watanabe, S., Laleu, B., Gaggini, F., Fioraso-Cartier, L., et al. (2012). Nicotinamide adenine dinucleotide phosphate oxidase in experimental liver fibrosis: GKT137831 as a novel potential therapeutic agent. *Hepatology*, *56*(6), 2316–2327.

Armstrong, P. W., Pieske, B., Anstrom, K. J., Ezekowitz, J., Hernandez, A. F., Butler, J., et al. (2020). Vericiguat in patients with heart failure and reduced ejection fraction. *New England Journal of Medicine*, *382*(20), 1883–1893.

Ataei Ataabadi, E., Golshiri, K., Juttner, A., Krenning, G., Danser, A. H. J., & Roks, A. J. M. (2020). Nitric oxide-cGMP signaling in hypertension: Current and future options for pharmacotherapy. *Hypertension*, *76*(4), 1055–1068.

Ataei Ataabadi, E., Golshiri, K., van der Linden, J., de Boer, M., Duncker, D. J., Juttner, A., et al. (2021). Vascular ageing features caused by selective DNA damage in smooth muscle cell. *Oxidative Medicine and Cellular Longevity*, *2021*, 2308317.

Baeyens, N., Bandyopadhyay, C., Coon, B. G., Yun, S., & Schwartz, M. A. (2016). Endothelial fluid shear stress sensing in vascular health and disease. *Journal of Clinical Investigation*, *126*(3), 821–828.

Bagnost, T., Ma, L., da Silva, R. F., Rezakhaniha, R., Houdayer, C., Stergiopulos, N., et al. (2010). Cardiovascular effects of arginase inhibition in spontaneously hypertensive rats with fully developed hypertension. *Cardiovascular Research*, *87*(3), 569–577.

Barton, M., Meyer, M. R., & Prossnitz, E. R. (2019). Nox1 downregulators: A new class of therapeutics. *Steroids*, *152*, 108494.

Beuve, A. (2017). Thiol-based redox modulation of soluble guanylyl cyclase, the nitric oxide receptor. *Antioxidants & Redox Signalling*, *26*(3), 137–149.

Botden, I. P., Oeseburg, H., Durik, M., Leijten, F. P., Van Vark-Van Der Zee, L. C., Musterd-Bhaggoe, U. M., et al. (2012). Red wine extract protects against oxidative-stress-induced endothelial senescence. *Clinical Science (London)*, *123*(8), 499–507.

Bottani, E., Lamperti, C., Prigione, A., Tiranti, V., Persico, N., & Brunetti, D. (2020). Therapeutic approaches to treat mitochondrial diseases: "One-size-fits-all" and "precision medicine" strategies. *Pharmaceutics*, *12*(11), 1083.

Boustany-Kari, C. M., Harrison, P. C., Chen, H., Lincoln, K. A., Qian, H. S., Clifford, H., et al. (2016). A soluble guanylate cyclase activator inhibits the progression of diabetic nephropathy in the ZSF1 rat. *Journal of Pharmacology and Experimental Therapeutics*, *356*(3), 712–719.

Bredemeier, M., Lopes, L. M., Eisenreich, M. A., Hickmann, S., Bongiorno, G. K., d'Avila, R., et al. (2018). Xanthine oxidase inhibitors for prevention of cardiovascular events: a systematic review and meta-analysis of randomized controlled trials. *BMC Cardiovascular Disorders*, *18*(1), 24.

Brown, D. I., & Griendling, K. K. (2015). Regulation of signal transduction by reactive oxygen species in the cardiovascular system. *Circulation Research*, *116*(3), 531–549.

Burgoyne, J. R., Prysyazhna, O., Richards, D. A., & Eaton, P. (2017). Proof-of-principle for a novel class of anti-hypertensives that target the oxidaive activation of protein kinase G 1α. *Hypertension*, *70*, 577–586.

Burgoyne, J. R., Prysyazhna, O., Rudyk, O., & Eaton, P. (2012). cGMP-dependent activation of protein kinase G precludes disulfide activation: implications for blood pressure control. *Hypertension*, *60*(5), 1301–1308.

Cernadas, M. R., Sanchez de Miguel, L., Garcia-Duran, M., Gonzalez-Fernandez, F., Millas, I., Monton, M., et al. (1998). Expression of constitutive and inducible nitric oxide synthases in the vascular wall of young and aging rats. *Circulation Research*, *83*(3), 279–286.

Chen, S., Knight, W. E., & Yan, C. (2018). Roles of PDE1 in pathological cardiac remodeling and dysfunction. *Journal of Cardiovascular Development and Disease*, *5*(2), 22.

Chen, Y. X., Zhang, M., Cai, Y., Zhao, Q., & Dai, W. (2015). The Sirt1 activator SRT1720 attenuates angiotensin II-induced atherosclerosis in apoE(-)/(-) mice through inhibiting vascular inflammatory response. *Biochemical and Biophysical Research Communications*, *465*(4), 732–738.

Chertow, G. M., Appel, G. B., Andreoli, S., Bangalore, S., Block, G. A., Chapman, A. B., et al. (2021). Study design and baseline characteristics of the CARDINAL trial: A phase 3 study of bardoxolone methyl in patients with Alport syndrome. *American Journal of Nephrology*, *52*(3), 180–189.

Choi, H., Allahdadi, K. J., Tostes, R. C., & Webb, R. C. (2011). Augmented S-nitrosylation contributes to impaired relaxation in angiotensin II hypertensive mouse aorta: Role of thioredoxin reductase. *Journal of Hypertension*, *29*(12), 2359–2368.

Choi, H., Tostes, R. C., & Webb, R. C. (2011). Thioredoxin reductase inhibition reduces relaxation by increasing oxidative stress and s-nitrosylation in mouse aorta. *Journal of Cardiovascular Pharmacology*, *58*(5), 522–527.

Coffey, M. J., Natarajan, R., Chumley, P. H., Coles, B., Thimmalapura, P. R., Nowell, M., et al. (2001). Catalytic consumption of nitric oxide by 12/15-lipoxygenase: Inhibition of monocyte soluble guanylate cyclase activation. *Proceedings of the National Academy of Sciences of the United States of America*, *98*(14), 8006–8011.

Collaborators, G. B. D. R. F. (2016). Global, regional, and national comparative risk assessment of 79 behavioural, environmental and occupational, and metabolic risks or clusters of risks, 1990-2015: A systematic analysis for the global burden of disease study 2015. *Lancet*, *388*(10053), 1659–1724.

Corbin, J. D., Beasley, A., Blount, M. A., & Francis, S. H. (2005). High lung PDE5: A strong basis for treating pulmonary hypertension with PDE5 inhibitors. *Biochemical and Biophysical Research Communications*, *334*(3), 930–938.

Cordwin, D. J., Berei, T. J., & Pogue, K. T. (2021). The role of sGC stimulators and activators in heart failure with reduced ejection fraction. *Journal of Cardiovascular Pharmacology and Therapeutics*, *26*(6), 593–600.
Dai, D. F., Chen, T., Szeto, H., Nieves-Cintrón, M., Kutyavin, V., Santana, L. F., et al. (2011). Mitochondrial targeted antioxidant peptide ameliorates hypertensive cardiomyopathy. *Journal of the American College of Cardiology*, *58*(1), 73–82.
Dai, Y., Sweeny, E. A., Schlanger, S., Ghosh, A., & Stuehr, D. J. (2020). GAPDH delivers heme to soluble guanylyl cyclase. *Journal of Biological Chemistry*, *295*(24), 8145–8154.
de Zeeuw, D., Akizawa, T., Audhya, P., Bakris, G. L., Chin, M., Christ-Schmidt, H., et al. (2013). Bardoxolone methyl in type 2 diabetes and stage 4 chronic kidney disease. *New England Journal of Medicine*, *369*(26), 2492–2503.
Dikalova, A. E., Bikineyeva, A. T., Budzyn, K., Nazarewicz, R. R., McCann, L., Lewis, W., et al. (2010). Therapeutic targeting of mitochondrial superoxide in hypertension. *Circulation Research*, *107*(1), 106–116.
Dikalova, A. E., Itani, H. A., Nazarewicz, R. R., McMaster, W. G., Flynn, C. R., Uzhachenko, R., et al. (2017). Sirt3 impairment and SOD2 hyperacetylation in vascular oxidative stress and hypertension. *Circulation Research*, *121*(5), 564–574.
Dikalova, A. E., Pandey, A., Xiao, L., Arslanbaeva, L., Sidorova, T., Lopez, M. G., et al. (2020). Mitochondrial deacetylase Sirt3 reduces vascular dysfunction and hypertension while Sirt3 depletion in essential hypertension is linked to vascular inflammation and oxidative stress. *Circulation Research*, *126*(4), 439–452.
Donato, A. J., Magerko, K. A., Lawson, B. R., Durrant, J. R., Lesniewski, L. A., & Seals, D. R. (2011). SIRT-1 and vascular endothelial dysfunction with ageing in mice and humans. *Journal of Physiology*, *589*(Pt 18), 4545–4554.
Eirin, A., Hedayat, A. F., Ferguson, C. M., Textor, S. C., Lerman, A., & Lerman, L. O. (2018). Mitoprotection preserves the renal vasculature in porcine metabolic syndrome. *Experimental Physiology*, *103*(7), 1020–1029.
Eisner, V., Picard, M., & Hajnoczky, G. (2018). Mitochondrial dynamics in adaptive and maladaptive cellular stress responses. *Nature Cell Biology*, *20*(7), 755–765.
Evgenov, O. V., Pacher, P., Schmidt, P. M., Hasko, G., Schmidt, H. H., & Stasch, J. P. (2006). NO-independent stimulators and activators of soluble guanylate cyclase: Discovery and therapeutic potential. *Nature Reviews. Drug Discovery*, *5*(9), 755–768.
Farquharson, C. A., Butler, R., Hill, A., Belch, J. J., & Struthers, A. D. (2002). Allopurinol improves endothelial dysfunction in chronic heart failure. *Circulation*, *106*(2), 221–226.
Feelisch, M., Akaike, T., Griffiths, K., Ida, T., Prysyazhna, O., Goodwin, J. J., et al. (2020). Long-lasting blood pressure lowering effects of nitrite are NO-independent and mediated by hydrogen peroxide, persulfides, and oxidation of protein kinase G1alpha redox signalling. *Cardiovascular Research*, *116*(1), 51–62.
Feig, D. I., Soletsky, B., & Johnson, R. J. (2008). Effect of allopurinol on blood pressure of adolescents with newly diagnosed essential hypertension: A randomized trial. *JAMA*, *300*(8), 924–932.
Feyz, L., Bahmany, S., Daemen, J., van den Meiracker, A. H., Koch, B. C. P., van Gelder, T., et al. (2018). Therapeutic drug monitoring to assess drug adherence in assumed resistant hypertension: A comparison with directly observed therapy in 3 nonadherent patients. *Journal of Cardiovascular Pharmacology*, *72*(2), 117–120.
Fiedorczuk, K., Letts, J. A., Degliesposti, G., Kaszuba, K., Skehel, M., & Sazanov, L. A. (2016). Atomic structure of the entire mammalian mitochondrial complex I. *Nature*, *538*(7625), 406–410.
Fogacci, F., Tocci, G., Presta, V., Fratter, A., Borghi, C., & Cicero, A. F. G. (2019). Effect of resveratrol on blood pressure: A systematic review and meta-analysis of randomized, controlled, clinical trials. *Critical Reviews in Food Science and Nutrition*, *59*(10), 1605–1618.

Forstermann, U., & Li, H. (2011). Therapeutic effect of enhancing endothelial nitric oxide synthase (eNOS) expression and preventing eNOS uncoupling. *British Journal of Pharmacology, 164*(2), 213–223.

Francis, S. H., Busch, J. L., Corbin, J. D., & Sibley, D. (2010). cGMP-dependent protein kinases and cGMP phosphodiesterases in nitric oxide and cGMP action. *Pharmacological Reviews, 62*(3), 525–563.

Galie, N., Ghofrani, H. A., Torbicki, A., Barst, R. J., Rubin, L. J., Badesch, D., et al. (2005). Sildenafil citrate therapy for pulmonary arterial hypertension. *New England Journal of Medicine, 353*(20), 2148–2157.

Gano, L. B., Donato, A. J., Pasha, H. M., Hearon, C. M., Jr., Sindler, A. L., & Seals, D. R. (2014). The SIRT1 activator SRT1720 reverses vascular endothelial dysfunction, excessive superoxide production, and inflammation with aging in mice. *American Journal of Physiology. Heart and Circulatory Physiology, 307*(12), H1754–H1763.

Gao, L., Chalupsky, K., Stefani, E., & Cai, H. (2009). Mechanistic insights into folic acid-dependent vascular protection: Dihydrofolate reductase (DHFR)-mediated reduction in oxidant stress in endothelial cells and angiotensin II-infused mice: A novel HPLC-based fluorescent assay for DHFR activity. *Journal of Molecular and Cellular Cardiology, 47*(6), 752–760.

Gao, L., Siu, K. L., Chalupsky, K., Nguyen, A., Chen, P., Weintraub, N. L., et al. (2012). Role of uncoupled endothelial nitric oxide synthase in abdominal aortic aneurysm formation: Treatment with folic acid. *Hypertension, 59*(1), 158–166.

Gao, D., Zuo, Z., Tian, J., Ali, Q., Lin, Y., Lei, H., et al. (2016). Activation of SIRT1 attenuates klotho deficiency-induced arterial stiffness and hypertension by enhancing AMP-activated protein kinase activity. *Hypertension, 68*(5), 1191–1199.

Gardiner, S. M., March, J. E., Kemp, P. A., Ballard, S. A., Hawkeswood, E., Hughes, B., et al. (2004). Haemodynamic effects of the selective phosphodiesterase 5 inhibitor, UK-357,903, in conscious SHR. *British Journal of Pharmacology, 141*(1), 114–122.

George, J., Carr, E., Davies, J., Belch, J. J., & Struthers, A. (2006). High-dose allopurinol improves endothelial function by profoundly reducing vascular oxidative stress and not by lowering uric acid. *Circulation, 114*(23), 2508–2516.

Ghosh, A., Koziol-White, C. J., Asosingh, K., Cheng, G., Ruple, L., Groneberg, D., et al. (2016). Soluble guanylate cyclase as an alternative target for bronchodilator therapy in asthma. *Proceedings of the National Academy of Sciences of the United States of America, 113*(17), E2355–E2362.

Ghosh, A., Stasch, J. P., Papapetropoulos, A., & Stuehr, D. J. (2014). Nitric oxide and heat shock protein 90 activate soluble guanylate cyclase by driving rapid change in its subunit interactions and heme content. *Journal of Biological Chemistry, 289*(22), 15259–15271.

Giannetta, E., Feola, T., Gianfrilli, D., Pofi, R., Dall'Armi, V., Badagliacca, R., et al. (2014). Is chronic inhibition of phosphodiesterase type 5 cardioprotective and safe? A meta-analysis of randomized controlled trials. *BMC Medicine, 12*, 185.

Gingles, C. R., Symon, R., Gandy, S. J., Struthers, A. D., Houston, G., MacDonald, T. M., et al. (2019). Allopurinol treatment adversely impacts left ventricular mass regression in patients with well-controlled hypertension. *Journal of Hypertension, 37*(12), 2481–2489.

Goldstein, S., & Czapski, G. (1995). The reaction of NO. with O_2.- and HO_2.: A pulse radiolysis study. *Free Radical Biology and Medicine, 19*(4), 505–510.

Goldstein, I., Lue, T. F., Padma-Nathan, H., Rosen, R. C., Steers, W. D., & Wicker, P. A. (1998). Oral sildenafil in the treatment of erectile dysfunction. Sildenafil Study Group. *New England Journal of Medicine, 338*(20), 1397–1404.

Golshiri, K., Ataei Ataabadi, E., Brandt, R., van der Pluijm, I., de Vries, R., Danser, J., et al. (2020). Chronic sildenafil treatment improves vasomotor function in a mouse model of accelerated aging. *International Journal of Molecular Sciences, 21*(13), 4667.

Golshiri, K., Ataei Ataabadi, E., Portilla Fernandez, E. C., Jan Danser, A. H., & Roks, A. J. M. (2019). The importance of the nitric oxide-cGMP pathway in age-related cardiovascular disease: Focus on phosphodiesterase-1 and soluble guanylate cyclase. *Basic & Clinical Pharmacology & Toxicology*, *127*(2), 14.

Golshiri, K., Ataei Ataabadi, E., Rubio-Beltran, E., Dutheil, S., Yao, W., Snyder, G. L., et al. (2021). Selective PDE1 inhibition ameliorates vascular function, reduces inflammatory response, and lowers blood pressure in ageing animals. *Journal of Pharmacology and Experimental Therapeutics*, *378*(2), 173–183.

Graham, D., Huynh, N. N., Hamilton, C. A., Beattie, E., Smith, R. A., Cocheme, H. M., et al. (2009). Mitochondria-targeted antioxidant MitoQ10 improves endothelial function and attenuates cardiac hypertrophy. *Hypertension*, *54*(2), 322–328.

Guthikonda, S., Sinkey, C., Barenz, T., & Haynes, W. G. (2003). Xanthine oxidase inhibition reverses endothelial dysfunction in heavy smokers. *Circulation*, *107*(3), 416–421.

Hajmousa, G., Vogelaar, P., Brouwer, L. A., van der Graaf, A. C., Henning, R. H., & Krenning, G. (2017). The 6-chromanol derivate SUL-109 enables prolonged hypothermic storage of adipose tissue-derived stem cells. *Biomaterials*, *119*, 43–52.

Han, B., Poppinga, W. J., Zuo, H., Zuidhof, A. B., Bos, I. S., Smit, M., et al. (2016). The novel compound Sul-121 inhibits airway inflammation and hyperresponsiveness in experimental models of chronic obstructive pulmonary disease. *Scientific Reports*, *6*, 26928.

Hanrahan, J. P., Seferovic, J. P., Wakefield, J. D., Wilson, P. J., Chickering, J. G., Jung, J., et al. (2020). An exploratory, randomised, placebo-controlled, 14 day trial of the soluble guanylate cyclase stimulator praliciguat in participants with type 2 diabetes and hypertension. *Diabtologia*, *63*(4), 733–743.

Hanrahan, J. P., Wakefield, J. D., Wilson, P. J., Mihova, M., Chickering, J. G., Ruff, D., et al. (2019). A randomized, placebo-controlled, multiple-ascending-dose study to assess the safety, tolerability, pharmacokinetics, and pharmacodynamics of the soluble guanylate cyclase stimulator praliciguat in healthy subjects. *Clinical Pharmacology in Drug Development*, *8*(5), 564–575.

Herrmann, H. C., Chang, G., Klugherz, B. D., & Mahoney, P. D. (2000). Hemodynamic effects of sildenafil in men with severe coronary artery disease. *New England Journal of Medicine*, *342*(22), 1622–1626.

Hink, U., Li, H., Mollnau, H., Oelze, M., Matheis, E., Hartmann, M., et al. (2001). Mechanisms underlying endothelial dysfunction in diabetes mellitus. *Circulation Research*, *88*(2), E14–E22.

Hirano, K., Chen, W. S., Chueng, A. L., Dunne, A. A., Seredenina, T., Filippova, A., et al. (2015). Discovery of GSK2795039, a novel small molecule NADPH oxidase 2 inhibitor. *Antioxidants & Redox Signalling*, *23*(5), 358–374.

Hoffmann, B., Stöckl, A., Schlame, M., Beyer, K., & Klingenberg, M. (1994). The reconstituted ADP/ATP carrier activity has an absolute requirement for cardiolipin as shown in cysteine mutants. *Journal of Biological Chemistry*, *269*(3), 1940–1944.

Hoffmann, E., Wald, J., Lavu, S., Roberts, J., Beaumont, C., Haddad, J., et al. (2013). Pharmacokinetics and tolerability of SRT2104, a first-in-class small molecule activator of SIRT1, after single and repeated oral administration in man. *British Journal of Clinical Pharmacology*, *75*(1), 186–196.

Hong, Q., Zhang, L., Das, B., Li, Z., Liu, B., Cai, G., et al. (2018). Increased podocyte Sirtuin-1 function attenuates diabetic kidney injury. *Kidney International*, *93*(6), 1330–1343.

Howitz, K. T., Bitterman, K. J., Cohen, H. Y., Lamming, D. W., Lavu, S., Wood, J. G., et al. (2003). Small molecule activators of sirtuins extend Saccharomyces cerevisiae lifespan. *Nature*, *425*(6954), 191–196.

Huynh, P. K., Wilder, J., Hiller, S., Hagaman, J., Takahashi, N., Maeda-Smithies, N., et al. (2020). Beneficial effects of nicotinamide on hypertensive mice with impaired endothelial nitric oxide function. *Journal of Experimental Nephrology*, *1*(1), 1–8.

James, A. M., Cochemé, H. M., Smith, R. A., & Murphy, M. P. (2005). Interactions of mitochondria-targeted and untargeted ubiquinones with the mitochondrial respiratory chain and reactive oxygen species. Implications for the use of exogenous ubiquinones as therapies and experimental tools. *Journal of Biological Chemistry*, *280*(22), 21295–21312.

Janssen, M., de Jong, J. W., Pasini, E., & Ferrari, R. (1993). Myocardial xanthine oxidoreductase activity in hypertensive and hypercholesterolemic rats. *Cardioscience*, *4*(1), 25–29.

Johnson, D. K., Schillinger, K. J., Kwait, D. M., Hughes, C. V., McNamara, E. J., Ishmael, F., et al. (2002). Inhibition of NADPH oxidase activation in endothelial cells by ortho-methoxy-substituted catechols. *Endothelium*, *9*(3), 191–203.

Kelso, G. F., Porteous, C. M., Coulter, C. V., Hughes, G., Porteous, W. K., Ledgerwood, E. C., et al. (2001). Selective targeting of a redox-active ubiquinone to mitochondria within cells: Antioxidant and antiapoptotic properties. *Journal of Biological Chemistry*, *276*(7), 4588–4596.

Kloner, R. A. (2005). Pharmacology and drug interaction effects of the phosphodiesterase 5 inhibitors: Focus on α-blocker interactions. *The American Journal of Cardiology*, *96*(12, Suppl. 2), 42–46.

Kokkonen, K., & Kass, D. A. (2017). Nanodomain regulation of cardiac cyclic nucleotide signaling by phosphodiesterases. *Annual Review of Pharmacology and Toxicology*, *57*, 455–479.

Kovamees, O., Shemyakin, A., & Pernow, J. (2014). Effect of arginase inhibition on ischemia-reperfusion injury in patients with coronary artery disease with and without diabetes mellitus. *PLoS One*, *9*(7), e103260.

Krueger, J. G., Suarez-Farinas, M., Cueto, I., Khacherian, A., Matheson, R., Parish, L. C., et al. (2015). A randomized, placebo-controlled study of SRT2104, a SIRT1 activator, in patients with moderate to severe psoriasis. *PLoS One*, *10*(11), e0142081.

Lakatta, E. G., & Levy, D. (2003). Arterial and cardiac aging: major shareholders in cardiovascular disease enterprises: Part I: aging arteries: A "set up" for vascular disease. *Circulation*, *107*(1), 139–146.

Lambooy, S. P. H., Bidadkosh, A., Nakladal, D., van Buiten, A., Girgis, R. A. T., van der Graaf, A. C., et al. (2017). The novel compound Sul-121 preserves endothelial function and inhibits progression of kidney damage in type 2 diabetes mellitus in mice. *Scientific Reports*, 7(1), 11165.

Landmesser, U., Dikalov, S., Price, S. R., McCann, L., Fukai, T., Holland, S. M., et al. (2003). Oxidation of tetrahydrobiopterin leads to uncoupling of endothelial cell nitric oxide synthase in hypertension. *Journal of Clinical Investigation*, *111*(8), 1201–1209.

Lange, C., Nett, J. H., Trumpower, B. L., & Hunte, C. (2001). Specific roles of protein-phospholipid interactions in the yeast cytochrome bc1 complex structure. *EMBO Journal*, *20*(23), 6591–6600.

Laursen, M., Beck, L., Kehler, J., Christoffersen, C. T., Bundgaard, C., Mogensen, S., et al. (2017). Novel selective PDE type 1 inhibitors cause vasodilatation and lower blood pressure in rats. *British Journal of Pharmacology*, *174*(15), 2563–2575.

Li, R. L., Lu, Z. Y., Huang, J. J., Qi, J., Hu, A., Su, Z. X., et al. (2016). SRT1720, a SIRT1 specific activator, protected H_2O_2-induced senescent endothelium. *American Journal of Translational Research*, *8*(7), 2876–2888.

Li, Q., Youn, J. Y., & Cai, H. (2015). Mechanisms and consequences of endothelial nitric oxide synthase dysfunction in hypertension. *Journal of Hypertension*, *33*(6), 1128–1136.

Lopes, R. A., Neves, K. B., Tostes, R. C., Montezano, A. C., & Touyz, R. M. (2015). Downregulation of nuclear factor erythroid 2-related factor and associated antioxidant genes contributes to redox-sensitive vascular dysfunction in hypertension. *Hypertension, 66*(6), 1240–1250.

Lopez-Otin, C., Blasco, M. A., Partridge, L., Serrano, M., & Kroemer, G. (2013). The hallmarks of aging. *Cell, 153*(6), 1194–1217.

Luo, Z., Aslam, S., Welch, W. J., & Wilcox, C. S. (2015). Activation of nuclear factor erythroid 2-related factor 2 coordinates dimethylarginine dimethylaminohydrolase/PPAR-γ/endothelial nitric oxide synthase pathways that enhance nitric oxide generation in human glomerular endothelial cells. *Hypertension, 65*(4), 896–902.

Manuel, T., Sema, H. S., Evanthia, M., Sebastian, A. P., Guang, Y., Lydia, H., et al. (2017). Phosphodiesterase 5 inhibition ameliorates angiotensin II-dependent hypertension and renal vascular dysfunction. *American Journal of Physiology-Renal Physiology, 312*(3), F474–F481.

Marinko, M., Novakovic, A., Nenezic, D., Stojanovic, I., Milojevic, P., Jovic, M., et al. (2015). Nicorandil directly and cyclic GMP-dependently opens K+ channels in human bypass grafts. *Journal of Pharmacological Sciences, 128*(2), 59–64.

Mashima, R., & Okuyama, T. (2015). The role of lipoxygenases in pathophysiology; new insights and future perspectives. *Redox Biology, 6*, 297–310.

Mattagajasingh, I., Kim, C. S., Naqvi, A., Yamamori, T., Hoffman, T. A., Jung, S. B., et al. (2007). SIRT1 promotes endothelium-dependent vascular relaxation by activating endothelial nitric oxide synthase. *Proceedings of the National Academy of Sciences of the United States of America, 104*(37), 14855–14860.

Mergia, E., & Stegbauer, J. (2016). Role of phosphodiesterase 5 and cyclic GMP in hypertension. *Current Hypertension Reports, 18*(5), 39.

Meyer, M. R., Fredette, N. C., Daniel, C., Sharma, G., Amann, K., Arterburn, J. B., et al. (2016). Obligatory role for GPER in cardiovascular aging and disease. *Science Signaling, 9*(452), ra105.

Mollsten, A., Jorsal, A., Lajer, M., Vionnet, N., & Tarnow, L. (2009). The V16A polymorphism in SOD2 is associated with increased risk of diabetic nephropathy and cardiovascular disease in type 1 diabetes. *Diabtologia, 52*(12), 2590–2593.

Myung, S.-K., Ju, W., Cho, B., Oh, S.-W., Park, S. M., Koo, B.-K., et al. (2013). Efficacy of vitamin and antioxidant supplements in prevention of cardiovascular disease: Systematic review and meta-analysis of randomised controlled trials. *British Medical Journal, 346*, f10.

Nakamura, T., Zhu, G., Ranek, M. J., Kokkonen-Simon, K., Zhang, M., Kim, G. E., et al. (2018). Prevention of PKG-1alpha oxidation suppresses antihypertrophic/antifibrotic effects from PDE5 inhibition but not sGC stimulation. *Circulation Heart Failure, 11*(3), e004740.

Nakladal, D., Buikema, H., Romero, A. R., Lambooy, S. P. H., Bouma, J., Krenning, G., et al. (2019). The (R)-enantiomer of the 6-chromanol derivate SUL-121 improves renal graft perfusion via antagonism of the alpha1-adrenoceptor. *Scientific Reports, 9*(1), 13.

Neves, K. B., Morris, H. E., Alves-Lopes, R., Muir, K. W., Moreton, F., Delles, C., et al. (2021). Peripheral arteriopathy caused by Notch3 gain-of-function mutation involves ER and oxidative stress and blunting of NO/sGC/cGMP pathway. *Clinical Science (London), 135*(6), 753–773.

Nosalski, R., Mikolajczyk, T., Siedlinski, M., Saju, B., Koziol, J., Maffia, P., et al. (2020). Nox1/4 inhibition exacerbates age dependent perivascular inflammation and fibrosis in a model of spontaneous hypertension. *Pharmacological Research, 161*, 105235.

Pacher, P., Nivorozhkin, A., & Szabo, C. (2006). Therapeutic effects of xanthine oxidase inhibitors: Renaissance half a century after the discovery of allopurinol. *Pharmacological Reviews, 58*(1), 87–114.

Pacholec, M., Bleasdale, J. E., Chrunyk, B., Cunningham, D., Flynn, D., Garofalo, R. S., et al. (2010). SRT1720, SRT2183, SRT1460, and resveratrol are not direct activators of SIRT1. *Journal of Biological Chemistry, 285*(11), 8340–8351.

Pak, K. J., Hu, T., Fee, C., Wang, R., Smith, M., & Bazzano, L. A. (2014). Acute hypertension: A systematic review and appraisal of guidelines. *The Ochsner Journal, 14*(4), 655–663.

Pankey, E. A., Bhartiya, M., Badejo, A. M., Jr., Haider, U., Stasch, J. P., Murthy, S. N., et al. (2011). Pulmonary and systemic vasodilator responses to the soluble guanylyl cyclase activator, BAY 60-2770, are not dependent on endogenous nitric oxide or reduced heme. *American Journal of Physiology. Heart and Circulatory Physiology, 300*(3), H792–H802.

Prysyazhna, O., Rudyk, O., & Eaton, P. (2012). Single atom substitution in mouse protein kinase G eliminates oxidant sensing to cause hypertension. *Nature Medicine, 18*(2), 286–290.

Prysyazhna, O., Wolhuter, K., Switzer, C., Santos, C., Yang, X., Lynham, S., et al. (2019). Blood pressure-lowering by the antioxidant resveratrol is counterintuitively mediated by oxidation of cGMP-dependent protein kinase. *Circulation, 140*(2), 126–137.

Qiao, Y. N., He, W. Q., Chen, C. P., Zhang, C. H., Zhao, W., Wang, P., et al. (2014). Myosin phosphatase target subunit 1 (MYPT1) regulates the contraction and relaxation of vascular smooth muscle and maintains blood pressure. *Journal of Biological Chemistry, 289*(32), 22512–22523.

Rahaman, M. M., Nguyen, A. T., Miller, M. P., Hahn, S. A., Sparacino-Watkins, C., Jobbagy, S., et al. (2017). Cytochrome b5 reductase 3 modulates soluble guanylate cyclase redox state and cGMP signaling. *Circulation Research, 121*(2), 137–148.

Rainer, P. P., & Kass, D. A. (2016). Old dog, new tricks: Novel cardiac targets and stress regulation by protein kinase G. *Cardiovascular Research, 111*(2), 154–162.

Robledinos-Anton, N., Fernandez-Gines, R., Manda, G., & Cuadrado, A. (2019). Activators and inhibitors of NRF2: A review of their potential for clinical development. *Oxidative Medicine and Cellular Longevity, 2019*, 9372182.

Rodriguez-Iturbe, B., Sepassi, L., Quiroz, Y., Ni, Z., Wallace, D. C., & Vaziri, N. D. (2007). Association of mitochondrial SOD deficiency with salt-sensitive hypertension and accelerated renal senescence. *Journal of Applied Physiology (1985), 102*(1), 255–260.

Rossman, M. J., Gioscia-Ryan, R. A., Santos-Parker, J. R., Ziemba, B. P., Lubieniecki, K. L., Johnson, L. C., et al. (2021). Inorganic nitrite supplementation improves endothelial function with aging: Translational evidence for suppression of mitochondria-derived oxidative stress. *Hypertension*, 77(4), 1212–1222.

Rossman, M. J., Santos-Parker, J. R., Steward, C. A. C., Bispham, N. Z., Cuevas, L. M., Rosenberg, H. L., et al. (2018). Chronic supplementation with a mitochondrial antioxidant (MitoQ) improves vascular function in healthy older adults. *Hypertension, 71*(6), 1056–1063.

Roy, S., Kloner, R. A., Salloum, F. N., & Jovin, I. S. (2021). Cardiac effects of phosphodiesterase-5 inhibitors: Efficacy and safety. *Cardiovascular Drugs and Therapy*. https://doi.org/10.1007/s10557-021-07275-y.

Rudyk, O., Prysyazhna, O., Burgoyne, J. R., & Eaton, P. (2012). Nitroglycerin fails to lower blood pressure in redox-dead Cys42Ser PKG1alpha knock-in mouse. *Circulation, 126*(3), 287–295.

Rybalkin, S. D., Rybalkina, I., Beavo, J. A., & Bornfeldt, K. E. (2002). Cyclic nucleotide phosphodiesterase 1C promotes human arterial smooth muscle cell proliferation. *Circulation Research, 90*(2), 151–157.

Rybalkin, S. D., Rybalkina, I. G., Shimizu-Albergine, M., Tang, X. B., & Beavo, J. A. (2003). PDE5 is converted to an activated state upon cGMP binding to the GAF A domain. *EMBO Journal, 22*(3), 469–478.

Saad, A., Herrmann, S. M. S., Eirin, A., Ferguson, C. M., Glockner, J. F., Bjarnason, H., et al. (2017). Phase 2a clinical trial of mitochondrial protection (Elamipretide) during stent revascularization in patients with atherosclerotic renal artery stenosis. *Circulation. Cardiovascular Interventions, 10*(9), e005487.

Sabbah, H. N., Gupta, R. C., Singh-Gupta, V., Zhang, K., & Lanfear, D. E. (2018). Abnormalities of mitochondrial dynamics in the failing heart: normalization following long-term therapy with elamipretide. *Cardiovascular Drugs and Therapy*, *32*(4), 319–328.

Sage, P. R., de la Lande, I. S., Stafford, I., Bennett, C. L., Phillipov, G., Stubberfield, J., et al. (2000). Nitroglycerin tolerance in human vessels: evidence for impaired nitroglycerin bioconversion. *Circulation*, *102*(23), 2810–2815.

Scalera, F., Fulge, B., Martens-Lobenhoffer, J., Heimburg, A., & Bode-Boger, S. M. (2009). Red wine decreases asymmetric dimethylarginine via SIRT1 induction in human endothelial cells. *Biochemical and Biophysical Research Communications*, *390*(3), 703–709.

Schafer, A., Burkhardt, M., Vollkommer, T., Bauersachs, J., Munzel, T., Walter, U., et al. (2003). Endothelium-dependent and -independent relaxation and VASP serines 157/239 phosphorylation by cyclic nucleotide-elevating vasodilators in rat aorta. *Biochemical Pharmacology*, *65*(3), 397–405.

Schuhmacher, S., Wenzel, P., Schulz, E., Oelze, M., Mang, C., Kamuf, J., et al. (2010). Pentaerythritol tetranitrate improves angiotensin II-induced vascular dysfunction via induction of heme oxygenase-1. *Hypertension*, *55*(4), 897–904.

Schulz, E., Tsilimingas, N., Rinze, R., Reiter, B., Wendt, M., Oelze, M., et al. (2002). Functional and biochemical analysis of endothelial (dys)function and NO/cGMP signaling in human blood vessels with and without nitroglycerin pretreatment. *Circulation*, *105*(10), 1170–1175.

Seifi, B., Kadkhodaee, M., Karimian, S. M., Zahmatkesh, M., Shams, S., & Bakhshi, E. (2009). Reduction of kidney damage by supplementation of vitamins C and E in rats with deoxycorticosterone-salt-induced hypertension. *Iranian Journal of Kidney Diseases*, *3*(4), 197–202.

Sheehe, J. L., Bonev, A. D., Schmoker, A. M., Ballif, B. A., Nelson, M. T., Moon, T. M., et al. (2018). Oxidation of cysteine 117 stimulates constitutive activation of the type Ialpha cGMP-dependent protein kinase. *Journal of Biological Chemistry*, *293*(43), 16791–16802.

Shinzawa-Itoh, K., Aoyama, H., Muramoto, K., Terada, H., Kurauchi, T., Tadehara, Y., et al. (2007). Structures and physiological roles of 13 integral lipids of bovine heart cytochrome c oxidase. *EMBO Journal*, *26*(6), 1713–1725.

Stanley, C. P., Maghzal, G. J., Ayer, A., Talib, J., Giltrap, A. M., Shengule, S., et al. (2019). Singlet molecular oxygen regulates vascular tone and blood pressure in inflammation. *Nature*, *566*(7745), 548–552.

Stuehr, D. J., Misra, S., Dai, Y., & Ghosh, A. (2021). Maturation, inactivation, and recovery mechanisms of soluble guanylyl cyclase. *The Journal of Biological Chemistry*, *296*, 100336.

Su, H., Zeng, H., Liu, B., & Chen, J. X. (2020). Sirtuin 3 is essential for hypertension-induced cardiac fibrosis via mediating pericyte transition. *Journal of Cellular and Molecular Medicine*, *24*(14), 8057–8068.

Sumi-Ichinose, C., Suganuma, Y., Kano, T., Ihira, N., Nomura, H., Ikemoto, K., et al. (2017). Sepiapterin reductase gene-disrupted mice suffer from hypertension with fluctuation and bradycardia. *Physiological Reports*, *5*(6).

Surmeli, N. B., & Marletta, M. A. (2012). Insight into the rescue of oxidized soluble guanylate cyclase by the activator cinaciguat. *Chembiochem*, *13*(7), 977–981.

Takimoto, E., Koitabashi, N., Hsu, S., Ketner, E. A., Zhang, M., Nagayama, T., et al. (2009). Regulator of G protein signaling 2 mediates cardiac compensation to pressure overload and antihypertrophic effects of PDE5 inhibition in mice. *Journal of Clinical Investigation*, *119*(2), 408–420.

Taylor, C. T., & Moncada, S. (2010). Nitric oxide, cytochrome C oxidase, and the cellular response to hypoxia. *Arteriosclerosis, Thrombosis, and Vascular Biology*, *30*(4), 643–647.

Tejero, J., Shiva, S., & Gladwin, M. T. (2019). Sources of vascular nitric oxide and reactive oxygen species and their regulation. *Physiological Reviews*, *99*(1), 311–379.

Thida, M., Earl, J., Zhao, Y., Wang, H., Tse, C. S., Vickers, J. J., et al. (2010). Effects of sepiapterin supplementation and NOS inhibition on glucocorticoid-induced hypertension. *American Journal of Hypertension, 23*(5), 569–574.

Thomas, M. K., Francis, S. H., & Corbin, J. D. (1990). Substrate- and kinase-directed regulation of phosphorylation of a cGMP-binding phosphodiesterase by cGMP. *Journal of Biological Chemistry, 265*(25), 14971–14978.

Tousoulis, D., Androulakis, E., Papageorgiou, N., & Stefanadis, C. (2012). Novel therapeutic strategies in the management of arterial hypertension. *Pharmacology and Therapeutics, 135*(2), 168–175.

Tousoulis, D., Georgakis, M. K., Oikonomou, E., Papageorgiou, N., Zaromitidou, M., Latsios, G., et al. (2015). Asymmetric dimethylarginine: Clinical significance and novel therapeutic approaches. *Current Medicinal Chemistry, 22*(24), 2871–2901.

Ungvari, Z., Bagi, Z., Feher, A., Recchia, F. A., Sonntag, W. E., Pearson, K., et al. (2010). Resveratrol confers endothelial protection via activation of the antioxidant transcription factor Nrf2. *American Journal of Physiology. Heart and Circulatory Physiology, 299*(1), H18–H24.

Vähäheikkilä, M., Peltomaa, T., Róg, T., Vazdar, M., Pöyry, S., & Vattulainen, I. (2018). How cardiolipin peroxidation alters the properties of the inner mitochondrial membrane? *Chemistry and Physics of Lipids, 214*, 15–23.

Versari, D., Daghini, E., Rodriguez-Porcel, M., Sattler, K., Galili, O., Pilarczyk, K., et al. (2006). Chronic antioxidant supplementation impairs coronary endothelial function and myocardial perfusion in normal pigs. *Hypertension, 47*(3), 475–481.

Virdis, A., Neves, M. F., Amiri, F., Touyz, R. M., & Schiffrin, E. L. (2004). Role of NAD(P)H oxidase on vascular alterations in angiotensin II-infused mice. *Journal of Hypertension, 22*(3), 535–542.

Wang, C., Luo, Z., Carter, G., Wellstein, A., Jose, P. A., Tomlinson, J., et al. (2018). NRF2 prevents hypertension, increased ADMA, microvascular oxidative stress, and dysfunction in mice with two weeks of ANG II infusion. *American Journal of Physiology. Regulatory, Integrative and Comparative Physiology, 314*(3), R399–R406.

Wang, X., Yamada, S., LaRiviere, W. B., Ye, H., Bakeberg, J. L., Irazabal, M. V., et al. (2017). Generation and phenotypic characterization of Pde1a mutant mice. *PLoS One, 12*(7), e0181087.

White, W. B., Saag, K. G., Becker, M. A., Borer, J. S., Gorelick, P. B., Whelton, A., et al. (2018). Cardiovascular safety of febuxostat or allopurinol in patients with gout. *New England Journal of Medicine, 378*(13), 1200–1210.

Wind, S., Beuerlein, K., Armitage, M. E., Taye, A., Kumar, A. H., Janowitz, D., et al. (2010). Oxidative stress and endothelial dysfunction in aortas of aged spontaneously hypertensive rats by NOX1/2 is reversed by NADPH oxidase inhibition. *Hypertension, 56*(3), 490–497.

Wind, S., Beuerlein, K., Eucker, T., Müller, H., Scheurer, P., Armitage, M. E., et al. (2010). Comparative pharmacology of chemically distinct NADPH oxidase inhibitors. *British Journal of Pharmacology, 161*(4), 885–898.

Wohlfart, P., Xu, H., Endlich, A., Habermeier, A., Closs, E. I., Hubschle, T., et al. (2008). Antiatherosclerotic effects of small-molecular-weight compounds enhancing endothelial nitric-oxide synthase (eNOS) expression and preventing eNOS uncoupling. *Journal of Pharmacology and Experimental Therapeutics, 325*(2), 370–379.

Yaguas, K., Bautista, R., Quiroz, Y., Ferrebuz, A., Pons, H., Franco, M., et al. (2010). Chronic sildenafil treatment corrects endothelial dysfunction and improves hypertension. *American Journal of Nephrology, 31*(4), 283–291.

Yan, C. (2015). Cyclic nucleotide phosphodiesterase 1 and vascular aging. *Clinical Science (London), 129*(12), 1077–1081.

Yao, J., Shi, X., Fan, S., Gao, Y., Hu, H., Wang, P., et al. (2020). Effect of febuxostat on blood pressure in hyperuricemic patients: A protocol for a systematic review and meta-analysis. *Medicine*, *99*(24), e20673.

Youn, J. Y., Wang, T., Blair, J., Laude, K. M., Oak, J. H., McCann, L. A., et al. (2012). Endothelium-specific sepiapterin reductase deficiency in DOCA-salt hypertension. *American Journal of Physiology. Heart and Circulatory Physiology*, *302*(11), H2243–H2249.

Yuan, F., Hedayat, A. F., Ferguson, C. M., Lerman, A., Lerman, L. O., & Eirin, A. (2018). Mitoprotection attenuates myocardial vascular impairment in porcine metabolic syndrome. *American Journal of Physiology. Heart and Circulatory Physiology*, *314*(3), H669–H680.

Zhang, Y., Murugesan, P., Huang, K., & Cai, H. (2020). NADPH oxidases and oxidase crosstalk in cardiovascular diseases: Novel therapeutic targets. *Nature Reviews. Cardiology*, *17*(3), 170–194.

CHAPTER FOUR

Sphingosine-1-phosphate and Sphingosine-1-phosphate receptors in the cardiovascular system: pharmacology and clinical implications

Simona Federica Spampinato, Maria Angela Sortino, and Salvatore Salomone*
Department of Biomedical and Biotechnological Science, University of Catania, Catania, Italy
*Corresponding author: e-mail address: salomone@unict.it

Contents

Abstract

Sphingosine-1-phosphate (S1P) is a lipid that binds and activates five distinct receptor subtypes, $S1P_1$, $S1P_2$, $S1P_3$, $S1P_4$, $S1P_5$, widely expressed in different cells, tissues and organs. In the cardiovascular system these receptors have been extensively studied,

Advances in Pharmacology, Volume 94
ISSN 1054-3589
https://doi.org/10.1016/bs.apha.2022.02.001

but no drug acting on them has been approved so far for treating cardiovascular diseases. In contrast, a number of S1P receptor agonists are approved as immunomodulators, mainly for multiple sclerosis, because of their action on lymphocyte trafficking. This chapter summarizes the available information on S1P receptors in the cardiovascular system and discusses their potential for treating cardiovascular conditions and/or their role on the clinical pharmacology of drugs so far approved for non-cardiovascular conditions. Basic research has recently produced data useful to understand the molecular pharmacology of S1P and S1P receptors, regarding biased agonism, S1P storage, release and vehiculation and chaperoning by lipoproteins, paracrine actions, intracellular non-receptorial S1P actions. On the other hand, the approval of fingolimod and newer generation S1P receptor ligands as immunomodulators, provides information on a number of clinical observations on the impact of these drugs on cardiovascular system which need to be integrated with preclinical data. S1P receptors are potential targets for prevention and treatment of major cardiovascular conditions, including hypertension, myocardial infarction, heart failure and stroke.

Abbreviations

AJ adherens junctions
ApoM apolipoprotein M
BBB blood-brain barrier
BNP brain natriuretic peptide
CNS central nervous system
DOCA deoxycorticosterone acetate
eNOS endothelial nitric oxide synthase
GPCR G protein-coupled receptors
HDACS histone deacetylases
HDL high-density lipoproteins
HUVEC human umbilical vascular endothelial cells
LDL low-density lipoproteins
MCAO middle cerebral artery occlusion
MS multiple sclerosis
NO nitric oxide
OGD/r oxygen glucose deprivation/re-oxygenation
PI3K phosphatidylinositol 3-kinases
SPHK sphingosine kinase
SHRSP stroke-prone, spontaneously hypertensive rat, Sphingosine-1-phosphate
SPNS$_2$ Spinster homolog 2
SPP sphingosine phosphatases
STING stimulator of interferon gene
TGF-$\beta 1$ transforming growth factor-β
TJ tight junctions
VEGFR$_2$ vascular endothelial growth factor receptor 2
VLDL very low-density lipoproteins
VSMC vascular smooth muscle cells

1. Introduction

In mammals, systemic arterial blood pressure is tightly regulated, mainly through the sympathetic system and the renin-angiotensin-aldosterone system. This regulation acts either for short-term adjustments, such that when moving from supine position to orthostatism (to maintain cerebral blood flow), or for more sustained periods of time, such that when blood volume is reduced due to dehydration or hemorrhage. Chronic hypertension is a condition in which systemic arterial blood pressure is persistently higher than normal range values. Primary hypertension, also termed "essential hypertension" is the most common form and is not attributable to a single cause/ mechanism, but, rather, to a number of genetic and acquired defects; for this reason, the pharmacological treatment, though controlling blood pressure levels, cannot remove the cause and is not curative, and needs to be continued lifelong. In contrast, secondary hypertension can be attributable to a specific cause (compression of renal artery, pheochromocytoma, etc.), which, in some instances can be removed, with ensuing resolution of the disorder. Hypertension at least within certain limits, is asymptomatic, but represents a major risk factor for arterial disease with ensuing vital organ damage, including stroke, myocardial ischemia and renal disease. Another distinct condition is pulmonary hypertension, e.g., chronic increase of blood pressure in the pulmonary arteries, which we also will discuss below. In terms of hydrodynamics (from Poiseuille's law), blood pressure is directly proportional to cardiac output, which, in turn depends on cardiac activity and blood volume, and to peripheral vascular resistance, e.g., the diameter of resistance arterioles, depending on contractile status of vascular smooth muscle cells (VSMC). Other factors, such as blood viscosity (which mainly depends on hematocrit), contribute to resistance, but are not object of physiological regulation and do not play a significant role in hypertension. Among the factors that can affect several of these mechanisms is sphingosine-1-phosphate (S1P). This is a bioactive metabolite of sphingolipids, ubiquitously expressed in our body, where it exerts several functions, particularly in the cardiovascular and immune systems. Interestingly, a very recent report highlighted the correlation between S1P circulating levels and blood pressure, indicating higher S1P plasma concentrations in patients with systolic blood pressure $>140\,mmHg$ (Jujic et al., 2021). This observation appears relevant since, up to now, definition of a role for S1P in the development of hypertensive disease, has been rather puzzling. Data are available regarding modifications of sphingolipid metabolism in different models of experimental hypertension (Chen et al., 2014; Gairhe et al., 2016; Meissner et al., 2017; Tabeling et al., 2015; Zhao et al., 2015), but results fail to identify a definite function for S1P.

Of note, a correlation has been suggested between S1P in hypertension and its regulatory function on vascular tone, inflammation and more general metabolic processes, so that its potential role as a suitable biomarker to identify selected patient population at risk for cardiovascular diseases has been also envisaged (Jujic et al., 2021).

Although direct evidence is limited, a large body of data from the literature indicates that S1P exerts a myriad of effects on several functions and parameters that can indirectly impact on, or be related to, blood pressure control. It is the aim of this review to analyze some of these issues in order to clarify the role of S1P in the more general context of hypertension.

2. S1P synthesis, kinetics and general function

S1P is the product of the metabolism of membrane sphingolipids: sphingosine is generated by the catalysis of sphingomyelin into ceramide, converted into sphingosine by a ceramidase that is then phosphorylated into S1P by two sphingosine kinases ($SPHK_1$ and $SPKH_2$). The two kinases are redundant in generating S1P, but the deletion of both of them causes embryo lethality due to severe hemorrhage (Mizugishi et al., 2005). SPHK1 is mainly expressed in the cytosol and upon stimulation it translocates to plasma membrane, while $SPHK_2$ is localized in intracellular compartments, endoplasmic reticulum, mitochondria and nucleus (Kunkel, Maceyka, Milstien, & Spiegel, 2013). SPHKs cellular localization strongly correlates with their functions: while $SPHK_1$-generated S1P stimulates S1P receptors, S1P produced by $SPHK_2$ appears more involved in gene transcription and other responses occurring inside the cell, independent of S1P receptors activation. Upon stimulation with cytokines and growth factors, SPHKs' activity may be enhanced, leading to increased S1P production and signaling. Degradation of S1P is the result of its dephosphorylation into sphingosine through two sphingosine phosphatases, SPP_1 and SPP_2, or it can be irreversibly cleaved by sphingosine lyase (Ikeda, Kihara, & Igarashi, 2004).

Although virtually every single cell is able to produce S1P, endothelial cells and erythrocytes are the major sources of the sphingolipid in the plasma and, in pathological conditions, like in sepsis, also platelets release S1P (Yatomi et al., 1997). In particular, erythrocytes and platelets, that lack S1P lyase, are considered to be the perfect storage pool of S1P (Ito et al., 2007; Urtz et al., 2015); nevertheless, in endothelial cells, the expression of S1P lyase is reduced in the presence of laminar shear forces, thus in physiological conditions, this cell type significantly contributes to the maintenance of plasmatic S1P levels (Venkataraman et al., 2008). A more detailed analysis of platelet-derived S1P and its function is reported in Box 1.

BOX 1 Platelets as an important source of S1P for autocrine/paracrine effects

Platelets are another important supplementary source of S1P. They express in fact the enzyme isoform $SPHK_2$ that can produce S1P and, similarly to erythrocytes, they do not contain S1P lyase, one of the key enzymes necessary to efficiently degrade S1P. This makes platelets an "ideal" store for the sphingolipid (Yatomi, Ruan, Hakomori, & Igarashi, 1995). The release of S1P from platelets is mainly dependent on prostaglandin/thromboxane formation and, accordingly, aspirin and other cyclooxygenase inhibitors may largely reduce it (Ulrych et al., 2011), although it is not completely clear whether S1P synthesis or release are significantly affected by these drugs. More recently, it has been shown that the transporter Mfsd2b contributes to S1P release, being one of the main S1P exporter in platelets (Chandrakanthan et al., 2021). Interestingly, although this transport has only a secondary role in S1P release from platelets, deletion of Mfsd2b, markedly impairs platelet function with resulting reduced thrombus formation (Chandrakanthan et al., 2021). The correlation between S1P levels and platelet function is supported by the observation that the concentration of serum S1P appears to be increased two- to threefold upon platelets aggregation and clot formation (Ono et al., 2013). Among blood cells, both erythrocytes and platelets produce S1P. However, while red cells-derived S1P is essential for endothelial S1P receptors activation, platelets do not sufficiently contribute to increase plasmatic S1P levels (Pappu et al., 2007). They contain up to nine times more S1P than red blood cells, but due to the higher number of erythrocytes, their contribution to the total S1P pool is limited (Ito et al., 2007). Evidence though shows that platelets-derived S1P pools are strikingly and transiently reduced in myocardial infarction in rats (Knapp et al., 2012), and it is known that in human platelets the release of S1P is increased after stimulation (Urtz et al., 2015). Platelets may thus increase S1P local concentrations, potentially inducing the activation of receptors not saturated by S1P plasmatic levels (Taha, Argraves, & Obeid, 2004).

Continued

BOX 1 Platelets as an important source of S1P for autocrine/paracrine effects—cont'd

S1P signaling through both $S1P_1$ and $S1P_4$ appears also important for platelets biogenesis and function (Golfier et al., 2010; Niazi et al., 2019). S1P produced by platelets may be relevant for the autocrine activation of their own S1P receptors playing a role in hemostasis and thrombosis (Urtz et al., 2015). Accordingly, in ex vivo experiments and animal models, it was demonstrated that S1P induces platelets shape change (Yatomi et al., 1995) and affects their spreading on fibrinogen, with lamellipodia formation, and their aggregation to collagen (Gazit et al., 2016). However, controversies still exist regarding platelet function, since S1P appears not to affect platelets adhesion properties (Urtz et al., 2015) and to modify bleeding time. Moreover, chronic treatment with S1P modulators, including fingolimod, does not exert a measurable effect on platelets counts or their functions (Kappos et al., 2010). On the other hand, S1P accumulation into the platelets may also contribute to disruption of platelet function. Deletion of the Mfsd2b S1P transporter in platelets that, as mentioned, induces S1P accumulation within the cell, causes the formation of multiple lesions and pores in membranes, probably due to lipotoxicity. These morphological modifications, that have also been described in the erythrocytes of *Mfsd2b* KO mice, affect platelets functions and their ability to induce the formation of venous thrombosis (Chandrakanthan et al., 2021). The reduced expression of the transporter does not affect systemic S1P levels, so targeting Mfsd2b functions has been proposed as a potential approach to prevent abnormal thrombotic conditions.

Platelets-derived S1P also affects endothelial properties, probably by stimulating $S1P_1$; it induces endothelial cell migration, a crucial mechanism in the context of angio- and vasculogenesis (Panetti, Nowlen, & Mosher, 2000); aspirin treatment, by reducing platelet S1P release, appears to strongly reduce these mechanisms (Polzin et al., 2018) that are important for the restoration of endothelial layer integrity after vessels damage. As already stated, S1P affects endothelial barrier functions also increasing the tightness of endothelial cell to cell junctions and platelets-derived S1P may act in a paracrine manner to increase endothelial VE-Cadherin expression (Herzog et al., 2013). Nevertheless, in physiological conditions, platelets- and erythrocytes-derived S1P appears to be redundant for homeostasis, thrombosis and vascular integrity (Gazit et al., 2016). The importance of platelets-derived S1P in specific roles during coagulation may be otherwise increased when other S1P sources are damaged or exhausted (as in systemic inflammation, sepsis or anaphylaxis; Gazit et al., 2016).

The S1P produced by erythrocytes and endothelial cells is then released by the transmembrane transporter Spinster homolog 2 ($SPNS_2$). Erythrocytes and platelets release S1P also through the transporter Mfsd2b (Vu et al., 2017). In physiological conditions, S1P concentrations are high in blood [ranges between 0.1 and 1.2 μM (Venkataraman et al., 2008)] and in lymph fluid [1/4 lower than in the plasma (Hla, Venkataraman, & Michaud, 2008)], while they are even more variable in tissues [0.5–75 pmol/mg, (Xiong & Hla, 2014)]: the maintenance of a gradient among tissues, lymph and plasma may have critical importance for S1P functions, allowing for instance the trafficking of immune cells from the lymphatic tissue and their role in immune surveillance (Pappu et al., 2007). In the plasma, almost the majority of S1P is bound to protein carriers, in particular to albumin [30–40%, (Diarte-Anazco et al., 2019)] and for the remaining, almost 60%, to the high-density lipoproteins (HDL). While reducing its bioavailability, binding of S1P to HDL prolongs its half-life and enhances its biological effects, including the reduction of inflammatory state (Obinata & Hla, 2019). See Box 2 for a more detailed description of this interaction.

BOX 2 HDL/apoM-bound S1P and its biological significance

As already described, S1P transport in the plasma is mediated by specific carriers, albumin and lipoproteins. S1P bound to lipoproteins initiates long-term responses, as this binding increases the stability of S1P and prolongs its presence in plasma (Sato & Okajima, 2010). Among the lipoproteins that overall bind almost 60–70% S1P, HDL are the ones carrying >55%, while others bind S1P to a lesser extent; in particular about 10%, LDL and only 2–3%, very low-density lipoproteins (VLDL) (Hammad, Al Gadban, Semler, & Klein, 2012). Despite this high presence in HDL, most S1P seems to be biologically inactive. Among various Apo, ApoM appears critical for S1P association to HDL, both *in vitro* (Kurano & Yatomi, 2018) and *in vivo* (Christoffersen et al., 2011) and protects S1P from degradation. However, controversies still exist on the real role of ApoM as the main carrier of S1P in plasma. Accordingly, experimental ApoM deficiency in animal models is linked to a concomitant decrease in S1P plasma levels (Christoffersen et al., 2011) that is only partial, suggesting that other factors can bind and act as carriers of S1P. This link seems however relevant since HDL not only transport S1P, but the binding between S1P and ApoM leads to S1P enrichment in HDL and enhancement of lipoprotein biological activity (Jiang & Zhang, 2019; Robert, Osto, & von Eckardstein, 2021). It is well known that HDL exert several vasoprotective functions on endothelium by promoting endothelial cells proliferation, migration and prevent their apoptosis (reviewed in Robert et al., 2021).

Continued

BOX 2 HDL/apoM-bound S1P and its biological significance—cont'd

HDL are also able to stimulate $S1P_3$-mediated vasodilatation (Yuhanna et al., 2001) and increase barrier tightness by inducing expression of endothelial AJ and TJ (Argraves et al., 2008) and reducing the adhesion molecules VCAM-1, ICAM-1 and E-Selectin, with ensuing limitation of leukocytes diapedesis. ApoM-bound S1P has a main role in HDL effects on endothelium, as pointed out by *in vitro* and *in vivo* studies. Thus, reduced S1P plasma levels in ApoM KO mice were associated to increased plasma exudation into extravascular tissues, like lungs and brown adipose tissue, indicating enhanced endothelial membrane permeability (Christensen et al., 2016; Christoffersen et al., 2018, 2011). Lack of ApoM also increases BBB permeability to small molecules, in particular in the arterial branch of cerebral vasculature, where endothelial expression of $S1P_1$ is higher (Mathiesen Janiurek, Soylu-Kucharz, Christoffersen, Kucharz, & Lauritzen, 2019), whereas pharmacological stimulation of the same receptor rescues BBB function (Mathiesen Janiurek et al., 2019). *In vitro* studies, carried out in HUVEC and in microvascular endothelial cells, confirm that HDL/ApoM increase the integrity of the endothelial layer in a process involving $S1P_1$, Akt activation as well as AMPK phosphorylation (Argraves et al., 2008; Dennhardt, Finke, Huwiler, & Coldewey, 2019). By acting on $S1P_1$ and $S1P_3$ expressed on endothelial cells, ApoM-bound S1P also reduces the phosphorylation of NF-kB and the expression of the adhesion molecules VCAM1, ICAM1 and E-selectin (Robert et al., 2021; Ruiz et al., 2017), as well as secretion of IL-8 and monocyte chemoattractant protein 1 (or CCL2) (Del Gaudio et al., 2020), thus reducing the infiltration of leukocytes. These effects have been observed in aortic, brain microvascular as well as placental endothelial cells. According to the supposed role of HDL-S1P in the maintenance of a functional endothelial barrier, in sepsis, low levels of both HDL and S1P have been described (Fan et al., 2020; Yang et al., 2020) and HDL-S1P injection significantly reduces pulmonary edema, endothelial leakage and leukocytes infiltration in septic rats (Fan et al., 2020). Interestingly, ApoM shows a weakened ability to bind to S1P under conditions of high-glucose, with resulting decrease of S1P plasma levels and HDL biological function (Kobayashi et al., 2021). Furthermore, HDL glycation reduces S1P content of HDL and there is an inverse correlation between S1P concentration in HDL and Hemoglobin A1c values, with a negative outcome on cardiomyocyte survival (Brinck et al., 2016). This effect may be reversed by replenishing S1P in HDL. Finally, HDL-associated S1P appears to be mainly involved in the antiatherogenic effects exerted by HDL, including the inhibition of endothelial and smooth muscle cell apoptosis (Poti, Simoni, & Nofer, 2014). Of note, S1P controls also macrophage degeneration, regardless of their cholesterol-loading status, an effect observed both in human and murine macrophages that represent a key element at all the stages of atherosclerotic lesion development (Feuerborn et al., 2017; Martinet, Coornaert, Puylaert, & De Meyer, 2019). In conclusion, many of the

BOX 2 HDL/apoM-bound S1P and its biological significance—cont'd

antiatherogenic and biological functions ascribed to HDL may be actually mediated by their S1P cargo. The interaction between HDL-bound S1P and S1P receptors expressed by endothelial cells may be facilitated by Scavenger Receptor Class B Type 1 (SR-B1), one of the major HDL binding receptors, that has been demonstrated to directly affect HDL-associated S1P biological functions (Lee et al., 2017). Interestingly, as mentioned above, HDL may be loaded both *in vitro* and *in vivo* with S1P (Sattler et al., 2015). *In vitro*, HDL has been supplemented with S1P and the molecule appeared biologically active (Lee et al., 2010). Studies on anemic patients receiving blood transfusion also show an elevation in HDL-bound S1P, but whether this molecule is biologically active has not been assessed (Selim et al., 2011). The notion that ApoM-S1P exerts several protective functions on endothelial cells and that the content of S1P in HDL from patients with mild coronary disease is 5 times less than in healthy individuals (Sattler et al., 2015), may lead to the possibility to increase HDL-S1P content, and open the door to novel interesting therapeutic strategies.

3. Receptor-mediated S1P signaling

S1P plays a fundamental role both as intracellular messenger and extracellular mediator, through the paracrine/autocrine stimulation of five distinct receptors, $S1P_1$–$S1P_5$. By stimulating its receptors, S1P modulates cell proliferation and migration, angiogenesis, self-immunity and cytokines production. As second messenger operating directly inside the cell, S1P regulates calcium levels, plays a role in DNA synthesis, suppresses apoptosis (Lu, She, Zeng, Yi, & Zhang, 2021) and modulates inflammatory responses, regulating the phosphorylation of IkB and the activation of NF-kB (Alvarez et al., 2010). S1P is also directly associated to specific intracellular targets, like the stimulator of interferon gene (STING) (Anwar & Mehta, 2020) or histone deacetylases (HDACS), therefore influencing the transcription of target genes (Hait et al., 2009).

S1P receptors belong to the family of G protein-coupled receptors (GPCRs): they are coupled to different G protein α subunits, often providing opposite signaling. While $S1P_1$ only stimulates a Gi/o protein, $S1P_2$ and $S1P_3$ couple to Gi/o, Gq and G12/13. $S1P_4$ and $S1P_5$ instead are associated to Gi/o and G12/13 (Kihara, Maceyka, Spiegel, & Chun, 2014).

$S1P_1$-$S1P_3$ are broadly expressed in various tissues, in particular in the cardiovascular system, in the central nervous system (CNS) and in the immune system. $S1P_4$ is mostly expressed in the immune system and hematopoietic tissues, while $S1P_5$ predominates in the CNS (Sanchez & Hla, 2004). Upon S1P binding, at least $S1P_1$ receptor is quickly desensitized. After activation of the Gi/o protein, the C terminal tail of $S1P_1$ is phosphorylated and binds to β-arrestin, leading to receptor endocytosis and desensitization (Liu et al., 1999; Oo et al., 2007). The receptor is then recycled back to the surface in the next 1–2 h. When overstimulated by supra-physiological S1P levels or by a functional antagonist (like fingolimod), the receptor is ubiquinated and undergoes proteosomal degradation (Oo et al., 2011). This represents the mechanism used by drugs like fingolimod in multiple sclerosis (MS): fingolimod induces persistent phosphorylation of the C-terminal domain of the receptor, causing $S1P_1$ internalization and degradation, thus preventing leukocytes egress from lymph tissues and limiting the infiltration of autoreactive immune cells in the CNS (Oo et al., 2011).

Recently, great interest arose for the molecular determinants of biased agonism toward S1P receptors and S1P receptor ligands, endogenous and exogenous as well. In this respect, it seems that the length of the hydrophobic chain critically affects the interaction with a given transducer; for e.g., in $S1P_3$, short lipidic agonists do not interact with Leu122, resulting in greater G12/13- and Gi/o-mediated activation rather than Gq/11 (Maeda et al., 2021). A recently published design and screening of $S1P_1$ ligands suggests similar structure requirements for biased agonism at $S1P_1$ (Gilmore et al., 2021). The chemical structures of S1P and S1P receptor agonists already in clinical use are reported in Fig. 1.

4. S1P function at the endothelium

The endothelium is a monolayer of cells located at the interface between the vascular wall and the blood components and exerts mechanical and metabolic functions. For its location, the endothelium is exposed to several injuries, but it undergoes a process of continuous repair: alterations in its properties may lead to cardiovascular events (Lerman & Zeiher, 2005). Endothelial cells constitute a barrier controlling the transport and movement of fluids, ions and leukocytes from the blood stream to the tissues. The passage is regulated by the presence of intercellular junctions, adherens junctions (AJ), gap and tight junctions (TJ), as well as by specific transporters and pumps. The permeability of the endothelial barrier may be very different

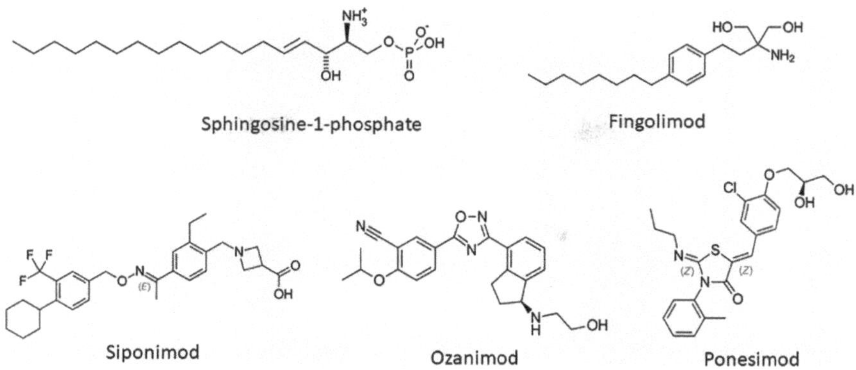

Fig. 1 Chemical structures of sphingosine-1-phosphate (S1P) and several S1P receptor agonists. Fingolimod binds S1P1, S1P3, S1P4 and S1P5; siponimod and ozanimod bind S1P1 and S1P5 whereas ponesimod is selective for S1P1.

according to the district, very loose in the hepatic district and very tight at the blood-brain barrier (BBB) and it may be affected in several pathological conditions. Inflammation, in particular, increases barrier leakage due to the destabilization of intercellular junctions. Increased endothelial leakage leads to serious consequences as hemorrhage, edema or inflammation (Xiong & Hla, 2014). Endothelial cells also express adhesion molecules that facilitate leukocytes rolling, adhesion, crawling and migration through the endothelial layer. Increased barrier leakage and leukocytes infiltration also represent a critical step in atherosclerosis (Kurano & Yatomi, 2018).

At endothelial level, the expression and the activity of S1P receptors, in particular $S1P_{1-3}$, play an important role in physiological vascular development and functions (Fig. 2). Deletion of *S1pr1–3* in triple knock out mice induces severe vessel abnormalities and subsequent embryonic lethality (Kono et al., 2004). In vascular physiology, $S1P_2$ and $S1P_3$ functions are redundant (Kono et al., 2004; Liu et al., 2000; Takuwa, Du, et al., 2010), while *S1pr1* deletion causes embryonic lethality due to defective vascular maturation and smooth muscle coverage, resulting in severe hemorrhage (Allende, Yamashita, & Proia, 2003; Liu et al., 2000). $S1P_1$ also reduces vascular endothelial growth factor receptor 2 ($VEGFR_2$) induced aberrant angiogenesis (Gaengel et al., 2012), though other data suggest that $S1P_1$ may also be involved in abnormal pathological angiogenesis, still by interacting with the same $VEGFR_2$ (Balaji Ragunathrao et al., 2019). Accordingly, mice lacking $S1P_1$, due to conditional excision of *S1pr1* in endothelial cells, undergo reduced tumor vascularization (Balaji Ragunathrao et al., 2019).

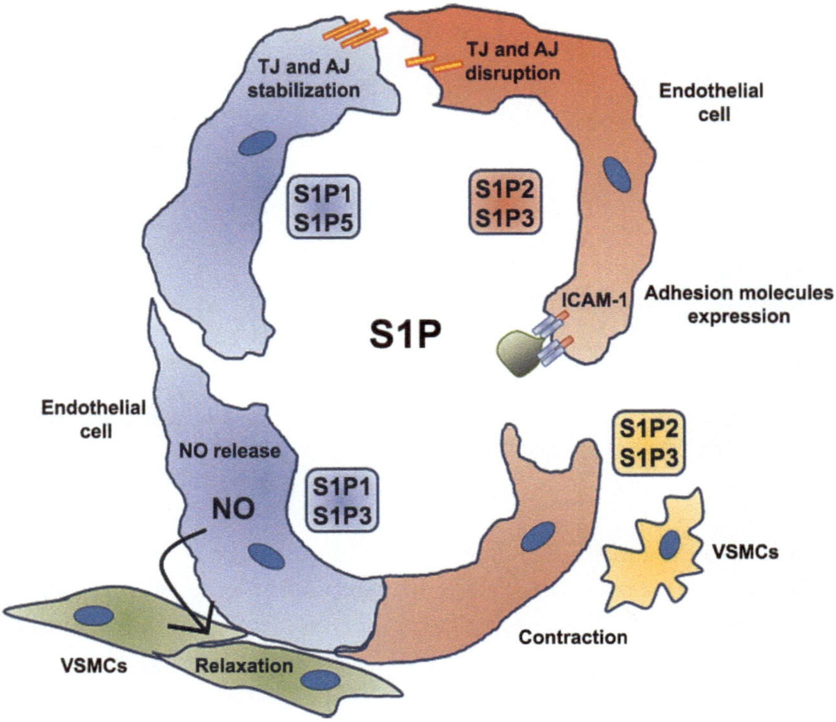

Fig. 2 Contrasting effects of S1P through different S1P receptors on endothelial cells and vascular smooth muscle cells (VSMCs). By interacting with S1P1 and S1P5, S1P stabilizes endothelial membranes, strengthening tight junctions (TJ) and adherens junctions (AJ), thus increasing cell-to-cell contacts. S1P binding to S1P1 and S1P3 promotes nitric oxide (NO) release that diffuses to vascular smooth muscle cells (VSMCs) causing relaxation. In contrast, activation of S1P2, as well as S1P3, on endothelial cells can cause TJ and AJ disruption and enhanced expression of adhesion molecules such as ICAM-1, with ensuing increase of endothelial leakiness and of leucocyte infiltration. Finally, S1P2 and S1P3 on VSMC can mediate a contractile response.

Barrier properties of endothelium, its permeability and leukocytes trans-endothelial migration, are as well affected by S1P signaling. By activating the small GTPase Rac1, Cdc42, PI3K and ERK pathways, $S1P_1$ induces endothelial cytoskeleton stabilization and cortical ring formation, resulting in cellular spreading, TJ and AJ stabilization and reduced endothelial permeability (Garcia et al., 2001; Mehta, Konstantoulaki, Ahmmed, & Malik, 2005). $S1P_1$ signaling at endothelial level is though highly heterogenous in multiple organs (Engelbrecht et al., 2020), and the effect of S1P on vascular permeability also strongly depends on its concentration. When at physiological concentrations, S1P acts as a barrier-protective agent, while higher S1P levels (e.g., >5 μM) cause endothelial barrier disruption, also due to the engagement of receptors other than $S1P_1$ (Prager, Spampinato, & Ransohoff, 2015; Xiong & Hla, 2014). This may also account for the different contribution of S1P to vascular permeability in various vascular beds. $S1P_1$ also cooperates in reducing endothelial response to inflammation: studies conducted on single cell RNA sequencing demonstrated that inflammation-related expression of mRNA was suppressed by $S1P_1$-dependent NF-kB pathway inhibition (Engelbrecht et al., 2020), thus contributing to reduced leukocytes trans-endothelial migration. In non-obese diabetic mice, the stimulation of $S1P_1$ reduces endothelial adhesion of monocytes (Whetzel et al., 2006) and endothelial expression of $S1P_1$ inversely correlates to the expression of the adhesion molecules ICAM-1 and VCAM-1, as observed in transgenic mice in which the receptor was either overexpressed or down regulated (Galvani et al., 2015).

$S1P_2$, as well as $S1P_3$, are not necessary to induce endothelial maturation (Kim et al., 2015), but are rather strongly involved in the regulation of vascular tone (Cardillo, Kilcoyne, Cannon, & Panza, 2000). Moreover, $S1P_1$ and $S1P_2$ induce contrasting endothelial response to inflammatory challenge. While $S1P_1$ prevents barrier damage, $S1P_2$ enhances its leakage: activating the Rho pathway, $S1P_2$ increases cytoskeleton contraction which weakens cell-to-cell junctions; VE-cadherin localization at the cell boundaries is reduced and barrier permeability to both blood solutes and leukocytes is increase (Sanchez et al., 2007). Thus, the inhibition of $S1P_2$ decreases endothelium permeability and expression of inflammatory markers, as observed in an in vivo model of endotoxemia (Zhang et al., 2013).

$S1P_3$ signaling synergizes with $S1P_1$ in the stimulation of endothelial cell progenitors' migration and proliferation, thus contributing to angiogenesis and vasculogenesis (Takuwa, Du, et al., 2010). $S1P_3$ seems also to enhance endothelial response to inflammatory stimuli. Pharmacological prevention of $S1P_3$ activity protected mice from lipopolysaccharide-induced endothelial damage (Niessen et al., 2008) and $S1P_3$ expression has been recently associated to increased mortality in septic patients in intensive care, following severe lung damage (Sun et al., 2012).

5. S1P at vascular level

As mentioned above, the tone of vascular smooth muscle cells in the media of arteries determines their caliber; vasoconstrictors, such as catecholamines are released from sympathetic nerve endings and also are transported through the bloodstream, in which they are secreted by adrenal medulla.

Other vasoconstrictors are released or locally converted from precursors, in a paracrine manner; these include endothelin-1 and angiotensin II. Vasodilators, such as brain natriuretic peptide (BNP), can also be secreted and transported through the bloodstream, but, more often, are produced locally, and exert their effects within a short range (paracrine). The most important paracrine vasodilator is, by far, nitric oxide (NO), which is produced in endothelium and diffuses in the surrounding smooth muscle cells, where it stimulates guanylyl cyclase, which produces cyclic GMP thereby activating G kinases and a vasodilating signaling pathway. Other vasodilators, such as bradykinin, are locally produced, but mostly act indirectly, by inducing NO release. The paracrine regulation of vascular tone has been recognized as a major mechanism adapting the caliber of vessels to the bloodstream velocity, shear stress being a physiological stimulator of bradykinin and/or NO production. Since S1P receptors discovery, S1P has been postulated to modulate vascular tone. Early studies showed that these effects where both direct, mediated by $S1P_2$ and $S1P_3$ on VSMC (Salomone et al., 2008, 2003), and indirect, mediated by $S1P_1$ and $S1P_3$ on endothelium, which induce NO release (Dantas, Igarashi, & Michel, 2003; Nofer et al., 2004). See Fig. 2 for a clear picture of S1P receptor distribution and function at the endothelium and in VSMCs. We were also able to show that vasoconstriction to S1P occurs maximally in isolated cerebral and coronary arteries (Salomone et al., 2003). Because such a vessel selectivity was observed in mouse, rat and rabbit, it seemed somehow species-independent. It appears that vasoconstriction is mediated via $S1P_2$ and $S1P_3$ expressed in VSMC (Fujii, Machida, Iizuka, & Hirafuji, 2014; Hoefer et al., 2010) and counteracted by $S1P_1$ and $S1P_3$ in endothelium (Dantas et al., 2003; Morales-Ruiz et al., 2001). Contractile status of VSMC is strictly related to the degree of myosin phosphorylation, which, in turn, depends on myosin light chain kinase (a Ca^{2+}/calmodulin dependent enzyme) and myosin light chain phosphatase (a Rho kinase regulated enzyme). S1P may act through both signaling mechanisms, because both $S1P_2$ and $S1P_3$ are coupled to Gq as well as to G12/13 (Takuwa, Okamoto, Yoshioka, & Takuwa, 2008; Waeber, Blondeau, & Salomone, 2004). Endothelium-dependent vasorelaxation might be mediated through phosphatidylinositol 3-kinases (PI3K)-Akt, which phosphorylates endothelial nitric oxide synthase (eNOS), increasing the NO production, with ensuing vasorelaxation (Atochin et al., 2007). PI3K/Akt are activated following $S1P_1$ stimulation (Morales-Ruiz et al., 2001; Takuwa et al., 2008). Systemic treatment with SEW2871, a $S1P_1$ agonist, induces a reduction of blood pressure in mice infused with angiotensin II (Cantalupo et al., 2015); on the other hand, specific deletion of endothelial $S1P_1$ decreases basal and stimulated NO production and increases blood pressure (Cantalupo et al., 2017). Of note, the endothelial NO release induced by $S1P_1$ stimulation might play a significant role in the vasodilatation and the subsequent reduction in vascular resistance and blood pressure determined by HDL; in fact, it has been showed that these HDL effects are potentiated by S1P (Persegol et al., 2018). Consistently, administration of the apolipoprotein M (ApoM), the major carrier of S1P in plasma associated to the HDL fraction, decreases blood pressure in mice infused with angiotensin II; worthy of note, this effect is associated to an increase in plasma nitrite concentration and blunted by W146, a $S1P_1$ antagonist (Swendeman et al., 2017). A recent study has further investigated the precise role of paracrine S1P produced by endothelium, which is exported extracellularly by Spinster-2, as well as the role of ApoM, in experimental hypertension. This study identifies an important role for Spinster-2 and ApoM-HDL in blood pressure homeostasis via S1P-NO signaling and shows that in KO mice for either gene, cardiac hypertrophy worsens compared to controls (Del Gaudio et al., 2021). For a deeper description of HDL/ApoM–S1P interaction and its biological significance, see Box 2.

The contraction of VSMC mediated by $S1P_3$ may have also a role in increasing vascular resistance and, thereby contribute to elevated blood pressure; in fact, continuous administration of S1P results in hypertension in conscious rats, as well as in wild-type mice, but not in *S1pr3* null mice (Forrest et al., 2004). However, mice lacking *S1pr2* have reduced vasoconstriction responses and are characterized by a decrease of peripheral vascular resistance (Lorenz, Arend, Robitz, Paul, & MacLennan, 2007), indicating a potential role also for $S1P_2$. The idea that hypertensive effects of S1P and/or S1P receptor agonists would be mainly due to increase in peripheral vascular resistance is consistent with the notion that cardiac effects of S1P (reduced heart rate and contractility), mediated by $S1P_1$, are not supposed to rise blood pressure values. Based on these premises, potential systemic effects need to be carefully considered when assessing cardiovascular effects and safety of S1P receptor agonists, including those acting as functional antagonists, used so far as immunomodulators in MS. Recently reported clinical observations confirm this dual, hemodynamically opposite effect of S1P receptor agonists such as siponimod (Habek et al., 2021) and ozanimod (Lassiter et al., 2020), i.e., slowing of heart rate and increase in blood pressure. The fact that these effects occur typically at the beginning of the treatment suggests that they are mediated through S1P receptor stimulation (mainly $S1P_1$ in heart and $S1P_3$ in vessels) rather than being due to down regulation (functional antagonism), which may require longer time intervals. Both the above mentioned compounds are selective agonists of $S1P_1$ and $S1P_5$, suggesting that these receptor subtypes are involved in the observed effects. However, beside direct systemic effects potentially exerted by S1P receptor ligands, other indirect, paracrine effects, mediated by local S1P production following activation of SPHKs are involved in regulation of vascular tone by a number of endogenous substances and drugs. For example, activation of the S1P/$SPHK_1$/$S1P_1$ by the endogenous cannabinoid anandamide induces a rapid decrease of blood pressure in anesthetized mice, related to endothelium-dependent NO-induced vasodilatation (Greig et al., 2019), but the opposite paracrine effect, i.e., $SPHK_1$-dependent increase in vascular tone, induced by various vasoconstrictors in cerebral arteries has also been reported (Salomone, Soydan, Ip, Hopson, & Waeber, 2010). In line with these observations, experimental hypertension is associated with altered $SPHK_1$ expression in VSMC and endothelium (Meissner et al., 2017; Siedlinski et al., 2017).

Other than receptor-mediated effects of S1P, some studies have reported (i) calcium mobilization regulated by S1P in a receptor-independent manner, which may affect the contractile status of VSMC (Hopson, Truelove, Chun, Wang, & Waeber, 2011), as well as (ii) endothelial effects of intracellular S1P, potentially affecting NO production (Roviezzo et al., 2006). We do not further discuss these observations, because they are not likely to be reproduced with S1P receptor ligands already approved and/or in preclinical and clinical development. In conclusion, the effect of S1P and S1P receptor agonists and/or functional antagonists on vascular tone are complex, being the result of the integration of effects, largely opposite, on endothelium and VSMC. A recent study further underlines this complexity, showing that as low as 0.1 μM S1P applied intraluminally in isolated pressurized arteries induces NO-dependent vasodilatation, while larger concentrations, above 1 μM, induce vasoconstriction (Kerage, Gombos, Wang, Brown, & Hemmings, 2021). Thus, precisely targeting S1P receptor-mediated effects on endothelium or on VSMC might have clinically relevant consequences.

6. S1P effects at the kidney

S1P can also directly affect kidney functioning, sodium handling and, thereby, systemic blood pressure. The relationship between sodium and pressure is only transiently linked to blood volume (which increases and decreases following diminished or augmented sodium excretion), but is rather linked to the tone of VSMC in the media of resistance arteries, which is sensitive to increased plasma sodium concentration (Wirth et al., 2008). Early studies showed that infusion of S1P in anaesthetized rats increased sodium excretion and urine volume, an effect attributed to tubular actions, because it was not accompanied by changes in creatinine clearance (Bischoff, Meyer Zu Heringdorf, Jakobs, & Michel, 2001). A very recent study, taking advantage of a selective deletion of $S1P_1$ in the collecting duct (cre-recombinase under control of acquaporin-2 promoter) showed that in this model there is reduced sodium excretion, increased sodium retention, and accelerated deoxycorticosterone acetate-(DOCA) salt-induced salt-sensitive hypertension. Importantly, the authors measured protein levels of renal medullary $S1P_1$, which were increased by 100% after high-salt intake, an effect not seen in animals treated with DOCA, which accelerates the development of hypertension (Hu et al., 2021). $S1P_1$ therefore critically controls sodium excretion and counteracts salt-induced hypertension. Interestingly, a previous study reported a twofold increased expression of $S1P_1$ mRNA in kidney of salt-loaded stroke-prone, spontaneously hypertensive rats (SHRSP) compared to their control Wistar Kyoto; this increase, however, was not paralleled by an increase in $S1P_1$ protein, which was rather reduced (Graham et al., 2007). We may speculate that a, not yet defined, post-transcriptional mechanism decreases $S1P_1$ protein levels in kidney, which reduces sodium excretion in hypertensive animal models.

Worthy of note, inducible deletion of *S1pr1* in endothelium has shown that this receptor subtype exerts a protective role against acute kidney ischemia-reperfusion injury, an effect somehow related to endothelial barrier integrity and endothelial HSP27 expression (Ham et al., 2014).

7. The hazy link between the immune system and hypertension and the role of S1P

During the last decade, several studies have underscored the potential role of inflammation and immune system activation in the pathophysiology of hypertension (for review see Norlander, Madhur, & Harrison, 2018). In this context, activated immune cells may enter the vasculature and the kidney, and release mediators, such as reactive oxygen species, metalloproteinases, cytokines and antibodies, promoting damage of these target organs. The ensuing dysfunction may affect vascular tone and remodeling, which increases peripheral vascular resistance, while, in the kidney, expression and/or activation of sodium transporters may change sodium balance, followed, in the mid/long term by interstitial fibrosis and glomerular injury. Therapeutic strategies targeting immune activation may theoretically prove beneficial in preventing the establishment of hypertension and even more to avoid its long-term sequelae and related cardiovascular complications. However, evidence of beneficial mechanisms linked to anti-inflammatory and immunomodulatory effects of S1P and S1P receptor ligands in experimental hypertension remains anecdotical (see for example, Meissner et al., 2017), while no clinical data support so far, an anti-hypertensive action of S1P receptor ligands used as immunomodulators in MS. All drugs currently approved to treat essential hypertension are not curative, i.e., they do not reverse the processes which lead to high blood pressure (including hypothetical inflammatory/immune-related mechanisms), and, for this reason, they need to be administered along lifetime. Furthermore, antihypertensive drug treatment initiated once the stable high blood pressure is already present; this means that the pathological mechanisms, including hypothetical inflammatory/immune-related mechanisms, preceded by month or even years the diagnosis and the ensuing drug prescription. Despite these considerations, antihypertensive drugs, are effective not only in reducing blood pressure, but, more importantly, in reducing the occurrence of major cardiovascular events; this action is linked only in part to the control of blood pressure, being also related, at least for some classes such as the RAAS inhibitors, to beneficial effects on cardiovascular remodeling. We may therefore hypothesize that modulators of inflammatory-immune mechanisms associated to hypertension might be also exploited to reduce the chronic cardiovascular risk. In this context, the recent evidence that HDL-bound S1P exerts significant effects, lead to the view that beside a paracrine mechanism regulating vascular tone, there must be a systemic effect of circulating S1P on blood pressure, somehow related also to inflammation, potentially targetable by antihypertensive drugs and usable as biomarker. Consistent with this prediction, a recent study (Jujic et al., 2021) explored the associations between plasma S1P and blood pressure in a family-based study cohort and in a longitudinally conducted murine hypertension cohort. In both humans and mice, linear multivariate regression analyses revealed a significant association of S1P plasma concentration with high blood pressure; further proteomic analysis showed some markers of inflammation, metabolism, and cardiovascular disease potentially associated to high S1P, suggesting S1P as a potential biomarker (Jujic et al., 2021).

8. A role for S1P also in pulmonary arterial hypertension

Beside systemic hypertension, a specific cardiovascular condition in which S1P and S1P receptor ligands may play a significant role is pulmonary arterial hypertension. This is a severe and progressive disease, characterized by increased pressure in pulmonary artery, related to increased vascular resistance. Chronic elevated pressure in the pulmonary arterial bed increases the afterload of the right ventricle which further induces cardiac remodeling and eventually right heart failure and death. While functional vasoconstriction may play a role in the initial, reversible phase of the disease, a major role is commonly attributed to the ensuing arterial remodeling, characterized by vascular wall thickening, largely due to VSMC proliferation and migration, with their transition from a contractile phenotype to a proliferative phenotype. An intermediate phenotype, including both contractile and proliferative, might also be present at some point. Transforming growth factor (TGF)-$\beta 1$ seems to be a central player in this process, being capable of inducing elevated expression of contractile genes, resulting in increased VSMC tone and hypertrophy (Qiu, Feng, & Li, 2003). Later on, a model where S1P participates as a paracrine actor has been postulated; according to this model, TGF-$\beta 1$ increases the level of S1P, by upregulating $SPHK_1$ (Cencetti, Bernacchioni, Nincheri, Donati, & Bruni, 2010); S1P, in turn, activates Rho signaling and stimulates expression of αSMA and CNN1 in VSMC. Consistent with this model, inhibition of $SPHK_1$ activity by either genetic or pharmacological approaches exerts protective effects in animal models of pulmonary hypertension (Chen et al., 2014; Gairhe et al., 2016). A recent study confirms that in human pulmonary arterial smooth muscle cells, TGF-β1 activates Rho/MRTF-A/SRF by potentiating an autocrine/paracrine S1P signaling mechanism through $SPHK_1$, and points to the importance of $S1P_3$, whose mRNA is induced by TGF-β1, as the receptor subtype targeted by autocrine/paracrine S1P (Ji, Lisabeth, & Neubig, 2021). Other recent studies carried out in pulmonary arterial VSMC point to some other pathways, such as YAP/Notch3 (Shi et al., 2021; Wang et al., 2021), which may still be linked to TGF-β1 signaling (Wang et al., 2019). Worthy of note, EMAP II, a pro-inflammatory signaling cytokine, has also been found to regulate expression and translocation of $SPHK_1$, highlighting the potential involvement of autocrine/paracrine S1P in inflammatory mechanisms that underlie vascular remodeling processes leading to pulmonary hypertension (Ranasinghe, Lee, & Schwarz, 2020).

9. Indirect effects of S1P on cardiovascular events that may impact the control of blood pressure

9.1 The dual role of S1P receptors in atherosclerosis lesion development

A healthy endothelium layer regulates vascular tone and promotes fibrinolytic properties, preventing abnormal coagulation. Increased endothelial permeability, inflammation, cytokines production, leukocytes adhesion and platelets aggregations are responsible for atherosclerotic lesions; atherosclerosis is a chronic, systemic disease affecting different vascular beds and is characterized by hardening and narrowing of the vascular lumen due to the formation of cholesterol-rich plaques in the vessel wall. A clear association between S1P levels and atherosclerosis needs to be fully elucidated, although it appears that S1P signaling may differently affect the onset of several atherogenic events. Modulation of S1P receptors interferes with macrophage migration, a mechanism that plays an important role in plaque regression (Feig et al., 2011), and is often impaired in atherosclerotic plaques. As mentioned, the role of S1P appears ambiguous, according to the different S1P receptor engaged. $S1P_2$ negatively modulates the involvement of macrophages favoring macrophages/foam cells retentions into atherosclerotic plaques and cytokines release (Michaud, Im, & Hla, 2010; Skoura et al., 2011). In contrast, $S1P_1$ mediates increased macrophage migration (Al-Jarallah, Chen, Gonzalez, & Trigatti, 2014), further preventing their apoptotic death induced by oxidized low-density lipoproteins (LDL) (Gonzalez, Qian, Tahir, Yu, & Trigatti, 2017). S1P receptors also interfere with vascular response to the atherogenic insult, but their role is again rather controversial. The $S1P_1$ agonist KRP-203 was described to prevent endothelial inflammatory response (Poti et al., 2013), but, at the same time, $S1P_1$ stimulation can induce the proliferation of VSMC (Holvoet & Sinnaeve, 2008) and the growth of neointima (Kitano et al., 2019), indispensable steps in the development of atherosclerosis. Accordingly, in areas highly prone to atheroprogression, like the femoral artery segment, the foam cell accumulation co-localizes with increased expression of $S1P_1$ (Liu et al., 2018). $S1P_2$ and $S1P_3$ mediate primarily pro-atherogenic events as their activation induces vascular inflammatory responses, as mentioned above (Kimura et al., 2006; Zhang et al., 2013). However, again, controversial data are available as they may also exert antiatherogenic effects by limiting the neointima formation and the appearance of atherosclerotic lesions

(Kimura et al., 2006; Takashima et al., 2008). We may conclude that the effects of S1P are mostly anti-atherosclerotic when mediated by $S1P_1$ and pro-atherosclerotic when mediated via $S1P_2$. Targeting selectively S1P receptors may thus interfere with the progression of atherosclerotic lesions. As reported in mice models, fingolimod treatment was able to reduce the size of atherosclerotic lesions in animals fed with a high cholesterol diet (Keul et al., 2007; Nofer et al., 2007), effect also observed when mice were treated with KRP-203, a $S1P_1$ selective agonist (Poti et al., 2013). At the moment, the use of these compounds in atherosclerosis is not fully ascertained due to the lack of data from human studies, but a better understanding of the dual role played by S1P receptors in the proatherogenic/antiatherogenic mechanisms, may provide a new potential tool in atherosclerosis treatment.

9.2 S1P and cardiac physiology

Several anecdotical reports have been produced since the 2000s on S1P receptor expression in heart and/or S1P specific effects on heart physiology (reviewed in Means & Brown, 2009). A systematic analysis of S1P receptor expression in heart has been carried out more recently (Ahmed et al., 2017), both at the mRNA level, by quantitative PCR, and at the protein level by western blot and immunohistochemistry. $S1P_1$, $S1P_2$ and $S1P_3$ show a similar expression level in atria and ventricles, more robust for $S1P_1$ and $S1P_3$ than for $S1P_2$, both in human and rat. Particularly useful are the immunohistochemical data, which demonstrate localization of these receptors in cardiomyocytes. In contrast, $S1P_4$ and $S1P_5$ are not detectable (Ahmed et al., 2017). Stimulation of $S1P_1$ (and possibly, with a minor role, of $S1P_3$) by S1P, may antagonize β-adrenergic responses by inhibiting adenylyl cyclase through $G\alpha_i$ and thereby decrease L-type calcium channel conductance, with ensuing negative inotropic effect. Additionally, $G_{\beta\gamma}$ subunit release may increase outward K^+ current, shorten the duration of the action potential and refractoriness time, and further decrease Ca^{2+} influx. Consistent with this assumption, S1P has been found to evoke negative inotropic effects associated with decreased cAMP and myocyte shortening (Landeen et al., 2008; Means, Miyamoto, Chun, & Brown, 2008). The importance of $S1P_1$ signaling in mediating negative inotropy has been further confirmed with the use of cardiomyocyte-specific *S1pr1* knockout mice (Keul et al., 2016).

S1P also acts as a negative chronotropic agent affecting heart rate. Early studies reported that $S1P_3$ may induce transient bradycardia in vivo, based on the observation that non-specific S1P receptor agonists induce bradycardia in wild type mice, but not in $S1P_3$ knockout mice, while a supposedly specific $S1P_1$ agonist did not appear to change heart rate (Sanna et al., 2004). However, subsequent studies demonstrated $S1P_1$ activation as responsible for the bradycardic effect in rats and humans (Camm, Hla, Bakshi, & Brinkmann, 2014; Fryer et al., 2012; Gergely et al., 2012). Importantly, fingolimod, when used as treatment in MS, is known to produce bradycardia as a side effect (Calabresi et al., 2014). The bradycardic effect of S1P or fingolimod is dependent on the $S1P_1/G_i$-protein–coupled inwardly rectifying potassium (GIRK) channels activation, which triggers membrane hyperpolarization and transiently reduces excitability (Koyrakh, Roman, Brinkmann, & Wickman, 2005). An expression pattern similar to that assessed in cardiomyocytes, has been observed for S1P receptors in sinoatrial node, both at the protein and mRNA level (Egom et al., 2010), which accounts for $G_{\beta\gamma}$ subunit release, induced by G_i-coupled $S1P_1$, and thereby increased outward K^+ current through GIRK. Furthermore, since fingolimod stimulates $S1P_1$ in ventricles by reducing cAMP, it also reduces left ventricular systolic function (Racca et al., 2016). A second-generation S1P-related immunomodulator siponimod, a selective agonist of $S1P_1$ and $S1P_5$ receptors, has been approved by FDA for the treatment of secondary progressive MS. At variance with fingolimod, siponimod does not activate $S1P_3$ signaling, but it still reduces heart rate (Gergely et al., 2012), as we may expect following $S1P_1$ stimulation (Calabresi et al., 2014; Legangneux, Gardin, & Johns, 2013). Other newer S1P receptor-targeting drugs, such as ozanimod, do not significantly affect heart rate (Comi et al., 2019); this in vivo effect, observed in chronic human therapy, might be related to the fact that, despite ozanimod shows a $S1P_1$ agonist potency similar to fingolimod when measured as cAMP reduction, it results about 10-fold more potent in inducing $S1P_1$ internalization and down regulation (Scott et al., 2016); the activation of $S1P_1/G_i$ signaling responsible for bradycardia would then be counterbalanced by the efficient down-regulation of $S1P_1$ induced by ozanimod through the activation of β-arrestin pathway.

9.3 S1P, cardiac hypertrophy and fibrosis

Physiological cardiac hypertrophy occurs as normal response to healthy exercise or pregnancy and is associated to increased pumping ability. Pathological hypertrophy occurs as a consequence of prolonged and abnormal hemodynamic stress or myocardial infarction, is accompanied by systolic and diastolic dysfunction, and eventually progresses to heart failure. This condition is characterized by an increase in thickness of the myocardium without a corresponding increase in ventricular size. Furthermore, there is not a corresponding proliferation of the vasculature, which results in reduced blood and oxygen supply. Thickening is caused by cardiomyocyte growth, with increase in sarcomers in series, enhanced proliferation and phenotype shift of cardiac fibroblast to myofibroblasts, leading to excessive production of extracellular matrix and interstitial fibrosis. In the more advanced stage, the cardiac wall becomes thinner, due to death of cardiac myocytes, which produces ventricular dilation.

Early studies did not report consistent data on S1P and heart hypertrophy, providing either no effect (Sekiguchi, Yokoyama, Kurabayashi, Okajima, & Nagai, 1999) or enhanced hypertrophy, mainly through $S1P_1/G_i$ (Robert et al., 2001). Later on, in vitro studies carried out in in murine cardiac fibroblasts showed that the TGF-β-induced production of extra-cellular matrix proteins depends on SPHK1 and occurs through $S1P_2/G_{12/13}$ and Rho kinase signaling, suggesting that S1P may mediate the pro-fibrotic effect of TGF-β in a paracrine manner (Gellings Lowe, Swaney, Moreno, & Sabbadini, 2009). Consistent with this observation, more recent studies show that genetic deletion or pharmacological blockade of $SPHK_1$ reduces cardiac hypertrophy following a 2 week-treatment with ATII (Jozefczuk et al., 2020; Siedlinski et al., 2017), while $SPHK_1$ overexpression is accompanied by increased cardiac interstitial fibrosis, with no effect on cardiomyocyte hypertrophy (Takuwa, Ohkura, et al., 2010). The profibrotic effect of paracrine S1P might be mediated through $S1P_3$ and/or $S1P_1$ in cardiomyocytes and/or fibroblast (Ohkura et al., 2017; Takuwa, Ohkura, et al., 2010). However, in apparent conflict with these data, fingolimod reverses cardiac hypertrophy and fibrosis, an effect attributed to $S1P_1/G_i$ and NFAT signaling, based on the inhibition by pertussis toxin and not related to S1P down regulation, (Liu et al., 2013). These data highlighted the complexity of this response and of the relationship between cardiac hypertrophy and S1P receptors involvement, pointing out that SIP_1 may play a dual role, stimulated by fingolimod when acting either as an agonist or as a functional antagonist. In addition, the involvement of other receptor subtypes such as $S1P_2$ and, in particular $S1P_3$, cannot be ruled out. On the other hand, the latter study did not analyze S1P receptor protein and/or mRNA, despite a 2-week in vivo treatment of mice with fingolimod, which is supposed to induce $S1P_1$ down regulation.

$SPHK_1$ expression and S1P level have also been found increased in post-myocardial infarction hearts (Zhang et al., 2016). The clinical relevance of this paradigm is further reinforced by the observation that circulating S1P positively correlates with cardiac mass in patients with Fabry disease (Brakch et al., 2010).

Taken together, the above data point to S1P receptor inhibition and/or down regulation as a promising new approach in the treatment of heart hypertrophic/fibrotic disease which may ultimately progress to heart failure. Thus, the available $S1P_1$ agonists (which act as functional antagonists) may offer a novel therapeutic approach for counteracting heart remodeling and deserve to be tested in suitable models, as long as they are demonstrated capable of inducing effective S1P receptor down regulation. Nevertheless, the complexity of the system and its regulation in its whole has always to be taken in mind and certainly still requires a deeper analysis to warrant a more precise knowledge.

9.4 S1P and myocardial infarction

Myocardial infarction occurs when oxygen supply to myocardium is substantially reduced, following a sudden impairment of coronary blood flow, often due to rupture of an atherosclerotic plaque, aggregation of platelets, formation of a thrombus and/or release of vasoconstrictors. While data reported above point to a detrimental impact of cardiac S1P stimulation on fibrosis, remodeling and, ultimately heart failure, available evidence indicates a protective role of S1P on cardiomyocyte, particularly in experimental paradigms of ischemia-reperfusion, as discussed below, suggesting that S1P receptor stimulation may be useful, particularly when recanalization can be achieved through angioplasty or thrombolysis (e.g., t-PA infusion).

Early studies showed that exogenous S1P exhibited protective effects in ischemia/reperfusion in isolated hearts from rodents (Jin et al., 2002; Lecour et al., 2002), an effect consistent with the observation that $SPHK_1$ activity played a critical role in reducing infarct size following ischemic injury (Jin, Goetzl, & Karliner, 2004; Jin et al., 2007). Studies in mouse cardiac myocyte indicate that S1P and S1P receptor agonists afford protection from apoptosis through activation of Akt, inhibition of glycogen synthase kinase-3 beta (GSK-3β) and reduction of cytochrome *c* release from the mitochondria (Means et al., 2007; Zhang et al., 2007).

Data obtained in *S1pr2* and *S1pr3* deficient mice indicate that cardioprotection following ischemia/reperfusion depends on $S1P_2$/$S1P_3$

(Means et al., 2007; Theilmeier et al., 2006). These data, taken all together, and considering that the expression of both $S1P_2$ and $S1P_3$ in human ventricles reaches comparable levels (Ahmed et al., 2017), suggest that $S1P_2$ and $S1P_3$ biased agonists (i.e., not inducing down regulation) might offer potential for treating coronary artery disease. An important caveat, however, concerns the potent vasoconstriction mediated by $S1P_3$ stimulation, as we demonstrated in vitro several years ago in various arteries, including rat coronary arteries (Salomone et al., 2003), an observation recently confirmed in Langendorff-perfused murine hearts (Wafa et al., 2020). Thus, the risk of coronary artery spasm associated with $S1P_3$ stimulation must be taken into account when considering the development of S1P receptor agonists as cardioprotective agents. The possibility that increases of S1P mediate also the cardiovascular protective effect associated with physical activity is briefly discussed in Box 3.

BOX 3 An interesting role for S1P in the cardioprotective effects of physical exercise

The importance of physical exercise in preventing cardiovascular diseases and atherosclerotic lesion is well known (Blair & Morris, 2009). Interestingly, it has been shown that physical exercise may also increase S1P levels in muscles, where the sphingolipid regulates several biological aspects including excitation-contraction coupling (Danieli-Betto et al., 2005), as well as in plasma. S1P levels were measured after physical exercises in athletes, obese individuals and patients with type 2 diabetes, and it appears that acute training increases S1P plasma levels more efficiently in untrained subjects (Bergman et al., 2015) compared to athletes, who need much higher intensity exercise to obtain the same induction (Baranowski et al., 2015). Enhanced S1P levels were observed during the exercise and within the first 30 min of recovery after the training, both locally in the active muscles (Bergman et al., 2016) as well as in the plasma of the subject, likely as a consequence of the increased production and release from erythrocytes (Baranowski, Charmas, Dlugolecka, & Gorski, 2011). The increase of S1P levels may have direct muscular implications, such as the reduction of muscular fatigue and a better recovery (Germinario et al., 2016). In addition, it is not possible to exclude that the beneficial effects observed after physical exercise in reducing cardiovascular diseases (anti-hypertensive, anti-atherosclerogenic and anti-inflammatory activity) may also depend on the training-induced S1P levels (Germinario et al., 2016).

An alternative and safer approach to exogenous S1P receptor agonists might be to implement strategies for increasing endogenous S1P, particularly that bound to HDL. Circulating S1P is in fact mainly bound to apolipoprotein M (ApoM), included in the high-density lipoprotein (HDL) (Christoffersen et al., 2011). ApoM contains a hydrophobic binding pocket for S1P; ApoM-bound S1P is involved in lymphocyte trafficking and inhibits lymphopoiesis (through $S1P_1$ receptor); furthermore, it stimulates S1P receptors on endothelial cells and cardiomyocytes (Blaho et al., 2015). Specific biological functions may be imparted by specific chaperones to S1P (Ding et al., 2020). ApoM and S1P affect the progression of heart ischemia injury and heart failure (Morel et al., 2016; Theilmeier et al., 2006). ApoM/S1P exerts a number of anti-inflammation actions, such as inhibition of the effect of tumor necrosis factor-α (TNF-α) on gene expression, of monocyte adhesion to the endothelium and preservation of endothelial barrier integrity (Ruiz et al., 2017). ApoM also increases cardiomyocyte survival (Sattler et al., 2015; Theilmeier et al., 2006). Based on the reported anti-inflammatory and cardioprotective role of ApoM/S1P (see Box 2), a recent study tested the hypothesis that reduced circulating ApoM might be associated to a worse outcome in patients with heart failure (Chirinos et al., 2020). This study showed that reduced circulating apoM is independently associated with adverse outcomes across the spectrum of human heart failure. The relationship between ApoM levels and inflammation was validated with multiple inflammatory markers measured using large-scale plasma proteomics (Chirinos et al., 2020). Whether or not S1P exerts a direct effect on cardiac cells, associated with an antifibrotic effect, or instead, it acts through modulation of lymphocyte trafficking is still unclear. A study with conditional T-cell *S1pr1* knockout mice in a model of streptozotocin-induced diabetic cardiomyopathy suggests that, in T-cell, $S1P_1$ signaling activation exerts antifibrotic effects in normoglycemia but exacerbates cardiac fibrosis under hyperglycemia (Abdullah & Jin, 2018).

9.5 A role for S1P and its receptors in cerebral ischemia

Stroke represents the second most common cause of death worldwide (Campbell et al., 2019) and may depend on ischemic event (ischemic stroke) or, conversely, be the consequence of an important bleeding (hemorrhagic stroke). The ischemic stroke is caused by thrombotic or embolic occlusion of a vessel reaching a specific area in the brain and is responsible for parenchymal cell death, inflammation, endothelial dysfunction and disruption of vascular integrity (Stokum, Gerzanich, & Simard, 2016). The BBB, the vascular structure that encloses, protects and tightly regulates the microenvironment to allow optimal *CNS activity,* is also severely impaired in ischemic conditions. Dysfunction at the BBB can lead to vasogenic edema and facilitate the access of leukocytes into the brain parenchyma, further enhancing neuronal damage (Obermeier, Verma, & Ransohoff, 2016).

S1P receptor expression and function are often modified in cerebral ischemia, and their dysfunction may be involved in the mechanisms leading to ischemic damage. Although there is not a consensus on the up- or down-regulation of $S1P_1$ in cerebral infarction (Lu et al., 2021). In animal models, the unilateral common carotid artery occlusion caused the increased expression of $S1P_1$ that is instrumental to collateral growth induced by shear stress (Ichijo et al., 2015); after stroke, the receptor was generally over-expressed in the leptomeninges of the peri-infarct area, whereas it was downregulated in the ischemic core (Iwasawa et al., 2018). Conversely, in vitro studies pointed out the decreased expression of $S1P_1$ after oxygen/glucose deprivation and reperfusion (OGD/r) (Lin et al., 2018). Overall, the stimulation of $S1P_1$ seems to play a beneficial role in the recovery from an ischemic damage. Several $S1P_1$ modulators (RP101075, LASW1238, SEW2871, FTY720) have been proven to significantly reduce cerebral infarct size, neuronal damage and improve neurobehavior in animal models (Brait, Tarrason, Gavalda, Godessart, & Planas, 2016; Ichijo et al., 2015; Li et al., 2019). In addition, the modulation of $S1P_1$ with selective agonists, like SEW2871, promptly increases cerebral blood flow, promoting neoangiogenesis and enhancing collateral branching and revascularization (Ichijo et al., 2015; Iwasawa et al., 2018). All these effects are likely due to $S1P_1$–induced phosphorylation of eNOS, as reported in mice subjected to permanent middle cerebral artery occlusion (MCAO) (Iwasawa et al., 2018). Drugs modulating the properties of S1P receptors have been mainly developed in the context of autoimmune disorders and, in particular, in the treatment of MS. Fingolimod, for example, was introduced in clinical practice for its ability to prevent leukocytes egress from lymph nodes (Brinkmann, 2009). However, fingolimod effects have been largely demonstrated to go well beyond its interaction with leukocytes. Interacting with endothelial $S1P_1$ at the BBB, fingolimod and other S1P1 modulators also reinforce barrier properties. Endothelial cells at the BBB are characterized by firm intercellular junctions (AJ and TJ) that prevent barrier permeability to blood borne solutes toward the CNS. In ischemic conditions, the junctions between endothelial cells are loosened, leading to edema formation.

S1P is able to affect the tightness of endothelial junctions and cytoskeleton organization, and its release by all the components of the BBB (endothelium, astrocytes and pericytes) is increased under ischemic condition, as shown in *in vivo* and *in vitro* studies (Nakagawa & Aruga, 2020; Salas-Perdomo et al., 2019). Several studies on human umbilical vascular endothelial cells (HUVEC) and human brain microvascular cells demonstrated that the modulation of S1P/S1P_1 signaling with drugs like fingolimod and the more recent analogs, siponimod and ozanimod, reduces endothelial barrier permeability after exposure to an inflammatory stimulus or following hypoxia plus glucose deprivation (Lee et al., 2006; Spampinato, Merlo, Sano, Kanda, & Sortino, 2021). These in vitro pieces of evidence were supported by in vivo studies where fingolimod and the S1P_1 selective agonist AUY954 attenuated BBB dysfunction in transient middle cerebral artery occlusion (MCAO) model, reducing brain edema formation following stroke (Wei et al., 2011). Leukocytes are important players in the pathogenesis of tissue injury in stroke and, by interacting with endothelial cells and platelets, they can foster vascular dysfunction and infarct growth (Kim, Park, Chang, Kim, & Lee, 2016). Of note, S1P_1-mediated modulation of BBB properties also involves the prevention of leukocytes migration toward the CNS. Accordingly, the use of fingolimod in animals exposed to transient MCAO, prevented leukocytes egress from lymph nodes, but also reduced their infiltration through the BBB (Kraft et al., 2013). The ability of this drug to prevent leukocytes infiltration is the consequence of the reduced number of activated leukocytes and neutrophils as well as of their reduced interaction with the endothelial adhesion molecule, ICAM-1. After MCAO and fingolimod treatment, positive ICAM-1 immunostaining in blood vessels was reduced (Wei et al., 2011). These data are supported also by results obtained in *in vitro* models, where S1P_1 modulators, like fingolimod and siponimod, prevented TNFα-induced endothelial expression of the adhesion molecule ICAM-1 and further reduced the expression of the chemoattractant factor CCL2 (Spampinato, Merlo, Costantino, et al., 2021; Spampinato et al., 2015; Wei et al., 2011). S1P receptors, in the CNS, are also expressed in astrocytes, microglia and neurons. Astrocytes and microglia behave as main actors in the inflammatory response that occurs in the brain after cerebral ischemia, a process that can further precipitate neuronal damage (Kraft et al., 2013). Stimulation of S1P_1 decreases neuroinflammation by reducing astrocytic activation (Brunkhorst et al., 2013; Spampinato, Merlo, Costantino, et al., 2021) and ponesimod, a S1P_1 specific modulator, prevents astrocyte polarization toward the detrimental A1 phenotype, as observed in subarachnoid hemorrhage (Zhang et al., 2021). In addition, fingolimod reduces microglia activation (Czech et al., 2009) and polarization, as shown by repression of inflammatory genes by transcriptomic analysis (Das et al., 2017) and activation of the STAT3 signaling pathway associated with M2 phenotype (Qin et al., 2017).

However, there is not total agreement on the role played by S1P in ischemia and contrasting data on the effects exerted by S1P in ischemic conditions have been reported. Thus, it has been described that the inhibition of S1P release reduced BBB impairment in a MCAO ischemia model and after oxygen glucose deprivation/re-oxygenation (OGD/r), in an *in vitro* BBB model (Nakagawa & Aruga, 2020). In the latter, all cellular elements, endothelial cells, astrocytes and pericytes, were able to produce and release S1P, and this was increased after OGD/r insult. By reducing S1P release, the endothelial barrier appeared more stable and TJ proteins were better organized (Nakagawa & Aruga, 2020). Although these data are in apparent contrast with those previously described, it is known that, at physiological concentrations, S1P more likely stimulates the activity of $S1P_1$. However, when S1P levels are increased, as occurs after the ischemic insult, other S1P receptors may be stimulated, in particular $S1P_2$, whose activity on endothelial barrier appears detrimental (reviewed in Prager et al., 2015). Accordingly, genetic deletion or pharmacological blockade of $S1P_2$ signaling reduces, in rodent models, cerebral edema and stroke injury by preventing BBB damage (Cao et al., 2019; Kim et al., 2015). Conversely, the role of $S1P_3$ in ischemic conditions is not fully elucidated: evidence points out that blockade of this receptor subtype may reduce the cerebral infarction area, dampening microglia activation and M1 polarization (Gaire, Song, & Choi, 2018). In line with this observation, in a mouse model of intra cerebral hemorrhage, $S1P_3$ mediates an increased expression of ICAM-1 by activating the CCL2-p38-MAPK signaling pathway (Xu et al., 2021). To contrast these data, $S1P_3$ stimulation appears important to prevent astrocytic injury after OGD/r and thus the receptor may reduce neuroinflammatory response (Dong et al., 2018).

To summarize, fingolimod, that mostly interacts with $S1P_1$ with no effect on $S1P_2$, appears a useful therapeutic tool in ischemic conditions, reducing the number of leukocytes and preserving BBB function. This results in limitation of brain edema and subsequent neuroinflammation and leads to a significant functional improvement (reviewed in Wang, Kawabori, & Houkin, 2020). Accordingly, two pilot studies evaluated the outcome of patients treated with fingolimod after ischemic stroke or intracerebral hemorrhage. Results showed fingolimod efficacy in reducing neurological impairment and increasing recovery both in ischemic (Fu, Zhang, et al., 2014; Zhu et al., 2015) and hemorrhagic stroke (Fu, Hao, et al., 2014).

10. Conclusion

The abundant preclinical data on S1P and cardiovascular system already available at the begin of the millennium, have been further enriched by clinical data after the approval of fingolimod and subsequent clinical development of new generation S1P receptor ligands. All these drugs have found, so far, application as immunomodulator only, based on their ability of down-regulating S1P receptors in lymphocytes. Their extensive use, however, has produced a number of clinical observations on the impact of these drugs on cardiovascular system which need to be integrated with preclinical data. On the other hand, ongoing basic research has fostered new hypotheses and ideas, particularly useful to understand the molecular pharmacology of S1P and S1P receptors, regarding biased agonism, S1P storage, release, vehiculation and chaperoning by lipoproteins, paracrine actions, intracellular non-receptorial actions. Precising the role of different receptor subtypes in different contexts, leads to the conclusion that $S1P_1$ agonism, associated or not to $S1P_2/_3$ antagonism might be exploitable as antihypertensive treatment, because $S1P_1$ stimulation promotes decrease of cardiac output (reduction of heart rate and contractility) and of peripheral vascular resistances (NO-induced vasorelaxation), while $S1P_{2/3}$ antagonism would inhibit potential contractile effects of endogenous S1P on VSMC, thereby reducing vascular resistance. In order to be clinically exploitable, however, a drug exerting such effects should produce stable and predictable effects, e.g., not associated to receptor down regulation. Novel compounds endowed with $S1P_1$ agonist activity and/or $S1P_{2/3}$ antagonism might result also useful in reducing the occurrence and the severity of major cardiovascular events such as myocardial infarction and stroke (both ischemic and hemorrhagic). A summary of S1P sources and targets, all related to control of hypertension and cardiovascular function is depicted in Fig. 3. A potential caveat to be considered when looking at S1P agonists as potential antihypertensive agents, however, is the effect of chronic $S1P_1$ stimulation on cardiac hypertrophy and fibrosis, which may accelerate heart failure, while a $S1P_1$ down regulation might be of benefit in halting/reversing cardiac remodeling.

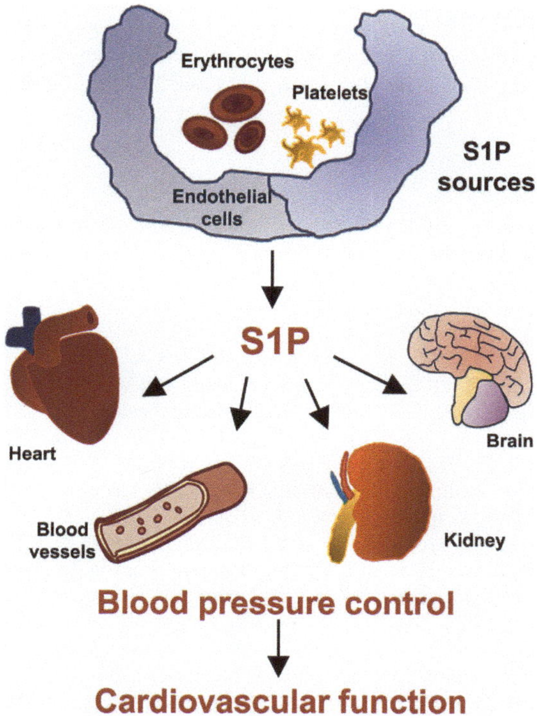

Fig. 3 Sphingosine-1-phosphate (S1P) acts at different levels to exert a control of cardioprotective function. S1P is produced by several cell types, endothelial cells representing one of the main sources. It is also produced by blood cells, mainly erythrocytes and platelets. It acts on several organs, including blood vessels, heart, kidney, brain, all involved, directly or indirectly, with the control of cardiovascular function (see text for details).

A deeper understanding of the systemic effects of SPHK inhibitors might be relevant in view of their development to inhibit paracrine, pro-fibrotic effects of S1P.

Finally, it is important to consider that cardiovascular therapy usually pursue several goals and, to do so, simultaneously uses drugs as diverse as vasodilators, diuretics, sympatholytics, renin-angiotensin-aldosterone inhibitors, etc. Thus, any pharmacological intervention on S1P and S1P receptors needs to be placed in this perspective, where the effects of different, unrelated drugs, may produce synergism or antagonism, and affect the overall safety of the therapy, with substantial impacts on the clinical outcome.

Acknowledgments

The contribution of PRIN 2017 from Italian Ministry of University (E64117000190001) and PIACERI grant from University of Catania, Italy (20722142135) is acknowledged.

Conflict of interest

The authors declare no conflicts of interest. All data reported in the present review are from the public scientific literature.

References

Abdullah, C. S., & Jin, Z. Q. (2018). Targeted deletion of T-cell S1P receptor 1 ameliorates cardiac fibrosis in streptozotocin-induced diabetic mice. *The FASEB Journal*, *32*, 5426–5435.

Ahmed, N., Linardi, D., Decimo, I., Mehboob, R., Gebrie, M. A., Innamorati, G., et al. (2017). Characterization and expression of sphingosine 1-phosphate receptors in human and rat heart. *Frontiers in Pharmacology*, *8*, 312.

Al-Jarallah, A., Chen, X., Gonzalez, L., & Trigatti, B. L. (2014). High density lipoprotein stimulated migration of macrophages depends on the scavenger receptor class B, type I, PDZK1 and Akt1 and is blocked by sphingosine 1 phosphate receptor antagonists. *PLoS One*, *9*, e106487.

Allende, M. L., Yamashita, T., & Proia, R. L. (2003). G-protein-coupled receptor S1P1 acts within endothelial cells to regulate vascular maturation. *Blood*, *102*, 3665–3667.

Alvarez, S. E., Harikumar, K. B., Hait, N. C., Allegood, J., Strub, G. M., Kim, E. Y., et al. (2010). Sphingosine-1-phosphate is a missing cofactor for the E3 ubiquitin ligase TRAF2. *Nature*, *465*, 1084–1088.

Anwar, M., & Mehta, D. (2020). Post-translational modifications of S1PR1 and endothelial barrier regulation. *Biochimica et Biophysica Acta - Molecular and Cell Biology of Lipids*, *1865*, 158760.

Argraves, K. M., Gazzolo, P. J., Groh, E. M., Wilkerson, B. A., Matsuura, B. S., Twal, W. O., et al. (2008). High density lipoprotein-associated sphingosine 1-phosphate promotes endothelial barrier function. *The Journal of Biological Chemistry*, *283*, 25074–25081.

Atochin, D. N., Wang, A., Liu, V. W., Critchlow, J. D., Dantas, A. P., Looft-Wilson, R., et al. (2007). The phosphorylation state of eNOS modulates vascular reactivity and outcome of cerebral ischemia in vivo. *The Journal of Clinical Investigation*, *117*, 1961–1967.

Balaji Ragunathrao, V. A., Anwar, M., Akhter, M. Z., Chavez, A., Mao, Y., Natarajan, V., et al. (2019). Sphingosine-1-phosphate receptor 1 activity promotes tumor growth by amplifying VEGF-VEGFR2 angiogenic signaling. *Cell Reports*, *29*. 3472-87.e4.

Baranowski, M., Blachnio-Zabielska, A. U., Charmas, M., Helge, J. W., Dela, F., Ksiazek, M., et al. (2015). Exercise increases sphingoid base-1-phosphate levels in human blood and skeletal muscle in a time- and intensity-dependent manner. *European Journal of Applied Physiology*, *115*, 993–1003.

Baranowski, M., Charmas, M., Dlugolecka, B., & Gorski, J. (2011). Exercise increases plasma levels of sphingoid base-1 phosphates in humans. *Acta Physiologica (Oxford, England)*, *203*, 373–380.

Bergman, B. C., Brozinick, J. T., Strauss, A., Bacon, S., Kerege, A., Bui, H. H., et al. (2015). Serum sphingolipids: Relationships to insulin sensitivity and changes with exercise in humans. *American Journal of Physiology. Endocrinology and Metabolism*, *309*, E398–E408.

Bergman, B. C., Brozinick, J. T., Strauss, A., Bacon, S., Kerege, A., Bui, H. H., et al. (2016). Muscle sphingolipids during rest and exercise: A C18:0 signature for insulin resistance in humans. *Diabetologia*, *59*, 785–798.

Bischoff, A., Meyer Zu Heringdorf, D., Jakobs, K. H., & Michel, M. C. (2001). Lysosphingolipid receptor-mediated diuresis and natriuresis in anaesthetized rats. *British Journal of Pharmacology*, *132*, 1925–1933.

Blaho, V. A., Galvani, S., Engelbrecht, E., Liu, C., Swendeman, S. L., Kono, M., et al. (2015). HDL-bound sphingosine-1-phosphate restrains lymphopoiesis and neuroinflammation. *Nature*, *523*, 342–346.

Blair, S. N., & Morris, J. N. (2009). Healthy hearts- -and the universal benefits of being physically active: Physical activity and health. *Annals of Epidemiology*, *19*, 253–256.

Brait, V. H., Tarrason, G., Gavalda, A., Godessart, N., & Planas, A. M. (2016). Selective sphingosine 1-phosphate receptor 1 agonist is protective against ischemia/reperfusion in mice. *Stroke*, *47*, 3053–3056.

Brakch, N., Dormond, O., Bekri, S., Golshayan, D., Correvon, M., Mazzolai, L., et al. (2010). Evidence for a role of sphingosine-1 phosphate in cardiovascular remodelling in Fabry disease. *European Heart Journal*, *31*, 67–76.

Brinck, J. W., Thomas, A., Lauer, E., Jornayvaz, F. R., Brulhart-Meynet, M. C., Prost, J. C., et al. (2016). Diabetes mellitus is associated with reduced high-density lipoprotein sphingosine-1-phosphate content and impaired high-density lipoprotein cardiac cell protection. *Arteriosclerosis, Thrombosis, and Vascular Biology*, *36*, 817–824.

Brinkmann, V. (2009). FTY720 (fingolimod) in multiple sclerosis: Therapeutic effects in the immune and the central nervous system. *British Journal of Pharmacology*, *158*, 1173–1182.

Brunkhorst, R., Kanaan, N., Koch, A., Ferreiros, N., Mirceska, A., Zeiner, P., et al. (2013). FTY720 treatment in the convalescence period improves functional recovery and reduces reactive astrogliosis in photothrombotic stroke. *PLoS One*, *8*, e70124.

Calabresi, P. A., Radue, E. W., Goodin, D., Jeffery, D., Rammohan, K. W., Reder, A. T., et al. (2014). Safety and efficacy of fingolimod in patients with relapsing-remitting multiple sclerosis (FREEDOMS II): A double-blind, randomised, placebo-controlled, phase 3 trial. *Lancet Neurology*, *13*, 545–556.

Camm, J., Hla, T., Bakshi, R., & Brinkmann, V. (2014). Cardiac and vascular effects of fingolimod: Mechanistic basis and clinical implications. *American Heart Journal*, *168*, 632–644.

Campbell, B. C. V., De Silva, D. A., Macleod, M. R., Coutts, S. B., Schwamm, L. H., Davis, S. M., et al. (2019). Ischaemic stroke. *Nature Reviews. Disease Primers*, *5*, 70.

Cantalupo, A., Gargiulo, A., Dautaj, E., Liu, C., Zhang, Y., Hla, T., et al. (2017). S1PR1 (Sphingosine-1-phosphate receptor 1) signaling regulates blood flow and pressure. *Hypertension*, *70*, 426–434.

Cantalupo, A., Zhang, Y., Kothiya, M., Galvani, S., Obinata, H., Bucci, M., et al. (2015). Nogo-B regulates endothelial sphingolipid homeostasis to control vascular function and blood pressure. *Nature Medicine*, *21*, 1028–1037.

Cao, C., Dai, L., Mu, J., Wang, X., Hong, Y., Zhu, C., et al. (2019). S1PR2 antagonist alleviates oxidative stress-enhanced brain endothelial permeability by attenuating p38 and Erk1/2-dependent cPLA2 phosphorylation. *Cellular Signalling*, *53*, 151–161.

Cardillo, C., Kilcoyne, C. M., Cannon, R. O., 3rd, & Panza, J. A. (2000). Interactions between nitric oxide and endothelin in the regulation of vascular tone of human resistance vessels in vivo. *Hypertension*, *35*, 1237–1241.

Cencetti, F., Bernacchioni, C., Nincheri, P., Donati, C., & Bruni, P. (2010). Transforming growth factor-beta1 induces transdifferentiation of myoblasts into myofibroblasts via up-regulation of sphingosine kinase-1/S1P3 axis. *Molecular Biology of the Cell*, *21*, 1111–1124.

Chandrakanthan, M., Nguyen, T. Q., Hasan, Z., Muralidharan, S., Vu, T. M., Li, A. W. L., et al. (2021). Deletion of Mfsd2b impairs thrombotic functions of platelets. *Nature Communications*, *12*, 2286.

Chen, J., Tang, H., Sysol, J. R., Moreno-Vinasco, L., Shioura, K. M., Chen, T., et al. (2014). The sphingosine kinase 1/sphingosine-1-phosphate pathway in pulmonary arterial hypertension. *American Journal of Respiratory and Critical Care Medicine*, *190*, 1032–1043.

Chirinos, J. A., Zhao, L., Jia, Y., Frej, C., Adamo, L., Mann, D., et al. (2020). Reduced apolipoprotein M and adverse outcomes across the spectrum of human heart failure. *Circulation*, *141*, 1463–1476.

Christensen, P. M., Liu, C. H., Swendeman, S. L., Obinata, H., Qvortrup, K., Nielsen, L. B., et al. (2016). Impaired endothelial barrier function in apolipoprotein M-deficient mice is dependent on sphingosine-1-phosphate receptor 1. *The FASEB Journal*, *30*, 2351–2359.

Christoffersen, C., Federspiel, C. K., Borup, A., Christensen, P. M., Madsen, A. N., Heine, M., et al. (2018). The apolipoprotein M/S1P axis controls triglyceride metabolism and brown fat activity. *Cell Reports*, *22*, 175–188.

Christoffersen, C., Obinata, H., Kumaraswamy, S. B., Galvani, S., Ahnstrom, J., Sevvana, M., et al. (2011). Endothelium-protective sphingosine-1-phosphate provided by HDL-associated apolipoprotein M. *Proceedings of the National Academy of Sciences of the United States of America*, *108*, 9613–9618.

Comi, G., Kappos, L., Selmaj, K. W., Bar-Or, A., Arnold, D. L., Steinman, L., et al. (2019). Safety and efficacy of ozanimod versus interferon beta-1a in relapsing multiple sclerosis (SUNBEAM): A multicentre, randomised, minimum 12-month, phase 3 trial. *Lancet Neurology*, *18*, 1009–1020.

Czech, B., Pfeilschifter, W., Mazaheri-Omrani, N., Strobel, M. A., Kahles, T., Neumann-Haefelin, T., et al. (2009). The immunomodulatory sphingosine 1-phosphate analog FTY720 reduces lesion size and improves neurological outcome in a mouse model of cerebral ischemia. *Biochemical and Biophysical Research Communications*, *389*, 251–256.

Danieli-Betto, D., Germinario, E., Esposito, A., Megighian, A., Midrio, M., Ravara, B., et al. (2005). Sphingosine 1-phosphate protects mouse extensor digitorum longus skeletal muscle during fatigue. *American Journal of Physiology. Cell Physiology*, *288*, C1367–C1373.

Dantas, A. P., Igarashi, J., & Michel, T. (2003). Sphingosine 1-phosphate and control of vascular tone. *American Journal of Physiology. Heart and Circulatory Physiology*, *284*, H2045–H2052.

Das, A., Arifuzzaman, S., Kim, S. H., Lee, Y. S., Jung, K. H., & Chai, Y. G. (2017). FTY720 (fingolimod) regulates key target genes essential for inflammation in microglial cells as defined by high-resolution mRNA sequencing. *Neuropharmacology*, *119*, 1–14.

Del Gaudio, I., Rubinelli, L., Sasset, L., Wadsack, C., Hla, T., & Di Lorenzo, A. (2021). Endothelial Spns2 and ApoM regulation of vascular tone and hypertension via sphingosine-1-phosphate. *Journal of the American Heart Association*, *10*, e021261.

Del Gaudio, I., Sreckovic, I., Zardoya-Laguardia, P., Bernhart, E., Christoffersen, C., Frank, S., et al. (2020). Circulating cord blood HDL-S1P complex preserves the integrity of the feto-placental vasculature. *Biochimica et Biophysica Acta - Molecular and Cell Biology of Lipids*, *1865*, 158632.

Dennhardt, S., Finke, K. R., Huwiler, A., & Coldewey, S. M. (2019). Sphingosine-1-phosphate promotes barrier-stabilizing effects in human microvascular endothelial cells via AMPK-dependent mechanisms. *Biochimica et Biophysica Acta - Molecular Basis of Disease*, *1865*, 774–781.

Diarte-Anazco, E. M. G., Mendez-Lara, K. A., Perez, A., Alonso, N., Blanco-Vaca, F., & Julve, J. (2019). Novel insights into the role of HDL-associated sphingosine-1-phosphate in cardiometabolic diseases. *International Journal of Molecular Sciences*, *20*, 6263.

Ding, B. S., Yang, D., Swendeman, S. L., Christoffersen, C., Nielsen, L. B., Friedman, S. L., et al. (2020). Aging suppresses sphingosine-1-phosphate chaperone ApoM in circulation resulting in maladaptive organ repair. *Developmental Cell*, *53*. 677-90.e4.

Dong, Y. F., Guo, R. B., Ji, J., Cao, L. L., Zhang, L., Chen, Z. Z., et al. (2018). S1PR3 is essential for phosphorylated fingolimod to protect astrocytes against oxygen-glucose deprivation-induced neuroinflammation via inhibiting TLR2/4-NFkappaB signalling. *Journal of Cellular and Molecular Medicine, 22*, 3159–3166.

Egom, E. E., Ke, Y., Musa, H., Mohamed, T. M., Wang, T., Cartwright, E., et al. (2010). FTY720 prevents ischemia/reperfusion injury-associated arrhythmias in an ex vivo rat heart model via activation of Pak1/Akt signaling. *Journal of Molecular and Cellular Cardiology, 48*, 406–414.

Engelbrecht, E., Levesque, M. V., He, L., Vanlandewijck, M., Nitzsche, A., Niazi, H., et al. (2020). Sphingosine 1-phosphate-regulated transcriptomes in heterogenous arterial and lymphatic endothelium of the aorta. *eLife, 9*, e52690.

Fan, Y., Chen, J., Liu, D., Li, W., Wang, H., Huang, Y., et al. (2020). HDL-S1P protects endothelial function and reduces lung injury during sepsis in vivo and in vitro. *The International Journal of Biochemistry & Cell Biology, 126*, 105819.

Feig, J. E., Rong, J. X., Shamir, R., Sanson, M., Vengrenyuk, Y., Liu, J., et al. (2011). HDL promotes rapid atherosclerosis regression in mice and alters inflammatory properties of plaque monocyte-derived cells. *Proceedings of the National Academy of Sciences of the United States of America, 108*, 7166–7171.

Feuerborn, R., Becker, S., Poti, F., Nagel, P., Brodde, M., Schmidt, H., et al. (2017). High density lipoprotein (HDL)-associated sphingosine 1-phosphate (S1P) inhibits macrophage apoptosis by stimulating STAT3 activity and survivin expression. *Atherosclerosis, 257*, 29–37.

Forrest, M., Sun, S. Y., Hajdu, R., Bergstrom, J., Card, D., Doherty, G., et al. (2004). Immune cell regulation and cardiovascular effects of sphingosine 1-phosphate receptor agonists in rodents are mediated via distinct receptor subtypes. *The Journal of Pharmacology and Experimental Therapeutics, 309*, 758–768.

Fryer, R. M., Muthukumarana, A., Harrison, P. C., Nodop Mazurek, S., Chen, R. R., Harrington, K. E., et al. (2012). The clinically-tested S1P receptor agonists, FTY720 and BAF312, demonstrate subtype-specific bradycardia (S1P(1)) and hypertension (S1P(3)) in rat. *PLoS One, 7*, e52985.

Fu, Y., Hao, J., Zhang, N., Ren, L., Sun, N., Li, Y. J., et al. (2014). Fingolimod for the treatment of intracerebral hemorrhage: A 2-arm proof-of-concept study. *JAMA Neurology, 71*, 1092–1101.

Fu, Y., Zhang, N., Ren, L., Yan, Y., Sun, N., Li, Y. J., et al. (2014). Impact of an immune modulator fingolimod on acute ischemic stroke. *Proceedings of the National Academy of Sciences of the United States of America, 111*, 18315–18320.

Fujii, K., Machida, T., Iizuka, K., & Hirafuji, M. (2014). Sphingosine 1-phosphate increases an intracellular Ca(2+) concentration via S1P3 receptor in cultured vascular smooth muscle cells. *The Journal of Pharmacy and Pharmacology, 66*, 802–810.

Gaengel, K., Niaudet, C., Hagikura, K., Lavina, B., Muhl, L., Hofmann, J. J., et al. (2012). The sphingosine-1-phosphate receptor S1PR1 restricts sprouting angiogenesis by regulating the interplay between VE-cadherin and VEGFR2. *Developmental Cell, 23*, 587–599.

Gaire, B. P., Song, M. R., & Choi, J. W. (2018). Sphingosine 1-phosphate receptor subtype 3 (S1P3) contributes to brain injury after transient focal cerebral ischemia via modulating microglial activation and their M1 polarization. *Journal of Neuroinflammation, 15*, 284.

Gairhe, S., Joshi, S. R., Bastola, M. M., McLendon, J. M., Oka, M., Fagan, K. A., et al. (2016). Sphingosine-1-phosphate is involved in the occlusive arteriopathy of pulmonary arterial hypertension. *Pulmonary Circulation, 6*, 369–380.

Galvani, S., Sanson, M., Blaho, V. A., Swendeman, S. L., Obinata, H., Conger, H., et al. (2015). HDL-bound sphingosine 1-phosphate acts as a biased agonist for the endothelial cell receptor S1P1 to limit vascular inflammation. *Science Signaling, 8*, ra79.

Garcia, J. G., Liu, F., Verin, A. D., Birukova, A., Dechert, M. A., Gerthoffer, W. T., et al. (2001). Sphingosine 1-phosphate promotes endothelial cell barrier integrity by Edg-dependent cytoskeletal rearrangement. *The Journal of Clinical Investigation, 108*, 689–701.
Gazit, S. L., Mariko, B., Therond, P., Decouture, B., Xiong, Y., Couty, L., et al. (2016). Platelet and erythrocyte sources of S1P are redundant for vascular development and homeostasis, but both rendered essential after plasma S1P depletion in anaphylactic shock. *Circulation Research, 119*, e110–e126.
Gellings Lowe, N., Swaney, J. S., Moreno, K. M., & Sabbadini, R. A. (2009). Sphingosine-1-phosphate and sphingosine kinase are critical for transforming growth factor-beta-stimulated collagen production by cardiac fibroblasts. *Cardiovascular Research, 82*, 303–312.
Gergely, P., Nuesslein-Hildesheim, B., Guerini, D., Brinkmann, V., Traebert, M., Bruns, C., et al. (2012). The selective sphingosine 1-phosphate receptor modulator BAF312 redirects lymphocyte distribution and has species-specific effects on heart rate. *British Journal of Pharmacology, 167*, 1035–1047.
Germinario, E., Bondi, M., Cencetti, F., Donati, C., Nocella, M., Colombini, B., et al. (2016). S1P3 receptor influences key physiological properties of fast-twitch extensor digitorum longus muscle. *Journal of Applied Physiology, 1985*(120), 1288–1300.
Gilmore, J. L., Xiao, H. Y., Dhar, T. G. M., Yang, M., Xiao, Z., Yang, X., et al. (2021). Bicyclic ligand-biased agonists of S1P1: Exploring side chain modifications to modulate the PK, PD, and safety profiles. *Journal of Medicinal Chemistry, 64*, 1454–1480.
Golfier, S., Kondo, S., Schulze, T., Takeuchi, T., Vassileva, G., Achtman, A. H., et al. (2010). Shaping of terminal megakaryocyte differentiation and proplatelet development by sphingosine-1-phosphate receptor S1P4. *The FASEB Journal, 24*, 4701–4710.
Gonzalez, L., Qian, A. S., Tahir, U., Yu, P., & Trigatti, B. L. (2017). Sphingosine-1-phosphate receptor 1, expressed in myeloid cells, slows diet-induced atherosclerosis and protects against macrophage apoptosis in Ldlr KO mice. *International Journal of Molecular Sciences, 18*, 2721.
Graham, D., McBride, M. W., Gaasenbeek, M., Gilday, K., Beattie, E., Miller, W. H., et al. (2007). Candidate genes that determine response to salt in the stroke-prone spontaneously hypertensive rat: Congenic analysis. *Hypertension, 50*, 1134–1141.
Greig, F. H., Nather, K., Ballantyne, M. D., Kazi, Z. H., Alganga, H., Ewart, M. A., et al. (2019). Requirement for sphingosine kinase 1 in mediating phase 1 of the hypotensive response to anandamide in the anaesthetised mouse. *European Journal of Pharmacology, 842*, 1–9.
Habek, M., Crnosija, L., Junakovic, A., Adamec, I., Barun, B., Gabelic, T., et al. (2021). Autonomic nervous system abnormalities predict cardiovascular changes after initiation of siponimod in secondary progressive multiple sclerosis. *Clinical Neurophysiology, 132*, 581–585.
Hait, N. C., Allegood, J., Maceyka, M., Strub, G. M., Harikumar, K. B., Singh, S. K., et al. (2009). Regulation of histone acetylation in the nucleus by sphingosine-1-phosphate. *Science, 325*, 1254–1257.
Ham, A., Kim, M., Kim, J. Y., Brown, K. M., Fruttiger, M., D'Agati, V. D., et al. (2014). Selective deletion of the endothelial sphingosine-1-phosphate 1 receptor exacerbates kidney ischemia-reperfusion injury. *Kidney International, 85*, 807–823.
Hammad, S. M., Al Gadban, M. M., Semler, A. J., & Klein, R. L. (2012). Sphingosine 1-phosphate distribution in human plasma: Associations with lipid profiles. *Journal of Lipids, 2012*, 180705.
Herzog, B. H., Fu, J., Wilson, S. J., Hess, P. R., Sen, A., McDaniel, J. M., et al. (2013). Podoplanin maintains high endothelial venule integrity by interacting with platelet CLEC-2. *Nature, 502*, 105–109.

Hla, T., Venkataraman, K., & Michaud, J. (2008). The vascular S1P gradient-cellular sources and biological significance. *Biochimica et Biophysica Acta, 1781*, 477–482.

Hoefer, J., Azam, M. A., Kroetsch, J. T., Leong-Poi, H., Momen, M. A., Voigtlaender-Bolz, J., et al. (2010). Sphingosine-1-phosphate-dependent activation of p38 MAPK maintains elevated peripheral resistance in heart failure through increased myogenic vasoconstriction. *Circulation Research, 107*, 923–933.

Holvoet, P., & Sinnaeve, P. (2008). Angio-associated migratory cell protein and smooth muscle cell migration in development of restenosis and atherosclerosis. *Journal of the American College of Cardiology, 52*, 312–314.

Hopson, K. P., Truelove, J., Chun, J., Wang, Y., & Waeber, C. (2011). S1P activates store-operated calcium entry via receptor- and non-receptor-mediated pathways in vascular smooth muscle cells. *American Journal of Physiology. Cell Physiology, 300*, C919–C926.

Hu, G., Zhu, Q., Wang, W., Xie, D., Chen, C., Li, P. L., et al. (2021). Collecting duct-specific knockout of sphingosine-1-phosphate receptor 1 aggravates DOCA-salt hypertension in mice. *Journal of Hypertension, 39*, 1559–1566.

Ichijo, M., Ishibashi, S., Li, F., Yui, D., Miki, K., Mizusawa, H., et al. (2015). Sphingosine-1-phosphate receptor-1 selective agonist enhances collateral growth and protects against subsequent stroke. *PLoS One, 10*, e0138029.

Ikeda, M., Kihara, A., & Igarashi, Y. (2004). Sphingosine-1-phosphate lyase SPL is an endoplasmic reticulum-resident, integral membrane protein with the pyridoxal 5'-phosphate binding domain exposed to the cytosol. *Biochemical and Biophysical Research Communications, 325*, 338–343.

Ito, K., Anada, Y., Tani, M., Ikeda, M., Sano, T., Kihara, A., et al. (2007). Lack of sphingosine 1-phosphate-degrading enzymes in erythrocytes. *Biochemical and Biophysical Research Communications, 357*, 212–217.

Iwasawa, E., Ishibashi, S., Suzuki, M., Li, F., Ichijo, M., Miki, K., et al. (2018). Sphingosine-1-phosphate receptor 1 activation enhances leptomeningeal collateral development and improves outcome after stroke in mice. *Journal of Stroke and Cerebrovascular Diseases, 27*, 1237–1251.

Ji, Y., Lisabeth, E. M., & Neubig, R. R. (2021). Transforming growth factor beta1 increases expression of contractile genes in human pulmonary arterial smooth muscle cells by potentiating sphingosine-1-phosphate signaling. *Molecular Pharmacology, 100*, 53–60.

Jiang, Z., & Zhang, H. (2019). Molecular mechanism of S1P binding and activation of the S1P1 receptor. *Journal of Chemical Information and Modeling, 59*, 4402–4412.

Jin, Z. Q., Goetzl, E. J., & Karliner, J. S. (2004). Sphingosine kinase activation mediates ischemic preconditioning in murine heart. *Circulation, 110*, 1980–1989.

Jin, Z. Q., Zhang, J., Huang, Y., Hoover, H. E., Vessey, D. A., & Karliner, J. S. (2007). A sphingosine kinase 1 mutation sensitizes the myocardium to ischemia/reperfusion injury. *Cardiovascular Research, 76*, 41–50.

Jin, Z. Q., Zhou, H. Z., Zhu, P., Honbo, N., Mochly-Rosen, D., Messing, R. O., et al. (2002). Cardioprotection mediated by sphingosine-1-phosphate and ganglioside GM-1 in wild-type and PKC epsilon knockout mouse hearts. *American Journal of Physiology. Heart and Circulatory Physiology, 282*, H1970–H1977.

Jozefczuk, E., Nosalski, R., Saju, B., Crespo, E., Szczepaniak, P., Guzik, T. J., et al. (2020). Cardiovascular effects of pharmacological targeting of sphingosine kinase 1. *Hypertension, 75*, 383–392.

Jujic, A., Matthes, F., Vanherle, L., Petzka, H., Orho-Melander, M., Nilsson, P. M., et al. (2021). Plasma S1P (sphingosine-1-phosphate) links to hypertension and biomarkers of inflammation and cardiovascular disease: Findings from a translational investigation. *Hypertension, 78*, 195–209.

Kappos, L., Radue, E. W., O'Connor, P., Polman, C., Hohlfeld, R., Calabresi, P., et al. (2010). A placebo-controlled trial of oral fingolimod in relapsing multiple sclerosis. *The New England Journal of Medicine*, *362*, 387–401.

Kerage, D., Gombos, R. B., Wang, S., Brown, M., & Hemmings, D. G. (2021). Sphingosine 1-phosphate-induced nitric oxide production simultaneously controls endothelial barrier function and vascular tone in resistance arteries. *Vascular Pharmacology*, *140*, 106874.

Keul, P., Tolle, M., Lucke, S., von Wnuck Lipinski, K., Heusch, G., Schuchardt, M., et al. (2007). The sphingosine-1-phosphate analogue FTY720 reduces atherosclerosis in apolipoprotein E-deficient mice. *Arteriosclerosis, Thrombosis, and Vascular Biology*, *27*, 607–613.

Keul, P., van Borren, M. M., Ghanem, A., Muller, F. U., Baartscheer, A., Verkerk, A. O., et al. (2016). Sphingosine-1-phosphate receptor 1 regulates cardiac function by modulating Ca2+ sensitivity and Na+/H+ exchange and mediates protection by ischemic preconditioning. *Journal of the American Heart Association*, *5*, e003393.

Kihara, Y., Maceyka, M., Spiegel, S., & Chun, J. (2014). Lysophospholipid receptor nomenclature review: IUPHAR Review 8. *British Journal of Pharmacology*, *171*, 3575–3594.

Kim, J. Y., Park, J., Chang, J. Y., Kim, S. H., & Lee, J. E. (2016). Inflammation after ischemic stroke: The role of leukocytes and glial cells. *Experimental Neurobiology*, *25*, 241–251.

Kim, G. S., Yang, L., Zhang, G., Zhao, H., Selim, M., McCullough, L. D., et al. (2015). Critical role of sphingosine-1-phosphate receptor-2 in the disruption of cerebrovascular integrity in experimental stroke. *Nature Communications*, *6*, 7893.

Kimura, T., Tomura, H., Mogi, C., Kuwabara, A., Ishiwara, M., Shibasawa, K., et al. (2006). Sphingosine 1-phosphate receptors mediate stimulatory and inhibitory signalings for expression of adhesion molecules in endothelial cells. *Cellular Signalling*, *18*, 841–850.

Kitano, T., Usui, S., Takashima, S. I., Inoue, O., Goten, C., Nomura, A., et al. (2019). Sphigosine-1-phosphate receptor 1 promotes neointimal hyperplasia in a mouse model of carotid artery injury. *Biochemical and Biophysical Research Communications*, *511*, 179–184.

Knapp, M., Zendzian-Piotrowska, M., Blachnio-Zabielska, A., Zabielski, P., Kurek, K., & Gorski, J. (2012). Myocardial infarction differentially alters sphingolipid levels in plasma, erythrocytes and platelets of the rat. *Basic Research in Cardiology*, *107*, 294.

Kobayashi, T., Kurano, M., Nanya, M., Shimizu, T., Ohkawa, R., Tozuka, M., et al. (2021). Glycation of HDL polymerizes apolipoprotein M and attenuates its capacity to bind to sphingosine 1-phosphate. *Journal of Atherosclerosis and Thrombosis*, *28*, 730–741.

Kono, M., Mi, Y., Liu, Y., Sasaki, T., Allende, M. L., Wu, Y. P., et al. (2004). The sphingosine-1-phosphate receptors S1P1, S1P2, and S1P3 function coordinately during embryonic angiogenesis. *The Journal of Biological Chemistry*, *279*, 29367–29373.

Koyrakh, L., Roman, M. I., Brinkmann, V., & Wickman, K. (2005). The heart rate decrease caused by acute FTY720 administration is mediated by the G protein-gated potassium channel I. *American Journal of Transplantation*, *5*, 529–536.

Kraft, P., Gob, E., Schuhmann, M. K., Gobel, K., Deppermann, C., Thielmann, I., et al. (2013). FTY720 ameliorates acute ischemic stroke in mice by reducing thrombo-inflammation but not by direct neuroprotection. *Stroke*, *44*, 3202–3210.

Kunkel, G. T., Maceyka, M., Milstien, S., & Spiegel, S. (2013). Targeting the sphingosine-1-phosphate axis in cancer, inflammation and beyond. *Nature Reviews. Drug Discovery*, *12*, 688–702.

Kurano, M., & Yatomi, Y. (2018). Sphingosine 1-phosphate and atherosclerosis. *Journal of Atherosclerosis and Thrombosis*, *25*, 16–26.

Landeen, L. K., Dederko, D. A., Kondo, C. S., Hu, B. S., Aroonsakool, N., Haga, J. H., et al. (2008). Mechanisms of the negative inotropic effects of sphingosine-1-phosphate on adult mouse ventricular myocytes. *American Journal of Physiology. Heart and Circulatory Physiology*, *294*, H736–H749.

Lassiter, G., Melancon, C., Rooney, T., Murat, A. M., Kaye, J. S., Kaye, A. M., et al. (2020). 'Ozanimod to treat relapsing forms of multiple sclerosis: A comprehensive review of disease, drug efficacy and side effects. *Neurology International, 12*, 89–108.

Lecour, S., Smith, R. M., Woodward, B., Opie, L. H., Rochette, L., & Sack, M. N. (2002). Identification of a novel role for sphingolipid signaling in TNF alpha and ischemic preconditioning mediated cardioprotection. *Journal of Molecular and Cellular Cardiology, 34*, 509–518.

Lee, M. H., Appleton, K. M., El-Shewy, H. M., Sorci-Thomas, M. G., Thomas, M. J., Lopes-Virella, M. F., et al. (2017). S1P in HDL promotes interaction between SR-BI and S1PR1 and activates S1PR1-mediated biological functions: Calcium flux and S1PR1 internalization. *Journal of Lipid Research, 58*, 325–338.

Lee, M. H., Hammad, S. M., Semler, A. J., Luttrell, L. M., Lopes-Virella, M. F., & Klein, R. L. (2010). HDL3, but not HDL2, stimulates plasminogen activator inhibitor-1 release from adipocytes: The role of sphingosine-1-phosphate. *Journal of Lipid Research, 51*, 2619–2628.

Lee, J. F., Zeng, Q., Ozaki, H., Wang, L., Hand, A. R., Hla, T., et al. (2006). Dual roles of tight junction-associated protein, zonula occludens-1, in sphingosine 1-phosphate-mediated endothelial chemotaxis and barrier integrity. *The Journal of Biological Chemistry, 281*, 29190–29200.

Legangneux, E., Gardin, A., & Johns, D. (2013). Dose titration of BAF312 attenuates the initial heart rate reducing effect in healthy subjects. *British Journal of Clinical Pharmacology, 75*, 831–841.

Lerman, A., & Zeiher, A. M. (2005). Endothelial function: Cardiac events. *Circulation, 111*, 363–368.

Li, H., Zhou, X., Li, Y., Ma, X., Gonzales, R. J., Qiu, S., et al. (2019). The selective sphingosine 1-phosphate receptor 1 modulator RP101075 improves microvascular circulation after cerebrovascular thrombosis. *The FASEB Journal, 33*, 10935–10941.

Lin, L., Wang, Q., Qian, K., Cao, Z., Xiao, J., Wang, X., et al. (2018). bFGF protects against oxygen glucose deprivation/reoxygenation-induced endothelial monolayer permeability via S1PR1-dependent mechanisms. *Molecular Neurobiology, 55*, 3131–3142.

Liu, H., Jin, H., Han, J., Yue, X., Yang, H., Zayed, M. A., et al. (2018). Upregulated sphingosine 1-phosphate receptor 1 expression in human and murine atherosclerotic plaques. *Molecular Imaging and Biology, 20*, 448–456.

Liu, C. H., Thangada, S., Lee, M. J., Van Brocklyn, J. R., Spiegel, S., & Hla, T. (1999). Ligand-induced trafficking of the sphingosine-1-phosphate receptor EDG-1. *Molecular Biology of the Cell, 10*, 1179–1190.

Liu, Y., Wada, R., Yamashita, T., Mi, Y., Deng, C. X., Hobson, J. P., et al. (2000). Edg-1, the G protein-coupled receptor for sphingosine-1-phosphate, is essential for vascular maturation. *The Journal of Clinical Investigation, 106*, 951–961.

Liu, W., Zi, M., Tsui, H., Chowdhury, S. K., Zeef, L., Meng, Q. J., et al. (2013). A novel immunomodulator, FTY-720 reverses existing cardiac hypertrophy and fibrosis from pressure overload by targeting NFAT (nuclear factor of activated T-cells) signaling and periostin. *Circulation. Heart Failure, 6*, 833–844.

Lorenz, J. N., Arend, L. J., Robitz, R., Paul, R. J., & MacLennan, A. J. (2007). Vascular dysfunction in S1P2 sphingosine 1-phosphate receptor knockout mice. *American Journal of Physiology. Regulatory, Integrative and Comparative Physiology, 292*, R440–R446.

Lu, S., She, M., Zeng, Q., Yi, G., & Zhang, J. (2021). Sphingosine 1-phosphate and its receptors in ischemia. *Clinica Chimica Acta, 521*, 25–33.

Maeda, S., Shiimura, Y., Asada, H., Hirata, K., Luo, F., Nango, E., et al. (2021). Endogenous agonist-bound S1PR3 structure reveals determinants of G protein-subtype bias. *Science Advances*, 7, eabf5325.

Martinet, W., Coornaert, I., Puylaert, P., & De Meyer, G. R. Y. (2019). Macrophage death as a pharmacological target in atherosclerosis. *Frontiers in Pharmacology*, *10*, 306.
Mathiesen Janiurek, M., Soylu-Kucharz, R., Christoffersen, C., Kucharz, K., & Lauritzen, M. (2019). Apolipoprotein M-bound sphingosine-1-phosphate regulates blood-brain barrier paracellular permeability and transcytosis. *eLife*, *8*, e49405.
Means, C. K., & Brown, J. H. (2009). Sphingosine-1-phosphate receptor signalling in the heart. *Cardiovascular Research*, *82*, 193–200.
Means, C. K., Miyamoto, S., Chun, J., & Brown, J. H. (2008). S1P1 receptor localization confers selectivity for Gi-mediated cAMP and contractile responses. *The Journal of Biological Chemistry*, *283*, 11954–11963.
Means, C. K., Xiao, C. Y., Li, Z., Zhang, T., Omens, J. H., Ishii, I., et al. (2007). Sphingosine 1-phosphate S1P2 and S1P3 receptor-mediated Akt activation protects against in vivo myocardial ischemia-reperfusion injury. *American Journal of Physiology. Heart and Circulatory Physiology*, *292*, H2944–H2951.
Mehta, D., Konstantoulaki, M., Ahmmed, G. U., & Malik, A. B. (2005). Sphingosine 1-phosphate-induced mobilization of intracellular Ca2+ mediates rac activation and adherens junction assembly in endothelial cells. *The Journal of Biological Chemistry*, *280*, 17320–17328.
Meissner, A., Miro, F., Jimenez-Altayo, F., Jurado, A., Vila, E., & Planas, A. M. (2017). Sphingosine-1-phosphate signalling-a key player in the pathogenesis of Angiotensin II-induced hypertension. *Cardiovascular Research*, *113*, 123–133.
Michaud, J., Im, D. S., & Hla, T. (2010). Inhibitory role of sphingosine 1-phosphate receptor 2 in macrophage recruitment during inflammation. *Journal of Immunology*, *184*, 1475–1483.
Mizugishi, K., Yamashita, T., Olivera, A., Miller, G. F., Spiegel, S., & Proia, R. L. (2005). Essential role for sphingosine kinases in neural and vascular development. *Molecular and Cellular Biology*, *25*, 11113–11121.
Morales-Ruiz, M., Lee, M. J., Zollner, S., Gratton, J. P., Scotland, R., Shiojima, I., et al. (2001). Sphingosine 1-phosphate activates Akt, nitric oxide production, and chemotaxis through a Gi protein/phosphoinositide 3-kinase pathway in endothelial cells. *The Journal of Biological Chemistry*, *276*, 19672–19677.
Morel, S., Christoffersen, C., Axelsen, L. N., Montecucco, F., Rochemont, V., Frias, M. A., et al. (2016). Sphingosine-1-phosphate reduces ischaemia-reperfusion injury by phosphorylating the gap junction protein Connexin43. *Cardiovascular Research*, *109*, 385–396.
Nakagawa, S., & Aruga, J. (2020). Sphingosine 1-phosphate signaling is involved in impaired blood-brain barrier function in ischemia-reperfusion injury. *Molecular Neurobiology*, *57*, 1594–1606.
Niazi, H., Zoghdani, N., Couty, L., Leuci, A., Nitzsche, A., Allende, M. L., et al. (2019). Murine platelet production is suppressed by S1P release in the hematopoietic niche, not facilitated by blood S1P sensing. *Blood Advances*, *3*, 1702–1713.
Niessen, F., Schaffner, F., Furlan-Freguia, C., Pawlinski, R., Bhattacharjee, G., Chun, J., et al. (2008). Dendritic cell PAR1-S1P3 signalling couples coagulation and inflammation. *Nature*, *452*, 654–658.
Nofer, J. R., Bot, M., Brodde, M., Taylor, P. J., Salm, P., Brinkmann, V., et al. (2007). FTY720, a synthetic sphingosine 1 phosphate analogue, inhibits development of atherosclerosis in low-density lipoprotein receptor-deficient mice. *Circulation*, *115*, 501–508.
Nofer, J. R., van der Giet, M., Tolle, M., Wolinska, I., von Wnuck Lipinski, K., Baba, H. A., et al. (2004). HDL induces NO-dependent vasorelaxation via the lysophospholipid receptor S1P3. *The Journal of Clinical Investigation*, *113*, 569–581.
Norlander, A. E., Madhur, M. S., & Harrison, D. G. (2018). The immunology of hypertension. *The Journal of Experimental Medicine*, *215*, 21–33.

Obermeier, B., Verma, A., & Ransohoff, R. M. (2016). The blood-brain barrier. *Handbook of Clinical Neurology*, *133*, 39–59.

Obinata, H., & Hla, T. (2019). Sphingosine 1-phosphate and inflammation. *International Immunology*, *31*, 617–625.

Ohkura, S. I., Usui, S., Takashima, S. I., Takuwa, N., Yoshioka, K., Okamoto, Y., et al. (2017). Augmented sphingosine 1 phosphate receptor-1 signaling in cardiac fibroblasts induces cardiac hypertrophy and fibrosis through angiotensin II and interleukin-6. *PLoS One*, *12*, e0182329.

Ono, Y., Kurano, M., Ohkawa, R., Yokota, H., Igarashi, K., Aoki, J., et al. (2013). Sphingosine 1-phosphate release from platelets during clot formation: Close correlation between platelet count and serum sphingosine 1-phosphate concentration. *Lipids in Health and Disease*, *12*, 20.

Oo, M. L., Chang, S. H., Thangada, S., Wu, M. T., Rezaul, K., Blaho, V., et al. (2011). Engagement of S1P(1)-degradative mechanisms leads to vascular leak in mice. *The Journal of Clinical Investigation*, *121*, 2290–2300.

Oo, M. L., Thangada, S., Wu, M. T., Liu, C. H., Macdonald, T. L., Lynch, K. R., et al. (2007). Immunosuppressive and anti-angiogenic sphingosine 1-phosphate receptor-1 agonists induce ubiquitinylation and proteasomal degradation of the receptor. *The Journal of Biological Chemistry*, *282*, 9082–9089.

Panetti, T. S., Nowlen, J., & Mosher, D. F. (2000). Sphingosine-1-phosphate and lysophosphatidic acid stimulate endothelial cell migration. *Arteriosclerosis, Thrombosis, and Vascular Biology*, *20*, 1013–1019.

Pappu, R., Schwab, S. R., Cornelissen, I., Pereira, J. P., Regard, J. B., Xu, Y., et al. (2007). Promotion of lymphocyte egress into blood and lymph by distinct sources of sphingosine-1-phosphate. *Science*, *316*, 295–298.

Persegol, L., Darabi, M., Dauteuille, C., Lhomme, M., Chantepie, S., Rye, K. A., et al. (2018). Small dense HDLs display potent vasorelaxing activity, reflecting their elevated content of sphingosine-1-phosphate. *Journal of Lipid Research*, *59*, 25–34.

Polzin, A., Knoop, B., Bohm, A., Dannenberg, L., Zurek, M., Zeus, T., et al. (2018). Aspirin inhibits platelet-derived sphingosine-1-phosphate induced endothelial cell migration. *Pharmacology*, *101*, 72–75.

Poti, F., Gualtieri, F., Sacchi, S., Weissen-Plenz, G., Varga, G., Brodde, M., et al. (2013). KRP-203, sphingosine 1-phosphate receptor type 1 agonist, ameliorates atherosclerosis in LDL-R-/- mice. *Arteriosclerosis, Thrombosis, and Vascular Biology*, *33*, 1505–1512.

Poti, F., Simoni, M., & Nofer, J. R. (2014). Atheroprotective role of high-density lipoprotein (HDL)-associated sphingosine-1-phosphate (S1P). *Cardiovascular Research*, *103*, 395–404.

Prager, B., Spampinato, S. F., & Ransohoff, R. M. (2015). Sphingosine 1-phosphate signaling at the blood-brain barrier. *Trends in Molecular Medicine*, *21*, 354–363.

Qin, C., Fan, W. H., Liu, Q., Shang, K., Murugan, M., Wu, L. J., et al. (2017). Fingolimod protects against ischemic white matter damage by modulating microglia toward M2 polarization via STAT3 pathway. *Stroke*, *48*, 3336–3346.

Qiu, P., Feng, X. H., & Li, L. (2003). Interaction of Smad3 and SRF-associated complex mediates TGF-beta1 signals to regulate SM22 transcription during myofibroblast differentiation. *Journal of Molecular and Cellular Cardiology*, *35*, 1407–1420.

Racca, V., Di Rienzo, M., Cavarretta, R., Toccafondi, A., Vaini, E., Ferratini, M., et al. (2016). Fingolimod effects on left ventricular function in multiple sclerosis. *Multiple Sclerosis*, *22*, 201–211.

Ranasinghe, A., Lee, D. D., & Schwarz, M. A. (2020). Mechanistic regulation of SPHK1 expression and translocation by EMAP II in pulmonary smooth muscle cells. *Biochimica et Biophysica Acta - Molecular and Cell Biology of Lipids*, *1865*, 158789.

Robert, J., Osto, E., & von Eckardstein, A. (2021). The endothelium is both a target and a barrier of HDL's protective functions. *Cell, 10*, 1041.

Robert, P., Tsui, P., Laville, M. P., Livi, G. P., Sarau, H. M., Bril, A., et al. (2001). EDG1 receptor stimulation leads to cardiac hypertrophy in rat neonatal myocytes. *Journal of Molecular and Cellular Cardiology, 33*, 1589–1606.

Roviezzo, F., Bucci, M., Delisle, C., Brancaleone, V., Di Lorenzo, A., Mayo, I. P., et al. (2006). Essential requirement for sphingosine kinase activity in eNOS-dependent NO release and vasorelaxation. *The FASEB Journal, 20*, 340–342.

Ruiz, M., Frej, C., Holmer, A., Guo, L. J., Tran, S., & Dahlback, B. (2017). High-density lipoprotein-associated apolipoprotein M limits endothelial inflammation by delivering sphingosine-1-phosphate to the sphingosine-1-phosphate receptor 1. *Arteriosclerosis, Thrombosis, and Vascular Biology, 37*, 118–129.

Salas-Perdomo, A., Miro-Mur, F., Gallizioli, M., Brait, V. H., Justicia, C., Meissner, A., et al. (2019). Role of the S1P pathway and inhibition by fingolimod in preventing hemorrhagic transformation after stroke. *Scientific Reports, 9*, 8309.

Salomone, S., Potts, E. M., Tyndall, S., Ip, P. C., Chun, J., Brinkmann, V., et al. (2008). Analysis of sphingosine 1-phosphate receptors involved in constriction of isolated cerebral arteries with receptor null mice and pharmacological tools. *British Journal of Pharmacology, 153*, 140–147.

Salomone, S., Soydan, G., Ip, P. C., Hopson, K. M., & Waeber, C. (2010). Vessel-specific role of sphingosine kinase 1 in the vasoconstriction of isolated basilar arteries. *Pharmacological Research, 62*, 465–474.

Salomone, S., Yoshimura, S., Reuter, U., Foley, M., Thomas, S. S., Moskowitz, M. A., et al. (2003). S1P3 receptors mediate the potent constriction of cerebral arteries by sphingosine-1-phosphate. *European Journal of Pharmacology, 469*, 125–134.

Sanchez, T., & Hla, T. (2004). Structural and functional characteristics of S1P receptors. *Journal of Cellular Biochemistry, 92*, 913–922.

Sanchez, T., Skoura, A., Wu, M. T., Casserly, B., Harrington, E. O., & Hla, T. (2007). Induction of vascular permeability by the sphingosine-1-phosphate receptor-2 (S1P2R) and its downstream effectors ROCK and PTEN. *Arteriosclerosis, Thrombosis, and Vascular Biology, 27*, 1312–1318.

Sanna, M. G., Liao, J., Jo, E., Alfonso, C., Ahn, M. Y., Peterson, M. S., et al. (2004). Sphingosine 1-phosphate (S1P) receptor subtypes S1P1 and S1P3, respectively, regulate lymphocyte recirculation and heart rate. *The Journal of Biological Chemistry, 279*, 13839–13848.

Sato, K., & Okajima, F. (2010). Role of sphingosine 1-phosphate in anti-atherogenic actions of high-density lipoprotein. *World Journal of Biological Chemistry, 1*, 327–337.

Sattler, K., Graler, M., Keul, P., Weske, S., Reimann, C. M., Jindrova, H., et al. (2015). Defects of high-density lipoproteins in coronary artery disease caused by low sphingosine-1-phosphate content: Correction by sphingosine-1-phosphate-loading. *Journal of the American College of Cardiology, 66*, 1470–1485.

Scott, F. L., Clemons, B., Brooks, J., Brahmachary, E., Powell, R., Dedman, H., et al. (2016). Ozanimod (RPC1063) is a potent sphingosine-1-phosphate receptor-1 (S1P1) and receptor-5 (S1P5) agonist with autoimmune disease-modifying activity. *British Journal of Pharmacology, 173*, 1778–1792.

Sekiguchi, K., Yokoyama, T., Kurabayashi, M., Okajima, F., & Nagai, R. (1999). Sphingosylphosphorylcholine induces a hypertrophic growth response through the mitogen-activated protein kinase signaling cascade in rat neonatal cardiac myocytes. *Circulation Research, 85*, 1000–1008.

Selim, S., Sunkara, M., Salous, A. K., Leung, S. W., Berdyshev, E. V., Bailey, A., et al. (2011). Plasma levels of sphingosine 1-phosphate are strongly correlated with haematocrit, but variably restored by red blood cell transfusions. *Clinical Science (London, England), 121*, 565–572.

Shi, W., Wang, Q., Wang, J., Yan, X., Feng, W., Zhang, Q., et al. (2021). Activation of yes-associated protein mediates sphingosine-1-phosphate-induced proliferation and migration of pulmonary artery smooth muscle cells and its potential mechanisms. *Journal of Cellular Physiology, 236*, 4694–4708.

Siedlinski, M., Nosalski, R., Szczepaniak, P., Ludwig-Galezowska, A. H., Mikolajczyk, T., Filip, M., et al. (2017). Vascular transcriptome profiling identifies Sphingosine kinase 1 as a modulator of angiotensin II-induced vascular dysfunction. *Scientific Reports*, 7, 44131.

Skoura, A., Michaud, J., Im, D. S., Thangada, S., Xiong, Y., Smith, J. D., et al. (2011). Sphingosine-1-phosphate receptor-2 function in myeloid cells regulates vascular inflammation and atherosclerosis. *Arteriosclerosis, Thrombosis, and Vascular Biology, 31*, 81–85.

Spampinato, S. F., Merlo, S., Costantino, G., Sano, Y., Kanda, T., & Sortino, M. A. (2021). Decreased astrocytic CCL2 accounts for BAF-312 effect on PBMCs transendothelial migration through a blood brain barrier in vitro model. *Journal of Neuroimmune Pharmacology* (Online ahead of print).

Spampinato, S. F., Merlo, S., Sano, Y., Kanda, T., & Sortino, M. A. (2021). Protective effect of the sphingosine-1 phosphate receptor agonist siponimod on disrupted blood brain barrier function. *Biochemical Pharmacology, 186*, 114465.

Spampinato, S. F., Obermeier, B., Cotleur, A., Love, A., Takeshita, Y., Sano, Y., et al. (2015). Sphingosine 1 phosphate at the blood brain barrier: Can the modulation of S1P receptor 1 influence the response of endothelial cells and astrocytes to inflammatory stimuli? *PLoS One, 10*, e0133392.

Stokum, J. A., Gerzanich, V., & Simard, J. M. (2016). Molecular pathophysiology of cerebral edema. *Journal of Cerebral Blood Flow and Metabolism, 36*, 513–538.

Sun, X., Singleton, P. A., Letsiou, E., Zhao, J., Belvitch, P., Sammani, S., et al. (2012). Sphingosine-1-phosphate receptor-3 is a novel biomarker in acute lung injury. *American Journal of Respiratory Cell and Molecular Biology, 47*, 628–636.

Swendeman, S. L., Xiong, Y., Cantalupo, A., Yuan, H., Burg, N., Hisano, Y., et al. (2017). An engineered S1P chaperone attenuates hypertension and ischemic injury. *Science Signaling, 10*, eaal2722.

Tabeling, C., Yu, H., Wang, L., Ranke, H., Goldenberg, N. M., Zabini, D., et al. (2015). CFTR and sphingolipids mediate hypoxic pulmonary vasoconstriction. *Proceedings of the National Academy of Sciences of the United States of America, 112*, E1614–E1623.

Taha, T. A., Argraves, K. M., & Obeid, L. M. (2004). Sphingosine-1-phosphate receptors: Receptor specificity versus functional redundancy. *Biochimica et Biophysica Acta, 1682*, 48–55.

Takashima, S., Sugimoto, N., Takuwa, N., Okamoto, Y., Yoshioka, K., Takamura, M., et al. (2008). G12/13 and Gq mediate S1P2-induced inhibition of Rac and migration in vascular smooth muscle in a manner dependent on Rho but not Rho kinase. *Cardiovascular Research, 79*, 689–697.

Takuwa, Y., Du, W., Qi, X., Okamoto, Y., Takuwa, N., & Yoshioka, K. (2010). Roles of sphingosine-1-phosphate signaling in angiogenesis. *World Journal of Biological Chemistry, 1*, 298–306.

Takuwa, N., Ohkura, S., Takashima, S., Ohtani, K., Okamoto, Y., Tanaka, T., et al. (2010). S1P3-mediated cardiac fibrosis in sphingosine kinase 1 transgenic mice involves reactive oxygen species. *Cardiovascular Research, 85*, 484–493.

Takuwa, Y., Okamoto, Y., Yoshioka, K., & Takuwa, N. (2008). Sphingosine-1-phosphate signaling and biological activities in the cardiovascular system. *Biochimica et Biophysica Acta, 1781*, 483–488.

Theilmeier, G., Schmidt, C., Herrmann, J., Keul, P., Schafers, M., Herrgott, I., et al. (2006). High-density lipoproteins and their constituent, sphingosine-1-phosphate, directly protect the heart against ischemia/reperfusion injury in vivo via the S1P3 lysophospholipid receptor. *Circulation, 114*, 1403–1409.

Ulrych, T., Bohm, A., Polzin, A., Daum, G., Nusing, R. M., Geisslinger, G., et al. (2011). Release of sphingosine-1-phosphate from human platelets is dependent on thromboxane formation. *Journal of Thrombosis and Haemostasis*, *9*, 790–798.

Urtz, N., Gaertner, F., von Bruehl, M. L., Chandraratne, S., Rahimi, F., Zhang, L., et al. (2015). Sphingosine 1-phosphate produced by sphingosine kinase 2 intrinsically controls platelet aggregation in vitro and in vivo. *Circulation Research*, *117*, 376–387.

Venkataraman, K., Lee, Y. M., Michaud, J., Thangada, S., Ai, Y., Bonkovsky, H. L., et al. (2008). Vascular endothelium as a contributor of plasma sphingosine 1-phosphate. *Circulation Research*, *102*, 669–676.

Vu, T. M., Ishizu, A. N., Foo, J. C., Toh, X. R., Zhang, F., Whee, D. M., et al. (2017). Mfsd2b is essential for the sphingosine-1-phosphate export in erythrocytes and platelets. *Nature*, *550*, 524–528.

Waeber, C., Blondeau, N., & Salomone, S. (2004). Vascular sphingosine-1-phosphate S1P1 and S1P3 receptors. *Drug News & Perspectives*, *17*, 365–382.

Wafa, D., Koch, N., Kovacs, J., Kerek, M., Proia, R. L., Tigyi, G. J., et al. (2020). Opposing roles of S1P3 receptors in myocardial function. *Cell*, *9*, 1770.

Wang, J., Feng, W., Li, F., Shi, W., Zhai, C., Li, S., et al. (2019). SphK1/S1P mediates TGF-beta1-induced proliferation of pulmonary artery smooth muscle cells and its potential mechanisms. *Pulmonary Circulation*, *9*, 2045894018816977.

Wang, Z., Kawabori, M., & Houkin, K. (2020). FTY720 (fingolimod) ameliorates brain injury through multiple mechanisms and is a strong candidate for stroke treatment. *Current Medicinal Chemistry*, *27*, 2979–2993.

Wang, J., Yan, X., Feng, W., Wang, Q., Shi, W., Chai, L., et al. (2021). S1P induces proliferation of pulmonary artery smooth muscle cells by promoting YAP-induced Notch3 expression and activation. *The Journal of Biological Chemistry*, *296*, 100599.

Wei, Y., Yemisci, M., Kim, H. H., Yung, L. M., Shin, H. K., Hwang, S. K., et al. (2011). Fingolimod provides long-term protection in rodent models of cerebral ischemia. *Annals of Neurology*, *69*, 119–129.

Whetzel, A. M., Bolick, D. T., Srinivasan, S., Macdonald, T. L., Morris, M. A., Ley, K., et al. (2006). Sphingosine-1 phosphate prevents monocyte/endothelial interactions in type 1 diabetic NOD mice through activation of the S1P1 receptor. *Circulation Research*, *99*, 731–739.

Wirth, A., Benyo, Z., Lukasova, M., Leutgeb, B., Wettschureck, N., Gorbey, S., et al. (2008). G12-G13-LARG-mediated signaling in vascular smooth muscle is required for salt-induced hypertension. *Nature Medicine*, *14*, 64–68.

Xiong, Y., & Hla, T. (2014). S1P control of endothelial integrity. *Current Topics in Microbiology and Immunology*, *378*, 85–105.

Xu, D., Gao, Q., Wang, F., Peng, Q., Wang, G., Wei, Q., et al. (2021). Sphingosine-1-phosphate receptor 3 is implicated in BBB injury via the CCL2-CCR2 axis following acute intracerebral hemorrhage. *CNS Neuroscience & Therapeutics*, *27*, 674–686.

Yang, L., Liu, S., Han, S., Hu, Y., Wu, Z., Shi, X., et al. (2020). The HDL from septic-ARDS patients with composition changes exacerbates pulmonary endothelial dysfunction and acute lung injury induced by cecal ligation and puncture (CLP) in mice. *Respiratory Research*, *21*, 293.

Yatomi, Y., Igarashi, Y., Yang, L., Hisano, N., Qi, R., Asazuma, N., et al. (1997). Sphingosine 1-phosphate, a bioactive sphingolipid abundantly stored in platelets, is a normal constituent of human plasma and serum. *Journal of Biochemistry*, *121*, 969–973.

Yatomi, Y., Ruan, F., Hakomori, S., & Igarashi, Y. (1995). Sphingosine-1-phosphate: A platelet-activating sphingolipid released from agonist-stimulated human platelets. *Blood*, *86*, 193–202.

Yuhanna, I. S., Zhu, Y., Cox, B. E., Hahner, L. D., Osborne-Lawrence, S., Lu, P., et al. (2001). High-density lipoprotein binding to scavenger receptor-BI activates endothelial nitric oxide synthase. *Nature Medicine*, *7*, 853–857.

Zhang, W., An, J., Jawadi, H., Siow, D. L., Lee, J. F., Zhao, J., et al. (2013). Sphingosine-1-phosphate receptor-2 mediated NFkappaB activation contributes to tumor necrosis factor-alpha induced VCAM-1 and ICAM-1 expression in endothelial cells. *Prostaglandins & Other Lipid Mediators, 106*, 62–71.

Zhang, L., Guo, K., Zhou, J., Zhang, X., Yin, S., Peng, J., et al. (2021). Ponesimod protects against neuronal death by suppressing the activation of A1 astrocytes in early brain injury after experimental subarachnoid hemorrhage. *Journal of Neurochemistry, 158*, 880–897.

Zhang, J., Honbo, N., Goetzl, E. J., Chatterjee, K., Karliner, J. S., & Gray, M. O. (2007). Signals from type 1 sphingosine 1-phosphate receptors enhance adult mouse cardiac myocyte survival during hypoxia. *American Journal of Physiology. Heart and Circulatory Physiology, 293*, H3150–H3158.

Zhang, F., Xia, Y., Yan, W., Zhang, H., Zhou, F., Zhao, S., et al. (2016). Sphingosine 1-phosphate signaling contributes to cardiac inflammation, dysfunction, and remodeling following myocardial infarction. *American Journal of Physiology. Heart and Circulatory Physiology, 310*, H250–H261.

Zhao, Y. D., Chu, L., Lin, K., Granton, E., Yin, L., Peng, J., et al. (2015). A biochemical approach to understand the pathogenesis of advanced pulmonary arterial hypertension: Metabolomic profiles of arginine, sphingosine-1-phosphate, and heme of human lung. *PLoS One, 10*, e0134958.

Zhu, Z., Fu, Y., Tian, D., Sun, N., Han, W., Chang, G., et al. (2015). Combination of the immune modulator fingolimod with alteplase in acute ischemic stroke: A pilot trial. *Circulation, 132*, 1104–1112.

CHAPTER FIVE

Polymorphisms in common antihypertensive targets: Pharmacogenomic implications for the treatment of cardiovascular disease

Dominique Brown, Heather Alcala, Peter Oelschlaeger, and Bradley T. Andresen*
Western University of Health Sciences, Pomona, CA, United States
*Corresponding author: e-mail address: bandresen@westernu.edu

Contents

Advances in Pharmacology, Volume 94
ISSN 1054-3589
https://doi.org/10.1016/bs.apha.2022.04.001

Abstract

The idea of personalized medicine came to fruition with sequencing the human genome; however, aside from a few cases, the genetic revolution has yet to materialize. Cardiovascular diseases are the leading cause of death globally, and hypertension is a common prelude to nearly all cardiovascular diseases. Thus, hypertension is an ideal candidate disease to apply tenants of personalized medicine to lessen cardiovascular disease. Herein is a survey that visually depicts the polymorphisms in the top eight anti-hypertensive targets. Although there are numerous genome-wide association studies regarding cardiovascular disease, few studies look at the effects of receptor polymorphisms on drug treatment. With 17,000+ polymorphisms in the combined target proteins examined, it is expected that some of the clinical variability in the treatment of hypertension is due to polymorphisms in the drug targets. Recent advances in techniques and technology, such as high throughput examination of single mutations, structure prediction, computational power for modeling, and CRISPR models of point mutations, allow for a relatively rapid and comprehensive examination of the effects of known and future polymorphisms on drug affinity and effects. As hypertension is easy to measure and has a plethora of clinically viable ligands, hypertension makes an excellent disease to study pharmacogenomics in the lab and the clinic. If the promises of personalized medicine are to materialize, a concerted effort to examine the effects polymorphisms have on drugs is required. A clinician with the knowledge of a patient's genotype can then prescribe drugs that are optimal for treating that specific patient.

Abbreviations

3' UTR 3′ untranslated region of the mRNA, which follows the coding region.

5' UTR 5′ untranslated region of the mRNA, which is found before the coding region.

a1-AR alpha-1 adrenergic receptor, also known as the alpha-1 adrenoceptor. The three family members include α_{1A}-, α_{1B}-, and α_{1D}-AR

a2-AR alpha-2 adrenergic receptor, also known as the alpha-2 adrenoceptor. The three family members include α_{2A}-, $\alpha_{2B\text{-}}$, and α_{2C}-AR

ACE angiotensin-converting enzyme

ACE I/D angiotensin-converting enzyme insertion/deletion polymorphism

ARB angiotensin II type 1 receptor antagonist (blocker)

AT1R angiotensin II type 1 receptor

b1-AR beta-1 adrenergic receptor, also known as the beta-1 adrenoceptor

b2-AR beta-2 adrenergic receptor, also known as the beta-2 adrenoceptor

BPH benign prostatic hyperplasia

BRET bioluminescence resonance energy transfer

Cav1.2α1c the alpha-1c subunit of the vascular L-type calcium channel.

CCB calcium channel blocker

cDNA complementary DNA. A DNA copy of a messenger RNA.

CFTR cystic fibrosis transmembrane conductance regulator

CK2 casein kinase 2

CRISPR clustered regularly interspaced short palindromic repeats; now used to represent the CRISPR/Cas9 gene editing.

CYP	cytochrome P450
EC_{50}	a pharmacological measure of the half-maximal effect of an agonist listed as a concentration of the agonist. EC50 is a constant for the specific ligand-receptor.
E_{max}	a pharmacological measure of the maximal effect of an agonist listed as a concentration of the agonist.
ER	endoplasmic reticulum
gACE	germinal angiotensin-converting enzyme, which is the same as tACE
GGCX	gene encoding gamma-glutamyl carboxylase
GPCR	G protein-coupled receptor
INR	international normalized ratio
K_i	affinity constant of an antagonist
L	ligand
LR	ligated receptor complex
MD	molecular dynamics
mRNA	messenger RNA
NCC	sodium chloride cotransporter, also known as solute carrier family 12 member 3
NKCC1	sodium-potassium-2 chloride cotransporter 1, officially called solute carrier family 12 member 2
NKCC2	sodium-potassium-2 chloride cotransporter 2, officially called solute carrier family 12 member 1
nsSNP	nonsynonymous single nucleotide polymorphism
PDB	Protein Data Bank
R	receptor
RCSB	Research Collaboratory for Structural Bioinformatics
sACE	somatic angiotensin-converting enzyme
SNP	single nucleotide polymorphism
sSNP	synonymous single nucleotide polymorphism
tACE	testicular angiotensin-converting enzyme
UTR	untranslated region
VKORC1	gene encoding Vitamin K epoxide reductase complex subunit 1
β-blocker	beta-adrenergic receptor antagonist (blocker)

1. Introduction

Variability in response to cardiovascular drugs is a well-known phenomenon with many potential contributors to the observed variability (El Desoky, Derendorf, & Klotz, 2006). Pharmacogenomics is one factor that contributes to the clinically observed variability in drug response. Pharmacogenomics arose from family-based studies that established a genetic disposition to drug responses (Weinshilboum & Wang, 2004).

Most research in the field has focused on metabolic enzymes' effect on pharmacokinetics (Ahmed, Zhou, Zhou, & Chen, 2016), and for a good reason, as described in the warfarin example listed below. However, all mutagenesis studies conducted in cell lines to identify drug binding sites, which are too numerous to cite, demonstrate that there is variability in drug effect when metabolic enzymes for a given drug are identical. Thus, one additional source of drug response variability is likely single nucleotide polymorphisms (SNPs) in target receptors (Hauser et al., 2018), which is the focus of this chapter.

1.1 Alterations in ligand affinity

Basic pharmacology indicates that there is an equilibrium between the drug, or ligand (L), plus receptor (R), and the receptor bound to the ligand (LR) (Fig. 1). Changes to either the ligand or receptor can change the equilibrium, increasing or decreasing drug affinity for the receptor. Changes to a ligand resulting in altered affinity are well known and are the basis of structure-activity relationship studies. With the advent of site-directed mutagenesis, many studies mutated receptors to identify ligand-binding pockets. Consequently, it is well accepted that a single amino acid change in a receptor can alter drug affinity. A nonsynonymous SNP (nsSNP) results in a change in the coded amino acid. Thus, natural amino acid sequence variability can result in changes to drug targets that may impact drug affinity (Morningstar-Kywi, Haworth, & Mosley, 2021).

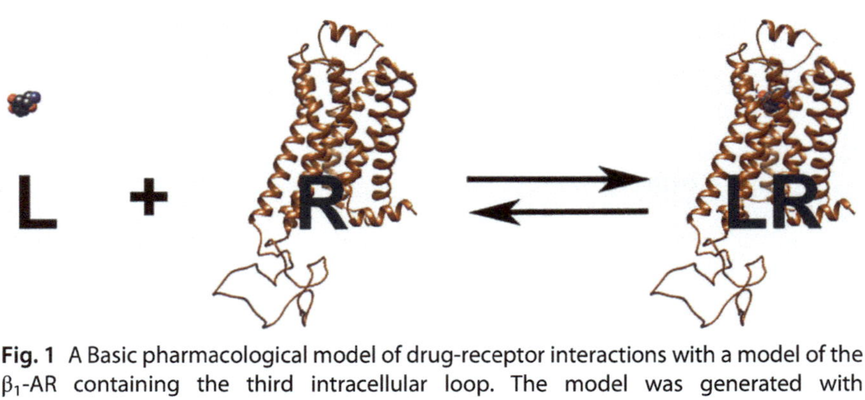

Fig. 1 A Basic pharmacological model of drug-receptor interactions with a model of the β_1-AR containing the third intracellular loop. The model was generated with Swiss-Model using PDB:7BU6 as a template (Xu et al., 2021).

1.2 Alterations in mRNA and protein translation

Polymorphisms within a gene can do more than affect the affinity of a ligand. Polymorphisms can alter mRNA levels as exemplified by the A1166C polymorphism of the Angiotensin II type 1 receptor (AT_1R) and mRNA translation as exemplified by the cystic fibrosis transmembrane conductance regulator (CFTR). The AT_1R A1166C polymorphism is located in the 3′ untranslated region (UTR) (Bonnardeaux et al., 1994). The CC genotype increases mRNA levels, likely via altering mRNA stability, and subsequently increases AT_1R translation (Bonnardeaux et al., 1994; Chandra et al., 2014). The increased translation of the AT_1R increases the endogenous ligand, Angiotensin II, mediated responses (van Geel et al., 2000). Increasing the concentration of a ligand or receptor will increase levels of the LR complex, resulting in greater effects (Fig. 2). Therefore, it is unsurprising that the A1166C polymorphism of the AT_1R is associated with increased blood pressure (Bonnardeaux et al., 1994; Chandra et al., 2014; Shamaa, Fouad, Haroun, & Shamaa, 2016), and it is likely that similar results occur for other drug targets.

Many CFTR polymorphisms result in misfolding and fewer channels at the cell surface (see below). The ΔF508 polymorphism also alters mRNA structure, decreasing the translational rate resulting in less protein production (Bartoszewski et al., 2010). Similarly, the synonymous SNP (sSNP) T2562G of CFTR, an sSNP alters codon usage but does not change the amino acid, changes translation velocity leading to reduced channels and altered regulation of expressed channels (Kirchner et al., 2017). Reducing receptor levels will reduce LR levels (Fig. 2B) and consequently reduce the effect of a steady-state agonist. However, reducing receptor numbers can also change the regulation of the receptor, as seen with CFTR T2562G. Therefore, there is a need for continued basic biology experiments designed to understand the control of receptors.

1.3 Alterations in protein folding and trafficking

Polymorphisms within the coding sequence can also alter protein folding and trafficking. Misfolded proteins are retained in the endoplasmic reticulum (ER) and degraded. Many polymorphisms involved in disease are the result of misfolded proteins. Examples include P23H rhodopsin leading to autosomal dominant retinitis pigmentosa (Illing, Rajan, Bence, & Kopito, 2002; Saliba, Munro, Luthert, & Cheetham, 2002), and multiple polymorphisms of CFTR, including ΔF508 CFTR, lead to misfolding and altered

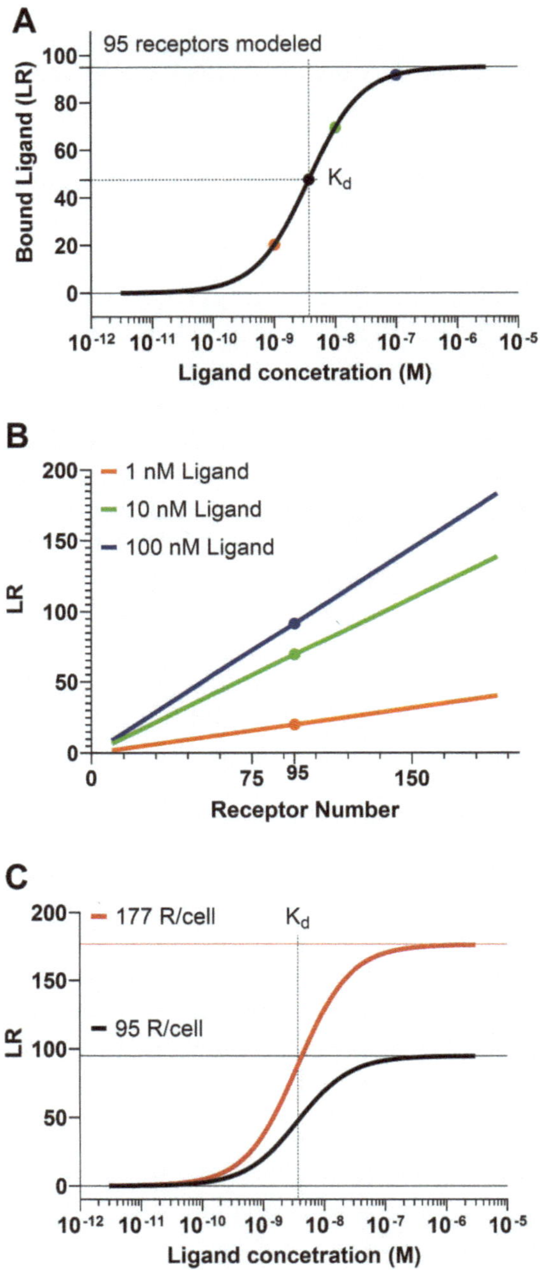

Fig. 2 Concentration-response models. (A) depicts a model of a classic concentration-response curve with ligand (L) concentration on the x-axis and number of receptors bound (LR) on the y-axis; total receptor number is 95, which can be calculated by the B_{max}. The colored dots correspond to the points on panel B. (B) depicts changing the receptor concentration on the x-axis while measuring LR with a constant ligand (L) concentration. (C) depicts a concentration-response curve with a 1.86-fold increase in the receptor to 177 receptors per cell (Chandra et al., 2014). For the formulas underlying the graphs see (Hunter & Cochran, 2016).

trafficking to the plasma membrane (van Willigen et al., 2019). However, receptor trafficking also includes compartmentalization of a receptor at the membrane and during endocytosis. The endocytic process is an essential component of receptor-mediated signaling (Andresen, Rizzo, Shome, & Romero, 2002; Tsvetanova & von Zastrow, 2014). As this process is further unraveled, proteins that interact with receptors and shepherd the receptors to their proper locations may also contain polymorphisms that alter receptor actions. The expanding understanding of compartment-dependent receptor signaling increases the scope of proteins that may harbor polymorphisms that affect receptor signaling and drug effects (Semesta, Tian, Kampmann, von Zastrow, & Tsvetanova, 2020).

1.4 Alterations in allosteric networks (change in effect)

Additionally, most receptors rely on a rearrangement of an internal allosteric network to transduce a signal from a ligand-binding pocket to an effector site, as exemplified by the adenosine A_{2A} receptor (Fernandes et al., 2021; Susac, Eddy, Didenko, Stevens, & Wuthrich, 2018) and β2-adrenergic receptor (β_2-AR) (Jones et al., 2020). Alterations in this allosteric network due to an nsSNP can change the effect of a drug with little to no change in affinity (Hauser et al., 2018; Jones et al., 2020). Therefore, as we learn about polymorphisms, it will become more important to screen patients for polymorphisms and understand how each polymorphism affects drug responses. Such an effort will bring personalized medicine to fruition with the current and future pharmacopeia.

2. Warfarin as a test case

The evolution of personalized medicine is well illustrated by pharmacogenomic guided dosing of warfarin. Warfarin was approved for human therapy in 1954 (Lim, 2017), and was the 52nd most prescribed drug within the US in 2018, with 14,772,355 prescriptions (Kane, 2020). Warfarin has a narrow therapeutic range; the risk of bleeding resulting in case fatality was 13.7% prior to current pharmacogenomic guidelines (Linkins, Choi, & Douketis, 2003). Bleeding occurs when the international normalized ratio of prothrombin clotting time (INR) is too large, while thromboembolic events occur with a low INR. When warfarin is metabolized slower or faster than average by polymorphic versions of Cytochrome P450 4F2 and 2C9 (CYP4F2 and CYP2C9), it will lead to a higher INR or lower INR, respectively. Similarly, polymorphisms in its target Vitamin K

Epoxide Reductase Complex Subunit 1 (VKORC1) as well as Gamma-Glutamyl Carboxylase (GGCX) can increase or decrease INR. Patients can have polymorphisms in more than one gene; thus, current warfarin dosing guidelines and dosing algorithms take into account the current INR, drug-drug interactions, patient physical characteristics, and polymorphisms within VKORC1, GGCX, CYP4F2, and CYP2C9 to maintain INR within a targeted range (Gage, 2016; Johnson et al., 2017; Jorgensen et al., 2019; Ravvaz, Weissert, Ruff, Chi, & Tonellato, 2017). Although these guidelines help patients maintain a healthy INR, current research aims to improve warfarin dosing (Asiimwe, Zhang, Osanlou, Jorgensen, & Pirmohamed, 2021; Sridharan et al., 2021). The evolution of the guidelines was slow. Genetic tests were recommended by the United States Food and Drug Administration in 2007, yet articles suggested a lack of evidence for basing warfarin dosing on genetics (Kangelaris, Bent, Nussbaum, Garcia, & Tice, 2009). More recent studies directly comparing genetic-based dosing to non-genetic based dosing of warfarin demonstrates that the guidelines reduces all adverse risks by nearly 4% (Gage et al., 2017). If, and likely when, pharmacogenomics is applied to hypertension and other disease treatments, the path to the common use of genomic information in prescribing "old" drugs will likely be a similarly long road as that of warfarin. However, recent advances in science greatly enhance the ease of genotyping drug targets and identifying polymorphisms that alter drug response.

3. Polymorphisms within receptors for antihypertensive drugs

Although the issues discussed in this article apply to all drug targets, as exemplified by the shift of pharmaceutical companies and clinical trials using genetics (Bienfait et al., 2021; Thase et al., 2019), only the targets of often prescribed drugs that lower blood pressure will be discussed herein. The data presented is collated from the GRCh38.p13 assembly from the human genome (Table 1) (Howe et al., 2021). The alterations to the coding sequence are displayed on models obtained from the AlphaFold project (Tunyasuvunakool et al., 2021). All unique alterations reported in the GRCh38.p13 assembly are summarized in tables designed to indicate the vast number of polymorphisms that may alter protein function and drug responses. nsSNPs, stop gained (nsSNPs resulting in a stop codon), in-frame deletion and addition (alterations that remove or add one or more amino acids, respectively, with no other changes to the sequence), frameshift

Table 1 Ensembl database sequences used to identify polymorphisms in antihypertensive targets.

Protein	Abbr.	Gene	Ensembl #
β_1-adrenergic receptor	β_1-AR	*adbr1*	ENSG00000043591
Angiotensin-converting enzyme	ACE	*ace1*	ENSG00000159640
Vascular L-type Ca^{2+} channel alpha 1c subunit	$Ca_v1.2$	*cacna1c*	ENSG00000151067
Sodium Chloride Cotransporter/Solute carrier family 12 member 3	NCC	*slc12a3*	ENSG00000070915
Angiotensin type 1 receptor	AT_1R	*agtr1*	ENSG00000144891
Na^+:K^+:$2Cl^-$ symporter/Solute carrier family 12 member 1	NKCC2	*slc12a1*	ENSG00000074803
α_{1A}-adrenergic receptor	α_{1A}-AR	*adra1a*	ENSG00000120907
α_{1B}-adrenergic receptor	α_{1B}-AR	*adra1b*	ENSG00000170214
α_{1D}-adrenergic receptor	α_{1D}-AR	*adra1d*	ENSG00000171873
α_{2A}-adrenergic receptor	α_{2A}-AR	*adra2a*	ENSG00000150594
α_{2B}-adrenergic receptor	α_{2B}-AR	*adra2b*	ENSG00000274286
α_{2C}-adrenergic receptor	α_{2C}-AR	*adra2c*	ENSG00000184160

(deletion or insertion of fewer than three nucleotides), and protein-altering variants (insertions that also add a novel amino acid to the sequence) are color-coded on each model.

The classes of drugs commonly used to lower blood pressure have been relatively constant over the last two decades. New drugs either fall into an accepted class, such as β-blockers, or are not used frequently, such as aliskiren (Tekturna® & Rasilez®). Prescription data from 2018, which is the most recent data available, indicate that in the United States, only a subset of each class of antihypertensive is commonly prescribed (Table 2). Ligand diversity to a single target may become more important as nsSNPs within the target may alter the effects of specific ligands (Anderson et al., 2020; Hauser et al., 2018). When combining the prescription data into pharmacological targets (Table 3), it becomes clear that the primary antihypertensive medications are highly prescribed, but so too are secondary medications such as β-blockers, NKCC2 inhibitors, α_1-adrenergic receptor blockers, and α_2-adrenergic receptor agonists (Whelton et al., 2018).

Table 2 List of antihypertensive drug targets and corresponding ligands.

Target	Target abbrev.	Drug classes	approx. # of drugs[a]	Drugs highly prescribed in the US	Total US prescriptions (2018)[b]
Na^+/Cl^- symporter	NCC	Thiazides	12	Hydrochlorothiazide	40,575,075
		Thiazide-like compounds	8	Chlorthalidone Metolazone	3,883,003 967,800
$Na^+:K^+:2Cl^-$ symporter	NKCC2	Loop Diuretics	7	Furosemide Bumetanide Torsemide	29,857,945 2,468,002 1,617,596
Epithelial sodium channel	ENaC	Potassium-sparing diuretics	3	–	–
Mineralocorticoid Receptor	MR	Potassium sparing diuretics	4	Spironolactone	12,260,624
Angiotensin converting enzyme	ACE	ACE inhibitors	16	Lisinopril Benazepril Enalapril Ramipril Quinapril	97,608,879 5,920,052 5,182,854 3,989,667 1,012,588
Angiotensin II type I receptor	AT_1R	AT_1R blockers (ARBs)	8	Losartan Valsartan Irbesartan Olmesartan Telmisartan	50,479,750 7,694,037 3,490,431 2,068,391 1,295,783

Vascular L-type Ca^{2+} channel	$Ca_v1.2$	Ca^{2+} Channel Blocker (LCCB)	14[c]	Amlodipine	75,811,947
				Diltiazem	10,505,373
				Nifedipine	5,649,892
β-Adrenergic receptors	β-AR[d]	β-blockers	19	Metoprolol	71,581,961
				Carvedilol	22,737,638
				Atenolol	18,644,884
				Propranolol	14,571,767
				Timolol	4,312,018
				Nebivolol	2,955,158
				Labetalol	2,297,672
				Sotalol	1,770,181
				Bisoprolol	1,396,798
α_1-Adrenergic receptors	α_1-AR	α-blockers	7	Tamsulosin	23,254,005
				Doxazosin	3,417,127
				Terazosin	2,954,414
				Prazosin	2,729,531
α_{2A}-Adrenergic receptors	α_{2A}-AR	α_{2A}-AR agonists	4[e]	Clonidine	11,141,934
				Tizanidine	8,901,700
				Guanfacine	5,429,776
Multiple targets	N/A	Vasodilators	4	Hydralazine	7,545,026

[a]The total number of drugs does not include discontinued medications or drugs used solely in animals. However, it does include drugs not available in the United States. When thinking of chemical space, all ligands in a class could, but unlikely, be used again in the future to circumvent polymorphisms altering the more often used drugs.
[b]Data obtained from (Kane, 2020).
[c]There is one LCCB no longer used for hypertension and a few others in development.
[d]β-Blockers are a large class with varying degrees of specificity to the β_1-, β_2-, and α_1-adrenergic receptors.
[e]Only α_{2A}-AR agonists used to treat blood pressure are listed; however, three drugs not included are used for other conditions.

However, the reason for each prescription is not known; only total prescriptions are reported (Kane, 2020). Multiple drugs on the list are used for conditions other than hypertension. For example, the α_1-adrenergic receptor (α_1-AR) blockers are long-standing medications for treating benign prostatic hyperplasia (BPH) (Caine, 1986); incidentally, a recent genetics study of BPH also examined α_1-adrenergic receptor blockade effects (Qian et al., 2017), further supporting the role of polymorphisms in modulating pharmacodynamics.

3.1 β-Blockers

The most prescribed class of drugs that lowers blood pressure are the β-blockers (Table 3). β-Blockers primarily target the beta-1-adrenergic receptor (β_1-AR); although, clinically used β-blockers also target β_2-ARs, as well as α_1-ARs. For simplicity, only the β_1-AR receptor will be discussed in this section as α_1-ARs are discussed below, and every residue of the β_2-AR was mutated to all possible residues, covering all possible single nsSNPs, displaying a range of alterations to normal receptor function (Jones et al., 2020).

The β_1-AR gene (*adrb1*) is located on chromosome 10 and has 1240 identified alterations from the reference sequence to date (Table 4). 417 of the nucleotide sequence changes alter the amino acid sequence of the gene product. As shown in Fig. 3, the amino acid sequence-altering

Table 3 Antihypertensives with the most prescriptions.

Pharmacology	Target family	Minimum # of prescriptions in USA[a]
β-AR blockers	GPCR	143,775,045
ACE inhibitors	Enzyme	133,932,448
LCCBs	Channel	95,251,390
NCC inhibitors	Channel	87,065,956
ARBs	GPCR	83,419,882
NKCC2 inhibitors	Channel	33,943,543
α_1-AR blockers	GPCR	33,514,445
α_{2A}-AR agonists	GPCR	25,473,410

[a]The table adds the numbers from Table 2 and all the drugs that contain a mix of two ligands to determine a minimum number of drugs prescribed per target.
Data was obtained from Kane, S. P. (2020). The Top 300 of 2021, ClinCalc DrugStats Database, Version 21.1. Retrieved from https://clincalc.com/DrugStats/Top300Drugs.aspx.

Table 4 Polymorphisms identified in GPCRs that are targets of antihypertensive drugs.

GPCR	β_1-AR	AT_1R	α_{1A}-AR	α_{1B}-AR	α_{1D}-AR	α_{2A}-AR	α_{2B}-AR	α_{2C}-AR[a]
Gene	*adrb1*	*agtr1*	*adra1a*	*adra1b*	*adra1d*	*adra2a*	*adra2b*	*adra2c*
nsSNP	369	243	491	352	568	338	361	686
Stop gained	12	9	22	8	22	11	19	27
In-frame deletion	11	3	0	18	12	8	14	16
In-frame addition	8	0	1	12	11	2	20	3
Frameshift	15	27	30	13	31	25	38	27
Protein-altering variant	2	0	0	2	4	0	1	0
sSNP	254	103	224	182	242	184	163	405
5'UTR	97	296	0	203	97	293	137	83
3'UTR	472	273	81	162	248	402	531	328
Totals	**1240**	**954**	**849**	**952**	**1235**	**1263**	**1284**	**1575**

[a]The numbers in α_{2C}-AR are likely not entirely accurate due to inaccuracies found in the GRCh38.p13 assembly.

polymorphisms cover the entire receptor. Although little is known regarding most of the alterations, two early identified nsSNPs, S49G and R389G, have been studied in vitro and in vivo (Filigheddu et al., 2004; Sandilands & O'Shaughnessy, 2005; Zhang & Steinberg, 2013). Serine at position 49 makes the β_1-AR resistant to agonist-promoted degradation (Levin, Marullo, Muntaner, Andersson, & Magnusson, 2002; Rathz, Brown, Kramer, & Liggett, 2002) but does not change clinical responses to atenolol (Filigheddu et al., 2004). Whereas

Glycine at position 389 results in reduced isoproterenol- and carvedilol-mediated phosphorylation of ERK (Zhang & Steinberg, 2013), and patients carrying G389 are resistant to propranolol and bucindolol treatment (Dorn & Liggett, 2008). However, as reviewed in A.J. Sandilands and K.M. O'Shaughnessy, the clinical data is mixed; moreover, clinical data may be complicated by other polymorphisms not examined (Filigheddu et al., 2004). Although not directly studied, the Y244D nsSNP occurring at the Ballesteros-Weinstein position 5.38 likely alters the ligand-binding pocket and affects signaling as an aromatic residue is conserved at position 5.38 (Sanchez-Soto et al., 2020). The sSNPs and alterations to the UTRs

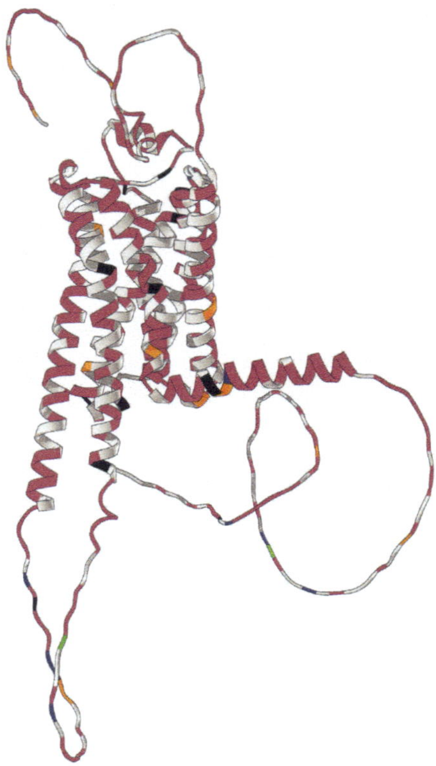

Fig. 3 AlphaFold model of the β_1-AR colored to display protein-altering polymorphisms. The reference sequence is gray, and colors are sequentially applied to changes in protein sequence: (1) nsSNPs are magenta, (2) in-frame deletions and additions are blue, (3) protein-altering variants are green, (4) frameshifts are orange, and (5) nsSNPs resulting in a stop codon are black. The colors applied first are replaced by later changes if they occur at identical residues.

could affect mRNA stability, and sSNPs can lead to less efficient codon usage; therefore, the silent changes could alter receptor number, which, as described, can alter drug response. Lastly, each of the identified and predicted glycosylation sites has a nsSNP that would ablate glycosylation (Park, Reddy, Wallukat, Xiang, & Steinberg, 2017), which may change drug effects.

Although many publications examine polymorphisms of the β_1-AR (at least 310 according to a PubMed search for "beta1 adrenergic receptor polymorphisms"), the discovery of polymorphisms has grown exponentially. In 2004 only 12 SNPs, of which 8 were nsSNPs, were known in the β_1-AR (Sandilands & O'Shaughnessy, 2005), compared to the 671 currently identified polymorphisms within the coding sequence (Table 4). Therefore, it will take a concerted effort by the scientific community to understand the physiological and pharmacological effects of each polymorphism. Identifying the clinical effects of each polymorphism will be even more difficult as the frequency of many polymorphisms is relatively low, making clinical studies difficult at best.

3.2 ACE inhibitors

Angiotensin-converting enzyme (ACE) inhibitors are the second most prescribed antihypertensive medication (Table 3). ACE, also known as CD143 and peptidyl-dipeptidase A, is a dipeptidase named for its role in converting angiotensin I to the bioactive hormone angiotensin II. However, ACE cleaves multiple other peptides in plasma (Semis, Gugiu, Bernstein, Bernstein, & Kalkum, 2019). The human ACE gene is located on chromosome 17 and has 2455 identified alterations to the reference sequence to date (Table 5). ACE is expressed in nearly every tissue, and there are two isoforms: somatic ACE (sACE), a 170 kDa protein, resulting from the transcription of the entire gene, and testicular ACE (tACE), also known as germinal ACE (gACE), a 100 kDa protein, resulting from transcription

Table 5 Polymorphisms identified in ACE and ion channels that are targets of antihypertensive drugs.

Protein	ACE[a]	$Ca_V1.2\alpha1C$	NCC	NKCC2
gene	*ace1*	*cacna1c*	*slc12a3*	*slc12a1*
nsSNP	1120	1299	846	746
Stop gained	63	356	29	36
In-frame deletion	25	23	11	11
In-frame addition	8	4	1	1
Frameshift	73	34	53	59
Protein-altering variant	9	5	4	0
sSNP	575	903	384	236
5'UTR	58	0	10	74
3'UTR	528	79	576	0
Totals	**2455**	**2703**	**1914**	**1253**

[a]The Ensembl database conflates tACE and sACE. Due to the conflation of the two transcripts, the numbers are highly likely an undercount of the polymorphisms.

from a promoter in intron 12. sACE contains two homologous domains called the N and C domains, corresponding to the N and C terminus. The two domains are likely the result of gene duplication, and both domains contain a zinc-bound active site (Sayed-Tabatabaei, Oostra, Isaacs, van Duijn, & Witteman, 2006). Apart from a divergent N-terminal portion of 67 amino acids, tACE corresponds to the C terminus of sACE. Both isoforms are dependent on zinc ions for activity, and ACE inhibitors block both domains (Riordan, 2003). 1294 Of the nucleotide changes alter the amino acid sequence. However, the GRCh38.p13 assembly appears to conflate the tACE and sACE sequences; therefore, Fig. 4 displays the polymorphisms only on tACE due to the sequence discrepancy in the GRCh38.p13 assembly.

Most studies into ACE polymorphisms involve the insertion/deletion (I/D) polymorphism in intron 16, where the deletion results in higher serum ACE levels (Rigat et al., 1990). Although many studies have examined ACE I/D association to disease, there is no association between ACE I/D and ACE inhibitor efficacy (Harrap et al., 2003). Fortunately, multiple molecular models (Brás, Fernandes, & Ramos, 2014; Fang et al., 2019) and a few

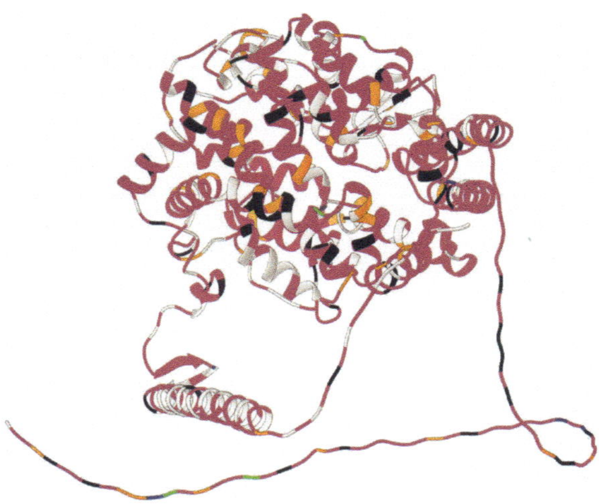

Fig. 4 AlphaFold model of tACE. The GRCh38.p13 assembly mixes tACE and sACE sequences. Therefore, tACE was modeled using AlphFold because it is more appropriate given the data. However, the representation may over-represent the polymorphisms due to the error in the GRCh38.p13 assembly. tACE is colored to display protein-altering polymorphisms. The reference sequence is gray, and colors are sequentially applied to changes in protein sequence: (1) nsSNPs are magenta, (2) in-frame deletions and additions are blue, (3) protein-altering variants are green, (4) frameshifts are orange, and (5) nsSNPs resulting in a stop codon are black. The colors applied first are replaced by later changes if they occur at identical residues.

crystal structures (Akif et al., 2011; Cozier et al., 2018) provide detailed identification of the ligand-binding sites and residues that interact with Zn^{2+}. In the following, we report the amino acid numbering corresponding to the reference sequence of tACE (Fig. 4), the N-terminal domain of sACE, and the C-terminal domain of sACE when first mentioned; subsequent discussion uses the tACE sequence. The standard binding site of ACE inhibitors contains ten residues, of which half have reported polymorphisms: A387/363/961P, H414/390/988R, H418/394/992D/R, H544/520/1118Y, and Y554/530/1128C. The histidine residues 414 and 418 are also involved in Zn^{2+} coordination; therefore, those polymorphisms will likely destroy ACE activity, and an ACE inhibitor would not be recommended. The H418D nsSNP reverses the charge, which likely affects substrate recognition, whereas the H418R may be tolerated, but the size is different. The H554Y nsSNP removes a charge and also likely affects substrate recognition. The A387P nsSNP resides in a β-sheet, and prolines disrupt β-sheets (Li, Goto, Williams, & Deber, 1996), suggesting that the A387P will structurally rearrange part of the ligand-binding site and likely abrogate substrate and ACE inhibitor recognition. The Y554C nsSNP removes a hydrogen bonding site but adds potential interesting chemistry due to the addition of a thiol. The secondary site identified by Akif et al. is composed of 11 residues and is only present in the C-terminal domain of sACE, which is identical in tACE. Although the functional effect of the secondary has not been elucidated, three residues contain nsSNPs (R155/729W/Q, R553/1127S, and N97/671T), numbering based on tACE and the C-terminal domain of sACE, respectfully. Asparagine 97 directly interacts with the ligand in the second site; thus, the N97T nsSNP likely ablates ligand binding. The R155W/Q and R553S change the charge around the ligand-binding pocket, which may disrupt ligand binding.

Lastly, sACE can dimerize and signal through CK2-mediated phosphorylation of S1270 (Kohlstedt et al., 2006; Kohlstedt, Shoghi, Muller-Esterl, Busse, & Fleming, 2002), which corresponds to S725 in tACE. CK2 cannot phosphorylate the nsSNP S1270F sACE and thus should prevent ACE inhibitor-mediated sACE shedding (Kohlstedt, Kellner, Busse, & Fleming, 2006). Although the long-term effects of ACE-medicated signaling remain unknown, the S1270F may have somatic and germinal effects. Furthermore, the dimerization interface is not fully understood, and polymorphisms that do not alter ACE inhibitor binding may interfere with the dimerization and consequently ACE-mediated signaling. There is an abundance of nsSNPs in ACE. However, their exact impact on ACE inhibitors' efficacy and cellular signaling remains unclear.

3.3 L-type calcium channel blockers (CCBs)

CCBs are a distant third in total prescriptions (Table 3); however, β-blockers and ACE inhibitors are frequently used in a wider variety of cardiovascular diseases than CCBs, suggesting that CCBs remain one of the most popular antihypertensive medications. The vascular L-type Ca^{2+} channel is critical to hormonal-mediated increases in blood pressure (Moosmang et al., 2003). Thus, inhibition of the vascular L-type Ca^{2+} channel results in significant reductions in blood pressure (Ghamami, Chiang, Dormuth, & Wright, 2014). The vascular L-type Ca^{2+} channel is composed of multiple subunits; however, the channel pore is located in the $Ca_v1.2\alpha1c$ subunit. CCBs also bind to residues within the channel pore (Hockerman, Peterson, Johnson, & Catterall, 1997; Nakayama & Kuniyasu, 1996). The $Ca_v1.2\alpha1c$ subunit is located on chromosome 12 and has 2703 identified alterations to the reference sequence to date (Table 5). 1721 of the alterations alter the protein sequence (Fig. 5). Due to CCBs interacting with the αlpha 1c subunit, only the αlpha 1c subunit was addressed in this manuscript.

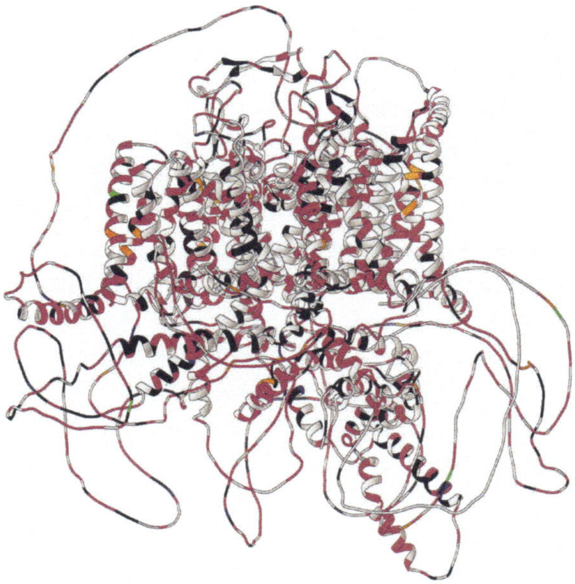

Fig. 5 AlphaFold model of $Ca_v1.2\alpha$ subunit colored to display protein-altering polymorphisms. The reference sequence is gray, and colors are sequentially applied to changes in protein sequence: (1) nsSNPs are magenta, (2) in-frame deletions and additions are blue, (3) protein-altering variants are green, (4) frameshifts are orange, and (5) nsSNPs resulting in a stop codon are black. The colors applied first are replaced by later changes if they occur at identical residues.

A few studies have identified patients that are non-responsive to CCBs and found multiple SNPs associated with diminished, or lack of, response (Bremer, Man, Kask, & Diamond, 2006; Kamide et al., 2009), and a SNP that tracks to specific treatment strategies (Beitelshees et al., 2009). The CCB binding site has been identified via crystallography, molecular modeling, and docking (Saddala, Kandimalla, Adi, Bhashyam, & Asupatri, 2017; Tang, Gamal El-Din, Lenaeus, Zheng, & Catterall, 2019), revealing that residues Ile 360, Ser 393, Asn 1179 (from the AlphaFold model), and Asn 740 are involved in dihydropine CCB binding. The I360V polymorphism may have minor effects on CCB binding, and there are multiple nsSNPs around Ser 393 and Asn 1179 that may alter dihydropine CCB interaction with the vascular L-type Ca^{2+} channel. For Diltiazem, the backbone of threonine in site 3 is important for binding. The corresponding threonine has an nsSNP that results in a methionine, which may alter the orientation of the protein backbone. Thus polymorphism within the ligand-binding site may result in altered CCB effects. Interestingly, not all of the SNPs identified in the clinical studies are within the binding site, the coding sequence, or even the alpha 1c subunit, strengthening the premise of this manuscript that all polymorphisms have the potential to alter drug effects.

3.4 NCC inhibitors

NCC inhibitors include the often prescribed hydrochlorothiazide, a thiazide drug class member, and the misnamed thiazide-like drugs that do not have a thiazide moiety. NCC inhibitors are the fourth most prescribed antihypertensive medication (Table 3) and are found co-formulated with multiple different antihypertensive medications. NCC, known as sodium-chloride cotransporter, officially named Solute carrier family 12 member 3 (SLC12A3), transports Na^+ and Cl^- from the distal tubule lumen into the cell and is responsible for $10.5\% \pm 1.8\%$ of the total filtered sodium load under standard sodium delivery to the distal tubule (Ellison, Velazquez, & Wright, 1987). NCC is located on chromosome 16 and has 1914 identified alterations to the reference sequence to date (Table 5). 1328 of the alterations alter the protein sequence (Fig. 6).

Polymorphisms in NCC are associated with Gitelman's syndrome (An, Liang, Zhang, & Su, 2016), and new polymorphisms associated with Gitelman's syndrome are still being discovered, suggesting that there may remain potential polymorphisms that can cause Gilerlman's syndrome

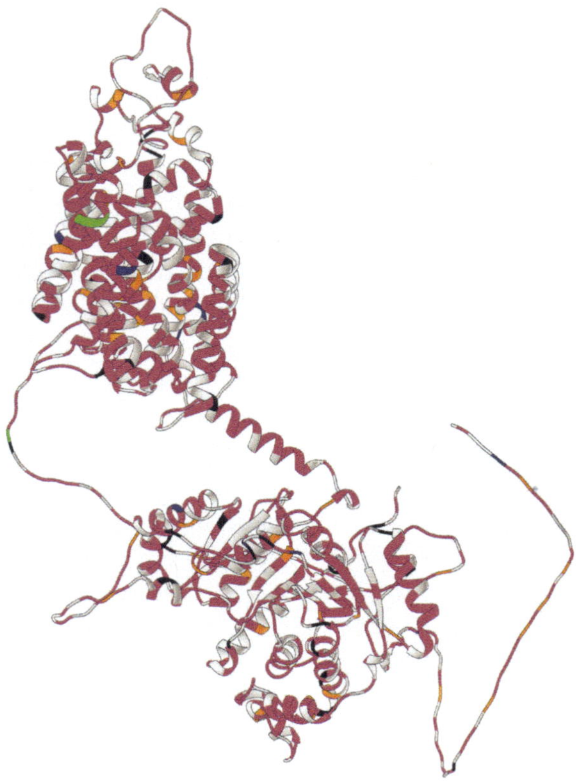

Fig. 6 AlphaFold model of NCC colored to display protein-altering polymorphisms. The reference sequence is gray, and colors are sequentially applied to changes in protein sequence: (1) nsSNPs are magenta, (2) in-frame deletions and additions are blue, (3) protein-altering variants are green, (4) frameshifts are orange, and (5) nsSNPs resulting in a stop codon are black. The colors applied first are replaced by later changes if they occur at identical residues.

(Wang, Chen, Yin, & Qiu, 2021; Zheng, Shang, Cai, Chen, & Li, 2021). Consequently, most genetic work is focused on Gitelman's syndrome. However, polymorphisms in NCC are associated with hypertension (An et al., 2016), and G264A is associated with a more significant loop diuretic effect (Vormfelde et al., 2007). Like most antihypertensive targets, few studies have examined the effect that polymorphisms of NCC have on the function of NCC inhibitors.

Furthermore, the binding site of NCC inhibitors is not fully elucidated; however, the binding site is between helixes 8 through 12 (Moreno et al., 2006). 19 nsSNPs and one insertion/deletion within this region may alter thiazide binding or effect. Additionally, alterations to glycosylation can increase thiazide binding (Hoover et al., 2003). However, these sites do not contain any known polymorphisms except frameshifts, which likely destroy NCC function. There is little information regarding polymorphisms in NCC that are not associated with Gitelman's syndrome.

3.5 ARBs

ARBs target the Angiotensin type 1 receptor (AT_1R) and are often prescribed (Table 3). The AT_1R is present in many tissues, including the brain, and although used primarily in cardiovascular and renal diseases, growing evidence suggests ARBs have further utility in diseases such as cancer (Coulson et al., 2017; Santala et al., 2020) and dementia (Li et al., 2010). The AT_1R gene is located on chromosome 3 and has 954 identified alterations to the reference sequence to date (Table 4). 282 alterations alter the protein sequence (Fig. 7), with multiple polymorphisms in the ligand-binding site (Zhang et al., 2015; Zhang et al., 2015).

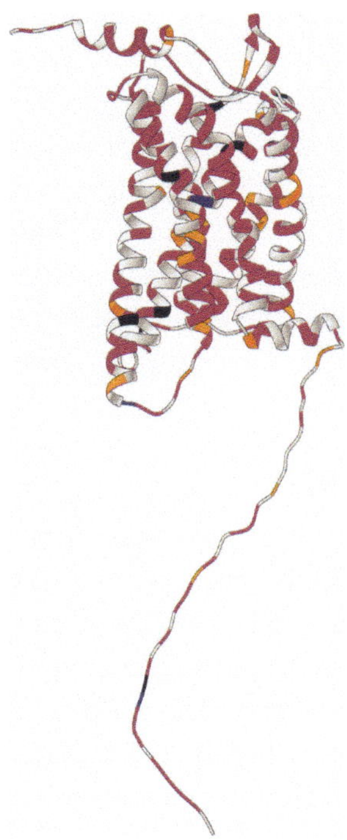

Fig. 7 AlphaFold model of the AT_1R colored to display protein-altering polymorphisms. The reference sequence is gray, and colors are sequentially applied to changes in protein sequence: (1) nsSNPs are magenta, (2) in-frame deletions and additions are blue, (3) frameshifts are orange, and (4) nsSNPs resulting in a stop codon are black. The colors applied first are replaced by later changes if they occur at identical residues.

Although there are numerous genetic studies of the AT_1R, few studies examine if polymorphisms alter ARB effects. A single study utilized a patient-derived nsSNP (A163T) to test the affinity of multiple ARBs (Arsenault et al., 2010). The threonine residue attenuated losartan and irbesartan binding but enhanced telmisartan binding while having no statistical effect on angiotensin II, valsartan, or candesartan binding, indicating that single changes can alter a subset of ligands. The AT_1R has been mutated to identify the ARB binding pocket (more times than cited here), but the mutations rarely match polymorphisms. When experimental mutations match polymorphisms, experimental, not clinical, ARBs were utilized (Ji, Leung, Zhang, Catt, & Sandberg, 1994; Ji, Zheng, Zhang, Catt, & Sandberg, 1995). As shown by Arsenault et al. and discussed in the introduction, affinity and drug effects are unique to a drug and receptor; any changes to either may alter drug affinity and effect. Therefore, experimental drugs may not predict clinically available drug effects. Molecular modeling has been used to predict ARB affinity (Anderson et al., 2020). However, some shortcomings prevent the direct application of the modeling data to the clinic. Like the β_1-AR, all the glycosylation sites within the AT_1R have an nsSNP that ablates glycosylation. In the AT_1R and the remaining G protein-coupled receptors (GPCRs) discussed, inhibition of glycosylation alters receptor trafficking. Specifically, single mutations to ablate glycosylation did not alter sarcosine^1-angiotensin II binding or signaling but are involved in receptor trafficking (Deslauriers et al., 1999). Collectively, the data is compelling that single alterations to the AT_1R sequence change ARB affinity, but little is known regarding identified polymorphisms.

3.6 NKCC2 inhibitors

NKCC2 inhibitors, called loop diuretics or water pills, target the Na^+:K^+:$2Cl^-$ symporter, officially called solute carrier family 12 member 1 (SLC12A1). NKCC2 is located in the loop of Henle. NKCC2 inhibitors are used primarily to reduce the extracellular fluid volume in cases of edema, chronic kidney disease, and heart failure; however, NKCC2 inhibitors will reduce blood pressure due to the decrease in volume (Malha & Mann, 2016). NKCC2 is located on chromosome 15 and has 1253 identified alterations to the reference sequence to date (Table 5). 853 Of the alterations alter the protein sequence (Fig. 8).

Polymorphisms in NKCC2 are primarily examined in Bartter's syndrome (Simon et al., 1996). Bartter's syndrome presents with hypokalaemic

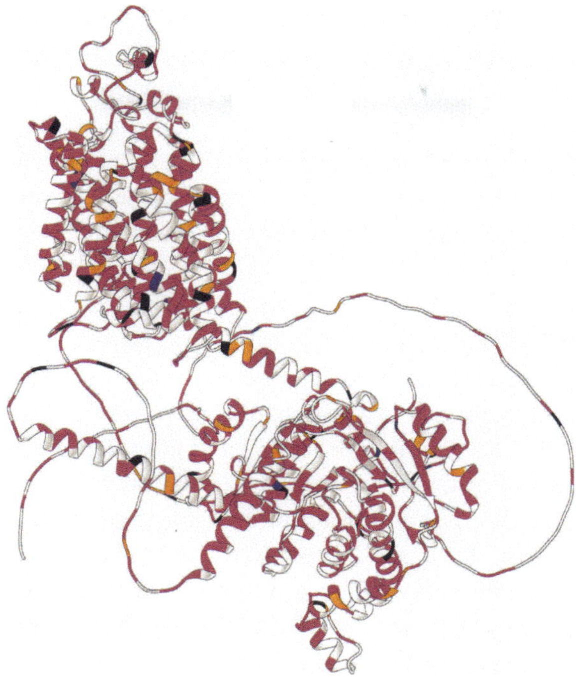

Fig. 8 AlphaFold model of NKCC2 colored to display protein-altering polymorphisms. The reference sequence is gray, and colors are sequentially applied to changes in protein sequence: (1) nsSNPs are magenta, (2) in-frame deletions and additions are blue, (3) frameshifts are orange, and (4) nsSNPs resulting in a stop codon are black. The colors applied first are replaced by later changes if they occur at identical residues.

alkalosis, which is a result of non-functional NKCC2. Few studies examine polymorphisms in NKCC2 affecting NKCC2 inhibitor function. Moreover, the limited polymorphisms studied within NKCC2 have not shown a direct effect on NKCC2 inhibitor function (Vormfelde et al., 2007; Vormfelde & Brockmoller, 2012). Modeling and mutagenesis studies indicate that alterations to transmembrane three of NKCC1 can alter the affinity (K_i) of bumetanide and furosemide (Somasekharan, Tanis, & Forbush, 2012). Translating the NKCC1 sequence to the NKCC2 AlphaFold model demonstrates a high degree of identity; however, the helix stretches longer than predicted, which may be an artifact of AlphaFold. Helix three of NKCC2 is predicted to be 35 amino acids long and contains 20 residues containing nsSNPs. None of the nsSNPs correspond to the cysteine and tryptophan mutations conducted. However, two residues examined by Somasekharan et al. that alter the K_i of the NKCC2 inhibitors are nsSNPs that introduce a lysine (I260K and N268K, corresponding to I368 and N376, respectively, in NKCC1). The two lysine residues may similarly alter binding due to the size and charge of lysine. Moreover, the AlphaFold modeled helix contains several nsSNPs that add a proline or change the charge, which could have similar effects on the K_i of NKCC2 inhibitors. As with most of the pharmacological targets discussed, further experimentation is necessary to draw clinically relevant conclusions.

3.7 α_1-AR blockers

Most α_1-AR antagonists are partially specific for two of the three subtypes: α_{1A}-AR, α_{1B}-AR, and α_{1D}-AR (Richardson, Donatucci, Page, Wilson, & Schwinn, 1997). The α_1-AR blockers are not considered first-line antihypertensive medications but are used for BPH, thus resulting in many prescriptions (Table 3). The three isoforms are located on chromosomes 8 (α_{1A}-AR), 5 (α_{1B}-AR), and 20 (α_{1D}-AR) and have 849, 952, and 1235 alterations to the reference sequence, respectively, to date (Table 4). The α_{1A}-, α_{1B}-, and α_{1D}-AR have 544, 405, and 648 alterations to the coding sequence, respectively (Fig. 9). It should be noted that there are discrepancies in the GRCh38.p13 assembly for parts of the α_{1A}-AR, but not α_{1B}-AR and α_{1D}-AR. The α_{1A}-AR sequence does not match the listed reference sequences at all points; therefore, the table and figure for the α_{1A}-AR should be used primarily for reference. The raw data (ENSG00000120907) should be used if the normal sequences in the GRCh38.p13 assembly match the accepted reference sequence.

The α_1-ARs are arguably the least studied of the nine adrenergic receptors. A few studies have examined the effect of α_1-ARs in disease, but few have examined polymorphisms in altering pharmacology. The data with polymorphisms and mutations are similar in that each alteration alters a subset of α_1-AR ligands. The α_{1A}-ARs nsSNP I200S reduces phentolamine affinity while having little effect on prazosin or agonist affinity. In contrast, the nsSNP V311I reduces agonist affinity but not phentolamine or prazosin (Lei et al., 2005). The α_{1A}-ARs nsSNPs I200S and V311I demonstrate the complex nature of polymorphisms. Agonist affinity should also be considered due to clinical drug efficacy being dependent, in part, on the ratio of the affinity of the endogenous agonist to the antagonist. Similar differential reductions in affinity are seen with antagonists, but not agonists, with mutations of F308 and F312 (Waugh et al., 2001). Residues 308 and 312 are indicated as sites of polymorphisms by the GRCh38.p13 assembly, but the normal residue is incorrect.

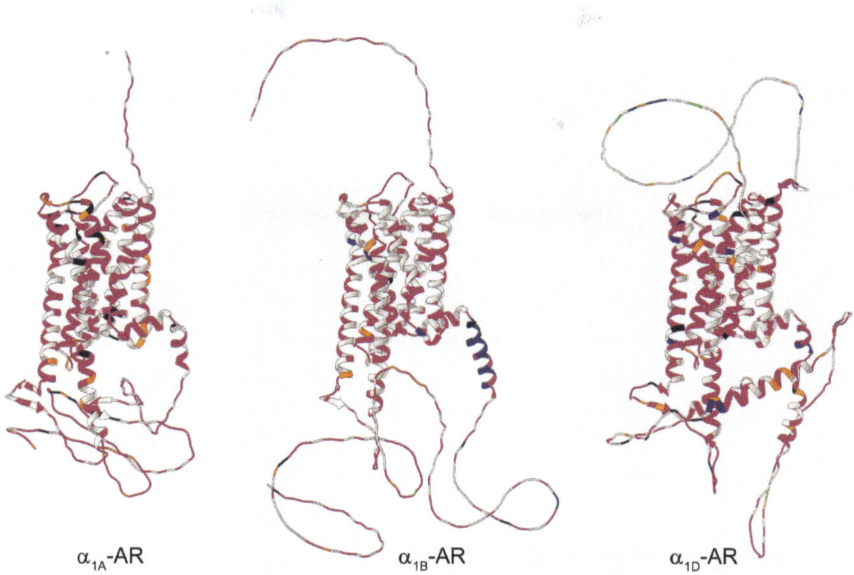

Fig. 9 AlphaFold models of the α_1-ARs aligned to each other and colored to display protein-altering polymorphisms. Discrepancies in the GRCh38.p13 assembly for a portion of the α_{1A}-AR, but not α_{1B}- and α_{1D}-AR, indicate that the α_{1A}-AR data should be viewed with caution. The reference sequence is gray, and colors are sequentially applied to changes in protein sequence: (1) nsSNPs are magenta, (2) in-frame deletions and additions are blue, (3) protein-altering variants are green, (4) frameshifts are orange, and (5) nsSNPs resulting in a stop codon are black. The colors applied first are replaced by later changes if they occur at identical residues.

Mutational studies of the α_{1B}-AR demonstrate that D125A, an nsSNP, drastically decreases the affinity for epinephrine and norepinephrine while decreasing the affinity for phentolamine but not prazosin (Porter, Hwa, & Perez, 1996). However, it is unlikely that patients with a D125A α_{1B}-AR would require an α_1-AR antagonist. Mutations of A204V and L314M in α_{1B}-AR convert agonist affinities similar to the α_{1A}-AR and individually result in constitutive active receptors (Hwa, Graham, & Perez, 1995, 1996). A204V is an nsSNP in the α_{1B}-AR, whereas L314V, not methionine, is also an nsSNP. Since phentolamine inhibits the constitutive activity of A204V (Hwa et al., 1996), patients carrying the A204V would likely benefit from phentolamine. Although other residues of the α_{1B}-AR alter antagonist affinity (Zhao, Hwa, & Perez, 1996), only G196R/E is an nsSNP. It is not clear what the addition of a charge will do to antagonist binding.

The α_{1D}-AR is much less studied than the other α_1-ARs. Unlike other α_1-ARs, the first 91 amino acids of the amino terminus of the α_{1D}-AR are cleaved. Mutation of the cleavage site to a series of bulky amino acids stopped the cleavage resulting in the expression of full-length α_{1D}-AR that has reduced agonist response (Kountz et al., 2016). Multiple in-frame deletions and nsSNPs around the cleavage site may abrogate cleavage; however, further experimentation is necessary. Alanine-based mutational studies of the α_{1D}-ARs indicate that D176, E237, and S258 are crucial for prazosin binding (Nagaoka et al., 2008). Based on the alanine mutagenesis, the α_{1D}-AR nsSNP D176G likely will not bind prazosin. Position 237 is the site of a frameshift, and the nsSNP E237K may abrogate binding due to a change in the change. Position 256 is the site of three nsSNPs (S258F/C/P) that may alter binding.

Molecular modeling of the α_{1A}-AR indicates that the binding sites for various antagonists are different, but include D106, C110, T111, R166, Q167, Q177, S188, S192, F193, S296, F312, F316 (Ishiguro et al., 2002; Pedretti, Elena Silva, Villa, & Vistoli, 2004). Of these 12 residues, five contain nsSNPs that may abrogate binding, and two contain a premature stop site that will ablate the α_{1A}-AR. Ishiguro et al. also examined the α_{1B}-AR and α_{1D}-AR. The antagonist binding sites in the α_{1B}-AR include D125, T130, K185, E186, S207, S211, and S318. Of these seven residues, three contain nsSNPs, which alters the charge of the residue, likely altering affinity. The antagonist binding sites in the α_{1D}-AR include D176, T181, K236, E237, S258, S262, and S372; however, a second modeling study indicates that (in updated numbering) D176, C180, W235, I248, F364, E381, and K385 are binding sites (Carrieri, Centeno, Rodrigo, Sanz, & Carotti, 2001). Of these 13 unique residues, eight contain nsSNPs, W235 is a premature stop site, and E237 and K385 are part of a frameshift. All but three nsSNPs change the charge or add/subtract significant bulk of the original residue, which would likely abrogate binding on the antagonists. The docking studies and the polymorphism studies strongly suggest that multiple nsSNPs will alter the affinity of α_1-AR antagonists but likely will not affect all ligands equally.

3.8 α_2-AR agonists

Although not first-line antihypertensive agents, α_2-AR agonists are often prescribed (Table 3). For hypertension, the α_{2A}-AR is specifically targeted, but most of the α_2-AR agonists target all three α_2-AR isoforms. Tizanidine is listed in Table 2 and is prescribed for muscle spasms associated with multiple sclerosis and neurological injury (Malanga, Reiter, & Garay, 2008); however, tizanidine does lower blood pressure, and blood pressure-lowering is a specific warning associated with the drug (Chaugai et al., 2019). The three isoforms are α_{2A}-, α_{2B}-, and α_{2C}-AR and are located on chromosomes 10, 2, and 4, respectively. The total number of reported polymorphisms is remarkably similar in the α_{2A}-AR and α_{2B}-AR at 1263 and 1284, respectively, but the α_{2C}-AR has 1575 identified polymorphisms (Table 4). The α_{2A}-, α_{2B}-, and α_{2C}-AR have 384, 453, and 759 polymorphisms, respectively, altering the protein sequence (Fig. 10).

As chronicled in each of the preceding sections, polymorphisms in the α_2-ARs are primarily examined in the context of disease, not pharmacogenomics. However, the D94N nsSNP (termed D79N in publications) of the α_{2A}-AR alters signaling and, when engineered into a mouse, prevents

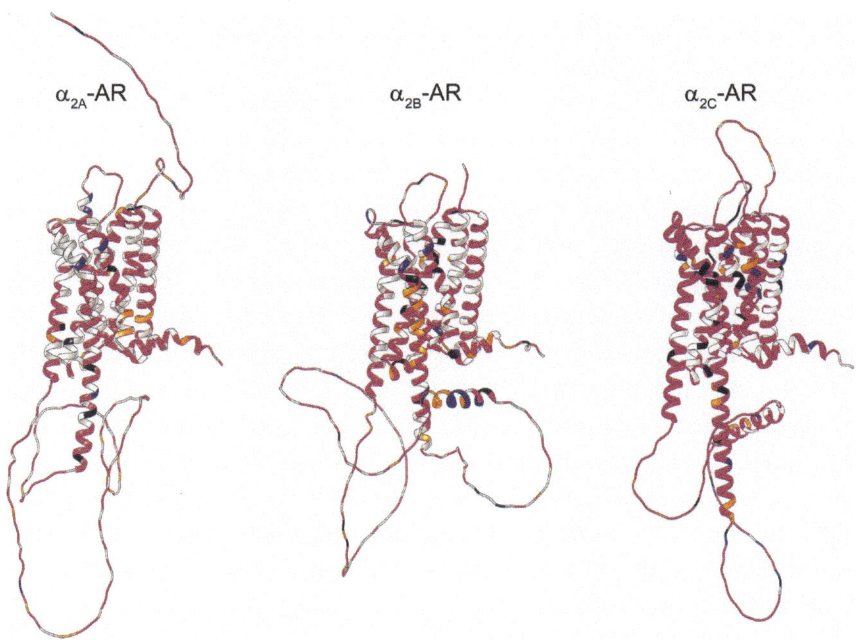

Fig. 10 AlphaFold models of the α_2-ARs aligned to each other and colored to display protein-altering polymorphisms. The α_{2C}-AR derived from the GRCh38.p13 assembly may have errors due to the appearance of two different proteins listed in the GRCh38.p13 assembly. Some single residues in the α_{2C}-AR GRCh38.p13 assembly are listed with two different wild-type amino acids, so the data cannot be easily untangled. The reference sequence is gray, and colors are sequentially applied to changes in protein sequence: (1) nsSNPs are magenta, (2) in-frame deletions and additions are blue, (3) protein-altering variants are green, (4) frameshifts are orange, and (5) nsSNPs resulting in a stop codon are black. The colors applied first are replaced by later changes if they occur at identical residues.

α_2-AR agonist-mediated reduction in blood pressure (MacMillan, Hein, Smith, Piascik, & Limbird, 1996; Surprenant, Horstman, Akbarali, & Limbird, 1992). D94 lies below the ligand-binding site according to the recent structures PDB:6KUY and 6KUX deposited on the Research Collaboratory for Structural Bioinformatics Protein Data Bank (RCSB PDB) site (Berman et al., 2000). Of the directly interacting α_{2A}-AR residues with the partial agonist (2∼{S})-4-fluoranyl-2-(1∼{H} -imidazol-5-yl)-1-propan-2-yl-2,3-dihydroindole three are nsSNPs sites: V129L, C132S, and S219Y. Aside from residues interacting with the partial agonist, numerous nsSNPs are lining the binding pocket. As shown with the AT_1R (Ji et al., 1994; Ji et al., 1995), changes distant from the binding pocket can also alter binding. The effects of distant polymorphisms can change the rotation of alpha helixes, which can alter the binding pocket. However, until tested, it is unknown how the clinically used agonists are affected by these polymorphisms.

The α_{2B}-AR has a string of 11 glutamic acid residues from residue 298 to 309 that also house six unique in-frame deletions. The residue 301–303 deletion, which corresponds to 300 to 303 in the GRCh38.p13 assembly, displays reduced agonist-mediated phosphorylation and consequently less desensitization in cells and people (Muszkat et al., 2010; Small, Brown, Forbes, & Liggett, 2001). It is likely that more than one of the deletions results in the same phenotype, but that has yet to be tested. The α_{2B}-AR agonist dexmedetomidine was used to capture a cryo-EM structure of the GPCR-G$\alpha\beta\gamma$ complex PDB:6K41 and 6K42 (Yuan et al., 2020). Of the six directly interacting residues, four residues are nsSNPs sites. All changes are rather drastic and will likely abrogate binding. W384 stop, Y416 stop, and a frameshift at V93 most likely result in a non-functional receptor. As with the α_{2A}-AR, the α_{2B}-AR binding pocket is surrounded by polymorphisms (Fig. 10). There are also polymorphisms in the transmembrane helixes, which may shift residues in the binding pocket (Fig. 10).

The α_{2C}-AR has an in-frame deletion involving residues 321–328 of the third intracellular loop that results in the deletion of the amino acids Gly-Ala-Gly-Pro. This deletion alters the efficacy and potency of multiple α_2-AR agonists (Small, Forbes, Rahman, Bridges, & Liggett, 2000), is found more frequently in African Americans (Feng et al., 2001), and has been linked to the altered clinical efficacy of bucindolol in heart failure patients (Bristow et al., 2010). According to the recent structure (PDB: 6KUW) of the α_{2C}-AR bound to the ligand (8Ar,12aS,13aR)-12-ethylsulfonyl-3-methoxy-5,6,8,8a,9,10,11,12a,13,13a-decahydroisoquinolino[2,1-g][1,6] naphthyridine deposited on the RCSB PDB site (Berman et al., 2000), the ligand directly interacts with eight residues. Due to errors in the GRCh38.p13 assembly, we can only positively identify four polymorphisms C135R, F398L, F399L, and F423L, all of which likely alter the ligand-binding pocket due to changes in charge and size. The data shown in Table 4 and Fig. 10 for the α_{2C}-AR may have errors from the GRCh38.p13 assembly. Thus, the data should be used only to display potential polymorphisms. In contrast, there are no problems with the GRCh38.p13 assembly of the α_{2A}-AR and α_{2B}-AR.

4. Future directions to functionalize personalized medicine

Personalized medicine can be described as medication that is specific to an individual's genetics. Therefore, in order to reach a point where personalized medicine is routinely practiced in the clinic, two changes are needed. First, genotyping will need to become more common. Second, experimental databases must be created to link each polymorphism within a receptor to drug affinity and action. Genotyping is not the focus of this manuscript. However, it is becoming less expensive, and multiple hospitals are offering, or conducting, whole-genome sequencing (Borrell, 2010; Marshall et al., 2020; Stranneheim et al., 2021). Although some groups are studying polymorphisms or mutating every amino acid in a receptor, a concerted pharmacogenomic examination of antihypertensive targets, or, more importantly, the entire pharmacopeia, is lacking. Therefore, future research into how known polymorphisms in drug targets alter drug effects is required to develop a program (an app) that will link a patient's genetic sequence to ideal drugs for that patient.

4.1 Modeling approaches

Molecular dynamics (MD) can be used to dock a flexible ligand to a mobile receptor and determine a relatively good approximation of ligand affinity (Lazim, Suh, & Choi, 2020). However, polymorphisms would have to be modeled without a ligand before docking the ligand. Unpublished data from our group demonstrates that modeling a single polymorphism in a GPCR from a wild-type structure takes 500 + ns of simulation time to reach equilibrium, on average; furthermore, it is not clear that the model is accurate. To circumvent this problem, AlphaFold may be able to predict the wild-type and polymorphic protein (Jumper et al., 2021), which would be very helpful as MD studies may not be able to push a wild-type structure over energy barriers to the polymorphic protein structure. However, such experiments with AlphaFold have yet to be published. Suppose AlphaFold can correctly predict the rotamer position of residues in an ordered structure. In that case, docking and MD studies can be initiated to determine ligand affinity, with the wild-type receptor used as a control. Such an approach answers most of the shorcomings discussed in modeling ARB affinity (Anderson et al., 2020). An AlphaFold-based MD approach may be appropriate for GPCRs as they are relatively small (less computational time) and function as monomers. However, for large multimeric proteins, such as $Ca_V1.2$, the complications of accurately modeling the protein-protein interactions in addition to the ligand-protein interactions make MD approaches challenging and less likely to be accurate due to the increased number of variables. Lastly, MD cannot model SNPs that do not alter the coding sequence, such as SNPs in the introns or sSNPs. Therefore, with current technology, MD studies are helpful for a subset of receptors and a subset of SNPs; however, all MD experiments should be confirmed with experimental results.

Similarly, data science-based approaches have successfully identified allosteric networks based on the crystal structures of inactive and active receptors (Venkatakrishnan et al., 2016). Furthermore, in conjunction with wet-lab studies, data sciences can be used to identify receptor regions involved in drug potency, efficacy, and drug potency and efficacy combined (Heydenreich et al., 2021). However, the limitation of these studies is that they rely on crystal structural comparison, and not all drug targets have representative structures, such as the lack of α_1-AR structures. Furthermore, crystalized drug targets with structures may not have all the subunits or structures of the active and inactive state. Perhaps cryo-EM or structure prediction will allow for the expanded application of data science-based approaches. However, as with MD experiments, wet-lab experimental results are required in data science-based approaches.

4.2 Experimental approaches

Given the vast number of polymorphisms that change the sequence of a receptor, high throughput systems are required. The system established by Jones et al. can be utilized to understand protein-altering SNPs-mediated alterations to the pharmacodynamics of prescribed drugs. Jones et al. mutated every residue of the β_2-AR to all possible residues and examined isoproterenol-mediated activity. The data provides mutation-dependent changes to the EC_{50} and E_{max} values of Isoproterenol (Jones et al., 2020). The addition of β-blockers would allow for the calculation of the K_i for each β-blocker matched to each polymorphism. Expanding this system for all drug targets would allow the measurement of polymorphism-dependent changes in EC_{50} and E_{max} for all agonists and K_i for all antagonists. Additionally, polymorphism-induced novel agonist properties can be examined by running the experiments with the drug alone (Hauser et al., 2018). However, expanding the system of Jones et al. to ion channels may pose a challenge, and such a system may not be feasible for enzymes. Therefore, further method development is necessary.

Activated receptors can display pluridimensional efficacy (Galandrin, Oligny-Longpre, & Bouvier, 2007), meaning a receptor can unequally signal to different signaling molecules. Due to an alteration in the allosteric network within the receptor, polymorphisms can change the signaling cascades. The new cascades may display an altered pluridimensional efficacy. Examination of pluridimensional efficacy requires multiple readouts (Galandrin et al., 2007), which can be obtained with multiple BRET sensors. Making all the receptors is time-consuming, but custom gene synthesis makes the process relatively simple. Additionally, adding receptor subunits to the cells allows for examining receptors with multiple subunits, such as ion channels. Furthermore, BRET sensors can be designed to recognize the product of enzymes. Although BRET sensor technology likely has broader utility, BRET sensors require multiple cell lines with a single receptor and one to two BRET sensors (Breton et al., 2010). Therefore, using BRET sensors to study polymorphisms in receptors will be significantly slower.

As more people undergo whole genome sequencing, the observance of novel and multiple polymorphisms in a single protein may increase. Assuming experimental systems for studying known polymorphisms are established, the novel patient data can be added to the experimental systems. Therefore, it is possible that rapid determination of K_i, EC_{50}, and E_{max} calculations can be achieved for every current and future drug to their respective protein-altering SNPs in a receptor.

Examining polymorphisms in the non-coding sequences is more challenging as cDNA expression constructs used in the assays discussed above are not appropriate. However, the non-coding changes are most likely to change receptor number, not receptor structure. Therefore, non-coding SNPs can be studied via CRISPR in either cells or a whole animal.

CRISPR-modified animal models may also prove to be essential for studying select polymorphisms that show either a gain of function or demonstrate pluridimensional efficacy. Polymorphisms leading to a gain of function are best exemplified by K235N and V302I mu-opioid receptors displaying increased efficacy of the weak partial agonist naloxone (Fukuda et al., 1998; Hauser et al., 2018). Many antagonists used in the clinic are not true antagonists but are incredibly weak partial agonists; therefore, it is possible that multiple drugs display increased efficacy in specific polymorphisms of a receptor that functionally turns a clinically identified antagonist into an agonist. Whole animal studies of such polymorphisms will allow for the safety of a drug-polymorphism combination to be thoroughly evaluated.

5. Conclusion

The majority of polymorphism in receptors to current antihypertensive drugs are not thoroughly studied. From the sample of studies discussed, it is clear that nsSNPs can alter drug effects. Most of the alterations to drug effects are likely going to be due to alterations in the affinity. For some drugs, this can be overcome by increasing the dosage of the drug; however, the dose changes may require a change in drug dispensing. To prescribe the optimum dose of a drug may require individualized compounding (packaging) by a pharmacist instead of standardized doses from the manufacturer. Many polymorphisms will be linked to diseases, as exemplified in genetic studies of specific diseases and the Framingham Heart Study (Surendran et al., 2020), which may, or may not, indicate that the receptor should be targeted to treat the disease. However, for personalized medicine to move from a buzzword to clinical practice, a concerted effort in examining the effect of polymorphisms on drug-receptor pairs is required. Such an effort will allow for tailored medication therapy for a patient that, in theory, should be better than current standards of care.

A move toward genomic-informed prescriptions will likely increase therapeutic effects and consequently reduce the consequences of the disease. In the current reimbursement climate, hospitals are paid for the quality of the care they provide, which is measured, in part, by keeping patients at goal and preventing their return to the hospital. A drug regimen tailored to a patient's genetics maximizes the likelihood that the drugs will be effective and the patient will remain controlled and out of the hospital. The design of the current reimbursement scheme is to reward providers for reducing medical costs. Therefore, moving to genomic-informed prescriptions has the potential to reduce overall healthcare costs.

Aside from a cost argument, moving toward genomic-informed prescriptions will aid in dealing with racial issues in prescribing drugs. A key example is an often and long-stated claim that African-Americans do not respond to β-blockers (Veiga & Taylor, 1986). Although there are race-based differences in antihypertensive therapies (Brewster & Seedat, 2013); the rationale for the differences remains unknown, but will be due to variables such as genetics, not a person's race, and may not apply to all members of a race or all conditions where a drug is used (Luzum et al., 2018). Moving toward genomic-informed prescriptions will also allow for the precise identification of non-responders. A priori prediction of the effectiveness of a drug will revolutionize race-based decisions, especially when a greater percentage of the population, at least in the United States, self-identifies as multi-racial.

Recent advances in science (detailed in this manuscript) allow for a comprehensive approach toward understanding the effects of polymorphisms in all proteins that interact with a drug or the drug target. Furthermore, the greater access to whole-genome sequencing and the reduced cost of sequencing facilitate the sequencing of more people. With more people being sequenced, more polymorphisms will be identified. As time progresses, more combinations of polymorphisms in a single protein will be identified. Thus, the goal of understanding how polymorphisms affect drug action will be an ongoing project that will continually obtain novel polymorphisms to examine. Therefore, there is an unmet and growing scientific need to understand how polymorphisms alter drug activity in patients. It is unclear if such an approach will be organized by a governmental agency, like the initial human genome project (Lander et al., 2001), which incidentally was recently completed (Nurk et al., 2021), or if companies will fill the void as Celera did to expedite the first draft human genome (Venter et al., 2001). As more data emerges regarding the effect of polymorphisms on clinical drug efficacy, there will be a move to translate the findings to patient care. The sooner a concerted effort is made to systematically examine how polymorphisms alter drug activity, the sooner the promises of personalized medicine will be realized.

Acknowledgments

Although acknowledged as authors, the data crunching by Dominique Brown and Heather Alcala to remove duplicates and categorize the GRCh38.p13 assembly was tremendously helpful; a few files totaled over 100,000 entries and were collated by hand.

Conflict of interest statement

The authors have no conflicts of interest to report.

References

Ahmed, S., Zhou, Z., Zhou, J., & Chen, S. Q. (2016). Pharmacogenomics of drug metabolizing enzymes and transporters: Relevance to precision medicine. *Genomics, Proteomics & Bioinformatics*, *14*(5), 298–313. https://doi.org/10.1016/j.gpb.2016.03.008.

Akif, M., Schwager, S. L., Anthony, C. S., Czarny, B., Beau, F., Dive, V., et al. (2011). Novel mechanism of inhibition of human angiotensin-I-converting enzyme (ACE) by a highly specific phosphinic tripeptide. *The Biochemical Journal*, *436*(1), 53–59. https://doi.org/10.1042/BJ20102123.

An, C., Liang, J., Zhang, K., & Su, X. (2016). Polymorphisms in the SLC12A3 gene encoding sodium-chloride cotransporter are associated with hypertension: A family-based study in the Mongolian population. *Kidney & Blood Pressure Research*, *41*(1), 18–28. https://doi.org/10.1159/000368543.

Anderson, S. D., Tabassum, A., Yeon, J. K., Sharma, G., Santos, P., Soong, T. H., et al. (2020). In silico prediction of ARB resistance: A first step in creating personalized ARB therapy. *PLoS Computational Biology*, *16*(11), e1007719. https://doi.org/10.1371/journal.pcbi.1007719.

Andresen, B. T., Rizzo, M. A., Shome, K., & Romero, G. (2002). The role of phosphatidic acid in the regulation of the Ras/MEK/Erk signaling cascade. *FEBS Letters*, *531*(1), 65–68 (Retrieved from PM:12401205).

Arsenault, J., Lehoux, J., Lanthier, L., Cabana, J., Guillemette, G., Lavigne, P., et al. (2010). A single-nucleotide polymorphism of alanine to threonine at position 163 of the human angiotensin II type 1 receptor impairs losartan affinity. *Pharmacogenetics and Genomics*, *20*(6), 377–388. https://doi.org/10.1097/FPC.0b013e32833a6d4a.

Asiimwe, I. G., Zhang, E. J., Osanlou, R., Jorgensen, A. L., & Pirmohamed, M. (2021). Warfarin dosing algorithms: A systematic review. *British Journal of Clinical Pharmacology*, *87*(4), 1717–1729. https://doi.org/10.1111/bcp.14608.

Bartoszewski, R. A., Jablonsky, M., Bartoszewska, S., Stevenson, L., Dai, Q., Kappes, J., et al. (2010). A synonymous single nucleotide polymorphism in DeltaF508 CFTR alters the secondary structure of the mRNA and the expression of the mutant protein. *The Journal of Biological Chemistry*, *285*(37), 28741–28748. https://doi.org/10.1074/jbc.M110.154575.

Beitelshees, A. L., Navare, H., Wang, D., Gong, Y., Wessel, J., Moss, J. I., et al. (2009). CACNA1C gene polymorphisms, cardiovascular disease outcomes, and treatment response. *Circulation. Cardiovascular Genetics*, *2*(4), 362–370. https://doi.org/10.1161/CIRCGENETICS.109.857839.

Berman, H. M., Westbrook, J., Feng, Z., Gilliland, G., Bhat, T. N., Weissig, H., et al. (2000). The Protein Data Bank. *Nucleic Acids Research*, *28*(1), 235–242. https://doi.org/10.1093/nar/28.1.235.

Bienfait, K., Chhibber, A., Marshall, J. C., Armstrong, M., Cox, C., Shaw, P. M., et al. (2021). Current challenges and opportunities for pharmacogenomics: Perspective of the industry pharmacogenomics working group (I-PWG). *Human Genetics*. https://doi.org/10.1007/s00439-021-02282-3.

Bonnardeaux, A., Davies, E., Jeunemaitre, X., Fery, I., Charru, A., Clauser, E., et al. (1994). Angiotensin II type 1 receptor gene polymorphisms in human essential hypertension. *Hypertension*, *24*(1), 63–69.

Borrell, B. (2010). US clinics quietly embrace whole-genome sequencing. *Nature*. https://doi.org/10.1038/news.2010.465.

Brás, N. F., Fernandes, P. A., & Ramos, M. J. (2014). QM/MM study and MD simulations on the hypertension regulator angiotensin-converting enzyme. *ACS Catalysis*, *4*(8), 2587–2597. https://doi.org/10.1021/cs500093h.

Bremer, T., Man, A., Kask, K., & Diamond, C. (2006). CACNA1C polymorphisms are associated with the efficacy of calcium channel blockers in the treatment of hypertension. *Pharmacogenomics*, 7(3), 271–279. https://doi.org/10.2217/14622416.7.3.271.

Breton, B., Sauvageau, E., Zhou, J., Bonin, H., Le Gouill, C., & Bouvier, M. (2010). Multiplexing of multicolor bioluminescence resonance energy transfer. *Biophysical Journal*, *99*(12), 4037–4046. https://doi.org/10.1016/j.bpj.2010.10.025.

Brewster, L. M., & Seedat, Y. K. (2013). Why do hypertensive patients of African ancestry respond better to calcium blockers and diuretics than to ACE inhibitors and beta-adrenergic blockers? A systematic review. *BMC Medicine*, *11*, 141. https://doi.org/10.1186/1741-7015-11-141.

Bristow, M. R., Murphy, G. A., Krause-Steinrauf, H., Anderson, J. L., Carlquist, J. F., Thaneemit-Chen, S., et al. (2010). An alpha2C-adrenergic receptor polymorphism alters the norepinephrine-lowering effects and therapeutic response of the beta-blocker bucindolol in chronic heart failure. *Circulation. Heart Failure*, *3*(1), 21–28. https://doi.org/10.1161/CIRCHEARTFAILURE.109.885962.

Caine, M. (1986). The present role of alpha-adrenergic blockers in the treatment of benign prostatic hypertrophy. *The Journal of Urology*, *136*(1), 1–4. https://doi.org/10.1016/s0022-5347(17)44709-4.

Carrieri, A., Centeno, N. B., Rodrigo, J., Sanz, F., & Carotti, A. (2001). Theoretical evidence of a salt bridge disruption as the initiating process for the alpha1d-adrenergic receptor activation: A molecular dynamics and docking study. *Proteins*, *43*(4), 382–394.

Chandra, S., Narang, R., Sreenivas, V., Bhatia, J., Saluja, D., & Srivastava, K. (2014). Association of angiotensin II type 1 receptor (A1166C) gene polymorphism and its increased expression in essential hypertension: A case-control study. *PLoS One*, *9*(7), e101502. https://doi.org/10.1371/journal.pone.0101502.

Chaugai, S., Dickson, A. L., Shuey, M. M., Feng, Q., Barker, K. A., Wei, W. Q., et al. (2019). Co-prescription of strong CYP1A2 inhibitors and the risk of Tizanidine-associated hypotension: A retrospective cohort study. *Clinical Pharmacology and Therapeutics*, *105*(3), 703–709. https://doi.org/10.1002/cpt.1233.

Coulson, R., Liew, S. H., Connelly, A. A., Yee, N. S., Deb, S., Kumar, B., et al. (2017). The angiotensin receptor blocker, losartan, inhibits mammary tumor development and progression to invasive carcinoma. *Oncotarget*, *8*(12), 18640–18656. https://doi.org/10.18632/oncotarget.15553.

Cozier, G. E., Schwager, S. L., Sharma, R. K., Chibale, K., Sturrock, E. D., & Acharya, K. R. (2018). Crystal structures of sampatrilat and sampatrilat-asp in complex with human ACE - a molecular basis for domain selectivity. *The FEBS Journal*, *285*(8), 1477–1490. https://doi.org/10.1111/febs.14421.

Deslauriers, B., Ponce, C., Lombard, C., Larguier, R., Bonnafous, J. C., & Marie, J. (1999). N-glycosylation requirements for the AT1a angiotensin II receptor delivery to the plasma membrane. *The Biochemical Journal*, *339*(Pt 2), 397–405.

Dorn, G. W., 2nd, & Liggett, S. B. (2008). Pharmacogenomics of beta-adrenergic receptors and their accessory signaling proteins in heart failure. *Clinical and Translational Science*, *1*(3), 255–262. https://doi.org/10.1111/j.1752-8062.2008.00059.x.

El Desoky, E. S., Derendorf, H., & Klotz, U. (2006). Variability in response to cardiovascular drugs. *Current Clinical Pharmacology*, *1*(1), 35–46. https://doi.org/10.2174/157488406775268273.

Ellison, D. H., Velazquez, H., & Wright, F. S. (1987). Thiazide-sensitive sodium chloride cotransport in early distal tubule. *The American Journal of Physiology*, *253*(3 Pt 2), F546–F554. https://doi.org/10.1152/ajprenal.1987.253.3.F546.

Fang, L., Geng, M., Liu, C., Wang, J., Min, W., & Liu, J. (2019). Structural and molecular basis of angiotensin-converting enzyme by computational modeling: Insights into the mechanisms of different inhibitors. *PLoS One*, *14*(4), e0215609. https://doi.org/10.1371/journal.pone.0215609.

Feng, J., Zheng, J., Gelernter, J., Kranzler, H., Cook, E., Goldman, D., et al. (2001). An in-frame deletion in the alpha(2C) adrenergic receptor is common in African--Americans. *Molecular Psychiatry*, *6*(2), 168–172. https://doi.org/10.1038/sj.mp.4000817.

Fernandes, D. D., Neale, C., Gomes, G. W., Li, Y., Malik, A., Pandey, A., et al. (2021). Ligand modulation of the conformational dynamics of the A2A adenosine receptor revealed by single-molecule fluorescence. *Scientific Reports*, *11*(1), 5910. https://doi.org/10.1038/s41598-021-84069-0.

Filigheddu, F., Reid, J. E., Troffa, C., PinnaParpaglia, P., Argiolas, G., Testa, A., et al. (2004). Genetic polymorphisms of the beta-adrenergic system: Association with essential hypertension and response to beta-blockade. *The Pharmacogenomics Journal*, *4*(3), 154–160. https://doi.org/10.1038/sj.tpj.6500247.

Fukuda, K., Kato, S., Shoda, T., Morikawa, H., Mima, H., & Mori, K. (1998). Partial agonistic activity of naloxone on the opioid receptors expressed from complementary deoxyribonucleic acids in Chinese hamster ovary cells. *Anesthesia and Analgesia*, *87*(2), 450–455. https://doi.org/10.1097/00000539-199808000-00041.

Gage, B. F. (2016). *WarfarinDosing Version 3.0*. Retrieved from http://www.warfarindosing.org.

Gage, B. F., Bass, A. R., Lin, H., Woller, S. C., Stevens, S. M., Al-Hammadi, N., et al. (2017). Effect of genotype-guided warfarin dosing on clinical events and anticoagulation control among patients undergoing hip or knee arthroplasty: The GIFT randomized clinical trial. *JAMA*, *318*(12), 1115–1124. https://doi.org/10.1001/jama.2017.11469.

Galandrin, S., Oligny-Longpre, G., & Bouvier, M. (2007). The evasive nature of drug efficacy: Implications for drug discovery. *Trends in Pharmacological Sciences*, *28*(8), 423–430. https://doi.org/10.1016/j.tips.2007.06.005.

Ghamami, N., Chiang, S. H., Dormuth, C., & Wright, J. M. (2014). Time course for blood pressure lowering of dihydropyridine calcium channel blockers. *Cochrane Database of Systematic Reviews*, *8*. https://doi.org/10.1002/14651858.CD010052.pub2. CD010052.

Harrap, S. B., Tzourio, C., Cambien, F., Poirier, O., Raoux, S., Chalmers, J., et al. (2003). The ACE gene I/D polymorphism is not associated with the blood pressure and cardiovascular benefits of ACE inhibition. *Hypertension*, *42*(3), 297–303. https://doi.org/10.1161/01.HYP.0000088322.85804.96.

Hauser, A. S., Chavali, S., Masuho, I., Jahn, L. J., Martemyanov, K. A., Gloriam, D. E., et al. (2018). Pharmacogenomics of GPCR drug targets. *Cell*, *172*(1–2), 41–54 e19. https://doi.org/10.1016/j.cell.2017.11.033.

Heydenreich, F. M., Marti-Solano, M., Sandhu, M., Kobilka, B. K., Bouvier, M., & Babu, M. M. (2021). Dissecting the allosteric networks governing agonist efficacy and potency in G protein-coupled receptors. *bioRxiv*.

Hockerman, G. H., Peterson, B. Z., Johnson, B. D., & Catterall, W. A. (1997). Molecular determinants of drug binding and action on L-type calcium channels. *Annual Review of Pharmacology and Toxicology*, *37*, 361–396. https://doi.org/10.1146/annurev.pharmtox.37.1.361.

Hoover, R. S., Poch, E., Monroy, A., Vazquez, N., Nishio, T., Gamba, G., et al. (2003). N-glycosylation at two sites critically alters thiazide binding and activity of the rat thiazide-sensitive Na(+):Cl(−) cotransporter. *Journal of the American Society of Nephrology*, *14*(2), 271–282. https://doi.org/10.1097/01.asn.0000043903.93452.d0.

Howe, K. L., Achuthan, P., Allen, J., Allen, J., Alvarez-Jarreta, J., Amode, M. R., et al. (2021). Ensembl 2021. *Nucleic Acids Research*, *49*(D1), D884–D891. https://doi.org/10.1093/nar/gkaa942.

Hunter, S. A., & Cochran, J. R. (2016). Cell-binding assays for determining the affinity of protein-protein interactions: Technologies and considerations. *Methods in Enzymology, 580*, 21–44. https://doi.org/10.1016/bs.mie.2016.05.002.

Hwa, J., Graham, R. M., & Perez, D. M. (1995). Identification of critical determinants of alpha 1-adrenergic receptor subtype selective agonist binding. *The Journal of Biological Chemistry, 270*(39), 23189–23195. https://doi.org/10.1074/jbc.270.39.23189.

Hwa, J., Graham, R. M., & Perez, D. M. (1996). Chimeras of alpha1-adrenergic receptor subtypes identify critical residues that modulate active state isomerization. *The Journal of Biological Chemistry, 271*(14), 7956–7964. https://doi.org/10.1074/jbc.271.14.7956.

Illing, M. E., Rajan, R. S., Bence, N. F., & Kopito, R. R. (2002). A rhodopsin mutant linked to autosomal dominant retinitis pigmentosa is prone to aggregate and interacts with the ubiquitin proteasome system. *The Journal of Biological Chemistry, 277*(37), 34150–34160. https://doi.org/10.1074/jbc.M204955200.

Ishiguro, M., Futabayashi, Y., Ohnuki, T., Ahmed, M., Muramatsu, I., & Nagatomo, T. (2002). Identification of binding sites of prazosin, tamsulosin and KMD-3213 with alpha(1)-adrenergic receptor subtypes by molecular modeling. *Life Sciences, 71*(21), 2531–2541. https://doi.org/10.1016/s0024-3205(02)02077-5.

Ji, H., Leung, M., Zhang, Y., Catt, K. J., & Sandberg, K. (1994). Differential structural requirements for specific binding of nonpeptide and peptide antagonists to the AT1 angiotensin receptor. Identification of amino acid residues that determine binding of the antihypertensive drug losartan. *Journal of Biological Chemistry, 269*(24), 16533–16536 (Retrieved from PM:8206967).

Ji, H., Zheng, W., Zhang, Y., Catt, K. J., & Sandberg, K. (1995). Genetic transfer of a nonpeptide antagonist binding site to a previously unresponsive angiotensin receptor. *Proceedings of the National Academy of Sciences of the United States of America, 92*(20), 9240–9244.

Johnson, J. A., Caudle, K. E., Gong, L., Whirl-Carrillo, M., Stein, C. M., Scott, S. A., et al. (2017). Clinical pharmacogenetics implementation consortium (CPIC) guideline for pharmacogenetics-guided warfarin dosing: 2017 update. *Clinical Pharmacology and Therapeutics, 102*(3), 397–404. https://doi.org/10.1002/cpt.668.

Jones, E. M., Lubock, N. B., Venkatakrishnan, A. J., Wang, J., Tseng, A. M., Paggi, J. M., et al. (2020). Structural and functional characterization of G protein-coupled receptors with deep mutational scanning. *eLife, 9*. https://doi.org/10.7554/eLife.54895.

Jorgensen, A. L., Prince, C., Fitzgerald, G., Hanson, A., Downing, J., Reynolds, J., et al. (2019). Implementation of genotype-guided dosing of warfarin with point-of-care genetic testing in three UK clinics: A matched cohort study. *BMC Medicine, 17*(1), 76. https://doi.org/10.1186/s12916-019-1308-7.

Jumper, J., Evans, R., Pritzel, A., Green, T., Figurnov, M., Ronneberger, O., et al. (2021). Highly accurate protein structure prediction with AlphaFold. *Nature*. https://doi.org/10.1038/s41586-021-03819-2.

Kamide, K., Yang, J., Matayoshi, T., Takiuchi, S., Horio, T., Yoshii, M., et al. (2009). Genetic polymorphisms of L-type calcium channel alpha1C and alpha1D subunit genes are associated with sensitivity to the antihypertensive effects of L-type dihydropyridine calcium-channel blockers. *Circulation Journal, 73*(4), 732–740. https://doi.org/10.1253/circj.cj-08-0761.

Kane, S. P. (2020). *The Top 300 of 2021, ClinCalc DrugStats Database, Version 21.1*. Retrieved from https://clincalc.com/DrugStats/Top300Drugs.aspx.

Kangelaris, K. N., Bent, S., Nussbaum, R. L., Garcia, D. A., & Tice, J. A. (2009). Genetic testing before anticoagulation? A systematic review of pharmacogenetic dosing of warfarin. *Journal of General Internal Medicine, 24*(5), 656–664. https://doi.org/10.1007/s11606-009-0949-1.

Kirchner, S., Cai, Z., Rauscher, R., Kastelic, N., Anding, M., Czech, A., et al. (2017). Alteration of protein function by a silent polymorphism linked to tRNA abundance. *PLoS Biology, 15*(5), e2000779. https://doi.org/10.1371/journal.pbio.2000779.

Kohlstedt, K., Gershome, C., Friedrich, M., Muller-Esterl, W., Alhenc-Gelas, F., Busse, R., et al. (2006). Angiotensin-converting enzyme (ACE) dimerization is the initial step in the ACE inhibitor-induced ACE signaling cascade in endothelial cells. *Molecular Pharmacology, 69*(5), 1725–1732. https://doi.org/10.1124/mol.105.020636.

Kohlstedt, K., Kellner, R., Busse, R., & Fleming, I. (2006). Signaling via the angiotensin-converting enzyme results in the phosphorylation of the nonmuscle myosin heavy chain IIA. *Molecular Pharmacology, 69*(1), 19–26. https://doi.org/10.1124/mol.105.016733.

Kohlstedt, K., Shoghi, F., Muller-Esterl, W., Busse, R., & Fleming, I. (2002). CK2 phosphorylates the angiotensin-converting enzyme and regulates its retention in the endothelial cell plasma membrane. *Circulation Research, 91*(8), 749–756. https://doi.org/10.1161/01.res.0000038114.17939.c8.

Kountz, T. S., Lee, K. S., Aggarwal-Howarth, S., Curran, E., Park, J. M., Harris, D. A., et al. (2016). Endogenous N-terminal domain cleavage modulates alpha1D-adrenergic receptor pharmacodynamics. *The Journal of Biological Chemistry, 291*(35), 18210–18221. https://doi.org/10.1074/jbc.M116.729517.

Lander, E. S., Linton, L. M., Birren, B., Nusbaum, C., Zody, M. C., Baldwin, J., et al. (2001). Initial sequencing and analysis of the human genome. *Nature, 409*(6822), 860–921.

Lazim, R., Suh, D., & Choi, S. (2020). Advances in molecular dynamics simulations and enhanced sampling methods for the study of protein systems. *International Journal of Molecular Sciences, 21*(17). https://doi.org/10.3390/ijms21176339.

Lei, B., Morris, D. P., Smith, M. P., Svetkey, L. P., Newman, M. F., Rotter, J. I., et al. (2005). Novel human alpha1a-adrenoceptor single nucleotide polymorphisms alter receptor pharmacology and biological function. *Naunyn-Schmiedeberg's Archives of Pharmacology, 371*(3), 229–239. https://doi.org/10.1007/s00210-005-1019-9.

Levin, M. C., Marullo, S., Muntaner, O., Andersson, B., & Magnusson, Y. (2002). The myocardium-protective Gly-49 variant of the beta 1-adrenergic receptor exhibits constitutive activity and increased desensitization and down-regulation. *The Journal of Biological Chemistry, 277*(34), 30429–30435. https://doi.org/10.1074/jbc.M200681200.

Li, S. C., Goto, N. K., Williams, K. A., & Deber, C. M. (1996). Alpha-helical, but not beta-sheet, propensity of proline is determined by peptide environment. *Proceedings of the National Academy of Sciences of the United States of America, 93*(13), 6676–6681. https://doi.org/10.1073/pnas.93.13.6676.

Li, N. C., Lee, A., Whitmer, R. A., Kivipelto, M., Lawler, E., Kazis, L. E., et al. (2010). Use of angiotensin receptor blockers and risk of dementia in a predominantly male population: Prospective cohort analysis. *BMJ, 340*, b5465. https://doi.org/10.1136/bmj.b5465.

Lim, G. B. (2017). Warfarin: From rat poison to clinical use. *Nature Reviews. Cardiology*. https://doi.org/10.1038/nrcardio.2017.172.

Linkins, L. A., Choi, P. T., & Douketis, J. D. (2003). Clinical impact of bleeding in patients taking oral anticoagulant therapy for venous thromboembolism: A meta-analysis. *Annals of Internal Medicine, 139*(11), 893–900. https://doi.org/10.7326/0003-4819-139-11-200312020-00007.

Luzum, J. A., Peterson, E., Li, J., She, R., Gui, H., Liu, B., et al. (2018). Race and Beta-blocker survival benefit in patients with heart failure: An investigation of self-reported race and proportion of African genetic ancestry. *Journal of the American Heart Association*, 7(10). https://doi.org/10.1161/JAHA.117.007956.

MacMillan, L. B., Hein, L., Smith, M. S., Piascik, M. T., & Limbird, L. E. (1996). Central hypotensive effects of the alpha2a-adrenergic receptor subtype. *Science, 273*(5276), 801–803. https://doi.org/10.1126/science.273.5276.801.

Malanga, G., Reiter, R. D., & Garay, E. (2008). Update on tizanidine for muscle spasticity and emerging indications. *Expert Opinion on Pharmacotherapy*, *9*(12), 2209–2215. https://doi.org/10.1517/14656566.9.12.2209.

Malha, L., & Mann, S. J. (2016). Loop diuretics in the treatment of hypertension. *Current Hypertension Reports*, *18*(4), 27. https://doi.org/10.1007/s11906-016-0636-7.

Marshall, C. R., Bick, D., Belmont, J. W., Taylor, S. L., Ashley, E., Dimmock, D., et al. (2020). The Medical Genome initiative: Moving whole-genome sequencing for rare disease diagnosis to the clinic. *Genome Medicine*, *12*(1), 48. https://doi.org/10.1186/s13073-020-00748-z.

Moosmang, S., Schulla, V., Welling, A., Feil, R., Feil, S., Wegener, J. W., et al. (2003). Dominant role of smooth muscle L-type calcium channel Cav1.2 for blood pressure regulation. *EMBO Journal*, *22*(22), 6027–6034. https://doi.org/10.1093/emboj/cdg583.

Moreno, E., Cristobal, P. S., Rivera, M., Vazquez, N., Bobadilla, N. A., & Gamba, G. (2006). Affinity-defining domains in the Na-cl cotransporter: A different location for cl- and thiazide binding. *The Journal of Biological Chemistry*, *281*(25), 17266–17275. https://doi.org/10.1074/jbc.M602614200.

Morningstar-Kywi, N., Haworth, I. S., & Mosley, S. A. (2021). Ligand-specific pharmacogenetic effects of nonsynonymous mutations. *Pharmacogenetics and Genomics*, *31*(4), 75–82. https://doi.org/10.1097/FPC.0000000000000424.

Muszkat, M., Kurnik, D., Sofowora, G. G., Solus, J., Xie, H. G., Harris, P. A., et al. (2010). Desensitization of vascular response in vivo: Contribution of genetic variation in the [alpha]2B-adrenergic receptor subtype. *Journal of Hypertension*, *28*(2), 278–284. https://doi.org/10.1097/HJH.0b013e328333d212.

Nagaoka, Y., Ahmed, M., Hossain, M., Bhuiyan, M. A., Ishiguro, M., Nakamura, T., et al. (2008). Amino acids of the human alpha1d-adrenergic receptor involved in antagonist binding. *Journal of Pharmacological Sciences*, *106*(1), 114–120. https://doi.org/10.1254/jphs.fp0071412.

Nakayama, H., & Kuniyasu, A. (1996). Identification of binding sites for calcium channel antagonists. *Japanese Heart Journal*, *37*(5), 643–650. https://doi.org/10.1536/ihj.37.643.

Nurk, S., Koren, S., Rhie, A., Rautiainen, M., Bzikadze, A. V., Mikheenko, A., et al. (2021). The complete sequence of a human genome. *bioRxiv*.

Park, M., Reddy, G. R., Wallukat, G., Xiang, Y. K., & Steinberg, S. F. (2017). beta1-adrenergic receptor O-glycosylation regulates N-terminal cleavage and signaling responses in cardiomyocytes. *Scientific Reports*, 7(1), 7890. https://doi.org/10.1038/s41598-017-06607-z.

Pedretti, A., Elena Silva, M., Villa, L., & Vistoli, G. (2004). Binding site analysis of full-length alpha1a adrenergic receptor using homology modeling and molecular docking. *Biochemical and Biophysical Research Communications*, *319*(2), 493–500. https://doi.org/10.1016/j.bbrc.2004.04.149.

Porter, J. E., Hwa, J., & Perez, D. M. (1996). Activation of the alpha1b-adrenergic receptor is initiated by disruption of an interhelical salt bridge constraint. *The Journal of Biological Chemistry*, *271*(45), 28318–28323. https://doi.org/10.1074/jbc.271.45.28318.

Qian, X., Xu, D., Liu, H., Lin, X., Yu, Y., Kang, J., et al. (2017). Genetic variants in 5p13.2 and 7q21.1 are associated with treatment for benign prostatic hyperplasia with the alpha-adrenergic receptor antagonist. *The Aging Male*, *20*(4), 250–256. https://doi.org/10.1080/13685538.2017.1358261.

Rathz, D. A., Brown, K. M., Kramer, L. A., & Liggett, S. B. (2002). Amino acid 49 polymorphisms of the human beta1-adrenergic receptor affect agonist-promoted trafficking. *Journal of Cardiovascular Pharmacology*, *39*(2), 155–160. https://doi.org/10.1097/00005344-200202000-00001.

Ravvaz, K., Weissert, J. A., Ruff, C. T., Chi, C. L., & Tonellato, P. J. (2017). Personalized anticoagulation: Optimizing warfarin management using genetics and simulated clinical trials. *Circulation. Cardiovascular Genetics*, *10*(6). https://doi.org/10.1161/CIRCGENETICS.117.001804.

Richardson, C. D., Donatucci, C. F., Page, S. O., Wilson, K. H., & Schwinn, D. A. (1997). Pharmacology of tamsulosin: Saturation-binding isotherms and competition analysis using cloned alpha 1-adrenergic receptor subtypes. *Prostate*, *33*(1), 55–59. https://doi.org/10.1002/(sici)1097-0045(19970915)33:1<55::aid-pros9>3.0.co;2-8.

Rigat, B., Hubert, C., Alhenc-Gelas, F., Cambien, F., Corvol, P., & Soubrier, F. (1990). An insertion/deletion polymorphism in the angiotensin I-converting enzyme gene accounting for half the variance of serum enzyme levels. *The Journal of Clinical Investigation*, *86*(4), 1343–1346. https://doi.org/10.1172/JCI114844.

Riordan, J. F. (2003). Angiotensin-I-converting enzyme and its relatives. *Genome Biology*, *4*(8), 225. https://doi.org/10.1186/gb-2003-4-8-225.

Saddala, M. S., Kandimalla, R., Adi, P. J., Bhashyam, S. S., & Asupatri, U. R. (2017). Novel 1, 4-dihydropyridines for L-type calcium channel as antagonists for cadmium toxicity. *Scientific Reports*, 7, 45211. https://doi.org/10.1038/srep45211.

Saliba, R. S., Munro, P. M., Luthert, P. J., & Cheetham, M. E. (2002). The cellular fate of mutant rhodopsin: Quality control, degradation and aggresome formation. *Journal of Cell Science*, *115*(Pt 14), 2907–2918.

Sanchez-Soto, M., Verma, R. K., Willette, B. K. A., Gonye, E. C., Moore, A. M., Moritz, A. E., et al. (2020). A structural basis for how ligand binding site changes can allosterically regulate GPCR signaling and engender functional selectivity. *Science Signaling*, *13*(617). https://doi.org/10.1126/scisignal.aaw5885.

Sandilands, A. J., & O'Shaughnessy, K. M. (2005). The functional significance of genetic variation within the beta-adrenoceptor. *British Journal of Clinical Pharmacology*, *60*(3), 235–243. https://doi.org/10.1111/j.1365-2125.2005.02438.x.

Santala, E. E. E., Murto, M. O., Artama, M., Pukkala, E., Visvanathan, K., & Murtola, T. J. (2020). Angiotensin receptor blockers associated with improved breast Cancer survival-a Nationwide cohort study from Finland. *Cancer Epidemiology, Biomarkers & Prevention*, *29*(11), 2376–2382. https://doi.org/10.1158/1055-9965.EPI-20-0711.

Sayed-Tabatabaei, F. A., Oostra, B. A., Isaacs, A., van Duijn, C. M., & Witteman, J. C. (2006). ACE polymorphisms. *Circulation Research*, *98*(9), 1123–1133. https://doi.org/10.1161/01.RES.0000223145.74217.e7.

Semesta, K. M., Tian, R., Kampmann, M., von Zastrow, M., & Tsvetanova, N. G. (2020). A high-throughput CRISPR interference screen for dissecting functional regulators of GPCR/cAMP signaling. *PLoS Genetics*, *16*(10), e1009103. https://doi.org/10.1371/journal.pgen.1009103.

Semis, M., Gugiu, G. B., Bernstein, E. A., Bernstein, K. E., & Kalkum, M. (2019). The plethora of angiotensin-converting enzyme-processed peptides in mouse plasma. *Analytical Chemistry*, *91*(10), 6440–6453. https://doi.org/10.1021/acs.analchem.8b03828.

Shamaa, M. M., Fouad, H., Haroun, M., & Shamaa, L. A. (2016). Angiotensin II type 1 receptor (A1166C) gene polymorphism and essential hypertension in Egyptian population. *The Egyptian Heart Journal*, *68*(3), 165–169. https://doi.org/10.1016/j.ehj.2016.02.004.

Simon, D. B., Karet, F. E., Hamdan, J. M., DiPietro, A., Sanjad, S. A., & Lifton, R. P. (1996). Bartter's syndrome, hypokalaemic alkalosis with hypercalciuria, is caused by mutations in the Na-K-2Cl cotransporter NKCC2. *Nature Genetics*, *13*(2), 183–188. https://doi.org/10.1038/ng0696-183.

Small, K. M., Brown, K. M., Forbes, S. L., & Liggett, S. B. (2001). Polymorphic deletion of three intracellular acidic residues of the alpha 2B-adrenergic receptor decreases G protein-coupled receptor kinase-mediated phosphorylation and desensitization. *The Journal of Biological Chemistry*, *276*(7), 4917–4922. https://doi.org/10.1074/jbc.M008118200.

Small, K. M., Forbes, S. L., Rahman, F. F., Bridges, K. M., & Liggett, S. B. (2000). A four amino acid deletion polymorphism in the third intracellular loop of the human alpha 2C-adrenergic receptor confers impaired coupling to multiple effectors. *The Journal of Biological Chemistry*, *275*(30), 23059–23064. https://doi.org/10.1074/jbc.M000796200.

Somasekharan, S., Tanis, J., & Forbush, B. (2012). Loop diuretic and ion-binding residues revealed by scanning mutagenesis of transmembrane helix 3 (TM3) of Na-K-cl cotransporter (NKCC1). *The Journal of Biological Chemistry*, *287*(21), 17308–17317. https://doi.org/10.1074/jbc.M112.356014.

Sridharan, K., Al Banna, R., Malalla, Z., Husain, A., Sater, M., Jassim, G., et al. (2021). Influence of CYP2C9, VKORC1, and CYP4F2 polymorphisms on the pharmacodynamic parameters of warfarin: A cross-sectional study. *Pharmacological Reports*. https://doi.org/10.1007/s43440-021-00256-w.

Stranneheim, H., Lagerstedt-Robinson, K., Magnusson, M., Kvarnung, M., Nilsson, D., Lesko, N., et al. (2021). Integration of whole genome sequencing into a healthcare setting: High diagnostic rates across multiple clinical entities in 3219 rare disease patients. *Genome Medicine*, *13*(1), 40. https://doi.org/10.1186/s13073-021-00855-5.

Surendran, P., Feofanova, E. V., Lahrouchi, N., Ntalla, I., Karthikeyan, S., Cook, J., et al. (2020). Discovery of rare variants associated with blood pressure regulation through meta-analysis of 1.3 million individuals. *Nature Genetics*, *52*(12), 1314–1332. https://doi.org/10.1038/s41588-020-00713-x.

Surprenant, A., Horstman, D. A., Akbarali, H., & Limbird, L. E. (1992). A point mutation of the alpha 2-adrenoceptor that blocks coupling to potassium but not calcium currents. *Science*, *257*(5072), 977–980. https://doi.org/10.1126/science.1354394.

Susac, L., Eddy, M. T., Didenko, T., Stevens, R. C., & Wuthrich, K. (2018). A2A adenosine receptor functional states characterized by (19)F-NMR. *Proceedings of the National Academy of Sciences of the United States of America*, *115*(50), 12733–12738. https://doi.org/10.1073/pnas.1813649115.

Tang, L., Gamal El-Din, T. M., Lenaeus, M. J., Zheng, N., & Catterall, W. A. (2019). Structural basis for diltiazem block of a voltage-gated ca(2+) channel. *Molecular Pharmacology*, *96*(4), 485–492. https://doi.org/10.1124/mol.119.117531.

Thase, M. E., Parikh, S. V., Rothschild, A. J., Dunlop, B. W., DeBattista, C., Conway, C. R., et al. (2019). Impact of pharmacogenomics on clinical outcomes for patients taking medications with gene-drug interactions in a randomized controlled trial. *The Journal of Clinical Psychiatry*, *80*(6). https://doi.org/10.4088/JCP.19m12910.

Tsvetanova, N. G., & von Zastrow, M. (2014). Spatial encoding of cyclic AMP signaling specificity by GPCR endocytosis. *Nature Chemical Biology*, *10*(12), 1061–1065. https://doi.org/10.1038/nchembio.1665.

Tunyasuvunakool, K., Adler, J., Wu, Z., Green, T., Zielinski, M., Zidek, A., et al. (2021). Highly accurate protein structure prediction for the human proteome. *Nature*. https://doi.org/10.1038/s41586-021-03828-1.

van Geel, P. P., Pinto, Y. M., Voors, A. A., Buikema, H., Oosterga, M., Crijns, H. J., et al. (2000). Angiotensin II type 1 receptor A1166C gene polymorphism is associated with an increased response to angiotensin II in human arteries. *Hypertension*, *35*(3), 717–721. https://doi.org/10.1161/01.hyp.35.3.717.

van Willigen, M., Vonk, A. M., Yeoh, H. Y., Kruisselbrink, E., Kleizen, B., van der Ent, C. K., et al. (2019). Folding-function relationship of the most common cystic fibrosis-causing CFTR conductance mutants. *Life Science Alliance*, *2*(1). https://doi.org/10.26508/lsa.201800172.

Veiga, R. V., & Taylor, R. E. (1986). Beta blockers, hypertension, and blacks- -is the answer really in? *Journal of the National Medical Association*, *78*(9), 851–856.

Venkatakrishnan, A. J., Deupi, X., Lebon, G., Heydenreich, F. M., Flock, T., Miljus, T., et al. (2016). Diverse activation pathways in class a GPCRs converge near the G-protein-coupling region. *Nature, 536*(7617), 484–487. https://doi.org/10.1038/nature19107.

Venter, J. C., Adams, M. D., Myers, E. W., Li, P. W., Mural, R. J., Sutton, G. G., et al. (2001). The sequence of the human genome. *Science, 291*(5507), 1304–1351.

Vormfelde, S. V., & Brockmoller, J. (2012). The genetics of loop diuretic effects. *The Pharmacogenomics Journal, 12*(1), 45–53. https://doi.org/10.1038/tpj.2010.68.

Vormfelde, S. V., Sehrt, D., Toliat, M. R., Schirmer, M., Meineke, I., Tzvetkov, M., et al. (2007). Genetic variation in the renal sodium transporters NKCC2, NCC, and ENaC in relation to the effects of loop diuretic drugs. *Clinical Pharmacology and Therapeutics, 82*(3), 300–309. https://doi.org/10.1038/sj.clpt.6100131.

Wang, T., Chen, Y., Yin, X., & Qiu, H. (2021). Novel heterozygous mutation of SLC12A3 gene in Gitelman syndrome. *QJM*. https://doi.org/10.1093/qjmed/hcab066.

Waugh, D. J., Gaivin, R. J., Zuscik, M. J., Gonzalez-Cabrera, P., Ross, S. A., Yun, J., et al. (2001). Phe-308 and Phe-312 in transmembrane domain 7 are major sites of alpha 1-adrenergic receptor antagonist binding. Imidazoline agonists bind like antagonists. *The Journal of Biological Chemistry, 276*(27), 25366–25371. https://doi.org/10.1074/jbc.M103152200.

Weinshilboum, R., & Wang, L. (2004). Pharmacogenomics: Bench to bedside. *Nature Reviews. Drug Discovery, 3*(9), 739–748. https://doi.org/10.1038/nrd1497.

Whelton, P. K., Carey, R. M., Aronow, W. S., Casey, D. E., Jr., Collins, K. J., Dennison Himmelfarb, C., et al. (2018). 2017 ACC/AHA/AAPA/ABC/ACPM/AGS/APhA/ASH/ASPC/NMA/PCNA guideline for the prevention, detection, evaluation, and Management of High Blood Pressure in adults: A report of the American College of Cardiology/American Heart Association task force on clinical practice guidelines. *Hypertension, 71*(6), e13–e115. https://doi.org/10.1161/HYP.0000000000000065.

Xu, X., Kaindl, J., Clark, M. J., Hubner, H., Hirata, K., Sunahara, R. K., et al. (2021). Binding pathway determines norepinephrine selectivity for the human beta1AR over beta2AR. *Cell Research, 31*(5), 569–579. https://doi.org/10.1038/s41422-020-00424-2.

Yuan, D., Liu, Z., Kaindl, J., Maeda, S., Zhao, J., Sun, X., et al. (2020). Activation of the alpha2B adrenoceptor by the sedative sympatholytic dexmedetomidine. *Nature Chemical Biology, 16*(5), 507–512. https://doi.org/10.1038/s41589-020-0492-2.

Zhang, F., & Steinberg, S. F. (2013). S49G and R389G polymorphisms of the beta(1)-adrenergic receptor influence signaling via the cAMP-PKA and ERK pathways. *Physiological Genomics, 45*(23), 1186–1192. https://doi.org/10.1152/physiolgenomics.00087.2013.

Zhang, H., Unal, H., Desnoyer, R., Han, G. W., Patel, N., Katritch, V., et al. (2015). Structural basis for ligand recognition and functional selectivity at angiotensin receptor. *The Journal of Biological Chemistry, 290*(49), 29127–29139. https://doi.org/10.1074/jbc.M115.689000.

Zhang, H., Unal, H., Gati, C., Han, G. W., Liu, W., Zatsepin, N. A., et al. (2015). Structure of the angiotensin receptor revealed by serial femtosecond crystallography. *Cell, 161*(4), 833–844. https://doi.org/10.1016/j.cell.2015.04.011.

Zhao, M. M., Hwa, J., & Perez, D. M. (1996). Identification of critical extracellular loop residues involved in alpha 1-adrenergic receptor subtype-selective antagonist binding. *Molecular Pharmacology, 50*(5), 1118–1126.

Zheng, X., Shang, S., Cai, G., Chen, X., & Li, Q. (2021). Genetic analysis of SLC12A3 gene and diagnostic process in patients with Gitelman syndrome. *Clinical Nephrology, 96*(3), 165–174. https://doi.org/10.5414/CN110425.

CHAPTER SIX

Relaxin/serelaxin for cardiac dysfunction and heart failure in hypertension

Prasad Chunduri[a], Shrey A. Patel[a], and Scott P. Levick[b,*]
[a]School of Biomedical Sciences, The University of Queensland, Brisbane, QLD, Australia
[b]Physiology and Pharmacology, West Virginia University, Morgantown, WV, United States
*Corresponding author: e-mail address: scott.levick@hsc.wvu.edu

Contents

Abstract

The pregnancy related hormone relaxin is produced throughout the reproductive system. However, relaxin also has important cardiovascular effects as part of the adaptation that the cardiovascular system undergoes in response to the extra demands of pregnancy. These effects are primarily mediated by the relaxin family peptide receptor 1, which is one of four known relaxin receptors. The effects of relaxin on the cardiovascular system during pregnancy, as well as its anti-fibrotic and anti-inflammatory properties, have led to extensive studies into the potential of relaxin therapy as an approach to treat heart failure. Cardiomyocytes, cardiac fibroblasts, and endothelial cells all possess

Advances in Pharmacology, Volume 94
ISSN 1054-3589
https://doi.org/10.1016/bs.apha.2022.04.002

relaxin family peptide receptor 1, allowing for direct effects of therapeutic relaxin on the heart. Many pre-clinical animal studies have demonstrated a beneficial effect of exogenous relaxin on adverse cardiac remodeling including inflammation, fibrosis, cardiomyocyte hypertrophy and apoptosis, as well as effects on cardiac contractile function. Despite this, clinical studies have yielded disappointing results for the synthetic seralaxin, even though seralaxin was well tolerated. This article will provide background on relaxin in the context of normal physiology, as well as the role of relaxin in pregnancy-related adaptations of the cardiovascular system. We will also present evidence from pre-clinical animal studies that demonstrate the potential benefits of relaxin therapy, as well as discussing the results from clinical trials. Finally, we will discuss possible reasons for the failure of these clinical trials as well as steps being taken to potentially improve relaxin therapy for heart failure.

Abbreviations

AHF	acute heart failure
AMI	acute myocardial infarction
cAMP	cyclic adenosine monophosphate
cGMP	cyclic guanosine monophosphate
ECM	extracellular matrix
eNOS	endothelial nitric oxide synthase
GC	guanylyl cyclase
HF	heart failure
HFpEF	heart failure with preserved ejection fraction
HFrEF	heart failure with reduced ejection fraction
HUVEC	human umbilical vein endothelial cell
iNOS	inducible nitric oxide synthase
INSL	insulin-like peptide
IV	intravenous
LVAD	left ventricular assist device
MAPK	mitogen activated kinase
MMP	matrix metalloproteinase
nNOS	neuronal nitric oxide synthase
NO	nitric oxide
PKA	protein kinase A
PUFA	polyunsaturated fatty acids
RLN	relaxin
RXFP	relaxin family peptide receptor
SRLN	serelaxin
TAC	transaortic constriction

1. Introduction

As has been detailed many times, relaxin (RLN) was first identified in 1926 when Frederick Hisaw observed that injection of serum from pregnant guinea pigs or rabbits caused relaxation of the pubic ligament of virgin guinea pigs, when given shortly after estrus (Hisaw, 1926). This did not occur when serum from males or non-pregnant females was administered. Subsequently in 1930, the hormone responsible for this effect was identified as RLN (Fevold, Hisaw, & Meyer, 1930). Given these observed effects, it is not surprising that RLN is widely distributed in the reproductive tissues, even in males, including the corpus luteum, uterus, mammary gland, testis, and prostate (Bathgate et al., 2013), where, due to the large increase in plasma concentrations, it acts as an endocrine factor. The endocrine actions of RLN are extensive and include inducing softening of the birth canal by regulating the extracellular matrix (ECM), decidualization, implantation, suppression of uterine contractility, and regulation of nipple development (Dschietzig, Bartsch, Baumann, & Stangl, 2006).

Although clearly a reproductive hormone, RLN has other roles in both females, as well as males, not related to reproduction. For example, as early as 1967, Hisaw and colleagues found a potential role for RLN in cardiovascular function, in which they used castrated monkeys and observed marked morphological changes in endometrial endothelial cells, suggestive of hyperplasia and hypertrophy (Hisaw, Hisaw, & Dawson, 1967). It is now known that RLN is widely distributed throughout the body, with expression in the brain as well as peripheral tissues including the heart, liver, lung, kidney, spleen, skin and pancreas (Bathgate et al., 2013). In these peripheral tissues, RLN functions as an autocrine or paracrine factor. For example, in pregnancy RLN acts on the cardiovascular system to increase maternal renal plasma flow and glomerular filtration, while also increasing cardiac output to meet increased demand (Martin, Romero, & Salama, 2019). The knowledge that the heart responds to RLN, together with the well-established roles of RLN to regulate the ECM and inflammation (Sarwar, Du, Dschietzig, & Summers, 2017), has fostered tremendous interest on the potential of RLN as a therapy for disease in the heart, particularly heart failure (HF). Like most molecules, RLN has both acute and chronic actions, with acute effects involving rapid activation of signaling pathways, while the chronic effects involve changes in gene patterns.

This chapter will begin by describing the basics of RLN physiology and pharmacology, including the various RLN isoforms, the receptors for RLN, and the signaling pathways initiated upon RLN receptor activation. We will then briefly describe the effects of RLN on the heart during pregnancy. Following that, we will discuss the broader cardiovascular-protective actions of RLN in the context of hypertension and HF. From this information we will propose future directions and draw conclusions.

1.1 Relaxin: Physiology and pharmacology

RLN was previously classed as a member of the insulin-like (INSL) family of peptides, but is now considered a distinct RLN family of peptides based on the two-chain structure, receptor binding motifs and activation of G protein-coupled receptors (Bathgate, Ivell, Sanborn, Sherwood, & Summers, 2006). Accordingly, RLN physiology and pharmacology are somewhat complex due to its structural similarity to insulin, a close association and interaction with INSL peptides, and the presence in mammals of three isoforms of RLN and four known RLN family peptide receptors (RXFP) (Bathgate et al., 2013; Chen et al., 2020; Nistor, Schmidt, & Schiffner, 2018; Sarwar et al., 2017).

1.1.1 Relaxin genes and peptides

Purification of RLN from animal sources allowed determination of the peptide structure. RLN is synthesized as a preprohormone with four distinct regions including a signal peptide, a B-chain, a C-chain, and a COOH-terminal A-chain (Bathgate et al., 2013). In humans and higher primates, two RLN peptides have been identified, RLN1 and RLN2, that share approximately 62% and 87% homology for the A- and B-chains, respectively (Bathgate et al., 2013; Hudson et al., 1983). The human *RLN1* and *RLN2* genes are located sequentially on chromosome 9 (Bathgate et al., 2013). While humans and higher primates express both *RLN1* and *RLN2*, other mammals only express *RLN1*. Interestingly, in humans, it is the peptide encoded by *RLN2* that is released during pregnancy, whereas in other mammals RLN1 is the pregnancy hormone (Bathgate et al., 2013). The function of RLN1 in humans is unknown. More recently, another gene encoding a RLN peptide was identified. Human gene *RLN3* has low sequence homology with *RLN1* and *RLN2* and is restricted to the brain and likely involved in functions related to stress, memory and appetite (Bathgate et al., 2013). RLN has a close structural relationship with INSL peptides-3, -4, -5, and -6 (Bathgate et al., 2013; Haley et al., 1982; Hudson, Haley, Cronk, Shine, & Niall, 1981; Sarwar et al., 2017). Serelaxin (SRLN) is a recombinant form of RLN2 used in clinical studies (Miyares & Davis, 2013). SRLN is administered as a continuous intravenous (IV) infusion over a period of 24 to 48 h.

1.1.2 Relaxin family peptide receptors

There are four RXFP members, all of which are G protein-coupled receptors numbered 1 through 4 (RXFP1, RXFP2, RXFP3, and RXFP4)

(Bathgate et al., 2013; Chen et al., 2020). RXFP1 and RXFP2 contain a leucine-rich repeat domain and a low-density lipoprotein class A module in their extracellular region (Bathgate et al., 2013; Chen et al., 2020). RXFP1 is the cognate receptor for RLN2 in humans, with RLN2 having roughly an order of magnitude higher affinity for RXFP1 (Halls, Bathgate, Sutton, Dschietzig, & Summers, 2015). RXFP1 has a much broader distribution than RXFP2 and there is no evidence that RXFP2 is activated by RLN in vivo (Bathgate et al., 2013; Chen et al., 2020). Therefore, the majority of RLN2 effects are believed to be mediated via RXFP1 even though RXFP2 shares very close structural similarity with RXFP1 (Bathgate et al., 2013; Chen et al., 2020). Although RXFP1 can interact with INSL3, it is the interaction between the extracellular domain of RXFP2 and INSL3 that makes RXFP2 the cognate receptor for INSL3, and plays a role in testicular descent, gonadal function, and bone metabolism (Bathgate et al., 2013; Chen et al., 2020). RXFP3 and RXFP4 are distinctly different in structure from RXFP1 and RXFP2 (Bathgate et al., 2013), with RLN3 and INSL-5 being the cognate ligands for RXFP3 and RXFP4, respectively (Sarwar et al., 2017).

Since RXFP1 is the receptor that mediates most of the effects of RLN2, including in the cardiovascular system, we will focus on this receptor. The gene for RXFP1 is located on chromosome 4 and encodes a 757 amino acid protein, although there are as many as 29 alternative splicing variants that have been identified (Chen et al., 2020). RXFP1 mRNA and protein are found in a wide range of reproductive tissues including the ovaries, uterus, placenta, mammary gland, prostate, and testis consistent with its role in reproduction (Bathgate et al., 2013). Beyond the reproductive system, RXFP1 is also found in the heart, kidney, lung, adrenal gland, intestines, liver, and blood cells as well as in a number of areas of brain such as cortex, organum vasculosum of the lamina terminalis, and subfornical organ (Bathgate et al., 2013; Chen et al., 2020).

1.1.3 RXFP1 signaling

The major second messenger system activated by RXFP1 is adenyl cyclase/cyclic adenosine monophosphate (cAMP) (Fig. 1). RXFP1 couples to at least three G proteins to modulate cAMP production (Bathgate et al., 2013; Chen et al., 2020; Nistor et al., 2018; Sarwar et al., 2017), with RLN2 capable of increasing cAMP in multiple cell types and organs, including the heart as a whole and cardiac fibroblasts more specifically (Halls et al., 2009; Kompa, Samuel, & Summers, 2002; Sarwar et al., 2017). Interestingly though, characteristics of RLN-mediated cAMP increases are dependent on

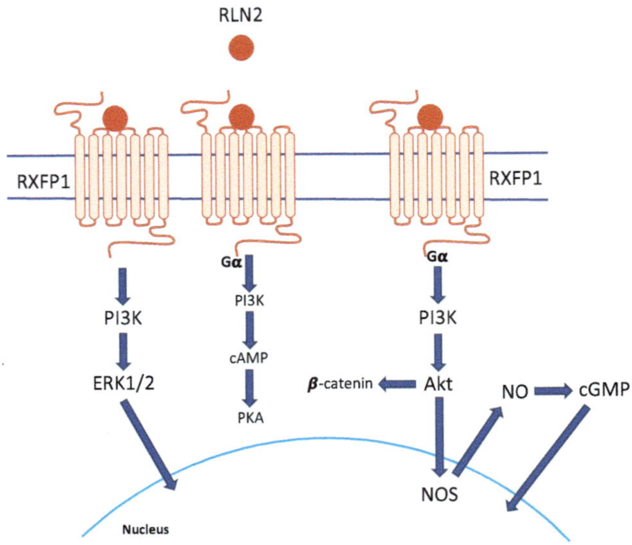

Fig. 1 Schematic depicting RXFP1-mediated signaling pathways.

cell type. In cardiac fibroblasts, RLN2 activation of RXFP1 induced the Gαi/PI3K/cAMP pathway, whereas RLN2 acts via Gαs in renal fibroblasts (Halls et al., 2009; Sarwar et al., 2017). cAMP activation seems counterintuitive for the cardioprotective actions of RLN2 observed in animal models because cAMP is the second messenger system activated by norepinephrine-induced β1-adrenergic receptor activation that has adverse impacts on cardiac remodeling and HF. However, cell-specific effects, as well as localization of cAMP, may be important. Also, in addition to cAMP, there are multiple other signaling pathways induced by RLN2/RXFP1 that have known beneficial effects on the cardiovascular system.

RLN2 can increase expression and activity of all three nitric oxide synthase (NOS) isoforms, endothelial NOS (eNOS), inducible NOS (iNOS) and neuronal NOS (nNOS), by a mechanism involving PI3K and Akt (Chow et al., 2012; Failli et al., 2002; McGuane et al., 2011; Mookerjee et al., 2009; Quattrone, Chiappini, Scapagnini, Bigazzi, & Bani, 2004) (Fig. 1). This has the effect of increasing nitric oxide (NO) production and cyclic guanosine monophosphate (cGMP) activation, which are known to be cardioprotective (Kingwell, 2000; Sarwar et al., 2017). cGMP is generated from guanylyl cyclases (GC) and GC activation is known to protect against ischemic injury, hypertrophy, and HF (Lukowski, Krieg, Rybalkin, Beavo, & Hofmann, 2014). NO induction of cGMP mediates RLN-induced smooth muscle cell relaxation (Lam et al., 2016). Further, RLN opposes TGF-β1-induced phosphorylation of Smad2 and subsequent myofibroblast conversion in renal cortical myofibroblasts by a mechanism involving NO activation of cGMP (C. Wang et al., 2016). There is also evidence that Akt activation by RLN2 induces cytoplasmic accumulation of β-catenin, indicative of modulation of canonical Wnt signaling by RLN2 (Liu et al., 2008) (Fig. 1). Although, RLN2 regulation of Wnt signaling may be complex with RLN2 reported to reduce Wnt activation leading to increased matrix metalloproteinase levels (Ho, Dilts, Bartol, & Bagnell, 2009).

Mitogen activated protein kinases (MAPK) are another signaling pathway invoked by RLN2/RXFP1 (Bathgate et al., 2013; Chen et al., 2020; Nistor et al., 2018; Sarwar et al., 2017). The major MAPK activated in response to RLN2 appears to be ERK1/2, with phosphorylation of ERK1/2 occurring in response to RLN2 in many cell types, including those of the cardiovascular system, rat renal fibroblasts (Chow et al., 2012), human smooth muscle cells (Zhang, Liu, Erikson, Lewis, & Unemori, 2002), and human umbilical vein endothelial cells (HUVECs) (Dschietzig et al., 2003). Similarly to NO, this at least in part involves PI3K (Sarwar, Samuel, Bathgate, Stewart, & Summers, 2015). Activation of other MAPKs such as p38 appears to be more cell type selective than ERK1/2 (Sarwar et al., 2017).

1.2 Relaxin and the cardiovascular system in pregnancy

Given that the primary functions of RLN are in reproduction, it is not surprising that the preliminary evidence of RLN's role in the cardiovascular system was linked to pregnancy. Pregnancy places a large burden on the cardiovascular system. To compensate and meet the need for pregnancy-induced increased blood flow, vascular resistance is reduced, which in turn leads to a reduction in cardiac afterload and preload (Fig. 2) (Conrad & Novak, 2004; Ramlakhan et al., 2020). This reduced vascular resistance is then compensated for by expansion of blood volume as well as increased heart rate, thereby increasing cardiac output (Fig. 2) (Ramlakhan et al., 2020). RLN is important in mediating these adaptations to the cardiovascular system including increasing endometrial and renal blood flow, general systemic vasodilation, and reduced vascular resistance (Conrad, 2011; Hisaw et al., 1967; Nistor et al., 2018). Interestingly, the effects of RLN to reduce vascular resistance also occur in non-pregnant females as well as

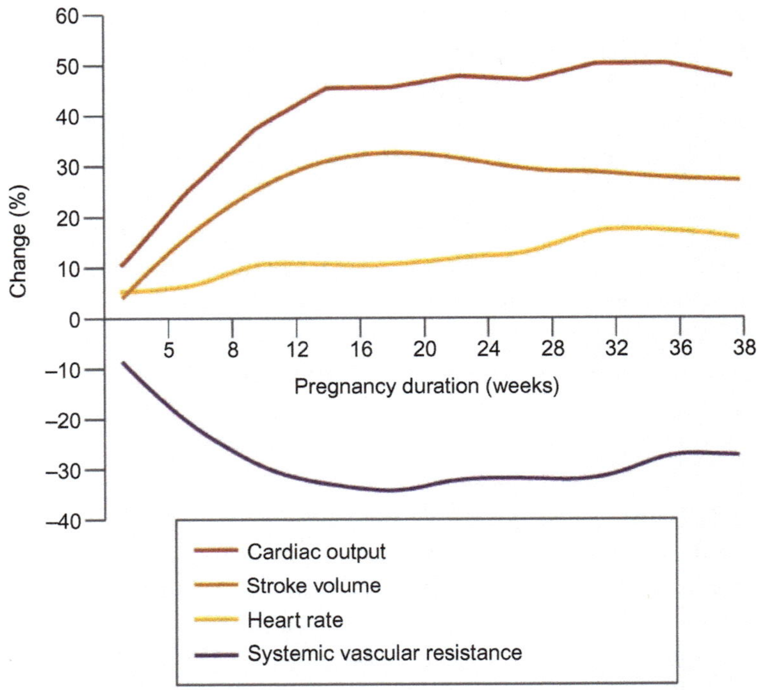

Fig. 2 Hemodynamic changes in pregnancy. A heavy burden is placed on the cardiovascular system during pregnancy due to increased blood supply demands. To meet this demand, systemic vasodilation occurs leading to reduced vascular resistance. This in turn results in an increase in heart rate and stroke volume in order to increase cardiac output. *Modified and published with permission Ramlakhan, K. P., Johnson, M. R., & Roos-Hesselink, J. W. (2020). Pregnancy and cardiovascular disease.* Nature Reviews. Cardiology, 17 *(11), 718–731.*

male rodents when exogenous RLN is administered (Conrad & Shroff, 2011). For example, exogenous RLN decreased arterial pressure in spontaneously hypertensive rats (SHR) (St-Louis & Massicotte, 1985), and increased coronary blood flow in isolated rat and guinea pig hearts (Bani-Sacchi, Bigazzi, Bani, Mannaioni, & Masini, 1995). Exogenous administration of RLN to non-pregnant rodents and humans has the effect of increasing cardiac output via an increase in stroke volume (Conrad & Shroff, 2011), likely a compensatory mechanism for the decreased vascular resistance (Fig. 2). Although, there are also direct effects of RLN on the heart. A 1996 study by Coulson et al., used isolated Langendorff hearts from pregnant and non-pregnant rats to examine the effects of pregnancy and SRLN treatment on heart function (Coulson, Thorp, Mayer, &

Cefalo, 1996). Coulson et al., demonstrated that SRLN has both inotropic and chronotropic effects – and that RLN is involved in the pregnancy-related changes in the cardiovascular system (Coulson et al., 1996). Furthermore, dose-dependent effects of SRLN to increase heart rate, contractile function, as well as left ventricular systolic pressure were observed in the rats; pregnancy did not modify outcomes (Coulson et al., 1996). Neutralizing antibodies to RLN prevented the reduced vascular resistance and the increase in cardiac output in pregnant rodents (Conrad & Shroff, 2011; Debrah et al., 2006). There are also direct actions of RLN on the sinoatrial-node to increase heart rate (Conrad & Novak, 2004). The general protective properties of RLN in vasculature and in cardiac disease, are discussed in the following sections.

2. Relaxin/serelaxin in hypertension and vascular cells

Initially, Novak and colleagues found RLN to mediate the changes in the maternal renal circulation during pregnancy in rats (Novak et al., 2001). Conrad, Debrah, Novak, Danielson, and Shroff (2004) subsequently conducted an experiment to determine whether SRLN had the potential to alter cardiovascular function in non-pregnant female rats. After SRLN administration for 10 days, circulating RLN levels were similar to pregnant rats during early to midterm pregnancy. Significant increases in global arterial compliance and cardiac output, as well as a decrease in systemic vascular resistance, were observed. Mean arterial pressure values did not change due to a compensatory increase in cardiac output. Furthermore, administered RLN has also been found to acutely dilate rat mesenteric arteries, rodent mesenteric and small renal arteries, and human subcutaneous and small gluteal arteries (McGuane et al., 2011). Emphasizing the importance of endogenous RLN, while mesenteric arteries from $RLN^{-/-}$ mice displayed no changes in passive circumferential wall stiffness, they did show reduced volume compliance (Leo, Jelinic, Gooi, Tare, & Parry, 2014). When the impact of aging on mesenteric arteries was assessed, an age-dependent increase in circumferential wall stiffness was observed with no additional detrimental effects of RLN deficiency (Jelinic, Tare, Conrad, & Parry, 2015). However, younger $RLN^{-/-}$ mice displayed an exacerbated vascular stiffness in the mesenteric arteries in comparison with wild type mice of equivalent age, indicating endogenous RLN to be important in the regulation of vascular function in arteries of younger animals (Jelinic et al., 2015). Superoxide dismutase production, but not NADPH oxidase expression, was shown to be increased in aorta of young RLN$^{-/-}$ mice along with significantly decreased levels of endogenous NOS and basal NO availability (Ng, Jelinic, Parry, & Leo, 2015), which could explain the effect of deletion of RLN in young mice. Especially since such vascular phenotypes were not observed in older RLN$^{-/-}$ mice (Ng et al., 2015). Vasodilatory effects of RLN in the presence of a functional NOS system were also observed in male Sprague-Dawley rats after a 2-week treatment, with reductions in mean arterial pressure and oxidative stress markers (Sasser, Cunningham, & Baylis, 2014; Sasser, Molnar, & Baylis, 2011). Clearly, endogenous RLN is vital for maintaining endothelial function and vasculature remodeling, particularly in smaller resistance arteries (Debrah et al., 2011; Jelinic et al., 2015). SRLN treatment for 4 weeks reduced atherosclerotic plaque size in the aorta of mice that are apolipoprotein-deficient and reversed endothelial dysfunction due to the reduction in production of vascular superoxide (Tiyerili et al., 2016). Similarly, 8-week long infusion of SRLN in the aorta of guinea pigs prevented endothelial dysfunction caused by cigarette smoke as it increased NO production and decreased the concentration of reactive oxygen species (Pini et al., 2016).

In rats with angiotensin II-induced hypertension, acute RLN administration (up to 6 h) increased cardiac output and global arterial compliance and significantly reduced systemic vascular resistance, albeit with no changes to mean arterial pressure (Debrah, Conrad, Jeyabalan, Danielson, & Shroff, 2005). While acute treatment with RLN had little effect in the SHR, chronic treatment (1 to 7 days) yielded the same outcomes as in rats with angiotensin-II induced hypertension (Debrah et al., 2005). The mechanism of RLN's action again included production of NO (Danielson, Sherwood, & Conrad, 1999). Thus, there is strong evidence that the protective vasodilatory actions of RLN in hypertension are via increased NO production and reduced oxidative stress. Some evidence also exists that RLN may facilitate vasodilation via the ET_B receptor (Danielson et al., 1999; Danielson, Kercher, & Conrad, 2000). In addition, it is also postulated that RLN stimulates the secretion of atrial natriuretic peptides based on previous research related to pulmonary vasorelaxation (Cargill & Lipworth, 1995). The anti-fibrotic effects of SRLN (discussed in later sections) also contribute to its therapeutic potential in hypertension (Lekgabe et al., 2005). Attributed to the decreases in cardiac and renal dysfunction via the prevention of fibrosis in both the heart and the kidney respectively, SRLN was also found to be effective in the DOCA-salt model of hypertension (Wang et al., 2017). Conversely, there are some examples where RLN is not effective. In a female mouse model of systemic lupus erythematosus, SRLN administration for 4 weeks did not improve vascular disease or hypertension, but instead worsened vascular endothelial dysfunction. This was also in agreement with another study in which RLN treatment did not alter development of hypertension in an angiotensin II model of preeclampsia (Haase et al., 2016).

3. Relaxin/serelaxin in the context of heart failure

SRLN treatment for patients with acute heart failure (AHF) had promising origins at the start of 21st century due to accumulating preclinical evidence, followed by support from Novartis Europharm Ltd. under the brand name Reasanz™ (Bani, 2020). This led to the first pilot study involving 234 patients with AHF in the Pre-RELAX-AHF trial published in 2009 (Teerlink et al., 2009). Results from this Phase IIb trial showed that RLN treatment had acceptable safety, and relieved dyspnoea as well as other clinical outcomes in patients with AHF (Teerlink et al., 2009). This was then followed by a promising Phase III clinical trial involving a larger group of 1161 hospitalized AHF patients in the RELAX-AHF study (Teerlink et al., 2013). Although RELAX-AHF confirmed RLN's safety and tolerance, as well as relief of dyspnoea, it did not find any positive effect on the subjects' readmission to hospital (Teerlink et al., 2013). In more recent times, a multi-center, double-blind, placebo-controlled RELAX-AHF-2 trial involving 6545 patients hospitalized due to AHF also failed to show improvements with SRLN treatment (Metra et al., 2019). In this trial, 48 h IV infusion of SRLN did not result in positive changes in any of the two primary end points, which included a lower incidence of death from cardiovascular disease within 180 days, or worsening HF at 5 days (Metra et al., 2019). While the designers of the trials mention the possibility that the positive outcomes from the previous RELAX-AHF trial could have been due to chance, and the previous RELAX-AHF trial being 5 times smaller than the 2019 RELAX-AHF-2 trial, it is to be recognized that there were some significant changes in the participant populations between these trials. Though the entry criteria remained nearly identical, the RELAX-AHF-2 trial included more patients with worse renal function and higher threshold for natriuretic peptides, which may explain the higher rates of non-cardiovascular mortality in the 2019 RELAX-AHF-2 trial compared to the 2013 RELAX-AHF trial (3% vs. 1.7%) (Metra et al., 2019). The percentage of patients with worsening HF was far less in the placebo group of the RELAX-AHF-2 trial compared to RELAX-AHF trial (7.7% vs. 12.2%) (Metra et al., 2019). In addition, a smaller number of patients received the full 48 h SRLN treatment in the RELAX-AHF-2 trial compared to the RELAX-AHF due to hypotension (18.5% vs. 12.5%) (Metra et al., 2019). Finally, other emerging evidence is also crucial in the context of these trials. For example, a recent study showed that angiotensin II type 1 receptor blockers such as candesartan inhibited the anti-fibrotic effects of SRLN in the heart and kidney, warning against their concomitant use (Chow et al., 2019). An overview of all HF-related human trials to-date with RLN is provided in Table 1. As a result of these trials, currently, recommendations of RLN treatment for AHF have halted almost everywhere in the world except Russia. Despite this, RLN research is still ongoing and treatment with RLN seems to be gaining support as a feasible therapeutic option for acute myocardial infarction (AMI) as opposed to AHF, the latter having received the most attention until now (Bani, 2020). RLN in AMI is beyond the scope of this article. Furthermore, whilst the results of the trials were not as favorable as hoped, several critical points have been raised about the protocols used in the trials. For example, McCullogh pointed out that the common 48 h infusion of therapy is not enough to reverse years of chronic disease, which applies to not only SLRN trials but also others such as PROTECT, SURVIVE and TRUE-HF (McCullough, 2017). While acknowledging the use of 48 h therapies to assess acute safety, MCullogh recommends that SRLN trials would need weeks-to-months of treatment to study their true efficacy (McCullough, 2017). In the sections below, we will explore evidence that supports a role for RLN in cardioprotection in models of hypertension and HF. These include both animal studies as well as clinical trials.

A pilot study in 2018 showed that the small proportion of AHF patients who were able to secrete RLN to the levels observed in pregnant women (20 out of total 814 patients) survived longer (Miró et al., 2018). Although most of the work to-date was conducted in relation to HF, it is of interest to note that RLN has been shown to be cardioprotective even within the healthy aging heart. A study by Martin et al. (2018) showed that 2-week treatment of aged (24 month old) F-344/Brown Norway rats with RLN (at doses of 0.4 mg/kg/day) suppressed transcription of multiple genes and pathways responsible for inflammation, fibrosis and HF in aging, but otherwise healthy, rats of both genders. Due to RLN's short half-life of 2–3 h, but long-lasting cardioprotective actions, it is suggested that RLN acts at the genomic level to reverse remodeling that is typical of HF, atrial fibrillation and aging (Romero & Salama, 2021).

Table 1 Patient characteristics and outcomes from major clinical trials.

Trial name/type	Year	Reference	No. of Patients	Patient Characteristics	Major outcomes
Pre-Relax-AHF Phase II Trial.	2009	Teerlink et al. (2009)	234 Patients with AHF.	International patient enrolment profile.	Improvement in dyspnoea along with length of stay and days alive out of hospital.
			62 Randomly assigned into placebo group.	Along with AHF, patients showed dyspnoea, congestion, increased BNP, renal insufficiency and systolic BP of more than 125 mmHg.	Readmission due to heart (or renal) failure or cardiovascular death were reduced at Day 60.
RELAX-AHF Phase III trial.	2013	Teerlink et al. (2013)	1161 Patients with AHF.	International patient enrolment profile.	Improvement in dyspnoea.
			580 Randomly assigned into placebo group.	Along with AHF, patients showed dyspnoea, congestion, increased BNP, renal insufficiency and systolic BP of more than 125 mmHg.	No other changes were significant especially secondary endpoints of death due to cardiovascular disease or readmission to hospital due to heart or renal failure.
RELAX-AHF-2 Phase III trial.	2019	Metra et al. (2019)	6545 Patients with AHF.	International patient enrolment profile.	No change in any of the 2 primary endpoints including lower incidence of death from cardiovascular causes at 180 days or worsening heart failure at 5 days.
			3271 Randomly assigned into placebo group.	Along with AHF, patients showed dyspnoea, vascular congestion, increased natriuretic peptides, renal insufficiency and systolic BP more than 125 mmHg.	

RLN has been shown to have positive effects on the myocardium in both HF with reduced ejection fraction (HFrEF) and HF with preserved ejection fraction (HFpEF). Although HFpEF was not the specific focus, a high proportion of patients in the RELAX-AHF trial (Teerlink et al., 2013) were cases with HFpEF (Wang et al., 2014). Although most studies focussed on RLN looked at fibrosis, it is important to note that RLN's positive effects on the heart are wide-ranging, as discussed in detail below, and these include protection against hypertrophy, apoptosis, arrhythmia, improving calcium dynamics and possessing positive chronotropic and inotropic properties as well as protection against inflammation and reactive oxygen species (Feijóo-Bandín et al., 2017).

3.1 Relaxin as an anti-fibrotic agent

Undoubtedly, cardiac fibrosis is a major player in the failing heart. Using two mouse models of cardiac fibrosis, Wilhelmi et al., have shown that RLN possesses a significant anti-fibrotic effect on the heart that is dose-dependent (Wilhelmi et al., 2020). This study for the first time also showed that RLN is able to increase the expression of its own receptor and that this precedes the mechanism by which RLN exerts it's anti-fibrotic effect—by inhibition of endothelial-to-mesenchymal transition (Wilhelmi et al., 2020). Five years before that, RLN was shown to suppress the transition of mouse fibroblasts or cardiac stromal cells to myofibroblasts (Squecco et al., 2015). Interestingly, in a β2-adrenergic receptor transgenic expression model, collagen concentration within the left ventricle was attenuated by RLN3 via TGFβ1 inhibition and increasing the ratio of pSmad2, and the effect was even more pronounced when RLN3 was combined with RLN2 (Hossain et al., 2011). The latter was shown in several studies, summarized in (Bathgate et al., 2008), to independently reduce collagen content when administered subcutaneously via implanted osmotic mini pumps. In the ischemic heart, Samuel et al., found that RLN2 treatment for 7 or 30 days in mice could reduce collagen content in the infarct itself as well as the border zone region, following permanent occlusion (Samuel et al., 2011). This likely contributed to the reduction in left ventricular end diastolic pressure observed, although relaxation and contractile properties of the heart were not improved. SRLN treatment has been found to suppress the ALK-5/Smad2/3 signaling pathway in cardiac fibroblasts isolated from adult rat hearts, thereby inhibiting their differentiation and collagen production (Wu, Wang, Wang, Shen, & Tan, 2018). RLN also exerted antifibrotic activity in isolated cardiac fibroblasts not only via the inhibition of Stat3/Smad3 signaling, but also through the attenuation of TGFβ1-induced autophagy (Yuan et al., 2017). Collectively, it was also postulated that RLN's anti-fibrotic effect involves an upregulation of Notch-1 signaling, which subsequently suppresses TGFβ1 expression/Smad3-induced transition of fibroblasts to myofibroblasts (Sassoli et al., 2013). In a broader context, RLN acting via RXFP1 can also regulate Smad2 activation via NO in fibroblasts. Collectively, using renal cortical fibroblasts isolated 3 days post-ureteric obstruction in Sprague-Dawley rats, several studies have clearly demonstrated that RLN up-regulates NO and cGMP to inhibit Smad2 activation, α-SMA levels, and collagen synthesis, indicative of a shift away from a profibrotic phenotype (Mookerjee et al., 2009; C. Wang, Kemp-Harper, et al., 2016). Increased production of NO is via phosphorylation of ERK to likely upregulate nNOS. There is also evidence that RLN opposes the profibrotic effects of TGFβ1 on cardiac fibroblasts also via activation of Wnt signaling. RLN up-regulated Wnt1 in cardiac fibroblasts isolated from adult F-344 rats, with Wnt signaling partially contributing to collagen synthesis by fibroblasts (Martin et al., 2019). This is interesting and warrants further exploring given that activation of Wnt signaling is typically considered to be profibrotic (Hu, Cao, Wu, Vaziri, & Zhao, 2020). Human fetal cardiac fibroblasts express RXFP1 (Sarwar et al., 2015); these human cardiac fibroblasts did not show cAMP accumulation in response to SRLN, but did show cGMP accumulation. This stands to reason since there was a substantial increase in nNOS in response to SRLN, and reinforces the likelihood that the RXFP1 > NO > cGMP pathway identified in rodents is relevant in humans.

An anti-fibrotic effect of RLN was also observed as an inverse relationship between RLN levels and myocardial fibrosis in patients with HFrEF and coronary artery disease (Simon et al., 2019). In an isoproterenol-induced cardiac damage model, SRLN was shown to be more effective than the ACE inhibitor enalapril in reducing cardiac fibrosis; and combining both SRLN and enalapril reduced cardiac fibrosis by at least twofold compared to administration of enalapril alone (Samuel et al., 2014). In vivo studies have shown that RLN modulates all aspects of cardiac fibroblast proliferation and differentiation, followed by decreased collagen expression and reversal of fibrosis (Samuel et al., 2004). Cardiac fibrosis, as well as renal fibrosis, was reversed in the SHR model (Lekgabe et al., 2005). Finally, RLN3 also decreased the levels of types I/II collagen and α-smooth muscle actin (α-SMA) as well as improving systolic and diastolic HF within the STZ-induced diabetic rats

(Zhang et al., 2017). Diastolic dysfunction, characterized by age-correlated increases in collagen within left ventricles of male mice, was more prominent in RLN-deficient male mice (Du et al., 2003). $RLN^{-/-}$ male mice displayed a progression of cardiac fibrosis with increases in pre-collagen type 1 mRNA gene expression, and collagen quantity in the ventricles (Du et al., 2003).

3.2 Relaxin as an anti-hypertrophic agent

Unlike fibrosis, the effect of RLN on cardiomyocyte hypertrophy is less clear and likely involves cell crosstalk. RLN was shown to reduce isoproterenol-induced cardiac hypertrophy in the mouse heart, by increasing endothelial NOS signaling (Sun et al., 2019). Treatment in this study was with RELAX10, a combination of human RLN2 and the Fc component of a human antibody (Sun et al., 2019). Furthermore, cardiac magnetic resonance studies in mice showed improvements in HF-related myocardial deformation parameters with SRLN treatment (Lapinskas et al., 2020). There were no decreases in stroke volume and ejection fraction of the left ventricle with SRLN treatment after transverse aortic constriction (TAC) compared to TAC mice receiving vehicle (Lapinskas et al., 2020). In a mouse model of permanent ischemia, Samuel et al., (Samuel et al., 2011) found no effect on overall hypertrophy (ventricular dilatation) of the heart with RLN2 treatment. Thus, the ability of RLN to exert effects on cardiomyocyte hypertrophy may be stimulus specific. To this end, it has been reported that RLN2 could not prevent phenylephrine-induced hypertrophy of isolated neonatal rat cardiomyocytes, however, RLN2 could prevent hypertrophy of cardiomyocytes induced by conditioned media from cardiac fibroblasts when fibroblasts were treated with RLN2 (Moore et al., 2007). Thus, while there are beneficial effects of RLN on hypertrophy in vivo in some cases, this may be through indirect actions rather than direct anti-hypertrophic effects on cardiomyocytes.

3.3 RLN as an anti-apoptotic agent

RLN has also been shown to possess anti-apoptotic properties. In ischemia, apoptosis of cardiomyocytes in the border zone of the infarct is critical to infarct expansion. RLN2 was able to reduce the number of apoptotic cells after 30 days in the infarct border zone in a mouse model of permanent coronary artery ligation (Samuel et al., 2011). Interestingly, in an aim to uncover the molecular mechanisms behind RLN protection from apoptosis,

You et al. (2018) have shown that ectopic expression of orphan nuclear receptor Nur77 increased the expression of RLN3 (but not RLN1) in neonatal rat cardiomyocytes as well as inhibiting isoproterenol-induced apoptosis of cardiomyocytes (You et al., 2018). RLN2 could also oppose the apoptotic effect of hydrogen peroxide on isolated rat neonatal cardiomyocytes by increasing Bcl-2 and decreasing Bax and ERK (Moore et al., 2007). RLN increased Akt activity, with Akt having known anti-apoptotic properties (New, Wu, Kwok, & Wong, 2007; Yang et al., 2004). Under high glucose conditions, RLN2 reduced apoptosis of H9c2 cardiomyocyte-like cells by a mechanism involving Notch-1 regulation of oxidative stress (Wei et al., 2018).

3.4 Relaxin improves calcium dynamics

Intramyocardial injection of adenoviral overexpressed RLN2 gene also improved diastolic function in a pressure-overloaded rat model, possibly through increased phosphorylation of phospholamban and Akt and thereby enhancing SERCA2 activity (Shuai et al., 2016). SRLN's cardiac stimulatory activity is further shown to be due to increasing sensitivity of cardiomyocytes to Ca^{2+} (Shaw et al., 2009). Rabbit sinoatrial node cells under voltage-clamp conditions displayed an increase in spontaneous action potentials and an increase in the L-type calcium current ($I_{Ca(L)}$) (Han, Habuchi, & Giles, 1994). It was found that the stimulation of $I_{Ca(L)}$ is similar to being induced by beta-adrenergic agonists as it is reliant on cAMP activity and cAMP-dependent protein kinase A (PKA) activity (Han et al., 1994).

3.5 Relaxin as a positive chronotropic and inotropic agent

The positive chronotropic effects of RLN have been detected in isolated right atria and perfused intact heart, and inotropic effects in left atria (Bani-Sacchi et al., 1995; Coulson et al., 1996; Kakouris, Eddie, & Summers, 1992). Similar to the outcomes in the Coulson et al. (1996) article described earlier, a 2011 study observed that RLN had positive inotropic effects in both failing and non-failing human hearts and that the mechanisms depend critically on the activation of PKA and inhibition of the transient K^+ outward current (Dschietzig et al., 2011). Furthermore, in murine myocardium, RLN was shown to have a positive inotropic effect via increasing myofilament phosphorylation by PKC and consequently the force generated by the myofilaments, with no increase in energy consumption

(Shaw et al., 2009). Kakouris and colleagues found that the potency of SRLN is even greater than endothelin-1, angiotensin II, adrenaline, histamine, isoprenaline, or serotonin in their isolated rat atria bioassay, with a mere nanomolar range concentration of human SRLN capable of generating the chronotropic and inotropic effects observed (Kakouris et al., 1992).

3.6 RLN as an anti-arrhythmic agent

Given that RLN receptors are primarily found in the atria, it is unsurprising that its cardioprotective role includes anti-arrhythmic properties. Through increasing Na^+ currents, RLN treatment reduced the occurrence of atrial fibrillation in the SHR (Parikh et al., 2013). Anti-apoptotic properties of RLN, in addition to antifibrotic properties, were shown to attenuate tachyarrythmia and improve cardiac function in a rat model of myocardial infarction (Wang, Zhu, Yang, & Sun, 2016). The combined antifibrotic and anti-inflammatory properties of RLN were also shown to reduce the susceptibility of mice to atrial fibrillation after being subjected to myocardial ischemia in addition to reducing the duration of fibrillation episodes (Beiert et al., 2017). Specifically within the atria, RLN increased conduction velocity as well as reducing hypertrophy and fibrosis (Beiert et al., 2017). Canonical Wnt signaling appears to be important in mediating the protective actions of RLN against arrythmias. This in part is likely via effects on fibrosis, but also through direct effects on cardiomyocytes whereby RLN increased β-catenin levels and promoted localization at the intercalated disks along with connexon 43 (Martin, Gabris, et al., 2019).

3.7 Other cardioprotective properties of relaxin including antioxidant and anti-inflammatory

A recently postulated mechanism for SRLN's positive effects on the cardiovascular system includes an increase in the endogenous synthesis of long chain polyunsaturated fatty acids (PUFA) (Aragón-Herrera et al., 2019). Sprague-Dawley rats in this study were treated with SRLN for 2 weeks at 0.4 mg/kg/day via osmotic minipumps and that resulted not only in changes to PUFA, but also to 5 amino acids of significance in the regulation of cardiac energy metabolism (Aragón-Herrera et al., 2019). These include glutamine, which has an important role in protecting the heart against ischemia-reperfusion as well as being a precursor for the antioxidant glutathione, and asparagine, which acts as a precursor for synthesis of non-essential amino acids and vasodilator NO during stress conditions

(Aragón-Herrera et al., 2019). In vitro experiments showed that RLN promotes growth and differentiation in myocardial cells (Nistri et al., 2012) and promotes metabolism through activating multiple regulators of cell homeostasis including ERK1/2, Akt and AMP-kinase (Aragón-Herrera et al., 2018). RLN was also shown to be cardioprotective in hypoxia/reoxygenation injury under in vitro conditions in the H9c2 cell line involving the activation of Nrf2/HO-1 signaling (Waza et al., 2018). In addition, RLN's antioxidant properties were also observed in the same study due to increases in the levels of antioxidant enzymes superoxide dismutase, catalase and glutathione peroxidase following SRLN treatment (Waza et al., 2018). In ischemia-reperfusion and oxidative damage, RLN upregulated Notch-1 signaling to increase cardiac muscle cell viability, decreased apoptosis as well as nitroxidative damage, and these positive effects were reduced in the presence of a Notch-1 inhibitor (Boccalini, Sassoli, Formigli, Bani, & Nistri, 2015). Several other studies have shown the cardioprotective role of RLN in ischemia-reperfusion injury suggesting a role for RLN in AMI (Bani, 2020). The broad ranging protective mechanisms include attenuating infarct size and the NLRP3 inflammasome (Valle Raleigh et al., 2017), reducing microvascular damage and inflammation (Gao et al., 2019).

Recently, it was also shown that left ventricular assist devices (LVAD) implanted in patients with end-stage heart disease trigger the RLN pathway showing potential for RLN to participate in myocardial recovery after HF (Cabiati, Botta, Caselli, & Del Ry, 2020). Using real-time PCR, this study demonstrated that RLN levels, along with the levels of endothelin-1 and inflammatory markers such as IL-6 and 8, increase significantly post-LVAD (Cabiati et al., 2020). In a very recent study mimicking decompensated HF, mice were subjected to pressure overload through TAC, followed by AAV9 treatment for expression of RXFP1 (Sasipong et al., 2021). Subsequent RLN administration not only slowed HF progression, but also restored systolic function of the left ventricle in vivo (Sasipong et al., 2021). Furthermore, the general upregulation of pathological markers of remodeling was also significantly reduced with RLN treatment (Sasipong et al., 2021).

4. Future directions

The numerous pre-clinical animal model studies that showed beneficial effects of RLN on tissue remodeling in general, and fibrosis and inflammation more specifically, continue to make RLN an attractive therapy for cardiovascular disease. However, this enthusiasm is dampened by poor clinical trial outcomes. Therefore, an understanding of the reasons for the discrepancy between pre-clinical and clinical findings is essential. Especially since RLN is safe and well-tolerated. Potential confounding factors in study participant composition has already been discussed in Section 3. However, probably the most critical factor is experimental design in pre-clinical studies versus clinical trial design. The RELAX-AHF-2 trial, the largest to date, administered RLN as IV infusion for just 48 h. It seems extremely unlikely that 2 days of RLN therapy would be able to reverse years of adverse remodeling of the heart. It takes time to reverse tissue remodeling. While RLN2 has been shown capable of reversing cardiac fibrosis in 9–10-month-old SHR for example, these hypertensive rats were treated for a two-week period (Lekgabe et al., 2005). It is unlikely that a two-day treatment would have been effective, even in rodents where timelines are typically compressed compared to humans. Matrix metalloproteinase (MMP)-2 was up-regulated by RLN2 in this study. Certain MMPs, including MMP-2, are capable of contributing to tissue remodeling through degradation of the ECM. Cardiac fibroblasts have been shown capable of increasing MMPs within days (Mookerjee, Unemori, Du, Tregear, & Samuel, 2005), however, it still takes time for ECM degradation to occur. Furthermore, if the long term beneficial effects of RLN are due to modifications at the gene level (Romero & Salama, 2021), then this too takes time to become established. Thus, a two-day infusion of RLN was likely doomed from the start. Future clinical trials would do well to incorporate substantially longer treatment periods.

The failure of Phase III clinical trials for RLN in HF may also in part be due to the short half-life of RLN, which then limits its therapeutic effectiveness. Thus, modified versions of RLN with increased half-life may prove more beneficial in a clinical setting. There have been numerous attempts to address this issue. Muppidi et al. (2019) took a semisynthetic approach of modifying the RLN A-chain to develop fatty acid-conjugated compounds with extended in vivo half-lives and improved in vivo efficacies. RLN activates RXFP1 primarily through the interaction of its B-chain. Accordingly, recent focus has been on exploiting this, with the recent identification of a single-chain peptide (B7-33), derived from this B-chain (Hossain et al., 2016). B7-33 is the first RXFP1 selective agonist. Despite lower potency than RLN (pKi of 5.54 vs 8.96), B7-33 was able to reverse both ischemia and isoprenaline-induced cardiac fibrosis to a level comparable to RLN. Very recently, Mallart et al., (Mallart et al., 2021) reported their efforts to identify a long-lasting B-chain RXFP1 agonist through a series of amino acid mutations, peptide length optimization, and fatty acid incorporation. Several agonists of increased potency and stability of the RLN B-chain were identified, with peptides displaying sub-nanomolar activity and high bioavailability, with extended half-lives (3–9 h) and in vivo efficacies.

A key finding in the RELAX-AHF trial was that RLN-induced changes in the first few days for biomarkers that reflect damage to the heart, kidney and liver have predictive value for 180 day prognosis in patients with AHF (Metra et al., 2013). Does this mean that for SRLN to be effective, it must be administered early in the disease state? That is, have clinical trials been less successful because enrolled individuals were of a population with late-stage disease, by which time SRLN is less effective? Endogenous expression of RLN is elevated in heart disease (Dschietzig et al., 2011). However, what happens to RXFP1 is less clear. Expression of RXFP1 has been shown to be decreased in the failing human myocardium (Dschietzig et al., 2011). Could the relative failure of SRLN clinical trials in relation to the extremely promising animal studies, in part be due to reduced levels of RXFP1? Administration of SRLN may be meaningless if there are not enough receptors available for activation. These are factors that should be considered and explored.

5. Conclusion

Although the 2009, 2013 and 2019 clinical trials have shown little promise for the treatment of HF with SRLN, taking all the available evidence, especially recently emerging, there is reason to pursue SRLN in more clinical trials. The positive effects of RLN in the cardiovascular system span a wide spectrum involving antifibrotic, antihypertrophic, anti-inflammatory, antiapoptotic, as well as antioxidant properties. Furthermore, it is important to note that, while varying results were obtained with various markers of HF disease progression, SRLN treatment was always shown to be well tolerated and safe. As discussed above, modifications to the original structure of the molecule to improve half-life holds great promise. Taken together, this might lead to the development of more clinical studies in the future especially with increased doses and/or modified versions of SRLN.

Acknowledgment

This work was supported in part by the George and Mary Thompson Fellowship (SPL).

Conflicts of interest

The authors have no conflicts of interest to declare.

References

Aragón-Herrera, A., Feijóo-Bandín, S., Abella, V., Álvarez, L., Roselló-Lletí, E., Portolés, M., et al. (2019). Serelaxin (recombinant human relaxin-2) treatment affects the endogenous synthesis of long chain poly-unsaturated fatty acids and induces substantial alterations of lipidome and metabolome profiles in rat cardiac tissue. *Pharmacological Research*, *144*, 51–65. https://doi.org/10.1016/j.phrs.2019.04.009.

Aragón-Herrera, A., Feijóo-Bandín, S., Rodríguez-Penas, D., Roselló-Lletí, E., Portolés, M., Rivera, M., et al. (2018). Relaxin activates AMPK-AKT signaling and increases glucose uptake by cultured cardiomyocytes. *Endocrine*, *60*(1), 103–111. https://doi.org/10.1007/s12020-018-1534-3.

Bani, D. (2020). Recombinant human H2 relaxin (serelaxin) as a cardiovascular drug: Aiming at the right target. *Drug Discovery Today*, *25*(7), 1239–1244. https://doi.org/10.1016/j.drudis.2020.04.014.

Bani-Sacchi, T., Bigazzi, M., Bani, D., Mannaioni, P. F., & Masini, E. (1995). Relaxin-induced increased coronary flow through stimulation of nitric oxide production. *British Journal of Pharmacology*, *116*(1), 1589–1594. https://doi.org/10.1111/j.1476-5381.1995.tb16377.x.

Bathgate, R. A., Halls, M. L., van der Westhuizen, E. T., Callander, G. E., Kocan, M., & Summers, R. J. (2013). Relaxin family peptides and their receptors. *Physiological Reviews*, *93*(1), 405–480. https://doi.org/10.1152/physrev.00001.2012.

Bathgate, R. A., Ivell, R., Sanborn, B. M., Sherwood, O. D., & Summers, R. J. (2006). International Union of Pharmacology LVII: Recommendations for the nomenclature of receptors for relaxin family peptides. *Pharmacological Reviews*, *58*(1), 7–31. https://doi.org/10.1124/pr.58.1.9.

Bathgate, R. A., Lekgabe, E. D., McGuane, J. T., Su, Y., Pham, T., Ferraro, T., et al. (2008). Adenovirus-mediated delivery of relaxin reverses cardiac fibrosis. *Molecular and Cellular Endocrinology*, *280*(1–2), 30–38. https://doi.org/10.1016/j.mce.2007.09.008.

Beiert, T., Tiyerili, V., Knappe, V., Effelsberg, V., Linhart, M., Stöckigt, F., et al. (2017). Relaxin reduces susceptibility to post-infarct atrial fibrillation in mice due to anti-fibrotic and anti-inflammatory properties. *Biochemical and Biophysical Research Communications*, *490*(3), 643–649. https://doi.org/10.1016/j.bbrc.2017.06.091.

Boccalini, G., Sassoli, C., Formigli, L., Bani, D., & Nistri, S. (2015). Relaxin protects cardiac muscle cells from hypoxia/reoxygenation injury: Involvement of the Notch-1 pathway. *The FASEB Journal*, *29*(1), 239–249. https://doi.org/10.1096/fj.14-254854.

Cabiati, M., Botta, L., Caselli, C., & Del Ry, S. (2020). Transcriptional evaluation of relaxin and endothelin-1 axis in heart failure patients: First evidence of its involvement during left ventricular assist device support. *International Journal of Cardiology*, *306*, 109–115. https://doi.org/10.1016/j.ijcard.2020.02.058.

Cargill, R. I., & Lipworth, B. J. (1995). The role of the renin-angiotensin and natriuretic peptide systems in the pulmonary vasculature. *British Journal of Clinical Pharmacology*, *40*(1), 11–18. https://doi.org/10.1111/j.1365-2125.1995.tb04528.x.

Chen, T. Y., Li, X., Hung, C. H., Bahudhanapati, H., Tan, J., Kass, D. J., et al. (2020). The relaxin family peptide receptor 1 (RXFP1): An emerging player in human health and disease. *Molecular Genetics & Genomic Medicine*, *8*(4), e1194. https://doi.org/10.1002/mgg3.1194.

Chow, B. S., Chew, E. G., Zhao, C., Bathgate, R. A., Hewitson, T. D., & Samuel, C. S. (2012). Relaxin signals through a RXFP1-pERK-nNOS-NO-cGMP-dependent pathway to up-regulate matrix metalloproteinases: The additional involvement of iNOS. *PLoS One*, 7(8), e42714. https://doi.org/10.1371/journal.pone.0042714.

Chow, B. S. M., Kocan, M., Shen, M., Wang, Y., Han, L., Chew, J. Y., et al. (2019). AT1R-AT2R-RXFP1 functional crosstalk in Myofibroblasts: Impact on the therapeutic targeting of renal and cardiac fibrosis. *Journal of the American Society of Nephrology*, *30*(11), 2191–2207. https://doi.org/10.1681/asn.2019060597.

Conrad, K. P. (2011). Emerging role of relaxin in the maternal adaptations to normal pregnancy: Implications for preeclampsia. *Seminars in Nephrology*, *31*(1), 15–32. https://doi.org/10.1016/j.semnephrol.2010.10.003.

Conrad, KP, Debrah, DO, Novak, J, Danielson, LA, & Shroff, SG. (2004). Relaxin modifies systemic arterial resistance and compliance in conscious, nonpregnant rats. *Endocrinology*, *145*, 3289–3296.

Conrad, K. P., & Novak, J. (2004). Emerging role of relaxin in renal and cardiovascular function. *American Journal of Physiology. Regulatory, Integrative and Comparative Physiology*, *287*(2), R250–R261. https://doi.org/10.1152/ajpregu.00672.2003.

Conrad, K. P., & Shroff, S. G. (2011). Effects of relaxin on arterial dilation, remodeling, and mechanical properties. *Current Hypertension Reports*, *13*(6), 409–420. https://doi.org/10.1007/s11906-011-0231-x.

Coulson, C. C., Thorp, J. M., Jr., Mayer, D. C., & Cefalo, R. C. (1996). Central hemodynamic effects of recombinant human relaxin in the isolated, perfused rat heart model. *Obstetrics and Gynecology*, *87*(4), 610–612. https://doi.org/10.1016/0029-7844(95)00493-9.

Danielson, L. A., Kercher, L. J., & Conrad, K. P. (2000). Impact of gender and endothelin on renal vasodilation and hyperfiltration induced by relaxin in conscious rats. *American Journal of Physiology. Regulatory, Integrative and Comparative Physiology*, *279*(4), R1298–R1304. https://doi.org/10.1152/ajpregu.2000.279.4.R1298.

Danielson, L. A., Sherwood, O. D., & Conrad, K. P. (1999). Relaxin is a potent renal vasodilator in conscious rats. *The Journal of Clinical Investigation*, *103*(4), 525–533. https://doi.org/10.1172/jci5630.

Debrah, D. O., Conrad, K. P., Jeyabalan, A., Danielson, L. A., & Shroff, S. G. (2005). Relaxin increases cardiac output and reduces systemic arterial load in hypertensive rats. *Hypertension*, *46*(4), 745–750. https://doi.org/10.1161/01.Hyp.0000184230.52059.33.

Debrah, D. O., Debrah, J. E., Haney, J. L., McGuane, J. T., Sacks, M. S., Conrad, K. P., et al. (2011). Relaxin regulates vascular wall remodeling and passive mechanical properties in mice. *Journal of Applied Physiology (Bethesda, MD: 1985)*, *111*(1), 260–271. https://doi.org/10.1152/japplphysiol.00845.2010.

Debrah, D. O., Novak, J., Matthews, J. E., Ramirez, R. J., Shroff, S. G., & Conrad, K. P. (2006). Relaxin is essential for systemic vasodilation and increased global arterial compliance during early pregnancy in conscious rats. *Endocrinology*, *147*(11), 5126–5131. https://doi.org/10.1210/en.2006-0567.

Dschietzig, T., Alexiou, K., Kinkel, H. T., Baumann, G., Matschke, K., & Stangl, K. (2011). The positive inotropic effect of relaxin-2 in human atrial myocardium is preserved in end-stage heart failure: Role of G(i)-phosphoinositide-3 kinase signaling. *Journal of Cardiac Failure*, *17*(2), 158–166. https://doi.org/10.1016/j.cardfail.2010.08.011.

Dschietzig, T., Bartsch, C., Baumann, G., & Stangl, K. (2006). Relaxin-a pleiotropic hormone and its emerging role for experimental and clinical therapeutics. *Pharmacology & Therapeutics*, *112*(1), 38–56. https://doi.org/10.1016/j.pharmthera.2006.03.004.

Dschietzig, T., Bartsch, C., Richter, C., Laule, M., Baumann, G., & Stangl, K. (2003). Relaxin, a pregnancy hormone, is a functional endothelin-1 antagonist: Attenuation of endothelin-1-mediated vasoconstriction by stimulation of endothelin type-B receptor expression via ERK-1/2 and nuclear factor-kappaB. *Circulation Research*, *92*(1), 32–40. https://doi.org/10.1161/01.res.0000051884.27117.7e.

Du, X. J., Samuel, C. S., Gao, X. M., Zhao, L., Parry, L. J., & Tregear, G. W. (2003). Increased myocardial collagen and ventricular diastolic dysfunction in relaxin deficient mice: A gender-specific phenotype. *Cardiovascular Research, 57*(2), 395–404. https://doi.org/10.1016/s0008-6363(02)00663-6.

Failli, P., Nistri, S., Quattrone, S., Mazzetti, L., Bigazzi, M., Sacchi, T. B., et al. (2002). Relaxin up-regulates inducible nitric oxide synthase expression and nitric oxide generation in rat coronary endothelial cells. *The FASEB Journal, 16*(2), 252–254. https://doi.org/10.1096/fj.01-0569fje.

Feijóo-Bandín, S., Aragón-Herrera, A., Rodríguez-Penas, D., Portolés, M., Roselló-Lletí, E., Rivera, M., et al. (2017). Relaxin-2 in Cardiometabolic diseases: Mechanisms of action and future perspectives. *Frontiers in Physiology, 8*, 599. https://doi.org/10.3389/fphys.2017.00599.

Fevold, H. L., Hisaw, F. L., & Meyer, R. K. (1930). The relaxative hormone of the corpus luteum. Its purification and concentration. *Journal of the American Chemistry Society, 52*, 3340–3348.

Gao, X. M., Su, Y., Moore, S., Han, L. P., Kiriazis, H., Lu, Q., et al. (2019). Relaxin mitigates microvascular damage and inflammation following cardiac ischemia-reperfusion. *Basic Research in Cardiology, 114*(4), 30. https://doi.org/10.1007/s00395-019-0739-9.

Haase, N., Golic, M., Herse, F., Rugor, J., Linz, D., Solano, M. E., et al. (2016). Relaxin treatment in an Ang-II-based transgenic Preeclamptic-rat model. *PLoS One, 11*(3), e0150743. https://doi.org/10.1371/journal.pone.0150743.

Haley, J., Hudson, P., Scanlon, D., John, M., Cronk, M., Shine, J., et al. (1982). Porcine relaxin: Molecular cloning and cDNA structure. *DNA, 1*(2), 155–162. https://doi.org/10.1089/dna.1.1982.1.155.

Halls, M. L., Bathgate, R. A., Sutton, S. W., Dschietzig, T. B., & Summers, R. J. (2015). International Union of Basic and Clinical Pharmacology. XCV. Recent advances in the understanding of the pharmacology and biological roles of relaxin family peptide receptors 1-4, the receptors for relaxin family peptides. *Pharmacological Reviews, 67*(2), 389–440. https://doi.org/10.1124/pr.114.009472.

Halls, M. L., Hewitson, T. D., Moore, X. L., Du, X. J., Bathgate, R. A., & Summers, R. J. (2009). Relaxin activates multiple cAMP signaling pathway profiles in different target cells. *Annals of the New York Academy of Sciences, 1160*, 108–111. https://doi.org/10.1111/j.1749-6632.2008.03814.x.

Han, X., Habuchi, Y., & Giles, W. R. (1994). Relaxin increases heart rate by modulating calcium current in cardiac pacemaker cells. *Circulation Research, 74*(3), 537–541. https://doi.org/10.1161/01.res.74.3.537.

Hisaw, F. L. (1926). Experimental relaxation of the pubic ligament of the guinea pig. *Proceedings of the Society for Experimental Biology and Medicine, 23*(8), 661–663. https://doi.org/10.3181/00379727-23-3107.

Hisaw, F. L., Hisaw, F. L., Jr., & Dawson, A. B. (1967). Effects of relaxin on the endothelium of endometrial blood vessels in monkeys (Macaca mulatta). *Endocrinology, 81*(2), 375–385. https://doi.org/10.1210/endo-81-2-375.

Ho, T. Y., Dilts, M. A., Bartol, F. F., & Bagnell, C. A. (2009). Relaxin promotes matrix metalloproteinase-2 and decreases Wnt/beta-catenin expression in the neonatal porcine heart. *Annals of the New York Academy of Sciences, 1160*, 287–288. https://doi.org/10.1111/j.1749-6632.2008.03810.x.

Hossain, M. A., Kocan, M., Yao, S. T., Royce, S. G., Nair, V. B., Siwek, C., et al. (2016). A single-chain derivative of the relaxin hormone is a functionally selective agonist of the G protein-coupled receptor, RXFP1. *Chemical Science, 7*(6), 3805–3819. https://doi.org/10.1039/c5sc04754d.

Hossain, M. A., Man, B. C., Zhao, C., Xu, Q., Du, X. J., Wade, J. D., et al. (2011). H3 relaxin demonstrates antifibrotic properties via the RXFP1 receptor. *Biochemistry, 50*(8), 1368–1375. https://doi.org/10.1021/bi1013968.

Hu, H. H., Cao, G., Wu, X. Q., Vaziri, N. D., & Zhao, Y. Y. (2020). Wnt signaling pathway in aging-related tissue fibrosis and therapies. *Ageing Research Reviews*, *60*, 101063. https://doi.org/10.1016/j.arr.2020.101063.

Hudson, P., Haley, J., Cronk, M., Shine, J., & Niall, H. (1981). Molecular cloning and characterization of cDNA sequences coding for rat relaxin. *Nature*, *291*(5811), 127–131. https://doi.org/10.1038/291127a0.

Hudson, P., Haley, J., John, M., Cronk, M., Crawford, R., Haralambidis, J., et al. (1983). Structure of a genomic clone encoding biologically active human relaxin. *Nature*, *301*(5901), 628–631. https://doi.org/10.1038/301628a0.

Jelinic, M., Tare, M., Conrad, K. P., & Parry, L. J. (2015). Differential effects of relaxin deficiency on vascular aging in arteries of male mice. *Age (Dordrecht, Netherlands)*, *37*(4), 9803. https://doi.org/10.1007/s11357-015-9803-z.

Kakouris, H., Eddie, L. W., & Summers, R. J. (1992). Cardiac effects of relaxin in rats. *Lancet*, *339*(8801), 1076–1078. https://doi.org/10.1016/0140-6736(92)90665-p.

Kingwell, B. A. (2000). Nitric oxide-mediated metabolic regulation during exercise: Effects of training in health and cardiovascular disease. *The FASEB Journal*, *14*(12), 1685–1696. https://doi.org/10.1096/fj.99-0896rev.

Kompa, A. R., Samuel, C. S., & Summers, R. J. (2002). Inotropic responses to human gene 2 (B29) relaxin in a rat model of myocardial infarction (MI): Effect of pertussis toxin. *British Journal of Pharmacology*, *137*(5), 710–718. https://doi.org/10.1038/sj.bjp.0704922.

Lam, M., Royce, S. G., Donovan, C., Jelinic, M., Parry, L. J., Samuel, C. S., et al. (2016). Serelaxin elicits bronchodilation and enhances β-adrenoceptor-mediated airway relaxation. *Frontiers in Pharmacology*, 7, 406. https://doi.org/10.3389/fphar.2016.00406.

Lapinskas, T., Kelle, S., Grune, J., Foryst-Ludwig, A., Meyborg, H., Jeuthe, S., et al. (2020). Serelaxin improves regional myocardial function in experimental heart failure: An in vivo cardiac magnetic resonance study. *Journal of the American Heart Association*, *9*(3), e013702. https://doi.org/10.1161/jaha.119.013702.

Lekgabe, E. D., Kiriazis, H., Zhao, C., Xu, Q., Moore, X. L., Su, Y., et al. (2005). Relaxin reverses cardiac and renal fibrosis in spontaneously hypertensive rats. *Hypertension*, *46*(2), 412–418. https://doi.org/10.1161/01.HYP.0000171930.00697.2f.

Leo, C. H., Jelinic, M., Gooi, J. H., Tare, M., & Parry, L. J. (2014). A vasoactive role for endogenous relaxin in mesenteric arteries of male mice. *PLoS One*, *9*(9), e107382. https://doi.org/10.1371/journal.pone.0107382.

Liu, S., Vinall, R. L., Tepper, C., Shi, X. B., Xue, L. R., Ma, A. H., et al. (2008). Inappropriate activation of androgen receptor by relaxin via beta-catenin pathway. *Oncogene*, *27*(4), 499–505. https://doi.org/10.1038/sj.onc.1210671.

Lukowski, R., Krieg, T., Rybalkin, S. D., Beavo, J., & Hofmann, F. (2014). Turning on cGMP-dependent pathways to treat cardiac dysfunctions: Boom, bust, and beyond. *Trends in Pharmacological Sciences*, *35*(8), 404–413. https://doi.org/10.1016/j.tips.2014.05.003.

Mallart, S., Ingenito, R., Bianchi, E., Bresciani, A., Esposito, S., Gallo, M., et al. (2021). Identification of potent and long-acting single-chain peptide mimetics of human Relaxin-2 for cardiovascular diseases. *Journal of Medicinal Chemistry*, *64*(4), 2139–2150. https://doi.org/10.1021/acs.jmedchem.0c01533.

Martin, B., Gabris, B., Barakat, A. F., Henry, B. L., Giannini, M., Reddy, R. P., et al. (2019). Relaxin reverses maladaptive remodeling of the aged heart through Wnt-signaling. *Scientific Reports*, *9*(1), 18545. https://doi.org/10.1038/s41598-019-53867-y.

Martin, B., Gabris-Weber, B. A., Reddy, R., Romero, G., Chattopadhyay, A., & Salama, G. (2018). Relaxin reverses inflammatory and immune signals in aged hearts. *PLoS One*, *13*(1), e0190935. https://doi.org/10.1371/journal.pone.0190935.

Martin, B., Romero, G., & Salama, G. (2019). Cardioprotective actions of relaxin. *Molecular and Cellular Endocrinology*, *487*, 45–53. https://doi.org/10.1016/j.mce.2018.12.016.

McCullough, P. A. (2017). How Trialists and pharmaceutical sponsors have failed us by thinking that acute heart failure is a 48-hour illness. *The American Journal of Cardiology, 120*(3), 505–508. https://doi.org/10.1016/j.amjcard.2017.04.056.

McGuane, J. T., Debrah, J. E., Sautina, L., Jarajapu, Y. P., Novak, J., Rubin, J. P., et al. (2011). Relaxin induces rapid dilation of rodent small renal and human subcutaneous arteries via PI3 kinase and nitric oxide. *Endocrinology, 152*(7), 2786–2796. https://doi.org/10.1210/en.2010-1126.

Metra, M., Cotter, G., Davison, B. A., Felker, G. M., Filippatos, G., Greenberg, B. H., et al. (2013). Effect of serelaxin on cardiac, renal, and hepatic biomarkers in the Relaxin in acute heart failure (RELAX-AHF) development program: Correlation with outcomes. *Journal of the American College of Cardiology, 61*(2), 196–206. Retrieved from http://www.ncbi.nlm.nih.gov/pubmed/23273292.

Metra, M., Teerlink, J. R., Cotter, G., Davison, B. A., Felker, G. M., Filippatos, G., et al. (2019). Effects of Serelaxin in patients with acute heart failure. *The New England Journal of Medicine, 381*(8), 716–726. https://doi.org/10.1056/NEJMoa1801291.

Miró, Ò., Herrero-Puente, P., Prieto, B., García-García, M., García-Hernández, P., Martín-Sánchez, F. J., et al. (2018). The subset of patients with acute heart failure able to secrete relaxin-2 at pregnancy concentrations could have a longer survival: A pilot study. *Biomarkers, 23*(6), 573–579. https://doi.org/10.1080/1354750x.2018.1463564.

Miyares, M. A., & Davis, K. A. (2013). Serelaxin, a 'breakthrough' investigational intravenous agent for acute heart failure. *Pharmacy and Therapeutics, 38*(10), 606–611.

Mookerjee, I., Hewitson, T. D., Halls, M. L., Summers, R. J., Mathai, M. L., Bathgate, R. A., et al. (2009). Relaxin inhibits renal myofibroblast differentiation via RXFP1, the nitric oxide pathway, and Smad2. *The FASEB Journal, 23*(4), 1219–1229. https://doi.org/10.1096/fj.08-120857.

Mookerjee, I., Unemori, E. N., Du, X. J., Tregear, G. W., & Samuel, C. S. (2005). Relaxin modulates fibroblast function, collagen production, and matrix metalloproteinase-2 expression by cardiac fibroblasts. *Annals of the New York Academy of Sciences, 1041*, 190–193. https://doi.org/10.1196/annals.1282.028.

Moore, X. L., Tan, S. L., Lo, C. Y., Fang, L., Su, Y. D., Gao, X. M., et al. (2007). Relaxin antagonizes hypertrophy and apoptosis in neonatal rat cardiomyocytes. *Endocrinology, 148*(4), 1582–1589. https://doi.org/10.1210/en.2006-1324.

Muppidi, A., Lee, S. J., Hsu, C. H., Zou, H., Lee, C., Pflimlin, E., et al. (2019). Design and synthesis of potent, long-acting Lipidated Relaxin-2 analogs. *Bioconjugate Chemistry, 30*(1), 83–89. https://doi.org/10.1021/acs.bioconjchem.8b00764.

New, D. C., Wu, K., Kwok, A. W., & Wong, Y. H. (2007). G protein-coupled receptor-induced Akt activity in cellular proliferation and apoptosis. *The FEBS Journal, 274*(23), 6025–6036. https://doi.org/10.1111/j.1742-4658.2007.06116.x.

Ng, H. H., Jelinic, M., Parry, L. J., & Leo, C. H. (2015). Increased superoxide production and altered nitric oxide-mediated relaxation in the aorta of young but not old male relaxin-deficient mice. *American Journal of Physiology. Heart and Circulatory Physiology, 309*(2), H285–H296. https://doi.org/10.1152/ajpheart.00786.2014.

Nistor, M., Schmidt, M., & Schiffner, R. (2018). The relaxin peptide family - potential future hope for neuroprotective therapy? A short review. *Neural Regeneration Research, 13*(3), 402–405. https://doi.org/10.4103/1673-5374.228713.

Nistri, S., Pini, A., Sassoli, C., Squecco, R., Francini, F., Formigli, L., et al. (2012). Relaxin promotes growth and maturation of mouse neonatal cardiomyocytes in vitro: Clues for cardiac regeneration. *Journal of Cellular and Molecular Medicine, 16*(3), 507–519. https://doi.org/10.1111/j.1582-4934.2011.01328.x.

Novak, J., Danielson, L. A., Kerchner, L. J., Sherwood, O. D., Ramirez, R. J., Moalli, P. A., et al. (2001). Relaxin is essential for renal vasodilation during pregnancy in conscious rats. *The Journal of Clinical Investigation, 107*(11), 1469–1475. https://doi.org/10.1172/jci11975.

Parikh, A., Patel, D., McTiernan, C. F., Xiang, W., Haney, J., Yang, L., et al. (2013). Relaxin suppresses atrial fibrillation by reversing fibrosis and myocyte hypertrophy and increasing conduction velocity and sodium current in spontaneously hypertensive rat hearts. *Circulation Research*, *113*(3), 313–321. https://doi.org/10.1161/circresaha.113.301646.

Pini, A., Boccalini, G., Baccari, M. C., Becatti, M., Garella, R., Fiorillo, C., et al. (2016). Protection from cigarette smoke-induced vascular injury by recombinant human relaxin-2 (serelaxin). *Journal of Cellular and Molecular Medicine*, *20*(5), 891–902. https://doi.org/10.1111/jcmm.12802.

Quattrone, S., Chiappini, L., Scapagnini, G., Bigazzi, B., & Bani, D. (2004). Relaxin potentiates the expression of inducible nitric oxide synthase by endothelial cells from human umbilical vein in in vitro culture. *Molecular Human Reproduction*, *10*(5), 325–330. https://doi.org/10.1093/molehr/gah040.

Ramlakhan, K. P., Johnson, M. R., & Roos-Hesselink, J. W. (2020). Pregnancy and cardiovascular disease. *Nature Reviews. Cardiology*, *17*(11), 718–731. https://doi.org/10.1038/s41569-020-0390-z.

Romero, G., & Salama, G. (2021). Relaxin abrogates genomic remodeling of the aged heart. *Vitamins and Hormones*, *115*, 419–448. https://doi.org/10.1016/bs.vh.2020.12.017.

Samuel, C. S., Bodaragama, H., Chew, J. Y., Widdop, R. E., Royce, S. G., & Hewitson, T. D. (2014). Serelaxin is a more efficacious antifibrotic than enalapril in an experimental model of heart disease. *Hypertension*, *64*(2), 315–322. https://doi.org/10.1161/hypertensionaha.114.03594.

Samuel, C. S., Cendrawan, S., Gao, X. M., Ming, Z., Zhao, C., Kiriazis, H., et al. (2011). Relaxin remodels fibrotic healing following myocardial infarction. *Laboratory Investigation*, *91*(5), 675–690. https://doi.org/10.1038/labinvest.2010.198.

Samuel, C. S., Unemori, E. N., Mookerjee, I., Bathgate, R. A., Layfield, S. L., Mak, J., et al. (2004). Relaxin modulates cardiac fibroblast proliferation, differentiation, and collagen production and reverses cardiac fibrosis in vivo. *Endocrinology*, *145*(9), 4125–4133. https://doi.org/10.1210/en.2004-0209.

Sarwar, M., Du, X. J., Dschietzig, T. B., & Summers, R. J. (2017). The actions of relaxin on the human cardiovascular system. *British Journal of Pharmacology*, *174*(10), 933–949. https://doi.org/10.1111/bph.13523.

Sarwar, M., Samuel, C. S., Bathgate, R. A., Stewart, D. R., & Summers, R. J. (2015). Serelaxin-mediated signal transduction in human vascular cells: Bell-shaped concentration-response curves reflect differential coupling to G proteins. *British Journal of Pharmacology*, *172*(4), 1005–1019. https://doi.org/10.1111/bph.12964.

Sasipong, N., Schlegel, P., Wingert, J., Lederer, C., Meinhardt, E., Ziefer, A., et al. (2021). Ligand-activated RXFP1 gene therapy ameliorates pressure overload-induced cardiac dysfunction. *Molecular Therapy*, *29*(8), 2499–2513. https://doi.org/10.1016/j.ymthe.2021.04.010.

Sasser, J. M., Cunningham, M. W., Jr., & Baylis, C. (2014). Serelaxin reduces oxidative stress and asymmetric dimethylarginine in angiotensin II-induced hypertension. *American Journal of Physiology. Renal Physiology*, *307*(12), F1355–F1362. https://doi.org/10.1152/ajprenal.00407.2014.

Sasser, J. M., Molnar, M., & Baylis, C. (2011). Relaxin ameliorates hypertension and increases nitric oxide metabolite excretion in angiotensin II but not N(ω)-nitro-L-arginine methyl ester hypertensive rats. *Hypertension*, *58*(2), 197–204. https://doi.org/10.1161/hypertensionaha.110.164392.

Sassoli, C., Chellini, F., Pini, A., Tani, A., Nistri, S., Nosi, D., et al. (2013). Relaxin prevents cardiac fibroblast-myofibroblast transition via notch-1-mediated inhibition of TGF-β/Smad3 signaling. *PLoS One*, *8*(5), e63896. https://doi.org/10.1371/journal.pone.0063896.

Shaw, E. E., Wood, P., Kulpa, J., Yang, F. H., Summerlee, A. J., & Pyle, W. G. (2009). Relaxin alters cardiac myofilament function through a PKC-dependent pathway. *American Journal of Physiology. Heart and Circulatory Physiology*, *297*(1), H29–H36. https://doi.org/10.1152/ajpheart.00482.2008.

Shuai, X. X., Meng, Y. D., Lu, Y. X., Su, G. H., Tao, X. F., Han, J., et al. (2016). Relaxin-2 improves diastolic function of pressure-overloaded rats via phospholamban by activating Akt. *International Journal of Cardiology*, *218*, 305–311. https://doi.org/10.1016/j.ijcard.2016.05.011.

Simon, J., Nemeth, E., Nemes, A., Husveth-Toth, M., Radovits, T., Foldes, G., et al. (2019). Circulating Relaxin-1 level is a surrogate marker of myocardial fibrosis in HFrEF. *Frontiers in Physiology*, *10*, 690. https://doi.org/10.3389/fphys.2019.00690.

Squecco, R., Sassoli, C., Garella, R., Chellini, F., Idrizaj, E., Nistri, S., et al. (2015). Inhibitory effects of relaxin on cardiac fibroblast-to-myofibroblast transition: An electrophysiological study. *Experimental Physiology*, *100*(6), 652–666. https://doi.org/10.1113/ep085178.

St-Louis, J., & Massicotte, G. (1985). Chronic decrease of blood pressure by rat relaxin in spontaneously hypertensive rats. *Life Sciences*, *37*(14), 1351–1357. https://doi.org/10.1016/0024-3205(85)90251-6.

Sun, J., Hao, W., Fillmore, N., Ma, H., Springer, D., Yu, Z. X., et al. (2019). Human Relaxin-2 fusion protein treatment prevents and reverses isoproterenol-induced hypertrophy and fibrosis in mouse heart. *Journal of the American Heart Association*, *8*(24), e013465. https://doi.org/10.1161/jaha.119.013465.

Teerlink, J. R., Cotter, G., Davison, B. A., Felker, G. M., Filippatos, G., Greenberg, B. H., et al. (2013). Serelaxin, recombinant human relaxin-2, for treatment of acute heart failure (RELAX-AHF): A randomised, placebo-controlled trial. *Lancet*, *381*(9860), 29–39. https://doi.org/10.1016/s0140-6736(12)61855-8.

Teerlink, J. R., Metra, M., Felker, G. M., Ponikowski, P., Voors, A. A., Weatherley, B. D., et al. (2009). Relaxin for the treatment of patients with acute heart failure (pre-RELAX-AHF): A multicentre, randomised, placebo-controlled, parallel-group, dose-finding phase IIb study. *Lancet*, *373*(9673), 1429–1439. https://doi.org/10.1016/s0140-6736(09)60622-x.

Tiyerili, V., Beiert, T., Schatten, H., Camara, B., Jehle, J., Schrickel, J. W., et al. (2016). Anti-atherosclerotic effects of serelaxin in apolipoprotein E-deficient mice. *Atherosclerosis*, *251*, 430–437. https://doi.org/10.1016/j.atherosclerosis.2016.06.008.

Valle Raleigh, J., Mauro, A. G., Devarakonda, T., Marchetti, C., He, J., Kim, E., et al. (2017). Reperfusion therapy with recombinant human relaxin-2 (Serelaxin) attenuates myocardial infarct size and NLRP3 inflammasome following ischemia/reperfusion injury via eNOS-dependent mechanism. *Cardiovascular Research*, *113*(6), 609–619. https://doi.org/10.1093/cvr/cvw246.

Wang, T. S., Hellkamp, A. S., Patel, C. B., Ezekowitz, J. A., Fonarow, G. C., & Hernandez, A. F. (2014). Representativeness of RELAX-AHF clinical trial population in acute heart failure. *Circulation. Cardiovascular Quality and Outcomes*, 7(2), 259–268. https://doi.org/10.1161/circoutcomes.113.000418.

Wang, C., Kemp-Harper, B. K., Kocan, M., Ang, S. Y., Hewitson, T. D., & Samuel, C. S. (2016). The anti-fibrotic actions of Relaxin are mediated through a NO-sGC-cGMP-dependent pathway in renal Myofibroblasts in vitro and enhanced by the NO donor, Diethylamine NONOate. *Frontiers in Pharmacology*, 7, 91. https://doi.org/10.3389/fphar.2016.00091.

Wang, D., Luo, Y., Myakala, K., Orlicky, D. J., Dobrinskikh, E., Wang, X., et al. (2017). Serelaxin improves cardiac and renal function in DOCA-salt hypertensive rats. *Scientific Reports*, 7(1), 9793. https://doi.org/10.1038/s41598-017-09470-0.

Wang, D., Zhu, H., Yang, Q., & Sun, Y. (2016). Effects of relaxin on cardiac fibrosis, apoptosis, and tachyarrhythmia in rats with myocardial infarction. *Biomedicine & Pharmacotherapy*, *84*, 348–355. https://doi.org/10.1016/j.biopha.2016.09.054.

Waza, A. A., Hamid, Z., Bhat, S. A., Shah, N. U. D., Bhat, M., & Ganai, B. (2018). Relaxin protects cardiomyocytes against hypoxia-induced damage in in-vitro conditions: Involvement of Nrf2/HO-1 signaling pathway. *Life Sciences*, *213*, 25–31. https://doi.org/10.1016/j.lfs.2018.08.059.

Wei, X., Yang, Y., Jiang, Y. J., Lei, J. M., Guo, J. W., & Xiao, H. (2018). Relaxin ameliorates high glucose-induced cardiomyocyte hypertrophy and apoptosis via the Notch1 pathway. *Experimental and Therapeutic Medicine*, *15*(1), 691–698. https://doi.org/10.3892/etm.2017.5448.

Wilhelmi, T., Xu, X., Tan, X., Hulshoff, M. S., Maamari, S., Sossalla, S., et al. (2020). Serelaxin alleviates cardiac fibrosis through inhibiting endothelial-to-mesenchymal transition via RXFP1. *Theranostics*, *10*(9), 3905–3924. https://doi.org/10.7150/thno.38640.

Wu, X. P., Wang, H. J., Wang, Y. L., Shen, H. R., & Tan, Y. Z. (2018). Serelaxin inhibits differentiation and fibrotic behaviors of cardiac fibroblasts by suppressing ALK-5/Smad2/3 signaling pathway. *Experimental Cell Research*, *362*(1), 17–27. https://doi.org/10.1016/j.yexcr.2017.10.004.

Yang, Z. Z., Tschopp, O., Baudry, A., Dümmler, B., Hynx, D., & Hemmings, B. A. (2004). Physiological functions of protein kinase B/Akt. *Biochemical Society Transactions*, *32*(Pt 2), 350–354. https://doi.org/10.1042/bst0320350.

You, X., Guo, Z. F., Cheng, F., Yi, B., Yang, F., Liu, X., et al. (2018). Transcriptional up-regulation of relaxin-3 by Nur77 attenuates β-adrenergic agonist-induced apoptosis in cardiomyocytes. *The Journal of Biological Chemistry*, *293*(36), 14001–14011. https://doi.org/10.1074/jbc.RA118.003099.

Yuan, Y., Zhang, Y., Han, X., Li, Y., Zhao, X., Sheng, L., et al. (2017). Relaxin alleviates TGFβ1-induced cardiac fibrosis via inhibition of Stat3-dependent autophagy. *Biochemical and Biophysical Research Communications*, *493*(4), 1601–1607. https://doi.org/10.1016/j.bbrc.2017.09.110.

Zhang, Q., Liu, S. H., Erikson, M., Lewis, M., & Unemori, E. (2002). Relaxin activates the MAP kinase pathway in human endometrial stromal cells. *Journal of Cellular Biochemistry*, *85*(3), 536–544. https://doi.org/10.1002/jcb.10150.

Zhang, X., Pan, L., Yang, K., Fu, Y., Liu, Y., Chi, J., et al. (2017). H3 Relaxin protects against myocardial injury in experimental diabetic cardiomyopathy by inhibiting myocardial apoptosis, fibrosis and inflammation. *Cellular Physiology and Biochemistry*, *43*(4), 1311–1324. https://doi.org/10.1159/000481843.

CHAPTER SEVEN

Cardiovascular effects of GLP-1 receptor agonism

Raymond J. Winquist[a,*] and Valentin K. Gribkoff[b,c]
[a]Alkermes Pharmaceuticals Inc., Waltham, MA, United States
[b]Section on Endocrinology, Department of Internal Medicine, Yale University School of Medicine, New Haven, CT, United States
[c]TheraStat LLC, Weston, MA, United States
*Corresponding author: e-mail address: winquist@aol.com

Contents

Abstract

Glucagon-like peptide-1 (GLP-1) receptor agonists are extensively used in type 2 diabetic patients for the effective control of hyperglycemia. It is now clear from outcomes trials that this class of drugs offers important additional benefits to these patients due to reducing the risk of developing major adverse cardiac events (MACE). This risk reduction is, in part, due to effective glycemic control in patients; however, the various outcomes trials, further validated by subsequent meta-analysis of the outcomes trials, suggest that the risk reduction in MACE is also dependent on glycemic-independent mechanisms

Advances in Pharmacology, Volume 94
ISSN 1054-3589
https://doi.org/10.1016/bs.apha.2022.02.005

operant in cardiovascular tissues. These glycemic-independent mechanisms are likely mediated by GLP-1 receptors found throughout the cardiovascular system and by the complex signaling cascades triggered by the binding of agonists to the G-protein coupled receptors. This heterogeneity of signaling pathways underlying different downstream effects of GLP-1 agonists, and the discovery of biased agonists favoring specific signaling pathways, may have import in the future treatment of MACE in these patients. We review the evidence supporting the glycemic-independent evidence for risk reduction of MACE by the GLP-1 receptor agonists and highlight the putative mechanisms underlying these benefits. We also comment on the different signaling pathways which appear important for mediating these effects.

Abbreviations

ANP	atrial natriuretic peptide
ASCVD	atherosclerotic cardiovascular disease
DMB	6,7-dichloro-2-methylsulfonyl-3-N-tert-butylaminoquinoxaline
E/A ratio	Ratio of the E wave (peak velocity of blood flow from the relaxation of the left ventricle) to A wave (peak velocity of blood flow from left atrial contraction).
ECD	extracellular domain
eNOS	endothelial nitric oxide synthase
ERK1/2	extracellular signal-regulated kinases 1 and 2
GPCR	G-protein coupled receptor
HAECs	human aortic endothelial cells
HbA_{1c}	glycated hemoglobin
JNK	c-Jun N-terminal kinase
K_{ATP}	ATP-dependent potassium channel
LPS	lipopolysaccharide
L-NAME	L-N^G-Nitro arginine methyl ester
MACE	major adverse cardiac events
mTOR	mammalian target of rapamycin
NF-κB	nuclear factor kappa-light-chain-enhancer of activated B cells
NO	nitric oxide
ODQ	1H-[1,2,4]Oxadiazolo[4,3-a]quinoxalin-1-one
ROCK	Rho-associated protein kinase
SGLT1	sodium-coupled glucose transporter 1
T2D	Type 2 diabetes
TMD	transmembrane domain
VCAM-1	vascular cell adhesion molecule-1

1. Introduction

Starting with the initial elucidation of the 2 glucagon-like peptides (GLP-1 and GLP-2) 4 decades ago there have been continual discoveries showcasing the complex biology and underlying pharmacology of these peptides (Drucker, 2018; Jones, 2021; Lund, 2005). Glucagon-like peptide-1 (7–36amide) (henceforth referred to as GLP-1) was found to be the major biologically active component of the 37 residue glucagon-like peptide-1 (see below). GLP-1 is secreted from the L cells in the small intestine postprandially as an insulinotropic hormone in response to oral glucose intake. Secreted GLP-1 acts on its Class B G-protein coupled receptor (GPCR) to stimulate insulin release and inhibit glucagon release from the pancreas. Subsequently GLP-1 was shown to slow gastric propulsions and promote satiety sensations in the brain. Not surprisingly these initial discoveries eventually triggered a huge investment by pharmaceutical companies for the development of GLP-1 receptor (GLP-1R) agonists (GLP-1RAs) for glycemic control and patient benefit in type 2 diabetes (T2D). The finding that subjects with T2D underwent significant weight loss during treatment with GLP-1 peptide agonists has resulted in significant efforts to quantify and extend these initial findings to classify GLP-1RAs as potential obesity drugs (Drucker, 2018; Jones, 2021; Rajeev & Wilding, 2016; Rotella, Pala, & Mannucci, 2005; Wren, 2008).

The large-scale clinical testing and widespread use of the approved drugs produced compelling but variable data suggesting that these GLP-1RAs exhibit additional beneficial effects in patients regarding neuroprotection, renoprotection, cardioprotection, memory enhancement and prevention of inflammatory-based pathologies, often independent of any obvious correlate to glycemic control. The pleotropic nature of this pharmacology was not surprisingly linked with observations consistent with distinct mechanisms of GLP-1R signaling in the associated tissues. More recent investigations have probed biased agonism at the GLP-1R assessing apparent signaling via G proteins and/or β-arrestin. These investigations have generated provocative data on spatio-temporal differences observed with the different GLP-1RAs but also with the same agonists in different tissues. Due to these findings GLP-1R pharmacology continues to be aggressively pursued with goals of developing GLP-1RAs with optimal combinations of biased signaling for improved therapeutic benefit and index.

In this chapter, we will briefly review the pleiotropic effects of GLP-1, critique the marketed GLP-1RAs and summarize the clinical findings supporting their cardiovascular (CV) protection. We will then list the mechanisms, both those dependent upon and independent of glycemic control, purported to underlie the protective effects of GLP-1RAs in CV tissues. We will also discuss more recent studies on biased agonism and how these studies may lead to the next generation of optimized GLP-1RAs for improved therapeutics having effective glycemic control along with minimizing risk of serious CV incidents.

2. Overview of GLP-1

The discussion of GLP-1, its receptor and mechanisms of signal transduction briefly provided below is not intended as an exhaustive review, which wouldn't be either appropriate or necessary for an analysis of the CV effects of GLP-1RAs. Rather, our intention is to provide some background for the discussion of the basis for the pleiotropic effects of GLP-1 agonist therapy. Activation of GLP-1 receptors by the endogenous peptide ligand GLP-1, or, therapeutically, by the growing number of GLP-1RAs approved for use in T2D, provides an effective feedback loop between glucose levels and insulin release from pancreatic β-cells (Drucker, 2018; Jones, 2021; Rajeev & Wilding, 2016; Reimann & Gribble, 2002; Rotella et al., 2005; Shigeto et al., 2015; Sun et al., 2017). In addition to what might be thought of as its primary function, however, it inhibits glucagon secretion, has diverse effects on β-cell mass and growth, inhibits food intake and increases satiety, enhances gastric motility, has many effects, mostly positive, on CV function (to be reviewed below) and possibly a number of central (CNS) effects (Drucker, 2018; Hölscher, 2014). All of these actions result from the interaction of a single peptide or close variant with a single receptor. To determine the source of these different effects, one has to consider the localization of the receptors for GLP-1, and the signaling cascade(s) that can be initiated by the interaction of GLP-1 or GLP-1RAs with the receptor. In the case of CV effects, it is also necessary to try and determine if the effects of GLP-1RA therapy are direct, via receptor-mediated direct action on cells of the CV system, or indirect, via benefits accrued by treatment of the primary target of the therapy, glycemic control in T2D.

2.1 Discovery and characterization of GLP-1

GLP-1 is a peptide hormone principally produced and released by L-cells of the intestine, but also from the central nervous system (CNS) and α-cells of the pancreas (Drucker, 2018; Edwards, 2005; Holst, 2007; Jones, Bloom, Buenaventura, Tomas, & Rutter, 2018; Müller et al., 2019; Rotella et al., 2005). Its discovery followed a step-wise path, from the concept of the hormone in general and secretins specifically, to its identification as an insulinotropic hormone, to the elucidation of its peptide structure and the characterization of its receptor. Bayliss and Starling discovered in 1902 that injection of acid into the denervated jejunum of the dog, isolated with respect to innervation from the pancreas (and therefore only connected via the blood stream), produced an output of secretions from the pancreas, suggesting the existence of "secretins," blood-borne substances from gut capable of acting on the distal pancreas. Secretin itself was subsequently shown to be a 27 amino acid peptide hormone with important physiological roles, including but not limited to pancreatic secretion (Adler & Beglinger, 1990; Bayliss & Starling, 1902; Chey & Chang, 2014; Henriksen & de Muckadell, 2000). This concept was later expanded to encompass any substance released from one site to act on a distal site, a hormone (Henriksen & de Muckadell, 2000; Starling, 1905, 1914). The identification of insulin as a major physiologically important regulator of glucose and a principal component of pancreatic secretions by Banting and Best in 1921 (Hegele & Maltman, 2020; Vecchio, Tornali, Bragazzi, & Martini, 2018), and the role of specific gut secretions as incretins (a contraction for intestinal secretion insulin) (Holst, 2019; Holst, Gasbjerg, & Rosenkilde, 2021; Lund, 2005; Tian & Jin, 2016), led to a decades-long search for the identity of important incretin hormones.

The first incretin identified was isolated and its amino acid sequence determined in the early 1970s (Brown & Dryburgh, 1971). Initially named gastric inhibitory peptide (GIP), it was later determined that the peptide had effects beyond gastric motility, and was insulinotropic, resulting in its renaming as glucose-dependent insulinotropic peptide (Brown, Dryburgh, Ross, & Dupré, 1975; Dupre, Ross, Watson, & Brown, 1973; Ebert & Creutzfeldt, 1980; Elahi et al., 1979; Taminato, Seino, Goto, Inoue, & Kadowaki, 1977); today the peptide is referred by either name, and retains its original acronym GIP.

Removal of GIP from gut extracts by immunoprecipitation only reduced the insulinotropic effects of these extracts by about 50%, suggesting that one or more other components of these extracts were equally effective at stimulating insulin release (Ebert, Unger, & Creutzfeldt, 1983). Proglucagon is a precursor of glucagon, as well as a large number of other bioactive peptides, including GLP-1 and GLP-2 (GLP-2 is not insulinotropic and will not be considered further in this review). Preproglucagons had been isolated from anglerfish islets and their amino acid sequences determined from the cDNAs (Lund, 2005; Lund, Goodman, & Habener, 1981; Lund, Goodman, Montminy, Dee, & Habener, 1983); this was closely followed by the isolation of 2 peptides, a 37 amino acid peptide, GLP-1 (1–37) and GLP-1(7–37) from the mammalian (including human) pancreas and intestine, and the subsequent demonstration that while the full-length peptide GLP-1(1–37) was not insulinotropic, the 31 amino acid GLP-1 (7–37) was a potent stimulator of insulin release (Mojsov, Weir, & Habener, 1987). It is now known that there are 3 predominant GLP-1 peptides, the full-length GLP-1(1–37), GLP-1(7–37, or glycine-extended GLP-1) and GLP-1(7–36 amide) (Orskov, Bersani, Johnsen, Højrup, & Holst, 1989). While both of the truncated and active GLP-1 peptides are insulinotropic, the majority of circulating GLP-1 is the GLP-1(7–36amide) (Orskov, Rabenhøj, Wettergren, Kofod, & Holst, 1994). Like GIP, these peptides are rapidly broken down in circulation by dipeptidyl peptidase IV (DPP IV) and neutral endopeptidase 24.11 (Deacon, 2004; Mentlein, Gallwitz, & Schmidt, 1993; Plamboeck, Holst, Carr, & Deacon, 2003, 2005), with a half-life of approximately 2 min, and while some GLP-1 breakdown products may have important biological activity, the rapid cleavage of the parent active peptide greatly limited its utility as a potential therapeutic. This was the basis for the development of GLP-1RAs that were superior, generally because of greater metabolic stability (see below).

The release of GLP-1 by glucose and other nutrients has been studied extensively. It has long been known that glucose delivered by oral administration was more effective in stimulating insulin release by the pancreas, relative to glucose introduced by intravenous injection/infusion (Perley & Kipnis, 1967). Fats, proteins and carbohydrates present in a meal are digested, and various components can directly act on the endocrine L cells of the small intestine and colon to induce GLP-1 release. In the case of glucose, the sodium-coupled glucose transporter SGLT1 has been shown to be critical in glucose-stimulated release, as have a number of ion channels (Kuhre, Frost, Svendsen, & Holst, 2015; Sun et al., 2017). Fat sensing depends on activation of GPCRs by short- and long-chain fatty acids, and proteins by a complex amalgam of mechanisms incorporating both the glucose release pathways and those of fats (Gribble & Reimann, 2017; Smith, Hackett, Galli, & Flynn, 2019). GLP-1 is often observed to be released biphasically, with a weaker initial phase followed by a more pronounced later phase in response to a meal, thought to result from its release by endocrine cells in the duodenum (Theodorakis et al., 2006). Once released, GLP-1 rapidly circulates and is available to interact with its receptors in a number of target tissues, including the pancreas and brain.

2.2 The GLP-1 receptor

The receptor for GLP-1was cloned from a cDNA library derived from rat β-cells from pancreatic islets (Thorens, 1992), closely followed by the cloning of the human β-cell homolog (Thorens et al., 1993) and its cloning from a number of other sources (Dillon et al., 1993; Dillon, Wheeler, Leng, Ligon, & Boyd, 1997; Graziano, Hey, Borkowski, Chicchi, & Strader, 1993; Lankat-Buttgereit & Göke, 1997; Lankat-Buttgereit, Göke, Fehmann, Richter, & Göke, 1994; MacNeil, Occi, Hey, Strader, & Graziano, 1994; Thorens et al., 1993; Volz et al., 1995). Previous evidence had demonstrated that a primary effect of ligand binding to GLP-1R was activation of adenylate cyclase and production of cAMP (Drucker, Philippe, Mojsov, Chick, & Habener, 1987), and heterologous expression of cloned GLP-1Rs demonstrated high-affinity activation of adenylate cyclase by GLP-1. The GLP-1R is a member of the Class B (secretin-like) family of GPCRs. First identified in 1993 (Segre & Goldring, 1993), they comprise a group of structurally-related receptors for at least 18 identified peptide hormones divided into a number of subgroups (de Graaf et al., 2017; Graaf et al., 2016; Hollenstein et al., 2014; Liapakis, Matsoukas, Karageorgos, Venihaki, & Mavromoustakos, 2017).

Similar to all GPCRs, class B GPCRs have a 7-transmembrane basic structure that forms a transmembrane domain (TMD), but also have a large N-terminal extracellular domain (ECD) (de Graaf et al., 2017; Hollenstein et al., 2014; Liang et al., 2020; Liapakis et al., 2017). The N-terminal ECD is critical for specific binding of the C-terminal portion of the peptide, GLP-1 in the case of the GLP-1R, and the N-terminal region of the ligand is bound to the TMD, and is the substrate of receptor activation (Cong et al., 2021; Hoare, 2005; Song et al., 2017; Underwood et al., 2010; Wootten, Reynolds, Smith, Mobarec, Koole, et al., 2016; Wu et al., 2020; Yang et al., 2016).

Class B GPCRs, including the GLP-1R, have complex signaling cascades that can extend far beyond the classical G-protein coupled activation of adenylate cyclase. All class B GPCRs, including GLP-1Rs, are $G\alpha_s$-coupled receptors, and binding of an agonist activates adenylate cyclase, resulting in an increase in cAMP (Jones, Bloom, et al., 2018; Rowlands, Heng, Newsholme, & Carlessi, 2018). While many of the signaling pathways of the GLP-1R and their relationship to physiological effects of GLP-1RA administration are not yet well understood, the canonical cAMP pathway leading to insulin synthesis and release from pancreatic beta cells has been characterized most fully. Upon receptor activation and stimulation of increased levels of intracellular cAMP via $G\alpha_s$ translocation and stimulation of adenylate cyclase, 2 primary downstream effectors, protein kinase A (PKA) and cAMP-regulated guanine nucleotide exchange factor II are responsible for regulation of proinsulin production and for creating the environment favorable for the release of vesicles containing insulin (Drucker et al., 1987; Fletcher, Halls, Christopoulos, Sexton, & Wootten, 2016; Holst, 2007; Jones, Bloom, et al., 2018). This latter function of directly promoting insulin release involves, among other things, alteration of critical ion channels, including phosphorylation-mediated inhibition of ATP-dependent potassium channel (K_{ATP}) opening and activation of voltage-gated calcium channels resulting from the subsequent depolarization (Kuhre et al., 2015; McClenaghan, Flatt, & Ball, 2006; Sun et al., 2017), which promote calcium-dependent insulin release. GLP-1R activation can have other important effects on β-cell mass, including longer-term effects on cell density and proliferation, and α- to β-cell conversion (Deng et al., 2020; Elahi et al., 1979; Popovic, Stokic, & Popovic, 2015). These effects, not yet completely characterized, may have implications for the use of GLP-1RAs in Type 1 diabetes.

2.3 Complexity of the signaling cascades and the concept of biased agonism

The canonical cAMP pathway is only one of several G-protein coupled and G-protein independent signaling cascades initiated by GLP-1R agonist binding. GLP-1R is coupled to (at least) $G\alpha_i$ and $G\alpha_q$ (Marzook, Tomas, & Jones, 2021). While the importance of the former is currently a point of debate, the latter can indirectly activate protein kinase C (PKC) leading to intracellular calcium increase and enhancement of GLP-1R-mediated insulin release (Shigeto, Cha, Rorsman, & Kaku, 2017; Shigeto et al., 2015). The GLP-1R inactivates following stimulation, a result of β-arrestin recruitment and signaling via extracellular signal-regulated kinases (ERK1/2) (Fletcher et al., 2018; Montrose-Rafizadeh et al., 1999; Quoyer et al., 2010; Roed et al., 2014; Sonoda et al., 2008). The complexity of these cascades, further discussion of which is beyond the scope of this review, and the elucidation of structural features of the GLP-1R that contribute to activation of specific downstream signaling cascades, is the genesis of the concept of biased agonism (or signal bias) in this system (Fletcher et al., 2018; Jones, 2021; Jones, Buenaventura, et al., 2018; Jones et al., 2021; Liang et al., 2018; Wootten, Christopoulos, Marti-Solano, Babu, & Sexton, 2018; Wootten et al., 2013; Zhao et al., 2020). Biased agonism encompasses the idea that in receptors with multiple downstream signaling cascades, it may be possible to design molecules that favor certain pathways over others, with beneficial effects. For example, in pancreatic β-cells, the release of insulin is largely under the control of G-protein-coupled increases in cAMP, but it is modulated (enhanced or decreased) also by other signaling pathways, for example receptor desensitization or internalization by β-arrestin. In the case of an agonist biased toward the cAMP-dependent pathways, minimizing activation of the β--arrestin pathway and thereby reducing receptor internalization could have value in further enhancement of any positive effects of a GLP-1RA. Is this possible? Yes, since we now know that specific receptor moieties are critical for specific signaling pathways (Liang et al., 2018; Wootten et al., 2018; Wootten, Reynolds, Koole, et al., 2016; Wootten, Reynolds, Smith, et al., 2016), and that specific peptide and non-peptide GLP-1RAs can display significant structurally detectable and physiologically relevant signal bias (Fang et al., 2020; Fremaux et al., 2019; Jones et al., 2018, 2021; Koole et al., 2013, 2010; Marzook, Tomas, & Jones, 2021; Zhao et al., 2020). While this is important for the use of GLP-1RAs in T2D, it may be as important or even more important in other GLP-1 targets and other diseases, such as neurodegenerative disorders and CV risk reduction in susceptible T2D patients, and may help to understand the differential effects of the various GLP-1RAs in the same target cells or tissue (Batista, Bodart-Santos, De Felice, & Ferreira, 2019; Hayes, 2012; Hölscher, 2014).

3. GLP-1 peptide agonists for use in type 2 diabetes

3.1 Marketed GLP-1RAs

Marketed GLP-1RAs comprise 2 general categories, analogs of exendin-4, an incretin discovered from the saliva of the Gila monster lizard, and analogs of GLP-1 (Graaf et al., 2016; Kalra, Bhattacharya, & Kapoor, 2021; Raufman, 1996). Analogs of exendin-4 tend to exhibit shorter half-lives while the GLP-1 analogs have additional groups for more sustained plasma exposures allowing for weekly administrations. Structures are shown in Fig. 1.

Exendin-4 has 53% amino acid homology to GLP-1 but due to its rapid breakdown by DPP IV served as the foundation for generation of more stable analogs to improve stability and plasma exposures. Exenatide, approved in 2005, is a 39 amino acid synthetic version of exendin-4 with 50% amino acid homology to GLP-1 in order to confer resistance to DPP IV. Still, the relatively short half-life of exenatide, reflected in its administration via a bid regimen, led to the eventual marketing of a long-acting release formulation Exenatide-LAR which is administered weekly. Lixisenatide is a 44 amino acid derivative of exendin-4 modifying the C-terminal with 6 lysine residues. Lixisenatide was approved in 2013 and is administered qd which was an improvement over the bid regimen for exenatide.

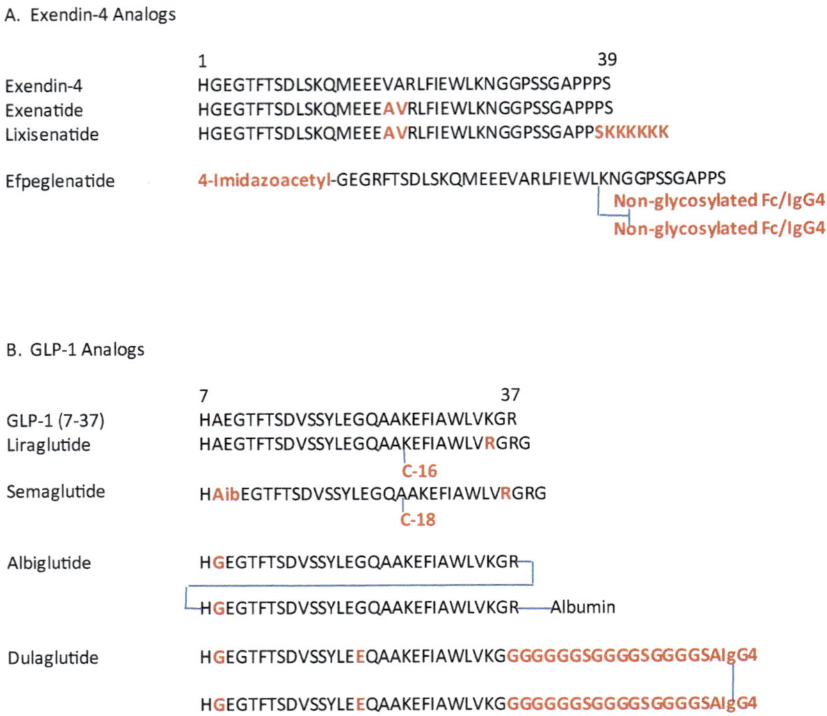

Fig. 1 2-D structures of peptide GLP-1 RAs. IgG4: Immunoglobulin subclass G4, C-16: acylated with palmitic acid; C-18: acylated with steric diacid.

Efforts to synthesize GLP-1 analogs with more sustained exposures resulted in the development of liraglutide, semaglutide, albiglutide, dulaglutide and efpeglenatide. Liraglutide shares a 97% amino acid identity to native GLP-1 but contains a C-16 fatty acid group appended to a lysine residue (lysine 26) and an arginine replacement for lysine 34. These substitutions lead to an increased binding to plasma albumin resulting in a longer half-life compared to exenatide and lixisenatide (approximately 12 h vs 4 h) and resistance to cleavage by DPP IV. Liraglutide is also administered daily and was approved for European/US markets in 2009/2010. Semaglutide, similar to liraglutide, is an acylated GLP-1RA with an arginine substitution at position 34. Semaglutide also has unique modifications at positions 8 (aminoisobutyric acid replacing alanine) and position 26 (C-18 diacid) which prolonged plasma exposures leading to once weekly dosing regimen. The once-weekly injectable form of semaglutide was approved for US and EU/Japanese/Canadian markets in 2017/2018. An oral form of semaglutide, administered daily utilizing an absorption enhancer was approved for US/European markets in 2019/2020. Albiglutide is a dimer of GLP-1 (7–36), covalently bound to albumin, which results in an extended half-life of 6–8 days. Albiglutide was withdrawn from prescription use in 2018. Dulaglutide is a GLP-1 (7–37) peptide attached to immunoglobulin G4 (IgG4) with a modified Fc domain which prevents binding to endogenous Fc receptors and allows for a dimerized molecule. This prevents cleavage by DPP IV and extends half-life to approximately 4 days. It is administered weekly and was approved for use in US/European markets in 2014.

Efpeglenatide is a GLP-1RA not yet approved but is discussed below due to being evaluated for CV protection in an outcomes trial (Gerstein et al., 2021). Efpeglenatide is an analog of exendin-4 fused to an IgG4 which affords stability and extended exposures, resulting in a once/weekly administration to patients.

3.2 GLP-1RAs: Future directions

A number of short peptides and non-peptidyl GLP-1RAs, as well as positive allosteric modulators, are in current preclinical and clinical development for use in T2D and other indications (Griffith et al., 2020; Haque et al., 2010; Knudsen et al., 2007; Malik & Li, 2021; Swedberg et al., 2015; Willard et al., 2021; Zhao et al., 2020; Zhou et al., 2021). Many of the short-peptide GLP-1RAs employ non-natural (non-proteinogenic) amino acids, including D-amino acids, which resist degradation by DPP IV and other pathways (Ding et al., 2020; Goldflam & Ullman, 2015; Rabideau & Pentelute, 2015). The potential of these compounds, if successful, is considerable since they can be more readily designed to avoid rapid metabolism, and they may also penetrate membranes more readily, making them more likely candidates for oral administration and brain targets (including central control of feeding) than long peptides, without the need for absorption enhancement as was employed in the development of oral semaglutide. Because of their mode of binding to the GLP-1R, they can be designed to be very biased agonists relative to existing peptide GLP-1RAs. Notable among these is LY3502970, an orally-active, potent and biased "small molecule" (M.W. 882.96; $C_{48}H_{48}F_2N_{10}O_5$) GLP-1RA (Kawai et al., 2020; Zhao et al., 2020). LY3502970 has completed a Phase 1 trial in healthy volunteers and a Phase 2 trial in subjects with T2D, and is recruiting for an additional Phase 2 trial in subjects with T2D (ClinicalTrials.gov; 2021).

4. Cardiovascular protection by GLP-1RA therapy in clinical trials

Regulatory agencies have mandated large CV outcomes trials for ascertaining CV safety for promising antihyperglycemic therapeutics for T2D patients (Pfeffer et al., 2015). Evaluations focus on both microvascular and macrovascular associated pathophysiologies as both such complications are associated with T2D patients (Mohammedi et al., 2017). At baseline enrollment, microvasular disease is typically assessed by macroalbuminuria (>300 mg/g albumin to creatinine ratio), retinal disease, e.g., retinopathy, macular edema or blindness and indices of end-stage renal disease. Macrovascular disease typical compasses myocardial infarction, stroke, coronary artery disease, unstable angina and revascularization procedures with the composite MACE serving as the common primary endpoint (Andrikou et al., 2019). This assessment of CV protection in T2D patients is a critical endeavor due to past data showing that some glucose-lowering medications can lead to a greater risk of heart failure (Udell et al., 2015). This meta-analysis showed a statistically significant risk of heart failure ($P = 0.04$) primarily associated with the use of peroxisome proliferation-activated receptor agonists but also with DPP IV inhibitors in patients with or at risk of T2D. Comparative analysis of these large outcomes trials are complicated by differences in comedications, percentage of enrolled patients harboring various CV risk factors or having prior serious CV events, differences in the duration of the various trials and differences amongst the GLP-1RAs duration of action. Nonetheless, the trials offer important insights into "real life" treatments where GLP-1RAs are added in combination with other medications to affect better control of hyperglycemia. GLP-1RAs such as liraglutide, semaglutide, exenatide, lixisenatide, albiglutide, dulaglutide and efpeglenatide have been examined in large, extended (e.g., 3–5 years follow-up) randomized clinical trials for their ability to confer protection against MACE when given in addition to standard of care anti-hyperglycemic drugs such as metformin, sulfonylureas, insulin or DPP-IV inhibitors. For this review, a key issue to determine is whether the CV protection is dependent or independent on glycemic control.

4.1 Cardiovascular outcomes trials

The LEADER trial (Marso et al., 2016) found that treatment with liraglutide (daily subcutaneous injection) led to a CV benefit in T2D patients, vs placebo, when added on to standard of care. Patients who had T2D along with either a coexisting CV condition (e.g., coronary heart disease) or at least one CV risk factor (e.g., hypertension) were enrolled. Treatment with liraglutide was associated with statistically significant decreases in the primary composite endpoint occurrence of CV-related death, non-fatal myocardial infarction or non-fatal stroke ($P < 0.001$ for noninferiority to placebo; $P = 0.01$ for superiority to placebo). Liraglutide was also associated with significant decreases in renal or retinal microvascular events compared to placebo ($P = 0.02$). This benefit was realized in both patient populations. The median duration of treatment was 3.5 years and the median duration of follow-up was 3.5 years. The significant effect on the primary endpoint was most pronounced in CV- or all-cause deaths as the changes in non-fatal myocardial infarction or non-fatal stroke were not different amongst the groups. At a prespecified timepoint of 36 months, the liraglutide group had a decrease of 0.4 percentage point in glycated hemoglobin (HbA_{1c}) compared to placebo. However, as Marso et al. point out, previous trials with other anti-diabetic medications in T2D patients that achieved similar levels of glycemic control lacked significant beneficial effects on CV outcomes. In addition, the authors suggest that the relatively delayed time to realize the beneficial effects of liraglutide may reflect halting progression of atherosclerotic vascular disease as opposed to changes in hemodynamics or HbA_{1c}. They note that patients receiving liraglutide actually had fewer hospitalizations for heart failure, compared to placebo, although this difference did not reach statistical significance. This same composite primary endpoint, as well as enrollment criteria, were used in a study evaluating the effects of semaglutide (SUSTAIN-6 study) (Marso et al., 2016) also added on to standard of care. Treatment with semaglutide also showed a statistically significant benefit compared to placebo for the primary composite endpoint with $P = 0.001$ for non-inferiority and $P = 0.02$ for superiority. There was also a significant ($P = 0.004$) decrease in indices of nephropathy. There were no differences among the treatment groups with regards to hospitalizations due to heart failure. The treatment groups of semaglutide were associated with a 0.7 (low dose) and 1.0 (high dose) percentage point decreases in HbA_{1c} compared to the placebo group, thus slightly larger than those reported in the liraglutide trial. The CV risk reductions were similar in both semaglutide treatment groups. The authors did conclude that several factors, including lowering of HbA_{1c} likely contributed to the CV protection in this trial. A more recent study evaluated semaglutide using a daily orally-bioavailable formulation (PIONEER-6 study; 14 mg daily) and having the same primary MACE composite endpoint as the above studies in T2D patients, and enrolled patients with either established CV or renal disease or exhibiting risk factors for adverse CV events (Husain et al., 2019). Median time in the trial for all patients was 15.9 months and oral semaglutide was also added on to standard of care. Treatment with oral semaglutide was shown to be non-inferior to placebo ($P = 0.001$) with respect to the primary endpoint. The rate of hospitalization due to heart failure was similar between the two groups as were indices of acute kidney injury. Results for the primary outcome were similar in both patient groups, i.-e., having established CV disease or harboring risk factors. Oral semaglutide also improved efficacy outcomes compared to placebo but these data were not assessed with corrections for multiple comparisons thus lacked appropriate statistical analyses. Nonetheless, patients receiving oral semaglutide had a mean decrease of 0.7 percentage points in HbA_{1c} compared to patients receiving placebo, similar to the changes reported in SUSTAIN-6. The authors did not comment on the importance of this decrease in HbA_{1c} for the primary outcome.

The EXSCEL study (Holman et al., 2017) also incorporated a similar primary composite outcome in a study examining the effects of extended release exenatide (subcutaneous injection weekly) with primary hypotheses of being non-inferior to placebo with respect to safety and superior to placebo with respect to efficacy. The study was designed to enroll T2D patients such that approximately 70% would have had a previous CV event and 30% with no such prior CV event. The median duration of treatment was 2.4 years for exenatide and 2.3 years for placebo, with the median duration of follow-up being 3.2 years. At the prespecified timepoint of 6 months, the exenatide treatment group had a 0.7 percentage point decrease in HbA_{1c} compared to placebo although this difference decreased with study duration (e.g., 0.53 percentage point decrease at study end). Exenatide was found to be non-inferior to placebo with respect to safety ($P < 0.001$). Although exenatide treatment appeared to exert a similar degree of benefit in the composite CV primary endpoint, as found in the LEADER and SUSTAIN-6 trials with liraglutide and semaglutide, this failed to reach statistical significance as being superior to placebo with respect to efficacy ($P = 0.06$). Several possible reasons for this lack of CV efficacy were discussed, including that patients enrolled in EXSCEL had lower baseline HbA_{1c} levels (8.0%) compared to the SUSTAIN-6 and PIONEER-6 trials (8.7%).

Pfeffer et al. (Pfeffer et al., 2015) reported on the effects of lixisenatide along with standard of care in T2D patients who had a recent incidence of an acute coronary syndrome, e.g., myocardial infarction, unstable angina (ELIXA study). Similar to the above studies, the primary composite endpoint was the first occurrence of CV death, non-fatal myocardial infarction, non-fatal stroke but also included hospitalization for unstable angina. Lixisenatide was administered subcutaneously daily and patients were followed for 25 months. And similar to the findings with exenatide in the EXSCEL study, lixisenatide was found to be non-inferior, but not superior to placebo with respect to the primary endpoint. A modest benefit in renal dynamics, urinary albumin to creatinine ratio, was observed in the lixisenatide group but statistical significance of this effect was lost in a post-hoc evaluation following adjustment for effects on HbA_{1c}. HbA_{1c} was significantly reduced in the lixisenatide (−0.6 percentage point) vs the placebo group (−0.2 percentage point) from baseline out to week 12 ($P=0.001$). Albeit modest, the significant effect on HbA_{1c} exerted by lixisenatide in this trial was associated with neutral effects (i.e., neither positive nor negative) on CV risk.

Hernandez et al. (HARMONY Study) (Hernandez et al., 2018) reported on the CV safety for albiglutide in T2D patients with CV disease as defined by having established coronary artery disease such as myocardial infarction or revascularization, stroke, or peripheral vascular event such as intermittent claudication. The HARMONY study utilized a similar MACE-composite primary endpoint of other outcomes trials focusing on the first occurrence of CV-related death, non-fatal myocardial infarction or non-fatal stroke. Secondary outcomes included a composite of the primary outcomes combined with initiation of procedures due to unstable angina, the individual components of the primary outcome composite, hospitalization due to heart failure, and safety outcomes including worsening renal function and death from any cause. Patients received albiglutide subcutaneously weekly but investigators could decide to increase the dose (from 30 to 50 mg) in order to obtain more acceptable glycemic control, in addition to standard of care. The median follow-up was 1.6 years for the primary outcome. Baseline levels of HbA_{1c} were 8.7% and treatment with albiglutide was associated with an approximate 0.6 percentage point decrease in HbA_{1c} compared to placebo at the 8 month timepoint. Examination of the primary outcome data showed that albiglutide was associated with a 22% reduced risk vs placebo, thus being non-inferior to placebo for CV safety ($P<0.0001$) and superior to placebo with respect to CV efficacy ($P=0.006$) with a benefit on myocardial infarction being the main finding driving the superiority to placebo. Treatment with albiglutide was similar to placebo with regards to CV-related deaths, hospitalizations due to heart failure or renal function during the trial. Investigators were allowed to use other glucose-lowering medications which was more common in the placebo group. It is important to note that the marketing of albiglutide was discontinued in 2018 (Giugliano et al., 2021).

The dulaglutide outcomes study (REWIND Study) (Dagenais et al., 2020; Gerstein et al., 2019a, 2019b) was randomized, double blind and placebo controlled, and enrolled patients, similar to the enrollment for the PIONEER-6 study, with T2D on a regimen of glucose-lowering drugs that had a previous CV event (e.g., myocardial infarction, ischemic stroke, unstable angina, myocardial ischemia) or exhibited risk factors (e.g., tobacco use, obesity, hypertension) for a cardiovascular adverse event. The study was designed to test superiority of dulaglutide vs placebo rather than testing for non-inferiority to placebo as with other trials. Approximately 30% of the enrolled patients had prior CV disease. The MACE composite primary endpoint included non-fatal myocardial infarction, non-fatal stroke or all-cause mortality with a median follow-up of 5.4 years. There was a small but significant ($P=0.026$) decrease in the percent occurrence of the composite endpoint in the dulaglutide (12%) vs the placebo (13.4%) group. Importantly, considering the meta-analysis by Zelniker et al. discussed below, the significant decrease in the primary composite endpoint was found in T2D patients with or without prior CV disease. The most pronounced difference was observed in the decreased incidence of non-fatal stroke. There was a trend for a decreased mortality in the dulaglutide (10.8%) vs placebo (12%) but this did not reach statistical significance ($P=0.067$). The secondary endpoint of composite renal microvascular outcomes was significantly decreased in the dulaglutide group compared to the placebo group ($P=0.0004$). The baseline value of HbA_{1c} was 7.2% and treatment with dulaglutide was associated with a significant lowering of HbA_{1c} vs placebo (0.6 percentage point, $P=0.0001$). Similar to other outcomes trials, the authors list several possible factors responsible for the CV efficacy including lowering of HbA_{1c}. However, the authors also point out that similar beneficial outcomes were achieved in patients with different levels of HbA_{1c} and compared to other trials with higher baseline values of HbA_{1c}.

The AMPLITUDE-O outcomes trial (Gerstein et al., 2021) examined the effects of efpeglenatide compared to placebo in T2D patients with a history of CV disease or renal disease in addition to at least 1 additional CV risk factor. Efpeglenatide was administered subcutaneously once weekly in patients continuing with standard of care with a composite MACE primary endpoint (first incidence of CV-related or non-related death, non-fatal myocardial infarction or non-fatal stroke) and a composite renal function secondary endpoint. Additional secondary endpoints included components of MACE and renal function, hospitalization for heart failure and levels of HbA_{1c}. The study had a mean follow-up of 1.81 years. Treatment with efpeglenatide decreased the composite MACE outcomes by 27% ($P < 0.001$ for non-inferiority; $P = 0.007$ for superiority) and decreased the occurrence of a renal outcome event by 32% ($P < 0.001$) compared to placebo. Patients treated with efpeglenatide had a significantly lower incidence of at least one of the MACE components ($P = 0.02$). Baseline levels of HbA_{1c} were 8.9% and treatment with efpeglenatide resulted in a reduction, compared to placebo, of 1.24 percentage points in the HbA_{1c} level. Lowering of HbA_{1c} was acknowledged as likely important for the CV efficacy, however, the authors comment that reductions in various parameters such as eGFR, pulse pressure and risk of renal dysfunction may be attributed to direct endothelial and microvascular effects. A summary of the CV outcomes trials is shown in Table 1.

4.2 Meta-analyses of outcomes trials

These protective effects against MACE and likely renal disease found in patients treated with GLP-1RAs, with respect to placebo, have been confirmed in several meta-analysis publications showing the benefit is an overall class effect. The published meta-analysis studies since 2019 examined trials which used MACE as the primary endpoint with the ELIXA trial (Kristensen et al., 2019; Pfeffer et al., 2015), adding hospitalization for unstable angina to the composite primary endpoint. Clear benefits on glycemic control, as evidenced by lowering of HbA_{1c} levels, was a common finding such that teasing out non-glycemic vs glycemic associated benefit is indeed challenging. Giugliano et al. (Giugliano, Chiodini, Maiorino, Bellastella, & Esposito, 2019) conducted a meta-regression analysis to examine whether the CV risk reduction benefits of the newer anti-hyperglycemic drugs (GLP-1RAs, sodium/glucose cotransporter 2 [SGLT-2] inhibitors and DPP IV inhibitors) was associated with the lowering of HbA_{1c}. The authors examined 11 outcomes trials of which 5 were with GLP-1RAs (ELIXA, LEADER, SUSTAIN-6, EXSCEL and HARMONY). They found that an improvement in the levels of HbA_{1c} may be important for achieving CV risk reduction. There is no question that glycemic control is of importance for CV protection; however, the conclusion from this study is based on an analysis of 3 different classes of anti-hyperglycemic drugs and that the 5 trials listed for the GLP-1RAs do not appear to show a correlation between

Table 1 CV outcomes trials for GLP-1RAs.

Authors/trial	Drug	Primary endpoint (vs placebo)	Patients enrolled	Percentage point decrease in % HbA_{1C} vs placebo	Suggested evidence for glycemic-independent efficacy by authors
Marso, Daniels, et al., 2016 LEADER	Liraglutide	Significantly superior to PL	Both coexisting CV condition or CV risk	0.4	Yes
Marso, Bain, et al., 2016 SUSTAIN-6	Semaglutide	Significantly superior to PL	Both coexisting CV condition or CV risk	0.7–1.0	No
Husain et al. PIONEER-6	Oral Semaglutide	Non-inferior to PL	Both coexisting CV condition or CV risk	0.7	No
Holman et al. EXSCEL	Exenatide LAR	Non-inferior to PL	Previous CV Event (70%) or no previous CV Event (30%)	0.7	Yes
Pfeffer et al. ELIXA	Lixisenatide	Non-inferior to PL	Recent Acute Coronary Syndrome	0.4	No
Hernandez et al. HARMONY	Albiglutide	Significantly superior to PL	Existing CV Disease	0.6	No
Gerstein et al. REWIND	Dulaglutide	Significantly superior to PL	Previous CV Event (30%) or CV Risk	0.6	No
Gerstein et al. AMPLITUDE-O	Efpeglenatide	Significantly superior to PL	History of CV event plus 1 Risk Factor	1.24	Yes

levels of HbA_{1c} and CV risk benefit (see Section 4). We assessed several meta-analyses for possible insight into this issue. Zelniker et al. (Zelniker et al., 2019) assessed clinical trial data for exenatide, lixisenatide, liraglutide, semaglutide and albiglutide with primary outcomes including a composite of MACE, hospitalization due to heart failure and indices of kidney disease. The 5 trials examined were ELIXA, EXSCEL, HARMONY, LEADER and SUSTAIN-6. There was an overall 12% decrease in MACE ($P < 0.001$) in the GLP-1RA treatment groups, however, this benefit was restricted to patients who presented with established atherosclerotic CV disease (ASCVD; range of 41–100% of all patients in the trials) at baseline whereas there was no such benefit in patients without established ASCVD but which exhibited multiple risk factors for ASCVD. It is of interest to note that the meta-analysis by Zelniker et al. did not include data from the REWIND trial described above (Gerstein, et al., 2019b) in which those authors found that the CV benefit using a composite primary endpoint was similar in T2D patients with or without prior CV disease. Treatment with GLP-1RAs was associated with a significant reduction in the risk of myocardial infarction (9%, $P = 0.012$) stroke (14%, $P = 0.012$) and CV-death (12%, $P = 0.004$). A composite endpoint was used for deterioration of kidney function which included occurrence of macroalbuminuria, degeneration of eGFR, development of end-stage renal disease or renal-associated death. Treatment with the GLP-1RAs exhibited a significant benefit on the composite endpoint for risk of progression of renal disease (18% reduction, $P < 0.001$). This benefit on kidney function was primarily due to a reduction in macroalbuminuria. Regarding the rate of hospitalization due to heart failure there was no difference between treatment with GLP-1RAs and placebo. The authors found no evidence for the findings being affected by trial duration. Although the range of decreases in HbA_{1c},were not specified, the beneficial CV effects were not obviously correlated with decreases in HbA_{1c}, suggesting the benefits were independent of control of hyperglycemia.

Kristensen et al. (Kristensen et al., 2019) conducted a meta-analysis of CV outcomes trials surveying 7 trials: ELIXA, EXSCEL, HARMONY, LEADER, PIONEER-6, REWIND and SUSTAIN-6, including 2 trials (REWIND and PIONEER-6) that were absent in the previously referenced meta-analysis (Zelniker et al., 2019). They estimated overall hazard ratios for MACE including the individual components, all-cause mortality, rate of hospitalizations due to heart failure and kidney function. Treatment with GLP-1RAs was associated with a 12% reduction in MACE ($P < 0.001$) without differences between patients having or not having prior CV disease.

Statistical significance was observed for the individual components: fatal or non-fatal myocardial infarction ($P = 0.043$), fatal or non-fatal stroke ($P < 0.001$) and CV-related death ($P = 0.003$). Treatment was also associated with a significant reduction in all-cause mortality (12% decrease, $P = 0.001$) and a significant decrease in the rate of hospitalization for heart failure (decrease of 9%, $P = 0.028$). There was also a significant benefit in assessing composite kidney function outcomes (new onset macroalbuminuria, decrease in the eGFR, development of end-stage kidney disease) where treatment with the GLP-1RAs led to a reduction of 17% ($P < 0.001$) primarily driven by a reduced urinary excretion of albumin. The range of decreases in HbA_{1c}, between treatment groups in the trials was 0.3–0.7 percentage points. Although the correlation between CV endpoints and changes in HbA_{1c} was not specified, the risk reduction in MACE and range of decrease in HbA_{1c}, was quite similar to that found in a meta-analysis with another anti-hyperglycemic class of drugs, SGLT-2 inhibitors (Zelniker et al., 2019). However, the cardioprotection associated with GLP-1RAs was suggested to be a residue of anti-atherothrombotic effects, due to the protection profile and the relatively long time course of protection compared to SGLT-2 inhibitors, suggesting that additional mechanisms for CV protection appear operant with the GLP-1RAs.

A meta-analysis of 8 trials, overlapping with the previous study (Kristensen et al., 2019), and with the addition of the AMPLITUDE-O trial, was largely consistent with regards to the class effect on CV risk reduction (Giugliano et al., 2021). It was concluded that GLP-1RAs provide significant cardioprotection against MACE (risk reduction of 14%, $P = 0.006$), with this benefit being significant in both T2D patients enrolled with CV disease and in T2D patients with only CV risk factors. There were statistically significant decreases in the risk associated with MACE components such as CV-related death (reduction of 13%, $P = 0.016$) and non-fatal stroke (reduction of 16%, $P = 0.007$). They also found that treatment with GLP-1RAs led to a statistically significant decrease in the rate of hospitalization due to heart failure (reduction of 10%, $P = 0.023$), a reduction in all-cause mortality (reduction of 12%, $P = 0.012$) and a reduction in a composite kidney outcomes endpoint (reduction of 17%, $P = 0.012$) primarily due to decreased macroalbuminuria. The analyses by Kristensen et al. and Giugliani et al. were consistent in their conclusions that several factors underlie the CV benefit including reductions in HbA_{1c} and blood pressure, and that reduction in composite renal outcomes suggests that GLP-1RAs may have additional direct effects on endothelial and microvascular-associated pathologies.

A meta-analysis of the effects of GLP-1RAs and SGLT-2 inhibitors was performed on the results of published trials (764 trials, including 421,326 patients) with CV outcomes in T2D patients which were at varying degrees of risk for developing CV and/or renal disease (Palmer et al., 2021). Defined important outcomes included all-cause and CV-related deaths, non-fatal myocardial infarction, non-fatal stroke, renal failure and hospitalization for heart failure. Both drug classes decreased the incidence of all-cause deaths in all risk groups, i.e., from very low risk to very high risk of developing CV/renal disease. SGLT-2 inhibitors decreased all-cause deaths when compared to treatment with GLP-1RAs in all the risk groups. Both treatments were similar in decreasing CV-related deaths, the incidence of myocardial infarction and renal failure but only GLP-1RAs reduced the incidence of non-fatal stroke in all risk groups. SGLT-2 inhibitors were associated with a greater decrease in the rate of hospitalization. Analysis of changes in HbA_{1c} showed that GLP-1RAs (−0.89 percentage point) reduced HbA_{1c} levels to a greater extent than SGLT-2 inhibitors (−0.60 percentage point). The authors did not address whether the differential protective effects between the 2 drug classes were possibly related to differences in the lowering of HbA_{1c} levels.

A recent meta-analysis (Alexander et al., 2021) examined cardioprotective effects of GLP-1RAs by including trials with more diverse anti-diabetic drug comparators and with longer follow-up times. This included 45 trials with at least a 52 week study duration, which resulted in a T2D patient database with 17 trials comparing a GLP-1RA to placebo and 30 trials comparing GLP-1RAs to other anti-glycemic drugs. The studies assessed at least 1 outcome related to CV risk, macro- or microvascular dysfunction, all-cause deaths or adverse events. Assessment of CV risk included levels of HbA_{1c}, systolic blood pressure, body weight and body mass index, serum lipoproteins and eGFR. Treatment with GLP-1RAs was associated with decreased levels of HbA_{1c} compared to placebo (MD = −0.67percentage point, 95% confidence intervals[CI] −0.77 to −0.58) but also compared to treatment with other anti-hyperglycemic medications (MD = −0.37 percentage point, 95% CI −0.53 to −0.22). GLP-1RAs were also associated with significant reductions in the CV risk factors of systolic blood pressure, body weight, body mass index and serum levels of low density lipoprotein compared to placebo and other medications. Evaluation of MACE composite endpoints showed that treatment with GLP-1RAs led to decreased MACE 3-component outcomes (RR = 0.87, 95% CI 0.82 to 0.93), strokes (RR = 0.86, 95% CI 0.82 to 0.93) and renal events (RR = 0.85, 95% CI 0.80 to 0.90) compared to placebo. Incidence of these macrovascular events was not different when comparing treatment with GLP-1RAs and other medications. Patients receiving GLP-1RAs had a lower risk of death compared to placebo but this risk was similar to that in patients receiving other medications. Insufficient data were included to compare between the drug classes and long-term effects on microvascular or macrovascular outcomes, leaving open the question as to whether the CV protection associated with administration of GLP-1RAs is clearly dependent on glycemic control.

The data from the 5 meta-analysis studies, summarized in Table 2, verified that as a class, GLP-1RAs provide a significant benefit when assessing composite MACE outcomes and most of its components. This CV protection was not restricted to the GLP-1RAs structurally similar to GLP-1 but was also observed with drugs of the exendin-4 subclass. These analyses were consistent in identifying significant benefits in CV-related death, incidence of myocardial infarction and incidence of stroke. In addition, the meta-analyses showed that this benefit is not clearly related to trial duration, degree of decrease in HbA_{1c} and includes beneficial effects on kidney function. The apparent independence of some aspects of CV protection from controlling hyperglycemia calls for an overview of putative CV mechanisms underlying the risk-reduction benefits of this drug class.

Table 2 Meta-analyses of GLP-1RA trials.

Meta-analysis study	Trials included	Percent change in primary endpoint (all statistically significant)	Percentage point decrease in % HbA_{1C} vs placebo	Suggested evidence for glycemic-independent efficacy by authors
Zelniker et al.	EXSCEL ELIXA LEADER SUSTAIN-6 HARMONY	12% decrease, only in patients with ASCVD	Not specified	Yes
Kristensen et al.	EXSCEL ELIXA LEADER SUSTAIN-6 HARMONY PIONEER-6 REWIND	12% decrease in patients with or without prior CV disease	0.3–0.7 decrease	Yes

Table 2 Meta-analyses of GLP-1RA trials.—cont'd

Meta-analysis study	Trials included	Percent change in primary endpoint (all statistically significant)	Percentage point decrease in % HbA_{1C} vs placebo	Suggested evidence for glycemic-independent efficacy by authors
Giugliano et al.	EXSCEL ELIXA LEADER SUSTAIN-6 HARMONY PIONEER-6 REWIND AMPLITUDE-O	14% decrease in patients with CV disease or CV disease risk factors	Not specified	Yes
Palmer et al.	764 trials for either GLP-1RAs or SCLT-2 inhibitors	Network Meta-analysis showed GLP-1RAs decreased all-cause and CV-mortality (odds ratio = 0.88), non-fatal MI (0.92), non-fatal stroke (0.84) and kidney failure (0.78)	0.89 decrease	Yes
Alexander et al.	45 trials	Weighted mean differences, pooled relative risk analysis showed GLP-1RAs reduced microvascular (RR = 0.85), macrovascular (RR = 0.86) complications and mortality (RR = 0.89)	Weighted mean difference of 0.67 decrease	No

5. Putative mechanisms underlying cardioprotection

GLP-1Rs are widely distributed throughout tissues associated with CV function (Almutairi, Al Batran, & Ussher, 2019; Baggio et al., 2017, 2018; Ban et al., 2008). As reviewed above, the CV protection associated with GLP-1RA treatment may reflect mechanisms of action distinct from the ability of these drugs to lower indices of hyperglycemia.

There are data in the literature to support the contention that GLP-1RAs exert CV benefits resulting from direct effects on cardiac and/or vascular wall function. Most of the reports utilize liraglutide for demonstrating apparent direct effects on cells/tissues, and the effective concentrations are in the 50–100 nM range. These concentrations are similar to the plasma exposures observed in T2D patients (Jiang, Zhang, Jacobsen, & Hu, 2011).

5.1 Effects on cardiovascular hemodynamics

Several groups have published that either GLP-1 (Yu et al., 2003) or GLP-1RAs (Fan, Xiong, Wang, Zhang, & Shi, 2020; Helmstädter et al., 2020) lower blood pressure in hypertensive models independent of effects on plasma glucose levels. Administration of liraglutide to spontaneously hypertensive rats (SHR) produced decreases in both systolic and diastolic blood pressures (Fan et al., 2020), while administration of liraglutide to mice made hypertensive by infusion of angiotensin II produced decreases in systolic blood pressure (Helmstädter et al., 2020). While exendin-4 increased mean arterial pressure in conscious rats following either intravenous or intracerebroventricular administration (Yamamoto et al., 2002), dosing regimens of exenatide in T2D patients resulted in modest but at times significant lowering of blood pressure (Brixner et al., 2009).

5.2 Direct effects on cardiac cells

GLP-1 as well as liraglutide caused the secretion of atrial natriuretic peptide (ANP) from mouse cardiac atria (Kim et al., 2013). The increased secretion of ANP, or the lowering of blood pressure to liraglutide did not occur in GLP-1R$^{-/-}$ mice and, consistent with the renal effects of ANP, liraglutide dosing resulted in increased natriuresis only in the wild type mice. Liraglutide also stimulated the release of ANP from isolated wild type mouse cardiomyocytes. In a Zucker rat model of diabetes, treatment with liraglutide improved cardiac function, serum biomarkers of cardiac muscle damage and cardiac fibrosis, and prevented the high glucose-induced decrease in viability and indices of apoptosis in isolated neonatal rat cardiomyocytes (Zhang et al., 2017). Exendin-4 prevented indices of cardiomyopathy, e.g., cardiac fibrosis, hypertrophy, in mice rendered diabetic by administration of streptozotocin with a high fat diet (Wu et al., 2018). Cardiac function, as measured by several variables including ejection fraction, cardiac fractional shortening, positive and negative dP/dt and myocardial ventricular filling velocities in early and late diastole (the E/A ratio) were also improved. The protective effect on cardiotoxicity was associated with a dampening of both the CD36-peroxisome proliferation-activated receptor α pathway and the Rho/ROCK pathway due to stimulation of protein kinase A. The streptozotocin/high fat diet-induced increases in blood glucose were normalized by treatment with exendin-4. They were also normalized in diabetic mice treated with insulin which failed to provide the protection against abnormal cardiac remodeling and dysfunction, which implies these beneficial effects in this model of diabetic cardiomyopathy may be independent of glycemic control.

Exogenously added liraglutide inhibited the high glucose-induced proliferation and fibrosis in human myocardial fibroblasts, associated with a down regulation of prolyl 4-hydroxylase subunit alpha-1 via inhibition of the CD36/p-JNK/AP-1 axis (Zhao et al., 2019). Liraglutide administration has also been shown to decrease the accumulation of collagen and reactive oxygen species elevated by angiotensin II in cultured mouse cardiac fibroblasts (Chen et al., 2021).

5.3 Direct effects on vascular function

5.3.1 Vascular Wall

Several studies have examined the apparent direct effects of GLP-1RAs on preventing inflammatory-associated pathophysiologies in the vascular wall. In one study intravascular ultrasound technology was used to image atherosclerotic plaques in the thoracic aortas of Watanabe heritable hyperlipidemic rabbits following treatment with the GLP-1RA lixisenatide or vehicle control, and found that the GLP-1RA-treated group exhibited decreased plaque progression (Sudo et al., 2017). The majority of studies on vascular function, however, have focused directly on the effects of GLP-1RAs on vascular endothelium and vascular smooth muscle.

5.3.2 Direct effects on vascular endothelium

It has been suggested that GLP-1RAs exert beneficial effects on CV outcomes due to halting progression of atherosclerotic vascular disease, which could implicate an anti-inflammatory action targeting the vascular endothelium (Marso, Bain, et al., 2016). Krasner et al. (Krasner, Ido, Ruderman, & Cacicedo, 2014) conducted experiments with liraglutide to identify possible mechanisms underlying this drug's anti-atherosclerotic efficacy by examining inflammatory-related indices using human aortic endothelial cells (HAECs). Liraglutide significantly decreased the expression of the adhesion glycoproteins E-selectin and VCAM-1, stimulated by the addition of TNF-α and lipopolysaccharide (LPS), in HAECs. Liraglutide also significantly inhibited the adhesion of monocytes to the HAECs which had been stimulated by either TNF-α or LPS. These effects were blocked by knockdown of AMP-activated protein kinase as well as by the addition of the calcium-calmodulin protein kinase kinase antagonist STO-609. Liraglutide also increased endothelial nitric oxide synthase (eNOS) mRNA and protein levels and decreased the mRNA and protein levels of the vasoconstrictor endothelin-1 in human umbilical vein endothelial cells, both activities being pro-vasorelaxant (Dai, Mehta, & Chen, 2013). The authors also showed that these effects were associated with inhibition of nuclear factor kappa-light-chain-enhancer of activated B cells (NF-κB) activation.

GLP-1 has also been shown to produce endothelium-dependent vascular relaxation, although there are conflicting data with regards to mechanism. Infusion of GLP-1 or saline was performed in T2D patients who were receiving secondary preventative medications for coronary artery disease due to a previous myocardial infarction, and endothelial function was evaluated by measuring post-ischemic flow-mediated dilation of the brachial artery which was relatively weak in the patients (Nyström et al., 2004). GLP-1 infusion in these T2D patients led to a significant increase in flow-mediated dilation compared to placebo but had no such effect in the healthy subjects. In a preclinical study GLP-1 and GLP-1 (9–36) elicited endothelial-dependent relaxations in rat small mesenteric arteries in vitro, which were blocked by the GLP-1R antagonist exendin 9–39 (Bayram, Nacitarhan, & Ozdem, 2014). The relaxations, albeit modest, were partially blocked by inhibitors of calcium-activated potassium channels and several inhibitors of endothelial-dependent vasodilatory pathways (e.g., L-NAME, ODQ), suggesting the involvement of multiple pathways. Liraglutide decreased blood pressure and provided CV protection largely mediated by GLP-1Rs existing on the vascular endothelium (Helmstädter et al., 2020). In these studies, hypertension was induced by angiotensin II (a non-diabetic model) in wild-type mice and various strains with altered expression of GLP-1Rs (global GLP-1R-, myeloid- or endothelial GLP-1R-null mice). Liraglutide decreased blood pressure, cardiac hypertrophy, vascular inflammation and fibrosis and endothelial dysfunction in wild type and myeloid GLP-1R deficient mice but not in global or endothelial GLP-1R deficient mice. Importantly, neither the infusion of angiotensin II nor the treatment with liraglutide had any effect on glucose homeostasis, e.g., blood glucose levels or insulin levels, associated with oral glucose tolerance tests.

5.3.3 Direct effects on vascular smooth muscle

As noted above liraglutide has been shown to decrease blood pressure in SHR (Fan et al., 2020). These authors also conducted in vitro experiments using rat aortic smooth muscle cells exposed to angiotensin II to assess direct effects of liraglutide on vascular remodeling. Liraglutide attenuated the angiotensin II induction of matrix metalloproteinase I. These authors included data using GLP-1 which exhibited similar effects on remodeling associated with down-regulation of ERK1/2 and NF-κB signaling. These results provide a new mechanistic understanding of key therapeutic strategies for the treatment of vascular remodeling-related diseases, and such mechanisms would be anticipated to positively influence CV risk protection in T2D patients.

Several studies have concluded that GLP-1 relaxes vascular smooth muscle via an endothelial-dependent mechanism. However, it has also been shown that GLP-1, GLP-1 (9–36), the non-peptidic GLP-1R allosteric agonist DMB and the antagonist exendin 9–39 all caused relaxations in isolated rat aortic rings, but that these responses were endothelium-independent (Green et al., 2008). This conclusion was supported by incubation of the aortic rings with antagonists of known endothelial vasodilatory substances (e.g., L-NAME to inhibit production of NO; indomethacin to inhibit prostanoids) but also by removal of the endothelial lining. These relaxation responses were partially inhibited by administration of glybenclamide, a selective inhibitor of K_{ATP} channels, and by the cAMP antagonist Rp-8-Br-cAMPS. GLP-1 has been reported to activate K_{ATP} channels in the pancreas which required intact PKA and PKC (McClenaghan et al., 2006). GLP-1 and the putative GLP-1R antagonist exendin 9–39 were found to increase the levels of cAMP in the aortic tissue. The marked relaxation to the allosteric agonist, DMB, the elevations in cAMP and the finding of clear mRNA for GLP-1R by real time RT-PCR in aortic tissue provide strong evidence for the functional expression of GLP-1R in this vascular preparation; however, the relaxations to the relatively inactive analog GLP-1 (9–36) and the antagonist exendin 9–39 argue for more non-conventional signaling dynamics for the vasodilation (Green et al., 2008). In support of this idea of pathway complexity, relaxation to GLP-1 in rat aortic rings was shown to be partially blocked by the glucagon antagonist hGCGR, further indicting multiple pathways underlying vascular relaxation by GLP-1 (Sélley et al., 2016). However, there is also evidence that GLP-1RAs produce endothelial-dependent relaxation largely due to increased activity of eNOS, the endothelial isozyme of nitric oxide (Liu, Liu, & Huang, 2015).

5.3.4 Stimulation of autophagy

A number of studies have implicated GLP-1RAs in the stimulation of autophagy. Kong et al. (Kong, Wan, Wang, Zhang, & Zhang, 2020) reported that low concentrations of liraglutide (10 nM) increased autophagy in cultured APPswe/SH-SY5Y cells, a cellular model of Alzheimer's disease, an effect mediated by the JNK pathway and not via inhibition of mTOR. Liraglutide also increased autophagic flux in isolated mouse hepatocytes as well as in the human hepatocyte cell line HepG2 (Fang et al., 2020). Using rat insulinoma INS-1 cells incubated with palmitate as a cellular model of T2D lipotoxicity, liraglutide increased viability and markers of autophagy and decreased cleaved caspase-3, a marker of apoptosis (Li, He, Wan, & Li, 2021). These protective effects of liraglutide were abolished by pretreatment with the autophagy inhibitor chloroquine. The in vitro and the in vivo cardioprotective effects reported by Zhang et al. (Zhang et al., 2017) were also significantly diminished by coadministration of chloroquine. Cardiomyocyte autophagy has been viewed as beneficial during stress conditions and hyperglycemia has been shown to exert an inhibitory effect on autophagy (Zech, Singh, Schlossarek, & Carrier, 2020). However, the role of autophagy in diabetic cardiomyopathy is complex with conflicted data supporting whether inhibition or stimulation is beneficial.

6. Biased agonism and GLP-1RA action: Future directions

As mentioned in Section 2.3, significant progress has been made in characterizing our understanding of biased agonism of GLP-1RAs (Lucey et al., 2021; Marzook et al., 2021) and also in the development of more selectively biased agonists (Kawai et al., 2020; van der Velden et al., 2021; Zhou, Guo, et al., 2021). A working hypothesis is that GLP-1RAs biased toward G-protein activation and thus minimal recruitment of β-arrestin, ostensibly leading to reduced receptor desensitization/internalization, will result in a more sustained insulinotropic therapeutic benefit (Drucker, 2018). Examples include the development of the exendin-4 analog AX09 (Zhou, Jiang, & Li, 2021) and the non-peptide agonist LY3502970 (Kawai et al., 2020). However, although biased agonism with respect to G-protein and β-arrestin signaling are the more commonly prosecuted phenomena, the composite signaling effects of ligated GLP-1R reflect additional phenomena including the action of β-arrestin on effector pathways, kinetics of GLP-1R internalization/recycling and the spatial (plasma membrane GLP-1R-triggered vs internalized GLP-1R-triggered pathways) and temporal (duration of activated pathways) dynamics affecting cellular function (Fletcher et al., 2018). Therefore, it would be anticipated that heterogeneity in the spatiotemporal kinetics for activation of pathways such as cAMP, ERK(1/2) and intracellular calcium amongst the different GLP-1RAs will translate into varied efficacy for CV risk reduction in outcomes trials.

With respect to the role of β-arrestin, liraglutide has been found to recruit both β-arrestin1 and 2 while exendin-4 is modestly biased toward β-arrestin2 signaling (Fletcher et al., 2018). The possible consequences of this difference in β-arrestin1 vs 2 recruitment on CV efficacy of GLP-1RAs are not currently clear nor are there any data to suggest this difference contributed to the significant effect of liraglutide, but not exenatide on CV efficacy (Section 4.1). However, these differences will likely affect the spatiotemporal dynamics noted above (Li et al., 2021). Regarding functional consequences of β-arrestin signaling, the protective effects of exendin-4 against hypoxia-reperfusion injury in isolated cardiomyocytes, either in normal or high glucose media, has been shown to be positively dependent on the presence of β-arrestin (Pan, Li, & Gao, 2021). The β-arrestin-dependent effect was associated with reversing mitochondrial dysfunction via PI3K/Akt pathway signaling. GLP-1 also restored dysfunctional endothelial-dependent relaxation in aortic rings prepared from obese/diabetic ob/ob mice, an effect that was blocked following RNAi knockdown of β-arrestin2 (Taguchi, Kaneko, Okudaira, Matsumoto, & Kobayashi, 2021). The relaxation response was associated with activation of both Akt and eNOS. Signaling via activated Akt and eNOS are noted above as potentially important mechanisms for improving CV function.

A key question is whether development of GLP-1RAs more strongly biased toward G-protein signaling, such as LY3502970, will be associated with similar CV risk protection as found with the currently marketed GLP-1RAs. Interestingly, modifications of GLP-1 which result in a clear G-protein bias, i.e., with no apparent internalization, can lead to diminished insulinotropic effects (van der Velden et al., 2021). LY3502970 has entered clinical trials and will be an important test case for whether a strongly G-protein biased GLP-1RA exhibits similar protective effects against MACE as found with the currently marketed drugs.

7. Conclusion

The clinically beneficial effects of the GLP-1RAs have been very favorably demonstrated in glycemic control in T2D since the launch of the first of the class, Byetta (Exenatide) in 2005 (Bridges, Bistas, & Jacobs, 2021; Gentilella, Pechtner, Corcos, & Consoli, 2019). As their use became more widespread it also became clear that they had significant effects in conditions that were frequent co-morbidities of T2D, such as CV disease (Andersen, Lund, Knop, & Vilsbøll, 2018; Seufert & Gallwitz, 2014; Wroge & Williams, 2016) and obesity (Andersen et al., 2018; Chia & Egan, 2020; Grill, 2020; Rajeev & Wilding, 2016; Rotella et al., 2005; Seufert & Gallwitz, 2014; Wren, 2008). In this review, we have examined the evidence for CV benefit of GLP-1RA therapies, and discussed the degree to which benefits are an indirect result of glycemic control in T2D, or a direct result of GLP-1R-mediated actions on cells of the CV system. While CV benefit no doubt accrues to the patient as a function of glycemic control, many of the CV benefits also appear to result from direct actions on component cells of the CV system. The pleiotropic nature of the pharmacotherapeutic effects of GLP-1RA administration results from the distribution of GLP-1Rs in different target tissues, the many different signaling pathways initiated by the interaction of the agonist with its receptor, and the structural differences between agonists that result in differential activation of downstream signaling pathways. While initial drug discovery efforts focused on finding peptide agonist homologs of GLP-1 that had better pharmacokinetic properties, recent efforts have explored structural means of preserving potency while designing agonists that specifically affect different signaling cascades. These new agonists, often shorter peptides or small molecules, or modified to enhance brain penetration, have enhanced potential for signal bias, as well as the potential for greater oral bioavailability. In the near future, GLP-1RAs will be created for specific target tissues, such as the CNS and perhaps cardiac or vascular smooth muscle, and specific disease modalities, including the central control of feeding, and neurodegenerative disorders and CV syndromes (Batista et al., 2019; During et al., 2003; Hayes, 2012; Hölscher, 2014; Sandoval, 2008).

Acknowledgment

The authors would like to acknowledge Ms. Patricia Reilly for her support in entering tabular data.

Conflict of interest statement

The authors declare no conflicts of interest. All data reported in the present review are from the public scientific literature.

References

Adler, G., & Beglinger, C. (1990). Hormones as regulators of pancreatic secretion in man. *European Journal of Clinical Investigation, 20*(Suppl 1), S27–S32. https://doi.org/10.1111/j.1365-2362.1990.tb01774.x.

Alexander, J. T., Staab, E. M., Wan, W., Franco, M., Knitter, A., Skandari, M. R., et al. (2021). The longer-term benefits and harms of glucagon-like Peptide-1 receptor agonists: A systematic review and meta-analysis. *Journal of General Internal Medicine*. https://doi.org/10.1007/s11606-021-07105-9.

Almutairi, M., Al Batran, R., & Ussher, J. R. (2019). Glucagon-like peptide-1 receptor action in the vasculature. *Peptides, 111*, 26–32. https://doi.org/10.1016/j.peptides.2018.09.002.

Andersen, A., Lund, A., Knop, F. K., & Vilsbøll, T. (2018). Glucagon-like peptide 1 in health and disease. *Nature Reviews. Endocrinology, 14*(7), 390–403. https://doi.org/10.1038/s41574-018-0016-2.

Andrikou, E., Tsioufis, C., Andrikou, I., Leontsinis, I., Tousoulis, D., & Papanas, N. (2019). GLP-1 receptor agonists and cardiovascular outcome trials: An update. *Hellenic Journal of Cardiology, 60*(6), 347–351. https://doi.org/10.1016/j.hjc.2018.11.008.

Baggio, L. L., Ussher, J. R., McLean, B. A., Cao, X., Kabir, M. G., Mulvihill, E. E., et al. (2017). The autonomic nervous system and cardiac GLP-1 receptors control heart rate in mice. *Molecular Metabolism, 6*(11), 1339–1349. https://doi.org/10.1016/j.molmet.2017.08.010.

Baggio, L. L., Yusta, B., Mulvihill, E. E., Cao, X., Streutker, C. J., Butany, J., et al. (2018). GLP-1 receptor expression within the human heart. *Endocrinology, 159*(4), 1570–1584. https://doi.org/10.1210/en.2018-00004.

Ban, K., Noyan-Ashraf, M. H., Hoefer, J., Bolz, S. S., Drucker, D. J., & Husain, M. (2008). Cardioprotective and vasodilatory actions of glucagon-like peptide 1 receptor are mediated through both glucagon-like peptide 1 receptor-dependent and -independent pathways. *Circulation, 117*(18), 2340–2350. https://doi.org/10.1161/circulationaha.107.739938.

Batista, A. F., Bodart-Santos, V., De Felice, F. G., & Ferreira, S. T. (2019). Neuroprotective actions of glucagon-like Peptide-1 (GLP-1) analogues in Alzheimer's and Parkinson's diseases. *CNS Drugs, 33*(3), 209–223. https://doi.org/10.1007/s40263-018-0593-6.

Bayliss, W. M., & Starling, E. H. (1902). The mechanism of pancreatic secretion. *The Journal of Physiology, 28*(5), 325–353. https://doi.org/10.1113/jphysiol.1902.sp000920.

Bayram, Z., Nacitarhan, C., & Ozdem, S. S. (2014). Effects of glucagon-like peptide-1 in diabetic rat small resistance arteries. *Journal of Cardiovascular Pharmacology*, *64*(3), 277–284. https://doi.org/10.1097/fjc.0000000000000120.

Bridges, A., Bistas, K. G., & Jacobs, T. F. (2021). Exenatide *StatPearls*. In *Treasure Island (FL): StatPearls publishing copyright © 2021*. LLC: StatPearls Publishing.

Brixner, D. I., McAdam-Marx, C., Ye, X., Boye, K. S., Nielsen, L. L., Wintle, M., et al. (2009). Six-month outcomes on A1C and cardiovascular risk factors in patients with type 2 diabetes treated with exenatide in an ambulatory care setting. *Diabetes, Obesity & Metabolism*, *11*(12), 1122–1130. https://doi.org/10.1111/j.1463-1326.2009.01081.x.

Brown, J. C., & Dryburgh, J. R. (1971). A gastric inhibitory polypeptide. II. The complete amino acid sequence. *Canadian Journal of Biochemistry*, *49*(8), 867–872. https://doi.org/10.1139/o71-122.

Brown, J. C., Dryburgh, J. R., Ross, S. A., & Dupré, J. (1975). Identification and actions of gastric inhibitory polypeptide. *Recent Progress in Hormone Research*, *31*, 487–532. https://doi.org/10.1016/b978-0-12-571131-9.50017-7.

Chen, P., Yang, F., Wang, W., Li, X., Liu, D., Zhang, Y., et al. (2021). Liraglutide attenuates myocardial fibrosis via inhibition of AT1R-mediated ROS production in hypertensive mice. *Journal of Cardiovascular Pharmacology and Therapeutics*, *26*(2), 179–188. https://doi.org/10.1177/1074248420942007.

Chey, W. Y., & Chang, T. M. (2014). Secretin: Historical perspective and current status. *Pancreas*, *43*(2), 162–182. https://doi.org/10.1097/01.mpa.0000437325.29728.d6.

Chia, C. W., & Egan, J. M. (2020). Incretins in obesity and diabetes. *Annals of the New York Academy of Sciences*, *1461*(1), 104–126. https://doi.org/10.1111/nyas.14211.

Cong, Z., Chen, L. N., Ma, H., Zhou, Q., Zou, X., Ye, C., et al. (2021). Molecular insights into ago-allosteric modulation of the human glucagon-like peptide-1 receptor. *Nature Communications*, *12*(1), 3763. https://doi.org/10.1038/s41467-021-24058-z.

Dagenais, G. R., Rydén, L., Leiter, L. A., Lakshmanan, M., Dyal, L., Probstfield, J. L., et al. (2020). Total cardiovascular or fatal events in people with type 2 diabetes and cardiovascular risk factors treated with dulaglutide in the REWIND trail: A post hoc analysis. *Cardiovascular Diabetology*, *19*(1), 199. https://doi.org/10.1186/s12933-020-01179-1.

Dai, Y., Mehta, J. L., & Chen, M. (2013). Glucagon-like peptide-1 receptor agonist liraglutide inhibits endothelin-1 in endothelial cell by repressing nuclear factor-kappa B activation. *Cardiovascular Drugs and Therapy*, *27*(5), 371–380. https://doi.org/10.1007/s10557-013-6463-z.

de Graaf, C., Song, G., Cao, C., Zhao, Q., Wang, M. W., Wu, B., et al. (2017). Extending the structural view of class B GPCRs. *Trends in Biochemical Sciences*, *42*(12), 946–960. https://doi.org/10.1016/j.tibs.2017.10.003.

Deacon, C. F. (2004). Circulation and degradation of GIP and GLP-1. *Hormone and Metabolic Research*, *36*(11 − 12), 761–765. https://doi.org/10.1055/s-2004-826160.

Deng, H., Yang, F., Ma, X., Wang, Y., Chen, Q., & Yuan, L. (2020). Long-term liraglutide administration induces pancreas neogenesis in adult T2DM mice. *Cell Transplantation*, *29*. https://doi.org/10.1177/0963689720927392.

Dillon, J. S., Tanizawa, Y., Wheeler, M. B., Leng, X. H., Ligon, B. B., Rabin, D. U., et al. (1993). Cloning and functional expression of the human glucagon-like peptide-1 (GLP-1) receptor. *Endocrinology*, *133*(4), 1907–1910. https://doi.org/10.1210/endo.133.4.8404634.

Dillon, J. S., Wheeler, M. B., Leng, X. H., Ligon, B. B., & Boyd, A. E., 3rd. (1997). The human glucagon-like peptide-1 (GLP-1) receptor. Cloning and functional expression. *Advances in Experimental Medicine and Biology*, *426*, 113–119. https://doi.org/10.1007/978-1-4899-1819-2_15.

Ding, Y., Ting, J. P., Liu, J., Al-Azzam, S., Pandya, P., & Afshar, S. (2020). Impact of non-proteinogenic amino acids in the discovery and development of peptide therapeutics. *Amino Acids*, *52*(9), 1207–1226. https://doi.org/10.1007/s00726-020-02890-9.

Drucker, D. J. (2018). Mechanisms of action and therapeutic application of glucagon-like Peptide-1. *Cell Metabolism*, *27*(4), 740–756. https://doi.org/10.1016/j.cmet.2018.03.001.
Drucker, D. J., Philippe, J., Mojsov, S., Chick, W. L., & Habener, J. F. (1987). Glucagon-like peptide I stimulates insulin gene expression and increases cyclic AMP levels in a rat islet cell line. *Proceedings of the National Academy of Sciences of the United States of America*, *84*(10), 3434–3438. https://doi.org/10.1073/pnas.84.10.3434.
Dupre, J., Ross, S. A., Watson, D., & Brown, J. C. (1973). Stimulation of insulin secretion by gastric inhibitory polypeptide in man. *The Journal of Clinical Endocrinology and Metabolism*, *37*(5), 826–828. https://doi.org/10.1210/jcem-37-5-826.
During, M. J., Cao, L., Zuzga, D. S., Francis, J. S., Fitzsimons, H. L., Jiao, X., et al. (2003). Glucagon-like peptide-1 receptor is involved in learning and neuroprotection. *Nature Medicine*, *9*(9), 1173–1179. https://doi.org/10.1038/nm919.
Ebert, R., & Creutzfeldt, W. (1980). Gastric inhibitory polypeptide. *Clinics in Gastroenterology*, *9*(3), 679–698.
Ebert, R., Unger, H., & Creutzfeldt, W. (1983). Preservation of incretin activity after removal of gastric inhibitory polypeptide (GIP) from rat gut extracts by immunoadsorption. *Diabetologia*, *24*(6), 449–454. https://doi.org/10.1007/bf00257346.
Edwards, C. M. (2005). The GLP-1 system as a therapeutic target. *Annals of Medicine*, *37*(5), 314–322. https://doi.org/10.1080/07853890510037400.
Elahi, D., Andersen, D. K., Brown, J. C., Debas, H. T., Hershcopf, R. J., Raizes, G. S., et al. (1979). Pancreatic alpha- and beta-cell responses to GIP infusion in normal man. *The American Journal of Physiology*, *237*(2), E185–E191. https://doi.org/10.1152/ajpendo.1979.237.2.E185.
Fan, S. H., Xiong, Q. F., Wang, L., Zhang, L. H., & Shi, Y. W. (2020). Glucagon-like peptide 1 treatment reverses vascular remodelling by downregulating matrix metalloproteinase 1 expression through inhibition of the ERK1/2/NF-κB signalling pathway. *Molecular and Cellular Endocrinology*, *518*, 111005. https://doi.org/10.1016/j.mce.2020.111005.
Fang, Z., Chen, S., Manchanda, Y., Bitsi, S., Pickford, P., David, A., et al. (2020). Ligand-specific factors influencing GLP-1 receptor post-endocytic trafficking and degradation in pancreatic Beta cells. *International Journal of Molecular Sciences*, *21*(21). https://doi.org/10.3390/ijms21218404.
Fang, Y., Ji, L., Zhu, C., Xiao, Y., Zhang, J., Lu, J., et al. (2020). Liraglutide alleviates hepatic steatosis by activating the TFEB-regulated autophagy-lysosomal pathway. *Frontiers in Cell and Development Biology*, *8*, 602574. https://doi.org/10.3389/fcell.2020.602574.
Fletcher, M. M., Halls, M. L., Christopoulos, A., Sexton, P. M., & Wootten, D. (2016). The complexity of signalling mediated by the glucagon-like peptide-1 receptor. *Biochemical Society Transactions*, *44*(2), 582–588. https://doi.org/10.1042/bst20150244.
Fletcher, M. M., Halls, M. L., Zhao, P., Clydesdale, L., Christopoulos, A., Sexton, P. M., et al. (2018). Glucagon-like peptide-1 receptor internalisation controls spatiotemporal signalling mediated by biased agonists. *Biochemical Pharmacology*, *156*, 406–419. https://doi.org/10.1016/j.bcp.2018.09.003.
Fremaux, J., Venin, C., Mauran, L., Zimmer, R., Koensgen, F., Rognan, D., et al. (2019). Ureidopeptide GLP-1 analogues with prolonged activity in vivo via signal bias and altered receptor trafficking. *Chemical Science*, *10*(42), 9872–9879. https://doi.org/10.1039/c9sc02079a.
Gentilella, R., Pechtner, V., Corcos, A., & Consoli, A. (2019). Glucagon-like peptide-1 receptor agonists in type 2 diabetes treatment: Are they all the same? *Diabetes/Metabolism Research and Reviews*, *35*(1), e3070. https://doi.org/10.1002/dmrr.3070.
Gerstein, H. C., Colhoun, H. M., Dagenais, G. R., Diaz, R., Lakshmanan, M., Pais, P., et al. (2019a). Dulaglutide and renal outcomes in type 2 diabetes: An exploratory analysis of the REWIND randomised, placebo-controlled trial. *Lancet*, *394*(10193), 131–138. https://doi.org/10.1016/s0140-6736(19)31150-x.

Gerstein, H. C., Colhoun, H. M., Dagenais, G. R., Diaz, R., Lakshmanan, M., Pais, P., et al. (2019b). Dulaglutide and cardiovascular outcomes in type 2 diabetes (REWIND): A double-blind, randomised placebo-controlled trial. *Lancet*, *394*(10193), 121–130. https://doi.org/10.1016/s0140-6736(19)31149-3.

Gerstein, H. C., Sattar, N., Rosenstock, J., Ramasundarahettige, C., Pratley, R., Lopes, R. D., et al. (2021). Cardiovascular and renal outcomes with Efpeglenatide in type 2 diabetes. *The New England Journal of Medicine*, *385*(10), 896–907. https://doi.org/10.1056/NEJMoa2108269.

Giugliano, D., Chiodini, P., Maiorino, M. I., Bellastella, G., & Esposito, K. (2019). Cardiovascular outcome trials and major cardiovascular events: Does glucose matter? A systematic review with meta-analysis. *Journal of Endocrinological Investigation*, *42*(10), 1165–1169. https://doi.org/10.1007/s40618-019-01047-0.

Giugliano, D., Scappaticcio, L., Longo, M., Caruso, P., Maiorino, M. I., Bellastella, G., et al. (2021). GLP-1 receptor agonists and cardiorenal outcomes in type 2 diabetes: An updated meta-analysis of eight CVOTs. *Cardiovascular Diabetology*, *20*(1), 189. https://doi.org/10.1186/s12933-021-01366-8.

Goldflam, M., & Ullman, C. G. (2015). Recent advances toward the discovery of drug-like peptides De novo. *Frontiers in Chemistry*, *3*, 69.

Graaf, C., Donnelly, D., Wootten, D., Lau, J., Sexton, P. M., Miller, L. J., et al. (2016). Glucagon-like Peptide-1 and its class B G protein-coupled receptors: A long march to therapeutic successes. *Pharmacological Reviews*, *68*(4), 954–1013. https://doi.org/10.1124/pr.115.011395.

Graziano, M. P., Hey, P. J., Borkowski, D., Chicchi, G. G., & Strader, C. D. (1993). Cloning and functional expression of a human glucagon-like peptide-1 receptor. *Biochemical and Biophysical Research Communications*, *196*(1), 141–146. https://doi.org/10.1006/bbrc.1993.2226.

Green, B. D., Hand, K. V., Dougan, J. E., McDonnell, B. M., Cassidy, R. S., & Grieve, D. J. (2008). GLP-1 and related peptides cause concentration-dependent relaxation of rat aorta through a pathway involving KATP and cAMP. *Archives of Biochemistry and Biophysics*, *478*(2), 136–142. https://doi.org/10.1016/j.abb.2008.08.001.

Gribble, F. M., & Reimann, F. (2017). Signalling in the gut endocrine axis. *Physiology & Behavior*, *176*, 183–188. https://doi.org/10.1016/j.physbeh.2017.02.039.

Griffith, D. A., Edmonds, D. J., Fortin, J.-P., Kalgutkar, A. S., Kuzmiski, J. B., Loria, P. M., et al. (2020). A small-molecule oral agonist of the human glucagon-like peptide-1 receptor. *bioRxiv*. https://doi.org/10.1101/2020.09.29.319483.

Grill, H. J. (2020). A role for GLP-1 in treating hyperphagia and obesity. *Endocrinology*, *161*-(8). https://doi.org/10.1210/endocr/bqaa093.

Haque, T. S., Lee, V. G., Riexinger, D., Lei, M., Malmstrom, S., Xin, L., et al. (2010). Identification of potent 11mer glucagon-like peptide-1 receptor agonist peptides with novel C-terminal amino acids: Homohomophenylalanine analogs. *Peptides*, *31*(5), 950–955. https://doi.org/10.1016/j.peptides.2010.01.008.

Hayes, M. R. (2012). Neuronal and intracellular signaling pathways mediating GLP-1 energy balance and glycemic effects. *Physiology & Behavior*, *106*(3), 413–416. https://doi.org/10.1016/j.physbeh.2012.02.017.

Hegele, R. A., & Maltman, G. M. (2020). Insulin's centenary: The birth of an idea. *The Lancet Diabetes and Endocrinology*, *8*(12), 971–977. https://doi.org/10.1016/s2213-8587(20)30337-5.

Helmstädter, J., Frenis, K., Filippou, K., Grill, A., Dib, M., Kalinovic, S., et al. (2020). Endothelial GLP-1 (glucagon-like Peptide-1) receptor mediates cardiovascular protection by liraglutide in mice with experimental arterial hypertension. *Arteriosclerosis, Thrombosis, and Vascular Biology*, *40*(1), 145–158. https://doi.org/10.1161/atv.0000615456.97862.30.

Henriksen, J. H., & de Muckadell, O. B. (2000). Secretin, its discovery, and the introduction of the hormone concept. *Scandinavian Journal of Clinical and Laboratory Investigation*, *60*(6), 463–471. https://doi.org/10.1080/003655100448446.

Hernandez, A. F., Green, J. B., Janmohamed, S., D'Agostino, R. B., Sr., Granger, C. B., Jones, N. P., et al. (2018). Albiglutide and cardiovascular outcomes in patients with type 2 diabetes and cardiovascular disease (Harmony outcomes): A double-blind, randomised placebo-controlled trial. *Lancet*, *392*(10157), 1519–1529. https://doi.org/10.1016/s0140-6736(18)32261-x.

Hoare, S. R. (2005). Mechanisms of peptide and nonpeptide ligand binding to class B G-protein-coupled receptors. *Drug Discovery Today*, *10*(6), 417–427. https://doi.org/10.1016/s1359-6446(05)03370-2.

Hollenstein, K., de Graaf, C., Bortolato, A., Wang, M. W., Marshall, F. H., & Stevens, R. C. (2014). Insights into the structure of class B GPCRs. *Trends in Pharmacological Sciences*, *35*(1), 12–22. https://doi.org/10.1016/j.tips.2013.11.001.

Holman, R. R., Bethel, M. A., Mentz, R. J., Thompson, V. P., Lokhnygina, Y., Buse, J. B., et al. (2017). Effects of once-weekly exenatide on cardiovascular outcomes in type 2 diabetes. *The New England Journal of Medicine*, *377*(13), 1228–1239. https://doi.org/10.1056/NEJMoa1612917.

Hölscher, C. (2014). Central effects of GLP-1: New opportunities for treatments of neurodegenerative diseases. *The Journal of Endocrinology*, *221*(1), T31–T41. https://doi.org/10.1530/joe-13-0221.

Holst, J. J. (2007). The physiology of glucagon-like peptide 1. *Physiological Reviews*, *87*(4), 1409–1439. https://doi.org/10.1152/physrev.00034.2006.

Holst, J. J. (2019). From the incretin concept and the discovery of GLP-1 to Today's diabetes therapy. *Frontiers in Endocrinology (Lausanne)*, *10*, 260. https://doi.org/10.3389/fendo.2019.00260.

Holst, J. J., Gasbjerg, L. S., & Rosenkilde, M. M. (2021). The role of incretins on insulin function and glucose homeostasis. *Endocrinology*, *162*(7). https://doi.org/10.1210/endocr/bqab065.

Husain, M., Birkenfeld, A. L., Donsmark, M., Dungan, K., Eliaschewitz, F. G., Franco, D. R., et al. (2019). Oral Semaglutide and cardiovascular outcomes in patients with type 2 diabetes. *The New England Journal of Medicine*, *381*(9), 841–851. https://doi.org/10.1056/NEJMoa1901118.

Jiang, J., Zhang, J., Jacobsen, L. V., & Hu, P. (2011). The pharmacokinetics, pharmacodynamics, and tolerability of liraglutide, a once-daily human GLP-1 analogue, after multiple subcutaneous administration in healthy Chinese male subjects. *Journal of Clinical Pharmacology*, *51*(12), 1620–1627. https://doi.org/10.1177/0091270010389468.

Jones, B. (2021). The therapeutic potential of GLP-1 receptor biased agonism. *British Journal of Pharmacology*. https://doi.org/10.1111/bph.15497.

Jones, B., Bloom, S. R., Buenaventura, T., Tomas, A., & Rutter, G. A. (2018). Control of insulin secretion by GLP-1. *Peptides*, *100*, 75–84. https://doi.org/10.1016/j.peptides.2017.12.013.

Jones, B., Buenaventura, T., Kanda, N., Chabosseau, P., Owen, B. M., Scott, R., et al. (2018). Targeting GLP-1 receptor trafficking to improve agonist efficacy. *Nature Communications*, *9*(1), 1602. https://doi.org/10.1038/s41467-018-03941-2.

Jones, B., McGlone, E. R., Fang, Z., Pickford, P., Corrêa, I. R., Jr., Oishi, A., et al. (2021). Genetic and biased agonist-mediated reductions in β-arrestin recruitment prolong cAMP signaling at glucagon family receptors. *The Journal of Biological Chemistry*, *296*, 100133. https://doi.org/10.1074/jbc.RA120.016334.

Kalra, S., Bhattacharya, S., & Kapoor, N. (2021). Contemporary classification of glucagon-like peptide 1 receptor agonists (GLP1RAs). *Diabetes Therapy*, *12*(8), 2133–2147. https://doi.org/10.1007/s13300-021-01113-y.

Kawai, T., Sun, B., Yoshino, H., Feng, D., Suzuki, Y., Fukazawa, M., et al. (2020). Structural basis for GLP-1 receptor activation by LY3502970, an orally active non-peptide agonist. *Proceedings of the National Academy of Sciences*, *117*(47), 29959. https://doi.org/10.1073/pnas.2014879117.

Kim, M., Platt, M. J., Shibasaki, T., Quaggin, S. E., Backx, P. H., Seino, S., et al. (2013). GLP-1 receptor activation and Epac2 link atrial natriuretic peptide secretion to control of blood pressure. *Nature Medicine*, *19*(5), 567–575. https://doi.org/10.1038/nm.3128.

Knudsen, L. B., Kiel, D., Teng, M., Behrens, C., Bhumralkar, D., Kodra, J. T., et al. (2007). Small-molecule agonists for the glucagon-like peptide 1 receptor. *Proceedings of the National Academy of Sciences of the United States of America*, *104*(3), 937–942. https://doi.org/10.1073/pnas.0605701104.

Kong, J., Wan, L., Wang, Y., Zhang, H., & Zhang, W. (2020). Liraglutide attenuates Aβ42 generation in APPswe/SH-SY5Y cells through the regulation of autophagy. *Neuropsychiatric Disease and Treatment*, *16*, 1817–1825. https://doi.org/10.2147/ndt.s260160.

Koole, C., Savage, E. E., Christopoulos, A., Miller, L. J., Sexton, P. M., & Wootten, D. (2013). Minireview: Signal bias, allosterism, and polymorphic variation at the GLP-1R: Implications for drug discovery. *Molecular Endocrinology*, *27*(8), 1234–1244. https://doi.org/10.1210/me.2013-1116.

Koole, C., Wootten, D., Simms, J., Valant, C., Sridhar, R., Woodman, O. L., et al. (2010). Allosteric ligands of the glucagon-like peptide 1 receptor (GLP-1R) differentially modulate endogenous and exogenous peptide responses in a pathway-selective manner: Implications for drug screening. *Molecular Pharmacology*, *78*(3), 456–465. https://doi.org/10.1124/mol.110.065664.

Krasner, N. M., Ido, Y., Ruderman, N. B., & Cacicedo, J. M. (2014). Glucagon-like peptide-1 (GLP-1) analog liraglutide inhibits endothelial cell inflammation through a calcium and AMPK dependent mechanism. *PLoS One*, *9*(5), e97554. https://doi.org/10.1371/journal.pone.0097554.

Kristensen, S. L., Rørth, R., Jhund, P. S., Docherty, K. F., Sattar, N., Preiss, D., et al. (2019). Cardiovascular, mortality, and kidney outcomes with GLP-1 receptor agonists in patients with type 2 diabetes: A systematic review and meta-analysis of cardiovascular outcome trials. *The Lancet Diabetes and Endocrinology*, 7(10), 776–785. https://doi.org/10.1016/s2213-8587(19)30249-9.

Kuhre, R. E., Frost, C. R., Svendsen, B., & Holst, J. J. (2015). Molecular mechanisms of glucose-stimulated GLP-1 secretion from perfused rat small intestine. *Diabetes*, *64*(2), 370. https://doi.org/10.2337/db14-0807.

Lankat-Buttgereit, B., & Göke, B. (1997). Cloning and characterization of the 5′ flanking sequences (promoter region) of the human GLP-1 receptor gene. *Peptides*, *18*(5), 617–624. https://doi.org/10.1016/s0196-9781(97)00001-6.

Lankat-Buttgereit, B., Göke, R., Fehmann, H. C., Richter, G., & Göke, B. (1994). Molecular cloning of a cDNA encoding for the GLP-1 receptor expressed in rat lung. *Experimental and Clinical Endocrinology*, *102*(4), 341–347. https://doi.org/10.1055/s-0029-1211301.

Li, X. D., He, S. S., Wan, T. T., & Li, Y. B. (2021). Liraglutide protects palmitate-induced INS-1 cell injury by enhancing autophagy mediated via FoxO1. *Molecular Medicine Reports*, *23*(2). https://doi.org/10.3892/mmr.2020.11786.

Li, Y., Xu, B., Yang, J., Wang, L., Tan, X., Hu, X., et al. (2021). Liraglutide protects against lethal renal ischemia-reperfusion injury by inhibiting high-mobility group box 1 nuclear-cytoplasmic translocation and release. *Pharmacological Research*, *173*, 105867. https://doi.org/10.1016/j.phrs.2021.105867.

Liang, Y.-L., Belousoff, M. J., Zhao, P., Koole, C., Fletcher, M. M., Truong, T. T., et al. (2020). Toward a structural understanding of class B GPCR peptide binding and activation. *Molecular Cell*, 77(3), 656–668. e655. https://doi.org/10.1016/j.molcel.2020.01.012.

Liang, Y. L., Khoshouei, M., Glukhova, A., Furness, S. G. B., Zhao, P., Clydesdale, L., et al. (2018). Phase-plate cryo-EM structure of a biased agonist-bound human GLP-1 receptor-Gs complex. *Nature, 555*(7694), 121–125. https://doi.org/10.1038/nature25773.

Liapakis, G., Matsoukas, M. T., Karageorgos, V., Venihaki, M., & Mavromoustakos, T. (2017). Family B G protein-coupled receptors and their ligands: From structure to function. *Current Medicinal Chemistry, 24*(31), 3323–3355. https://doi.org/10.2174/0929867324666170303162416.

Liu, L., Liu, J., & Huang, Y. (2015). Protective effects of glucagon-like peptide 1 on endothelial function in hypertension. *Journal of Cardiovascular Pharmacology, 65*(5), 399–405. https://doi.org/10.1097/fjc.0000000000000176.

Lucey, M., Ashik, T., Marzook, A., Wang, Y., Goulding, J., Oishi, A., et al. (2021). Acylation of the incretin peptide Exendin-4 directly impacts glucagon-like Peptide-1 receptor signaling and trafficking. *Molecular Pharmacology, 100*(4), 319–334. https://doi.org/10.1124/molpharm.121.000270.

Lund, P. K. (2005). The discovery of glucagon-like peptide 1. *Regulatory Peptides, 128*(2), 93–96. https://doi.org/10.1016/j.regpep.2004.09.001.

Lund, P. K., Goodman, R. H., & Habener, J. F. (1981). Pancreatic pre-proglucagons are encoded by two separate mRNAs. *The Journal of Biological Chemistry, 256*(13), 6515–6518.

Lund, P. K., Goodman, R. H., Montminy, M. R., Dee, P. C., & Habener, J. F. (1983). Anglerfish islet pre-proglucagon II. Nucleotide and corresponding amino acid sequence of the cDNA. *The Journal of Biological Chemistry, 258*(5), 3280–3284.

MacNeil, D. J., Occi, J. L., Hey, P. J., Strader, C. D., & Graziano, M. P. (1994). Cloning and expression of a human glucagon receptor. *Biochemical and Biophysical Research Communications, 198*(1), 328–334. https://doi.org/10.1006/bbrc.1994.1046.

Malik, F., & Li, Z. (2021). Non-peptide agonists and positive allosteric modulators of glucagon-like peptide-1 receptors: Alternative approaches for treatment of type 2 diabetes. *British Journal of Pharmacology*. https://doi.org/10.1111/bph.15446.

Marso, S. P., Bain, S. C., Consoli, A., Eliaschewitz, F. G., Jódar, E., Leiter, L. A., et al. (2016). Semaglutide and cardiovascular outcomes in patients with type 2 diabetes. *The New England Journal of Medicine, 375*(19), 1834–1844. https://doi.org/10.1056/NEJMoa1607141.

Marso, S. P., Daniels, G. H., Brown-Frandsen, K., Kristensen, P., Mann, J. F., Nauck, M. A., et al. (2016). Liraglutide and cardiovascular outcomes in type 2 diabetes. *The New England Journal of Medicine, 375*(4), 311–322. https://doi.org/10.1056/NEJMoa1603827.

Marzook, A., Chen, S., Pickford, P., Lucey, M., Wang, Y., Corrêa, I. R., Jr., et al. (2021). Evaluation of efficacy- versus affinity-driven agonism with biased GLP-1R ligands P5 and exendin-F1. *Biochemical Pharmacology, 190*. https://doi.org/10.1016/j.bcp.2021.114656, 114656.

Marzook, A., Tomas, A., & Jones, B. (2021). The interplay of glucagon-like Peptide-1 receptor trafficking and Signalling in pancreatic Beta cells. *Frontiers in Endocrinology (Lausanne), 12*. https://doi.org/10.3389/fendo.2021.678055, 678055.

McClenaghan, N. H., Flatt, P. R., & Ball, A. J. (2006). Actions of glucagon-like peptide-1 on KATP channel-dependent and -independent effects of glucose, sulphonylureas and nateglinide. *The Journal of Endocrinology, 190*(3), 889–896. https://doi.org/10.1677/joe.1.06949.

Mentlein, R., Gallwitz, B., & Schmidt, W. E. (1993). Dipeptidyl-peptidase IV hydrolyses gastric inhibitory polypeptide, glucagon-like peptide-1(7-36)amide, peptide histidine methionine and is responsible for their degradation in human serum. *European Journal of Biochemistry, 214*(3), 829–835. https://doi.org/10.1111/j.1432-1033.1993.tb17986.x.

Mohammedi, K., Woodward, M., Marre, M., Colagiuri, S., Cooper, M., Harrap, S., et al. (2017). Comparative effects of microvascular and macrovascular disease on the risk of major outcomes in patients with type 2 diabetes. *Cardiovascular Diabetology, 16*(1), 95. https://doi.org/10.1186/s12933-017-0574-y.

Mojsov, S., Weir, G. C., & Habener, J. F. (1987). Insulinotropin: Glucagon-like peptide I (7-37) co-encoded in the glucagon gene is a potent stimulator of insulin release in the perfused rat pancreas. *The Journal of Clinical Investigation, 79*(2), 616–619. https://doi.org/10.1172/jci112855.

Montrose-Rafizadeh, C., Avdonin, P., Garant, M. J., Rodgers, B. D., Kole, S., Yang, H., et al. (1999). Pancreatic glucagon-like peptide-1 receptor couples to multiple G proteins and activates mitogen-activated protein kinase pathways in Chinese hamster ovary cells. *Endocrinology, 140*(3), 1132–1140. https://doi.org/10.1210/endo.140.3.6550.

Müller, T. D., Finan, B., Bloom, S. R., D'Alessio, D., Drucker, D. J., Flatt, P. R., et al. (2019). Glucagon-like peptide 1 (GLP-1). *Molecular Metabolism, 30*, 72–130. https://doi.org/10.1016/j.molmet.2019.09.010.

Nyström, T., Gutniak, M. K., Zhang, Q., Zhang, F., Holst, J. J., Ahrén, B., et al. (2004). Effects of glucagon-like peptide-1 on endothelial function in type 2 diabetes patients with stable coronary artery disease. *American Journal of Physiology. Endocrinology and Metabolism, 287*(6), E1209–E1215. https://doi.org/10.1152/ajpendo.00237.2004.

Orskov, C., Bersani, M., Johnsen, A. H., Højrup, P., & Holst, J. J. (1989). Complete sequences of glucagon-like Peptide-1 from human and pig small intestine. *Journal of Biological Chemistry, 264*(22), 12826–12829. https://doi.org/10.1016/S0021-9258(18)51561-1.

Orskov, C., Rabenhøj, L., Wettergren, A., Kofod, H., & Holst, J. J. (1994). Tissue and plasma concentrations of amidated and glycine-extended glucagon-like peptide I in humans. *Diabetes, 43*(4), 535–539. https://doi.org/10.2337/diab.43.4.535.

Palmer, S. C., Tendal, B., Mustafa, R. A., Vandvik, P. O., Li, S., Hao, Q., et al. (2021). Sodium-glucose cotransporter protein-2 (SGLT-2) inhibitors and glucagon-like peptide-1 (GLP-1) receptor agonists for type 2 diabetes: Systematic review and network meta-analysis of randomised controlled trials. *BMJ, 372*, m4573. https://doi.org/10.1136/bmj.m4573.

Pan, X., Li, C., & Gao, H. (2021). High glucose attenuates cardioprotective effects of glucagon-like Peptide-1 through induction of mitochondria dysfunction via inhibition of β-Arrestin-signaling. *Frontiers in Physiology, 12*, 648399. https://doi.org/10.3389/fphys.2021.648399.

Perley, M. J., & Kipnis, D. M. (1967). Plasma insulin responses to oral and intravenous glucose: Studies in normal and diabetic sujbjects. *The Journal of Clinical Investigation, 46*(12), 1954–1962. https://doi.org/10.1172/jci105685.

Pfeffer, M. A., Claggett, B., Diaz, R., Dickstein, K., Gerstein, H. C., Køber, L. V., et al. (2015). Lixisenatide in patients with type 2 diabetes and acute coronary syndrome. *The New England Journal of Medicine, 373*(23), 2247–2257. https://doi.org/10.1056/NEJMoa1509225.

Plamboeck, A., Holst, J. J., Carr, R. D., & Deacon, C. F. (2003). Neutral endopeptidase 24.11 and dipeptidyl peptidase IV are both involved in regulating the metabolic stability of glucagon-like peptide-1 in vivo. *Advances in Experimental Medicine and Biology, 524*, 303–312. https://doi.org/10.1007/0-306-47920-6_36.

Plamboeck, A., Holst, J. J., Carr, R. D., & Deacon, C. F. (2005). Neutral endopeptidase 24.11 and dipeptidyl peptidase IV are both mediators of the degradation of glucagon-like peptide 1 in the anaesthetised pig. *Diabetologia, 48*(9), 1882–1890. https://doi.org/10.1007/s00125-005-1847-7.

Popovic, D. S., Stokic, E., & Popovic, S. L. (2015). GLP-1 receptor agonists and type 1 diabetes - where do we stand? *Current Pharmaceutical Design, 21*(36), 5292–5298. https://doi.org/10.2174/0929867322666151006142224.

Quoyer, J., Longuet, C., Broca, C., Linck, N., Costes, S., Varin, E., et al. (2010). GLP-1 mediates antiapoptotic effect by phosphorylating bad through a beta-arrestin 1-mediated ERK1/2 activation in pancreatic beta-cells. *The Journal of Biological Chemistry, 285*(3), 1989–2002. https://doi.org/10.1074/jbc.M109.067207.

Rabideau, A. E., & Pentelute, B. L. (2015). A d-amino acid at the N-terminus of a protein abrogates its degradation by the N-end rule pathway. *ACS Central Science*, *1*(8), 423–430. https://doi.org/10.1021/acscentsci.5b00308.

Rajeev, S. P., & Wilding, J. (2016). GLP-1 as a target for therapeutic intervention. *Current Opinion in Pharmacology*, *31*, 44–49. https://doi.org/10.1016/j.coph.2016.08.005.

Raufman, J. P. (1996). Bioactive peptides from lizard venoms. *Regulatory Peptides*, *61*(1), 1–18. https://doi.org/10.1016/0167-0115(96)00135-8.

Reimann, F., & Gribble, F. M. (2002). Glucose-sensing in glucagon-like Peptide-1-secreting cells. *Diabetes*, *51*(9), 2757. https://doi.org/10.2337/diabetes.51.9.2757.

Roed, S. N., Wismann, P., Underwood, C. R., Kulahin, N., Iversen, H., Cappelen, K. A., et al. (2014). Real-time trafficking and signaling of the glucagon-like peptide-1 receptor. *Molecular and Cellular Endocrinology*, *382*(2), 938–949. https://doi.org/10.1016/j.mce.2013.11.010.

Rotella, C. M., Pala, L., & Mannucci, E. (2005). Glucagon-like peptide 1 (GLP-1) and metabolic diseases. *Journal of Endocrinological Investigation*, *28*(8), 746–758. https://doi.org/10.1007/bf03347560.

Rowlands, J., Heng, J., Newsholme, P., & Carlessi, R. (2018). Pleiotropic effects of GLP-1 and analogs on cell signaling, metabolism, and function. *Frontiers in Endocrinology (Lausanne)*, *9*, 672.

Sandoval, D. (2008). CNS GLP-1 regulation of peripheral glucose homeostasis. *Physiology & Behavior*, *94*(5), 670–674. https://doi.org/10.1016/j.physbeh.2008.04.018.

Segre, G. V., & Goldring, S. R. (1993). Receptors for secretin, calcitonin, parathyroid hormone (PTH)/PTH-related peptide, vasoactive intestinal peptide, glucagonlike peptide 1, growth hormone-releasing hormone, and glucagon belong to a newly discovered G-protein-linked receptor family. *Trends in Endocrinology and Metabolism*, *4*(10), 309–314. https://doi.org/10.1016/1043-2760(93)90071-l.

Sélley, E., Kun, S., Szijártó, I. A., Kertész, M., Wittmann, I., & Molnár, G. A. (2016). Vasodilator effect of glucagon: Receptorial crosstalk among glucagon, GLP-1, and receptor for glucagon and GLP-1. *Hormone and Metabolic Research*, *48*(7), 476–483. https://doi.org/10.1055/s-0042-101794.

Seufert, J., & Gallwitz, B. (2014). The extra-pancreatic effects of GLP-1 receptor agonists: A focus on the cardiovascular, gastrointestinal and central nervous systems. *Diabetes, Obesity & Metabolism*, *16*(8), 673–688. https://doi.org/10.1111/dom.12251.

Shigeto, M., Cha, C. Y., Rorsman, P., & Kaku, K. (2017). A role of PLC/PKC-dependent pathway in GLP-1-stimulated insulin secretion. *Journal of Molecular Medicine (Berlin, Germany)*, *95*(4), 361–368. https://doi.org/10.1007/s00109-017-1508-6.

Shigeto, M., Ramracheya, R., Tarasov, A. I., Cha, C. Y., Chibalina, M. V., Hastoy, B., et al. (2015). GLP-1 stimulates insulin secretion by PKC-dependent TRPM4 and TRPM5 activation. *The Journal of Clinical Investigation*, *125*(12), 4714–4728. https://doi.org/10.1172/jci81975.

Smith, N. K., Hackett, T. A., Galli, A., & Flynn, C. R. (2019). GLP-1: Molecular mechanisms and outcomes of a complex signaling system. *Neurochemistry International*, *128*, 94–105. https://doi.org/10.1016/j.neuint.2019.04.010.

Song, G., Yang, D., Wang, Y., de Graaf, C., Zhou, Q., Jiang, S., et al. (2017). Human GLP-1 receptor transmembrane domain structure in complex with allosteric modulators. *Nature*, *546*(7657), 312–315. https://doi.org/10.1038/nature22378.

Sonoda, N., Imamura, T., Yoshizaki, T., Babendure, J. L., Lu, J. C., & Olefsky, J. M. (2008). Beta-Arrestin-1 mediates glucagon-like peptide-1 signaling to insulin secretion in cultured pancreatic beta cells. *Proceedings of the National Academy of Sciences of the United States of America*, *105*(18), 6614–6619. https://doi.org/10.1073/pnas.0710402105.

Starling, E. H. (1905). The Croonian lectures. I. on the chemical correlation of the functions of the body. *Lancet*, *166*, 339–341.

Starling, E. H. (1914). Discussion on the therapeutic value of hormones. *Proceedings of the Royal Society of Medicine 7(Ther Pharmacol Sect)*, 29–31.
Sudo, M., Li, Y., Hiro, T., Takayama, T., Mitsumata, M., Shiomi, M., et al. (2017). Inhibition of plaque progression and promotion of plaque stability by glucagon-like peptide-1 receptor agonist: Serial in vivo findings from iMap-IVUS in Watanabe heritable hyperlipidemic rabbits. *Atherosclerosis*, *265*, 283–291. https://doi.org/10.1016/j.atherosclerosis.2017.06.920.
Sun, E. W., de Fontgalland, D., Rabbitt, P., Hollington, P., Sposato, L., Due, S. L., et al. (2017). Mechanisms controlling glucose-induced GLP-1 secretion in human small intestine. *Diabetes*, *66*(8), 2144. https://doi.org/10.2337/db17-0058.
Swedberg, J. E., Schroeder, C. I., Mitchell, J. M., Durek, T., Fairlie, D. P., Edmonds, D. J., et al. (2015). Cyclic alpha-conotoxin peptidomimetic chimeras as potent GLP-1R agonists. *European Journal of Medicinal Chemistry*, *103*, 175–184. https://doi.org/10.1016/j.ejmech.2015.08.046.
Taguchi, K., Kaneko, N., Okudaira, K., Matsumoto, T., & Kobayashi, T. (2021). GLP-1 modulates insulin-induced relaxation response through β-arrestin2 regulation in diabetic mice aortas. *Acta Physiologica (Oxford, England)*, *231*(3), e13573. https://doi.org/10.1111/apha.13573.
Taminato, T., Seino, Y., Goto, Y., Inoue, Y., & Kadowaki, S. (1977). Synthetic gastric inhibitory polypeptide. Stimulatory effect on insulin and glucagon secretion in the rat. *Diabetes*, *26*(5), 480–484. https://doi.org/10.2337/diab.26.5.480.
Theodorakis, M. J., Carlson, O., Michopoulos, S., Doyle, M. E., Juhaszova, M., Petraki, K., et al. (2006). Human duodenal enteroendocrine cells: Source of both incretin peptides, GLP-1 and GIP. *American Journal of Physiology. Endocrinology and Metabolism*, *290*(3), E550–E559. https://doi.org/10.1152/ajpendo.00326.2004.
Thorens, B. (1992). Expression cloning of the pancreatic beta cell receptor for the gluco-incretin hormone glucagon-like peptide 1. *Proceedings of the National Academy of Sciences of the United States of America*, *89*(18), 8641–8645. https://doi.org/10.1073/pnas.89.18.8641.
Thorens, B., Porret, A., Bühler, L., Deng, S. P., Morel, P., & Widmann, C. (1993). Cloning and functional expression of the human islet GLP-1 receptor. Demonstration that exendin-4 is an agonist and exendin-(9-39) an antagonist of the receptor. *Diabetes*, *42*(11), 1678–1682. https://doi.org/10.2337/diab.42.11.1678.
Tian, L., & Jin, T. (2016). The incretin hormone GLP-1 and mechanisms underlying its secretion. *Journal of Diabetes*, *8*(6), 753–765. https://doi.org/10.1111/1753-0407.12439.
Udell, J. A., Cavender, M. A., Bhatt, D. L., Chatterjee, S., Farkouh, M. E., & Scirica, B. M. (2015). Glucose-lowering drugs or strategies and cardiovascular outcomes in patients with or at risk for type 2 diabetes: A meta-analysis of randomised controlled trials. *The Lancet Diabetes and Endocrinology*, *3*(5), 356–366. https://doi.org/10.1016/s2213-8587(15)00044-3.
Underwood, C. R., Garibay, P., Knudsen, L. B., Hastrup, S., Peters, G. H., Rudolph, R., et al. (2010). Crystal structure of glucagon-like peptide-1 in complex with the extracellular domain of the glucagon-like peptide-1 receptor. *The Journal of Biological Chemistry*, *285*(1), 723–730. https://doi.org/10.1074/jbc.M109.033829.
van der Velden, W. J. C., Smit, F. X., Christiansen, C. B., Møller, T. C., Hjortø, G. M., Larsen, O., et al. (2021). GLP-1 Val8: A biased GLP-1R agonist with altered binding kinetics and impaired release of pancreatic hormones in rats. *ACS Pharmacology & Translational Science*, *4*(1), 296–313. https://doi.org/10.1021/acsptsci.0c00193.
Vecchio, I., Tornali, C., Bragazzi, N. L., & Martini, M. (2018). The discovery of insulin: An important milestone in the history of medicine. *Frontiers in Endocrinology (Lausanne)*, *9*, 613. https://doi.org/10.3389/fendo.2018.00613.

Volz, A., Göke, R., Lankat-Buttgereit, B., Fehmann, H. C., Bode, H. P., & Göke, B. (1995). Molecular cloning, functional expression, and signal transduction of the GIP-receptor cloned from a human insulinoma. *FEBS Letters*, *373*(1), 23–29. https://doi.org/10.1016/0014-5793(95)01006-z.

Willard, F. S., Wainscott, D. B., Showalter, A. D., Stutsman, C., Ma, W., Cardona, G. R., et al. (2021). Discovery of an orally efficacious positive allosteric modulator of the glucagon-like Peptide-1 receptor. *Journal of Medicinal Chemistry*, *64*(6), 3439–3448. https://doi.org/10.1021/acs.jmedchem.1c00029.

Wootten, D., Christopoulos, A., Marti-Solano, M., Babu, M. M., & Sexton, P. M. (2018). Mechanisms of signalling and biased agonism in G protein-coupled receptors. *Nature Reviews. Molecular Cell Biology*, *19*(10), 638–653. https://doi.org/10.1038/s41580-018-0049-3.

Wootten, D., Reynolds, C. A., Koole, C., Smith, K. J., Mobarec, J. C., Simms, J., et al. (2016). A hydrogen-bonded polar network in the Core of the glucagon-like Peptide-1 receptor is a fulcrum for biased agonism: Lessons from class B crystal structures. *Molecular Pharmacology*, *89*(3), 335–347. https://doi.org/10.1124/mol.115.101246.

Wootten, D., Reynolds, C. A., Smith, K. J., Mobarec, J. C., Furness, S. G. B., Miller, L. J., et al. (2016a). Key interactions by conserved polar amino acids located at the transmembrane helical boundaries in class B GPCRs modulate activation, effector specificity and biased signalling in the glucagon-like peptide-1 receptor. *Biochemical Pharmacology*, *118*, 68–87. https://doi.org/10.1016/j.bcp.2016.08.015.

Wootten, D., Reynolds, C. A., Smith, K. J., Mobarec, J. C., Koole, C., Savage, E. E., et al. (2016b). The extracellular surface of the GLP-1 receptor is a molecular trigger for biased agonism. *Cell*, *165*(7), 1632–1643. https://doi.org/10.1016/j.cell.2016.05.023.

Wootten, D., Savage, E. E., Willard, F. S., Bueno, A. B., Sloop, K. W., Christopoulos, A., et al. (2013). Differential activation and modulation of the glucagon-like peptide-1 receptor by small molecule ligands. *Molecular Pharmacology*, *83*(4), 822–834. https://doi.org/10.1124/mol.112.084525.

Wren, A. M. (2008). Gut and hormones and obesity. *Frontiers of Hormone Research*, *36*, 165–181. https://doi.org/10.1159/000115364.

Wroge, J., & Williams, N. T. (2016). Glucagon-like Peptide-1 (GLP-1) receptor agonists in cardiac disorders. *The Annals of Pharmacotherapy*, *50*(12), 1041–1050. https://doi.org/10.1177/1060028016663218.

Wu, L., Wang, K., Wang, W., Wen, Z., Wang, P., Liu, L., et al. (2018). Glucagon-like peptide-1 ameliorates cardiac lipotoxicity in diabetic cardiomyopathy via the PPARα pathway. *Aging Cell*, *17*(4), e12763. https://doi.org/10.1111/acel.12763.

Wu, F., Yang, L., Hang, K., Laursen, M., Wu, L., Han, G. W., et al. (2020). Full-length human GLP-1 receptor structure without orthosteric ligands. *Nature Communications*, *11*(1), 1272. https://doi.org/10.1038/s41467-020-14934-5.

Yamamoto, H., Lee, C. E., Marcus, J. N., Williams, T. D., Overton, J. M., Lopez, M. E., et al. (2002). Glucagon-like peptide-1 receptor stimulation increases blood pressure and heart rate and activates autonomic regulatory neurons. *The Journal of Clinical Investigation*, *110*(1), 43–52. https://doi.org/10.1172/jci15595.

Yang, D., de Graaf, C., Yang, L., Song, G., Dai, A., Cai, X., et al. (2016). Structural determinants of binding the seven-transmembrane domain of the glucagon-like Peptide-1 receptor (GLP-1R). *The Journal of Biological Chemistry*, *291*(25), 12991–13004. https://doi.org/10.1074/jbc.M116.721977.

Yu, M., Moreno, C., Hoagland, K. M., Dahly, A., Ditter, K., Mistry, M., et al. (2003). Antihypertensive effect of glucagon-like peptide 1 in dahl salt-sensitive rats. *Journal of Hypertension*, *21*(6), 1125–1135. https://doi.org/10.1097/00004872-200306000-00012.

Zech, A. T. L., Singh, S. R., Schlossarek, S., & Carrier, L. (2020). Autophagy in cardiomyopathies. *Biochimica et Biophysica Acta, Molecular Cell Research*, *1867*(3), 118432. https://doi.org/10.1016/j.bbamcr.2019.01.013.

Zelniker, T. A., Wiviott, S. D., Raz, I., Im, K., Goodrich, E. L., Furtado, R. H. M., et al. (2019). Comparison of the effects of glucagon-like peptide receptor agonists and sodium-glucose cotransporter 2 inhibitors for prevention of major adverse cardiovascular and renal outcomes in type 2 diabetes mellitus. *Circulation*, *139*(17), 2022–2031. https://doi.org/10.1161/circulationaha.118.038868.

Zhang, Y., Ling, Y., Yang, L., Cheng, Y., Yang, P., Song, X., et al. (2017). Liraglutide relieves myocardial damage by promoting autophagy via AMPK-mTOR signaling pathway in zucker diabetic fatty rat. *Molecular and Cellular Endocrinology*, *448*, 98–107. https://doi.org/10.1016/j.mce.2017.03.029.

Zhao, T., Chen, H., Cheng, C., Zhang, J., Yan, Z., Kuang, J., et al. (2019). Liraglutide protects high-glucose-stimulated fibroblasts by activating the CD36-JNK-AP1 pathway to downregulate P4HA1. *Biomedicine & Pharmacotherapy*, *118*, 109224. https://doi.org/10.1016/j.biopha.2019.109224.

Zhao, P., Liang, Y. L., Belousoff, M. J., Deganutti, G., Fletcher, M. M., Willard, F. S., et al. (2020). Activation of the GLP-1 receptor by a non-peptidic agonist. *Nature*, *577*(7790), 432–436. https://doi.org/10.1038/s41586-019-1902-z.

Zhou, Q., Guo, W., Dai, A., Cai, X., Vass, M., de Graaf, C., et al. (2021). Discovery of novel allosteric modulators targeting an extra-helical binding site of GLP-1R using structure- and ligand-based virtual screening. *Biomolecules*, *11*(7). https://doi.org/10.3390/biom11070929.

Zhou, P., Jiang, X., & Li, X. (2021). Design and evaluation of GLP-1 receptor G-protein biased agonist with prolonged efficacy on diabetes. *Life Sciences*, *119844*. https://doi.org/10.1016/j.lfs.2021.119844.

CHAPTER EIGHT

ADAM and ADAMTS disintegrin and metalloproteinases as major factors and molecular targets in vascular malfunction and disease

HaiFeng Yang and Raouf A. Khalil*
Vascular Surgery Research Laboratories, Division of Vascular and Endovascular Surgery, Brigham and Women's Hospital, Harvard Medical School, Boston, MA, United States
*Corresponding author: e-mail address: raouf_khalil@hms.harvard.edu

Contents

Advances in Pharmacology, Volume 94
ISSN 1054-3589
https://doi.org/10.1016/bs.apha.2021.11.002

Abstract

A Disintegrin and Metalloproteinase (ADAM) and A Disintegrin and Metalloproteinase with Thrombospondin Motifs (ADAMTS) are two closely related families of proteolytic enzymes. ADAMs are largely membrane-bound enzymes that act as molecular scissors or sheddases of membrane-bound proteins, growth factors, cytokines, receptors and ligands, whereas ADAMTS are mainly secreted enzymes. ADAMs have a pro-domain, and a metalloproteinase, disintegrin, cysteine-rich and transmembrane domain. Similarly, ADAMTS family members have a pro-domain, and a metalloproteinase, disintegrin, and cysteine-rich domain, but instead of a transmembrane domain they have thrombospondin motifs. Most ADAMs and ADAMTS are activated by pro-protein convertases, and can be regulated by G-protein coupled receptor agonists, Ca^{2+} ionophores and protein kinase C. Activated ADAMs and ADAMTS participate in numerous vascular processes including angiogenesis, vascular smooth muscle cell proliferation and migration, vascular cell apoptosis, cell survival, tissue repair, and wound healing. ADAMs and ADAMTS also play a role in vascular malfunction and cardiovascular diseases such as hypertension, atherosclerosis, coronary artery disease, myocardial infarction, heart failure, peripheral artery disease, and vascular aneurysm. Decreased ADAMTS13 is involved in thrombotic thrombocytopenic purpura and microangiopathies. The activity of ADAMs and ADAMTS can be regulated by endogenous tissue inhibitors of metalloproteinases and other synthetic small molecule inhibitors. ADAMs and ADAMTS can be used as diagnostic biomarkers and molecular targets in cardiovascular disease, and modulators of ADAMs and ADAMTS activity may provide potential new approaches for the management of cardiovascular disorders.

Abbreviations

aa	amino acid
AAA	abdominal aortic aneurysm
ACE	angiotensin-I converting enzyme
ACE2	angiotensin-converting enzyme-2
ADAM	A Disintegrin and Metalloproteinase
ADAMTS	A Disintegrin and Metalloproteinase with Thrombospondin Motifs
AngII	angiotensin II
$ApoE^{-/-}$	apolipoprotein E deficient
APP	amyloid precursor protein
CABG	coronary artery bypass graft
CAD	coronary artery disease
C-domain	cysteine-rich domain
CHF	congestive heart failure

CNS	central nervous system
COMP	cartilage oligomeric matrix protein
CUB	C1r/C1s Uegf Bmp1
CVD	cardiovascular disease
D-domain	disintegrin domain
DOCA	deoxycorticosterone acetate
Dll4	delta-like 4
EC	endothelial cell
E-cadherin	epithelial cadherin
ECM	extracellular matrix
EGF	epidermal growth factor
EGFR	EGF receptor
ERK	extracellular signal-regulated protein kinase
GPCR	G-protein coupled receptor
GPIb	platelet glycoprotein Ib
GWAS	genome-wide association studies
HB-EGF	heparin-binding EGF-like growth factor
HUVECs	human umbilical vein endothelial cells
HTN	hypertension
HVR	highly variable region
ICAM-1	intercellular adhesion molecule-1
IL-6	interleukin 6
I/R	ischemia-reperfusion
JAM-A	junctional adhesion molecule A
KO	knockout
M-domain	metalloproteinase domain
LDL	low density lipoprotein
LPS	lipopolysaccharide
MAPK	mitogen activated protein kinase
MCP-1	monocyte chemoattractant protein-1
MDC	metalloproteinase/disintegrin/cysteine-rich
MI	myocardial infarction
MMP	matrix metalloproteinase
NSTEMI	non-ST-segment elevation MI
PAD	peripheral artery disease
PAI-1	plasminogen activator inhibitor-1
PE	preeclampsia
PLAC	protease and lacunin
RAGE	receptors-for-advanced-glycation-end-products
RGD	Arg-Gly-Asp
rh	recombinant human
SMC	smooth muscle cell
SNP	single nucleotide polymorphism
SVM	snake venom metalloproteinase
STEMI	ST-segment elevation MI
TAA	thoracic aortic aneurysm
Tie-2	tyrosine-protein kinase receptor

TIMP	tissue inhibitor of metalloproteinases
TNFα	tumor necrosis factor-α
TACE	TNFα-converting enzyme
tPA	tissue plasminogen activator
Tspan	tetraspanin
TSP1	thrombospondin 1
TSR	thrombospondin repeat
TTP	thrombotic thrombocytopenic purpura
uPA	urokinase plasminogen activator
VCAM-1	vascular cell adhesion molecule-1
VE-cadherin	vascular endothelial cadherin
VEGF	vascular endothelial growth factor
VEGFR	VEGF receptor
VSM	vascular smooth muscle
VSMC	VSM cell
VTE	venous thromboembolism
vWF	von Willebrand factor
WT	wild-type

1. Introduction

A disintegrin and metalloproteinase (ADAM) and a disintegrin and metalloproteinase with thrombospondin motifs (ADAMTS) are two families of proteolytic enzymes implicated in the regulation of extracellular matrix (ECM) proteins, cell-associated proteins, growth factors and cytokines, and modulation of numerous biological processes. ADAMs and ADAMTS share a highly conserved structure and protein homology in the form of a pro-domain, and a metalloproteinase, disintegrin and cysteine-rich domain. ADAMs are largely membrane-anchored by a transmembrane domain connected to a cytoplasmic tail, although some secreted ADAMs are generated by alternative splicing or cleavage. Through binding of the disintegrin domain to integrins together with the proteolytic activity of the metalloproteinase domain, ADAMs function as molecular scissors or sheddases of membrane-bound growth factors, cytokines and receptors. In contrast, ADAMTS family members are mainly secreted enzymes that lack the transmembrane domain and cytoplasmic tail, and instead have ancillary thrombospondin motifs, which structurally resemble thrombospondin 1 or 2, homotrimeric adhesive glycoproteins involved in cell-to-cell and cell-to-matrix interactions.

Several research articles have provided details of ADAMs and ADAMTS structure and function and their role in different biological processes including the regulation of the reproductive system, embryo development, central nervous system (CNS) and cell growth (Colige et al., 2005; Lemarchant et al., 2013; Mead & Apte, 2018; Porter, Clark, Kevorkian, & Edwards, 2005; Seals & Courtneidge, 2003; Stone, Kroeger, & Sang, 1999; Takeda, 2016; van der Vorst, Weber, & Donners, 2018). ADAMs and ADAMTS are also involved in pathological conditions such as inflammation, autoimmune disease and cancer (Mead & Apte, 2018). ADAMs and ADAMTS also participate in vascular processes such as angiogenesis, vascular smooth muscle cell (VSMC) proliferation and migration, and play a role in the vascular malfunction associated with cardiovascular disease (CVD) including hypertension (HTN), atherosclerosis, coronary artery disease (CAD) and dilated cardiomyopathy (Fedak et al., 2006; Santamaria & de Groot, 2020). Highlighting the role of ADAMs and ADAMTS in vascular malfunction should help to further understand the mechanisms of CVD.

In this review, we will use data published in PubMed and Web of Science to describe the biochemical and biological aspects of ADAMs and ADAMTS and their role in vascular malfunction and CVD. We will briefly describe ADAMs and ADAMTS structure, activators, targets, substrates, and inhibitors. We will introduce the general functions of representative ADAMs and ADAMTS and their mouse knockout phenotypes, then describe their specific roles in vascular processes such as angiogenesis, VSMC proliferation and migration, intimal hyperplasia and neointima formation, vascular cell apoptosis, and tissue repair and wound healing. We will follow with description of the role of ADAMs and ADAMTS in CVD such as HTN, atherosclerosis, CAD, myocardial infarction (MI), heart failure, ischemia-reperfusion (I/R) injury, peripheral artery disease (PAD), and vascular aneurysm. We will conclude with a perspective on how ADAMs and ADAMTS can be used as potential biomarkers and molecular targets in the diagnosis and management of CVD.

2. ADAMs and ADAMTS structure

ADAMs, formerly known as metalloproteinase/disintegrin/cysteine-rich (MDC) proteins, are zinc (Zn^{2+})-dependent proteolytic enzymes (Fig. 1). ADAMs and ADAMTS are members of the adamalysin subfamily, and they share similar structure and protein sequence including a pro-domain, a metalloproteinase, disintegrin, and cysteine-rich domain (Takeda, 2016).

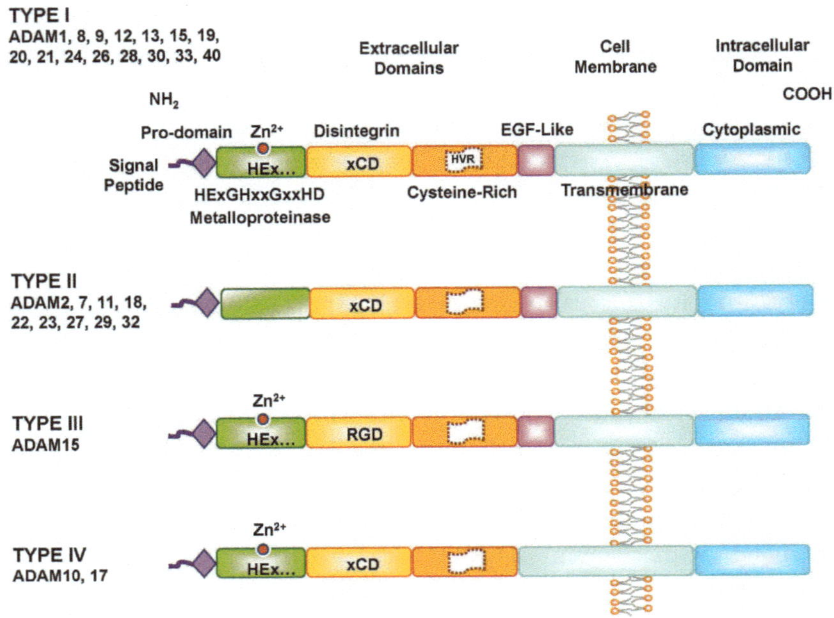

Fig. 1 ADAMs structure. Like MMPs, ADAMs have a signal peptide, pro-domain, and metalloproteinase domain. Also, like snake venom metalloproteinases (SVM), ADAMs have a disintegrin domain and cysteine-rich domain. Compared to SVM, ADAMs have a highly variable region in the cysteine-rich domain, and an additional epidermal growth factor (EGF)-like region, transmembrane domain and cytoplasmic tail. ADAMs have four types. Type I ADAMs have typical metalloprotease M-domain with the characteristic catalytic Zn^{2+} binding signature (HExGHxxGxxHD), and their disintegrin D-domain is based on xCD sequence. In Type II ADAMs the M-domain differs from that of Type I ADAMs, and lacks the catalytic-Zn^{2+} binding signature. In Type III ADAMs the M-domain contains the catalytic-Zn^{2+} binding signature, but the D-domain is based on RGD sequence rather than the xCD sequence in most ADAMs. In Type IV ADAMs the D-domain is based on xCD sequence, but they lack the EGF-like region found in Type I, II, and III.

The ADAM molecule starts with an N-terminus signal peptide which directs the enzyme to carry out its function, followed by the pro-domain which serves to correct protein folding, stabilize the protein and maintain enzyme latency via a "cysteine switch" that blocks the catalytic Zn^{2+} activation site. The cysteine switch in the pro-domain is different from the cysteine-rich domain (Bode, Gomis-Ruth, & Stockler, 1993; Van Wart & Birkedal-Hansen, 1990; Zhang, Shen, Fernandez-Patron, & Kassiri, 2016).

ADAMs have a C-shape arm that comprises a metalloproteinase (M), a disintegrin (D), and a cysteine-rich (C) domain with a Highly Variable Region (HVR) (Takeda, Igarashi, Mori, & Araki, 2006). The C-shape arm is essential for target recognition, protein interaction, and proteolytic activity.

The metalloproteinase or M-domain proteolytically interacts with various ligands, receptors and ion channels on the same cell or neighboring cell surface. The M-domain contains the catalytic Zn^{2+} binding signature (HExGHxxGxxHD), where H denotes histidine, E glutamic acid, G glycine, D aspartic acid, and x variable amino acid (aa). Through the M-domain, ADAMs serve as molecular scissors and sheddases of various ligands and receptors, and participate in cell signaling, proliferation, apoptosis, differentiation, tissue organization and organ function (Saha, Robev, Himanen, & Nikolov, 2019).

The disintegrin or D-domain follows the M-domain. The term "disintegrin" originated from its high similarity to the Arg-Gly-Asp (RGD)-containing sequence in snake venom proteins, which binds to integrins in snake bite victims, inhibits platelet aggregation and causes hemorrhage (Gould et al., 1990). Oddly, only ADAM15 still conserve the RGD sequence, while other ADAMs have a Glu-Cys-Asp (ECD) or xCD sequence, hence the more accurate term "disintegrin-like domain" (Blobel, 1997). ADAMs present their disintegrin domain on the cell surface where they interact with integrins (Blobel & White, 1992).

The cysteine-rich or C-domain has cell adhesive and fusogenic properties. Along with the cell surface protein syndecan, the C-domain of ADAM12 regulates inflammatory cell adhesion and tissue distribution in an integrin-dependent manner (Iba et al., 2000). The C-domain of ADAM13 is also involved in cell adhesion as it binds to the basement membrane proteins laminin and fibronectin (Smith et al., 2002). ADAM10 and 17 have less sequence similarities in the C-domain with other canonical ADAMs, allowing them to have a distinct but related role in specific pathological conditions and in CVD (Takeda et al., 2006). The highly variable region (HVR) of the C-domain also acts as a protein-protein adhesive interface (Takeda et al., 2006).

The epidermal growth factor (EGF)-like region, transmembrane domain and cytoplasmic tail connect the extracellular and intracellular components of ADAMs together, help to fix the C-shape arm to the cell membrane, and transmit the extracellular signal into the cell in order to regulate mRNA expression and protein phosphorylation (Stone et al., 1999).

Currently, 37 ADAMs have been identified in rats, 34 in mice, and 22 in the human genome, of which 13 proteins are proteolytically active (Edwards, Handsley, & Pennington, 2008; Zhang et al., 2016). ADAMs share common domains, but have some differences shown in four types (Fig. 1). Type I is the most common with the classic domain structure, and it includes ADAM1, 8, 9, 12, 13, 15, 19, 20, 21, 24, 26, 28, 30, 33, 40. In type I, the M-domain has the characteristic catalytic Zn^{2+} binding signature (HExGHxxGxxHD), the D-domain is based on xCD sequence, and the EGF-like region is present. Type II includes ADAM2, 7, 11, 18, 22, 23, 27, 29, 32, where the M-domain does not have the catalytic-Zn^{2+} binding signature, and is more variable. Type III is unique for ADAM15, where the M-domain contains the catalytic-Zn^{2+} binding signature, but the D-domain uniquely contains RGD sequence. Type IV is unique for ADAM10 and 17, where the D-domain is based on xCD sequence, but they lack the EGF-like region. The high similarity in the structure of ADAM10 and 17 may explain the similarities in some of their functions.

ADAMTS are multidomain extracellular proteases. Like ADAMs, ADAMTS have the common signal peptide, pro-domain, metalloproteinase M-domain, disintegrin D-domain and cysteine-rich C-domain. The main difference is that ADAMTS lack the EGF-like region, transmembrane domain and cytoplasmic tail, but have thrombospondin repeats (TSR) and spacer (Fig. 2). This makes secreted ADAMTS more soluble in the circulation, and enables them to function in remote tissues.

The ADAMTS ancillary TSR are critical for interaction with ECM, substrate recognition, and regulation of the enzyme activity. ADAMTS have a 50 aa TSR highly similar to thrombospondins 1, 2 (Adams & Lawler, 2011), followed by a cysteine-rich domain of more than 100 aa, and a cysteine-free spacer of 103–160 aa. The spacer is followed by 0–14 TSR modules, which in some ADAMTS are connected to GON-1 domain (present in the ADAMTS GON-1 identified in *C. elegans*), CUB (complement C1r/C1s, Uegf, Bmp1) domain, or PLAC (protease and lacunin) domain (Fig. 2).

There are 19 ADAMTS genes in mammalian genomes designated 1–20, except ADAMTS11 which was assigned a gene previously identified for ADAMTS5. Therefore, there are 19 ADAMTS proteins in humans, divided into six types. Type I has the basic structure and includes several members of ADAMTS family. Type II ADAMTS has a unique GON-1 domain, type III has a procollagen N-propeptidase, Type IV has CUB domains, type V has a PLAC domain and mucin/proteoglycan domain, and type VI has only a PLAC domain.

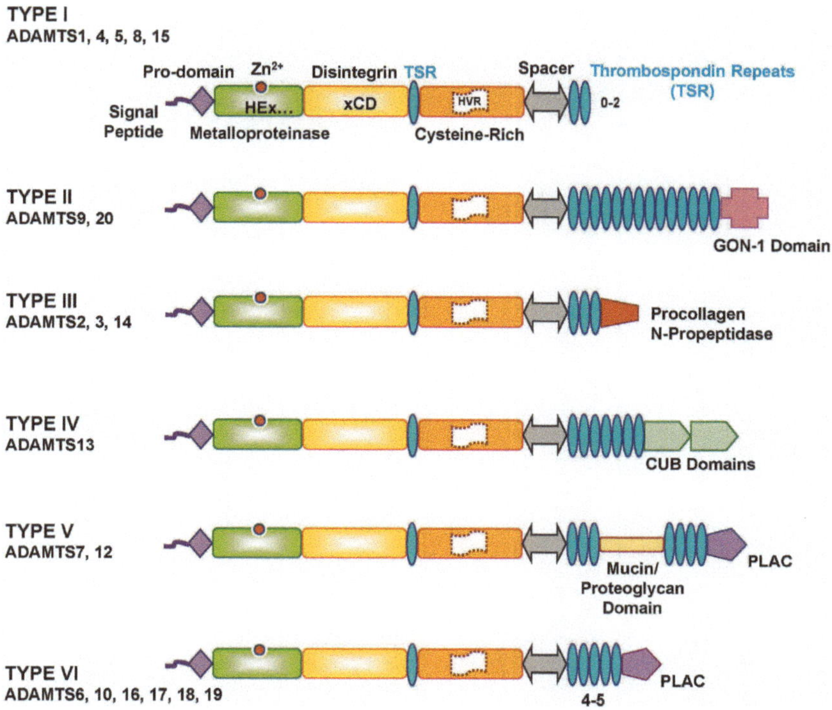

Fig. 2 Structure of different types of ADAMTS. ADAMTS have similar structure to ADAMs, but they lack the EGF-like region, transmembrane domain and cytoplasmic tail, and instead have thrombospondin repeats (TSR) and spacer. ADAMTS members have six types. Type I includes several members of ADAMTS and the protein structure comprises the basic pro-domain, metalloproteinase, disintegrin, cysteine-rich domain, thrombospondin repeats (TSR) and spacer. Type II ADAMTS has a unique GON-1 domain, type III has a procollagen N propeptidase, Type IV has a complement C1r/C1s, Uegf, Bmp1 (CUB) domain, Type V has a protease and lacunin (PLAC) region and mucin/proteoglycan domain, and Type VI has only PLAC region. The number of TSR varies among different ADAMTS types and within type I and type VI ADAMTS.

3. Sources and tissue distribution of ADAM and ADAMTS family

ADAMs are produced by different cells and have wide tissue distribution (Table 1). Many ADAMs, including ADAM1, 2, 3, 4, 5, 6, 7, 20, 21, 24 (testase 1), 25, 26, 27, 28, 29, 30, 32 and 34 are involved in reproduction processes such as spermatogenesis in the testis, sperm maturation and gain of fertilizing ability in the epididymis, and sperm migration from the uterus to

Table 1 Human ADAM family members, gene locus, molecular weight (MW) of full-length protein, source/tissue distribution, targets/substrates, and implications in biology or disease.

ADAM Other name	Gene Locus	MW kDa	Source/tissue distribution	Target/substrate	Implications in biology or disease	Reference
1 **(a & b)** Fertilin α, PH-30α	12q24.12	84	Sperm head surface, testis, epididymis, vas deferens	Integrins, ADAM3	Spermatogenesis, sperm maturation, sperm-egg interaction	Cho (2012)
2 Fertilin β, PH-30β, Cancer/testis antigen 15	8p11.22	82	Sperm head, surface, testis, epididymis, vas deferens	Integrin α6β1, epididymal protein DE (CRISP-1), intracellular chaperone calnexin, oocyte CD9, ADAM3	Sperm maturation & migration in female reproductive tract, sperm-egg interaction	Cho (2012)
3 Cyritestin, sperm surface antigen tMDC I, CYRN	8p11.22	80	Sperm surface, testis, epididymis	Integrins, testis-expressed gene 101, epididymal protein DE (CRISP-1), chaperones calnexin & calreticulin	Sperm maturation, sperm migration, sperm-egg interaction	Cho (2012)
6 Testis-derived tMDC IV	14q32.33	60	Testis	Integrins	Sperm maturation, sperm-egg interaction	Cho (2012)
7 EAPI, Sperm maturation-related glycoprotein GP-83	8p21.2	86	Sperm plasma membrane, testis, epididymis	Integrin α4β1 & α9β1, intracellular chaperone calnexin, heat shock protein 5, integral membrane protein 2B	Sperm maturation, sperm-egg interaction, melanoma progression	Cho (2012)

8 Cell surface antigen MS2, CD156a	10q26.3	90	Lung epithelium, ECs, SMCs, immune B cells, eosinophils, neutrophils, monocytes, macrophages, dendritic cells, invasive HLA-G-trophoblasts, intervertebral discs, joints, osteoclasts, neurons	Integrin β1, neural cell adhesion molecule close homologue of L1 (CHL-1), L-selectin, P-selectin glycoprotein ligand (PSGL-1), low-affinity IgE receptor CD23, low-affinity receptor FcεRII, CD-30-ligand, amyloid precursor protein (APP), fibronectin, myelin basic protein (MBP), brevican, vitronectin, VCAM-1, ADAM17	Angiogenesis, cell adhesion, neutrophil rolling, trans-endothelial extravasation, atherosclerosis, CAD, MI, ascending aortic dissection, ovulation, placental development, trophoblast migration, allergy, asthma, chronic obstructive pulmonary disease neurodegeneration, neuroinflammation, neoplastic meningitis, osteoclast differentiation, rheumatoid arthritis, breast, gastric, pancreatic, colorectal & brain cancer	Hsia et al. (2019), Kelly et al. (2005), Klein and Bischoff (2011), Le et al. (2018), Levula et al. (2011), Polverino et al. (2018), Schick et al. (2019), Vuohelainen et al. (2011)
9 MDC9, Meltrin-γ, γ Myeloma cell metalloprotease	8p11.22	91	Lung epithelium, muscle, brain, neutrophils, monocytes, macrophages	Pro-heparin-binding EGF-like growth factor (Pro-HB-EGF), EGF, FGFR2IIIb, VEGF, integrin αvβ3, α6β1 & α9β1, APP, fibronectin, tenascin, vitronectin, gelatin, collagen XVII, ACE, laminin, delta-like ligand 1, insulin-B chain, insulin-like growth factor binding protein-5, IL-11R	α-Secretase, angiogenesis, retinal neovascularization, endocardial cushion development, myogenesis, formation of myotubes, wound healing, bone formation, fertilization, cell proliferation & /migration, cell-cell interactions, AAA, lung inflammation, chronic obstructive pulmonary disease, chondrocyte differentiation and proliferation, osteoarthritis, gastric pancreatic, colorectal and ovarian cancer. Decreased in anterior polar cataract	Hodgkinson, Wang, Duncan, Edwards, and Wormstone (2010), Horiuchi, Zhou, Kelly, Manova, and Blobel (2005), Roychaudhuri et al. (2014), Shen et al. (2020)

Continued

Table 1 Human ADAM family members, gene locus, molecular weight (MW) of full-length protein, source/tissue distribution, targets/substrates, and implications in biology or disease.—cont'd

ADAM Other name	Gene Locus	MW kDa	Source/tissue distribution	Target/substrate	Implications in biology or disease	Reference
10 Kuzbanian protein homologue, CD156c, MDAM	15q21.3	84	Embryonic fibroblast, ECs, SMCs, cardiomyocytes, blood eosinophils, monocytes, macrophages, lung epithelium	Pro-HB-EGF, pro-TNFα, Notch, APP, cellular prion precursor, gelatin, DDR-1, β-cellulin, CD23, CD30, CD44, collagen IV & XVII, fractalkine, delta-like ligand 1, desmoglein, E-cadherin, N-cadherin, VE-cadherin, EGF, ephrin-A2 & A5, ErbB2 ligands, Fas-L, IL-6R, IL-11R, IL-23R, Klotho, LAG-3, MICA, Pcdh-γ, fibronectin, cystatin C, type I & II single membrane-spanning proteins, RAGE, JAM-A, ICAM-1	α-Secretase, Notch signaling, SMC proliferation, leukocyte migration, vascular cell apoptosis, wound healing, AAA, unstable atherosclerotic plaques, dilated cardiomyopathy, atrial fibrillation. Acute lung inflammation, asthma, nervous system development, Alzheimer's disease, chondrocyte proliferation & differentiation, osteoarthritis, colorectal cancer. Deficiency causes embryonic lethality	Duru, Fu, and Davies (2014), Hartmann et al. (2002), Hodgkinson et al. (2010), Hsia et al. (2019), Mehta et al. (2018), Pelisek et al. (2012), Raucci et al. (2008), Schulz et al. (2008), Shen et al. (2020), Speck et al. (2015), Zhang et al. (2010)
11 MDC11	17q21.31	83	Brain Hippocampus, cerebellum, brown fat	Integrin α4. Non-proteolytic	Neural development, myelination, synaptic transmission, epilepsy, breast cancer suppression. ADAM11$^{-/-}$ mice show learning deficiencies	Hsia et al. (2019), Takahashi et al. (2006), Wang, Hoggard, et al. (2018)

12 Meltrin-α, MLTN, MLTNA	10q26.2	100	SMCs, blood monocytes, macrophages, placenta	Insulin growth factor binding protein-3 (IGFBP-3), IGFBP-5, pro-HB-EGF, integrin α9β1, EGF, betacellulin, Delta-like1, gelatin, collagen IV, placental leucine aminopeptidase (P-LAP)	SMC proliferation, unstable atherosclerotic plaques, hypertrophic cardiomyopathy, bronchial asthma, breast, bladder & colorectal cancer, chondrocyte differentiation and proliferation, osteoarthritis, Down syndrome	Asakura et al. (2002), Duru et al. (2014), Kurisaki et al. (2003), Nyren-Erickson, Jones, Srivastava, and Mallik (2013), Pelisek et al. (2012), Smiljanic et al. (2011)
15 Metargidin, MDC15, AD56, CR II-7	1q21.3	93	Testis, ECs, SMCs, cardiomyocytes, blood monocytes, macrophages	Acrogranin, collagen IV, gelatin, amphiregulin, CD23, E-cadherin, HB-EGF, integrins α9β1 & αvβ3, Src family protein-tyrosine kinases, CD23, ADAM10	Sperm-egg interaction, cell-cell adhesion, angiogenesis, retinal neovascularization, vascular cell apoptosis, neointima formation, wound healing, atrial fibrillation, dilated cardiomyopathy, atherosclerosis, ascending aortic dissection, inflammation, rheumatoid arthritis, meningioma	Charrier-Hisamuddin, Laboisse, and Merlin (2008), Chung et al. (2016), Hodgkinson et al. (2010), Horiuchi et al. (2003), Hou et al. (2015), Levula et al. (2011)
17 TACE, CD156b, Snake venom-like protease, cSVP	2p25.1	93	Embryonic fibroblasts, SMCs, cardiomyocytes, blood monocytes, macrophages, lung epithelium	ECM, collagen, pro-TNFα, pro-TGF-α, pro-HB-EGF, EGFR ligand pro-amphiregulin, ACE2, TRANCE, pro-neuregulin-a-2C, Notch,	α-Secretase, TNFα processing, angiogenesis, EC and epithelial permeability, trans-endothelial leukocyte migration, SMC proliferation, vascular cell apoptosis. Wound healing,	Bertram et al. (2015), Caolo et al. (2015), Fan et al. (2016), Hodgkinson et al. (2010), Hsia et al. (2019), Jackson et al.

Continued

Table 1 Human ADAM family members, gene locus, molecular weight (MW) of full-length protein, source/tissue distribution, targets/substrates, and implications in biology or disease.—cont'd

ADAM Other name	Gene Locus	MW kDa	Source/tissue distribution	Target/substrate	Implications in biology or disease	Reference
				Fas ligand, fractalkine, L-selectin, collagen XVII, TNFR I & II, IL-1R II, IL-6R, IL-11R, IL-23R, Erb-B4/HER4, macrophage colony-stimulating factor receptor I, nerve growth factor receptor (TrkA), growth hormone receptor MUC1, APP, cellular prion precursor, fibronectin, cystatin C, β1 integrin, N-cadherin, VE-cadherin, JAM-A, ICAM-1, VCAM-1, syndecan-1, α-Klotho	Kawasaki disease, lung inflammation, neurite outgrowth and myelination, neuroinflammation, neoplastic meningitis, gastric and colorectal cancer. Knockout mice die perinatally with thickened and mis-shaped semilunar and atrioventricular valves, ventricular septal defect. Cardiomyocyte-specific knockout show reduced angiogenesis, post-MI left ventricle dilation & dysfunction	(2003), Jin et al. (2013), Mukerjee et al. (2019), Peng et al. (2016), Perna et al. (2017), Rizza et al. (2015), Sahin et al. (2004), Shen, Morton, Davidge, and Kassiri (2017), Speck et al. (2015), Wang, Li, et al. (2018)
18 tMDC III, ADAM27	8p11.22	83	Testis, sperm surface protein	Conotruncus (superior end of bulbus cordis of heart)	Endocardial cushion and heart development	Cho (2012)

19 Adamalysin19, Meltrin-β, MADDAM, Metalloprotease and disintegrin dendritic antigen marker, FKSG34	5q33.3	105	Heart, SMCs, lung epithelium, kidney, eosinophils, brain, peripheral nervous system, skeletal muscle, bone, testis	Pro-HB-EGF, ErbB ligands, NGR-β1 & β4, neuregulin, TNFα. Constitutive α-secretase activity that promotes processing of APP and could protect against Alzheimer's disease	Cell adhesion, cell-cell & cell-matrix interactions, embryo implantation, cardiovascular morphogenesis and neurogenesis, endocardial cushion development, endocardial epithelial-to-mesenchymal transformation, formation of cardiac septa and valves, dendritic cell differentiation. Brain astrocytoma and glioblastoma, lung, colon and ovarian cancer, lung and kidney inflammation. ADAM19$^{-/-}$ mice show ventricular septum defect, immature valves, neuronal defects, and die soon after birth	Kurisaki, Masuda, Osumi, Nabeshima, and Fujisawa-Sehara (1998), Kurohara et al. (2004), Qi, Newcomer, and Sang (2009), Yagami-Hiromasa et al. (1995), Zhou et al. (2004)
20	14q24.2	82	Testis, monocytes	Integrins	Embryo development	Blobel (1997)
21 ADAM31	14q24.2	81	Testis, blood monocytes, glia	Integrins	Sperm maturation, neurogenesis	Blobel (1997), Blobel and White (1992)
22 MDC2	7q21.12	100	Reproductive system, brain	Brain integrins. Non-proteolytic	Neural development, myelination, synaptic transmission, epilepsy, neointima formation	Blobel (1997), Hsia et al. (2019), Zhang, Jiang, et al. (2019)

Continued

Table 1 Human ADAM family members, gene locus, molecular weight (MW) of full-length protein, source/tissue distribution, targets/substrates, and implications in biology or disease.—cont'd

ADAM Other name	Gene Locus	MW kDa	Source/tissue distribution	Target/substrate	Implications in biology or disease	Reference
28 e-MDC II, MDC-L	8p21.2	87	Epididymis, brain, lymphocytes	Integrins $\alpha4\beta1$, $\alpha4\beta7$ & $\alpha9\beta1$, CD23	Sperm maturation, cancer	Blobel (1997)
29 Cancer/testis antigen 73, svph 1	4q34.1	93	Testis	Integrin $\alpha4$	Sperm maturation, melanoma progression	Blobel (1997), Smith et al. (2002), Wang, Hoggard, et al. (2018)
30 svph 4	1p12	89	Sperm, testis	APP metabolism	Embryo development. Loss linked to amyloid-β deposition & Alzheimer	Cho (2012), Letronne et al. (2016)
32	8p11.22	88	Sperm surface, testis, epididymis	Hyaluronic acid	Sperm development, egg fertilization	Cho (2012), Torabi, Bogle, Estanyol, Oliva, and Miller (2017)
33	20p13	88	Testis, epididymis lung epithelium	Integrin $\alpha9\beta1$	Embryo development, SMC proliferation, bronchial asthma	Cho (2012), Kim et al. (2017)

the oviducts where it fuses with the oocyte (Cho, 2012). ADAM8, 9, 10, 12, 15, 17 and 19 are involved in cardiovascular development, and the abnormal expression or function of these ADAMs may lead to CVD.

ADAMTS members are widely distributed in different tissues (Table 2), and play a role in multiple physiological and pathological processes including CVD.

4. ADAMs and ADAMTS activation

ADAMs can be activated by cytokines, proteinases, G-protein coupled receptor (GPCR) agonists, Ca^{2+} ionophores and protein kinase C activators. Compared to MMPs, whose activation occurs in ECM (Takawale, Sakamuri, & Kassiri, 2015), ADAMs activation occurs intracellularly where their pro-domain is removed by pro-protein convertases in the Golgi system during the transit process. The pro-protein convertase cleaves the Arg-Xaa-(Arg/Lys)-Arg or Rx(R/K)R motif of the pro-domain, allowing Zn^{2+} coordination to the metalloprotease domain so that ADAM can be catalytically activated and perform its sheddase activity and biological function (Anders, Gilbert, Garten, Postina, & Fahrenholz, 2001).

Several factors regulate ADAMs' processing. ADAM8 processing by autocatalysis produces a sheddase form that can contribute to cell adhesion (Schlomann et al., 2002). N-glycosylation is also important for processing, localization, stability, and activity of ADAM8 (Srinivasan, Romagnoli, Bohm, & Sonenshein, 2014). Tumor necrosis factor-α (TNFα) upregulates ADAM9 expression at the transcriptional level (Schouten et al., 2016). Meprin-β is a membrane-bound metalloprotease that processes ADAM9, 10 and 17, and plays a role in ECM assembly and inflammation (Wichert et al., 2019). Transforming growth factor-β (TGF-β) stimulates renal cells and causes upregulation of Adam10, 12, 17 and 19 (Ramdas, McBride, Denby, & Baker, 2013).

ADAM10 is a ubiquitous transmembrane metalloprotease that cleaves the ectodomain of transmembrane proteins such as Notch and amyloid precursor protein (APP). ADAM10 is compartmentalized into membrane microdomains by tetraspanins (Tspan), a family of 33 four-transmembrane proteins that regulate clustering and intracellular trafficking of other "partner" proteins. ADAM10 co-immunoprecipitates and interacts with the TspanC8 subgroup including Tspan5, 10, 14, 15, 17 and 33/Penumbra, all six are required for ADAM10 trafficking from the endoplasmic reticulum and its enzymatic maturation. ADAM10 could function as six different molecular scissors with

Table 2 Human ADAMTS family members, gene locus, molecular weight (MW) of full-length protein, tissue distribution, targets/substrates, and implications in biology or disease.

ADAMTS	Gene locus	MW (kDa)	Tissue distribution	Target/substrate	Implications in biology or disease	Reference
1 METH1	21q21.3	105	Heart, aorta, smooth muscle, bronchial epithelial cells, fetal lung, liver, colon, kidney, adrenal gland, bladder, prostate, ovary, uterus, placenta, spinal cord, ciliary ganglion, olfactory bulb, adipocytes, breast stromal fibroblasts, myoepithelial cells	Aggrecan, versican, syndecan 4, dystroglycan, mac-2, gelatin (denatured collagen type I), amphiregulin, TGF-α, HB-EGF, VEGF, TFPI-2, semaphorin 3C, nidogen-1 & −2, desmocollin-3	Embryogenesis. organ development, VSMC proliferation, inflammation, anti-angiogenic, cancer cachexia, gastric cancer & lymph node metastasis, lung cancer	Chen, Zhi, Chang, Zhang, and Dai (2013), Gunther, Skaftnesmo, Arnold, Bjerkvig, and Terzis (2005), Kelwick, Desanlis, Wheeler, and Edwards (2015), Kilic, Aynekin, Kara, Icen, and Demircan (2017), Kuno et al. (1997), Qu and Zhang (2018), Tang, Zhang, Zhang, and Zhang (2017), Toba et al. (2016), Vazquez et al. (1999)
2	5q35.3	135	Aorta, smooth muscle, heart, lung, liver, kidney, bladder, skeletal muscle, tendon, bone, skin, retina, superior cervical ganglion, breast stromal fibroblasts adipocytes, uterus, placenta	Fibrillar procollagen type I, II, III & V, N-propeptide	Anti-angiogenic, cartilage matrix anabolism, procollagen N-proteinase, osteoarthritis, Ehlers-Danlos syndrome type VIIc	Bekhouche and Colige (2015), Colige et al. (1997), Dubail et al. (2010), Kelwick, Desanlis, et al. (2015)

3	4q13.3	136	CD105 + ECs, CD34 + cells, heart, lung, pineal gland, cartilage, bone, skeletal muscle, tendon, breast myoepithelial cells, testis, ovary, placenta, brain	Fibrillar procollagen type II N-propeptide, biglycan, pro-VEGF-C, reelin	Procollagen N-proteinase, angiogenesis, lymphangiogenesis, placental & brain functions, cartilage matrix anabolism, osteoarthritis	Bekhouche and Colige (2015), Fernandes et al. (2001), Janssen et al. (2016), Jeltsch et al. (2014), Jha et al. (2017), Kelwick, Desanlis, et al. (2015), Ogino et al. (2017)
4 Aggrecanase-1, ADMP-1	1q23.3	90	Ovary, adrenal cortex, ciliary ganglion, trigeminal ganglion, brain, spinal cord, retina, heart, fetal lung, appendix, gall bladder, pancreas islets, skeletal muscle, uterus, breast myoepithelial cells, synovial fluid	Aggrecan, versican, neurocan, reelin, biglycan, brevican, matrilin-3, α2-macroglobulin, COMP	VSMC apoptosis, vascular inflammation, matrix degradation, sporadic aortic aneurysm and dissections, osteoarthritis	Boerboom et al. (2011), Dubail and Apte (2015), Kelwick, Desanlis, et al. (2015), Ren et al. (2017)
5 ADAMTS11, Aggrecanase-2, ADMP-2	21q21.3	102	Ovary, uterus, placenta, breast myoepithelial cells, bladder, adipocytes	Aggrecan, versican, reelin, biglycan, matrilin-4, brevican, α2-macroglobulin	Osteoarthritis, cancer (anti-tumorigenic, anti-angiogenic)	Abbaszade et al. (1999), Dubail and Apte (2015), Hurskainen, Hirohata, Seldin, and Apte (1999), Kelwick, Desanlis, et al. (2015)

Continued

Table 2 Human ADAMTS family members, gene locus, molecular weight (MW) of full-length protein, tissue distribution, targets/substrates, and implications in biology or disease.—cont'd

ADAMTS	Gene locus	MW (kDa)	Tissue distribution	Target/substrate	Implications in biology or disease	Reference
6	5q12.3	125	Heart, appendix, gall bladder, superior cervical ganglion, trigeminal ganglion, breast myoepithelial cells, placenta	Fibrillin-1, LTBP1, syndecan 4	Altered ventricular conduction, prolonged QRS interval	Hurskainen et al. (1999), Karoulias, Taye, Stanley, and Hubmacher (2020), Kelwick, Desanlis, et al. (2015), Prins et al. (2018)
7	15q25.1	182	Heart, smooth muscle, liver, pancreas, kidney, adrenal cortex, skeletal muscle, intervertebral disc, trigeminal ganglion, uterus, breast stromal fibroblasts	COMP, TSP-1	Atherosclerosis, CAD, VSMC migration, neointima formation, cartilage catabolism, osteoarthritis	Hanby and Zheng (2013), Hurskainen et al. (1999), Kelwick, Desanlis, et al. (2015), Wang et al. (2009)
8 METH2	11q24.3	96	Skeletal muscle, heart, lung, appendix, liver, adrenal cortex, breast stromal fibroblasts and luminal epithelial cells, placenta, brain, superior cervical ganglion	Aggrecan	Anti-angiogenic	Georgiadis, Hirohata, Seldin, and Apte (1999), Kelwick, Desanlis, et al. (2015), Vazquez et al. (1999)

9	3p14.1	217	Capillary ECs, heart, lung, kidney, pancreas, colon, ovary, skeletal muscle, dorsal root ganglion, breast myoepithelial cells, uterus, placenta	Aggrecan, versican	Cancer	Desanlis, Felstead, Edwards, and Wheeler (2018), Kelwick, Desanlis, et al. (2015), Koo et al. (2010), Somerville et al. (2003)
10	19p13.2	121	Heart, lung, liver, pancreas, kidney, brain, adipose tissue, CD8+ T-cells, breast stromal fibroblasts, uterus, placenta	Fibrillin-1	Weill-Marchesani syndrome (short stature, acromelic dysplasia, disproportionate distal limb shortening)	Hubmacher and Apte (2015), Kelwick, Desanlis, et al. (2015), Kutz et al. (2011), Le Goff and Cormier-Daire (2009), Mead and Apte (2018), Somerville, Jungers, and Apte (2004)
12	5p13.3	178	Atrioventricular node, smooth muscle, liver, gall bladder, bone marrow, adipose tissue, intervertebral disc, breast stromal fibroblasts and myoepithelial cells	COMP	Anti-angiogenic. Cell adhesion, cancer, osteoarthritis	Bai, Wang, Luan, Yu, and Liu (2009), El Hour et al. (2010), Kelwick, Desanlis, et al. (2015)

Continued

Table 2 Human ADAMTS family members, gene locus, molecular weight (MW) of full-length protein, tissue distribution, targets/substrates, and implications in biology or disease.—cont'd

ADAMTS	Gene locus	MW (kDa)	Tissue distribution	Target/substrate	Implications in biology or disease	Reference
13	9q34.2	154	ECs, heart, lung, liver, hepatic stellate cells, pancreas, kidney podocytes, brain, testis, breast myoepithelial cells, placenta, CD71 + early erythroid cells, thyroid	von Willebrand factor (vWF)	Deficiency leads to thrombotic thrombocytopenic purpura (TTP)	Cal et al. (2002), Kelwick, Desanlis, et al. (2015), Lopez and Dong (2004), Mead and Apte (2018), Moake (2004), Zheng et al. (2001), Zheng (2015)
14	10q22.1	134	Fibroblasts, lung, liver, gall bladder, prostate, retina, cerebellum, thalamus, fetal thyroid, adipocytes, bone marrow, skin, breast myoepithelial and luminal epithelial cells, placenta	Fibrillar procollagen type I N-propeptide (pNα1 and pNα2 chains)	Procollagen N-proteinase, cartilage matrix anabolism, osteoarthritis, multiple sclerosis	Bekhouche and Colige (2015), Cal et al. (2002), Goertsches, Comabella, Navarro, Perkal, and Montalban (2005), Kelwick, Desanlis, et al. (2015), Poonpet, Honsawek, Tammachote, Kanitnate, and Tammachote (2013), Rodriguez-Lopez et al. (2009)

15	11q24.3	103	Heart, colon, brain, musculoskeletal system, adipose tissue, breast myoepithelial cells, uterus, placenta	Aggrecan, versican	Anti-angiogenic, anti-tumorigenic	Dancevic et al. (2013), Kelwick, Desanlis, et al. (2015)
16	5p15.32	136	Aorta, gall bladder, brain, ovary, breast myoepithelial cells	ECM proteins, latency-associated peptide (LAP)-TGF-β complex	Hypertension, cardiac fibrosis and hypertrophy, heart failure. Loss linked to congenital undescended testes	Cal et al. (2002), Kelwick, Desanlis, et al. (2015), Sarila et al. (2020), Yao et al. (2020)
17	15q26.3	121	Ovary, breast myoepithelial cells	Fibrillin-1 & -2, fibronectin	Weill-Marchesani-like syndrome	Cal et al. (2002), Hubmacher and Apte (2015), Karoulias et al. (2020), Kelwick, Desanlis, et al. (2015), Mead and Apte (2018)
18	16q23.1	135	Endothelium, heart, brain, ciliary ganglion, skin, prostate, breast myoepithelial cells, uterus, placenta	Basal membrane-specific proteoglycan Col18a1, fibronectin	Microcornea, myopic chorioretinal atrophy and telecanthus	Ataca et al. (2020), Cal et al. (2002), Dubail and Apte (2015), Kelwick, Desanlis, et al. (2015), Mead and Apte (2018), Zhu et al. (2018)

Continued

Table 2 Human ADAMTS family members, gene locus, molecular weight (MW) of full-length protein, tissue distribution, targets/substrates, and implications in biology or disease.—cont'd

ADAMTS	Gene locus	MW (kDa)	Tissue distribution	Target/substrate	Implications in biology or disease	Reference
19	5q23.3	134	Dorsal root ganglion, breast myoepithelial cells, uterus, placenta	ECM Proteins	Loss causes non-syndromic heart valve disease	Karoulias et al. (2020), Kelwick, Desanlis, et al. (2015), Wunnemann et al. (2020)
20	12q12	215	Heart, lung, appendix, liver, pancreas, brain, skeletal muscle, pituitary, trigeminal ganglion, prostate, testis, breast myoepithelial cells, ovary, placenta	Versican	Colorectal, brain and breast cancer. Cleft lip and palate	Kelwick, Desanlis, et al. (2015), Llamazares, Cal, Quesada, and Lopez-Otin (2003), Somerville et al. (2003), Wolf et al. (2015)

different substrate specificities, depending on which of the six TspanC8s it is associated with. For example, human umbilical vein endothelial cells (HUVECs) express Tspan14, the knockdown of which reduces ADAM10 surface expression and activity (Haining et al., 2012). ADAM10 is also implicated in leukocyte transmigration by cleaving vascular endothelial cadherin (VE-cadherin), which regulates endothelial barrier function. ADAM10 knockdown on HUVECs impairs transmigration of peripheral blood T lymphocytes. The formation of endothelial Tspan5- and Tspan17-ADAM10 complexes may regulate inflammation by maintaining VE-cadherin expression and promoting T lymphocyte transmigration (Reyat et al., 2017). Mouse erythrocytes express mainly Tspan33, and ADAM10 expression is reduced in the absence of Tspan33. In contrast, ADAM10 expression is normal on Tspan33-deficient mouse platelets in which Tspan14 is the major TspanC8. In platelets, ADAM10-induced cleavage of the platelet collagen receptor GPVI is regulated by Tspan14, 15, and 33, leading to inhibition of GPVI receptor function and anti-thrombotic effects. Thus, TspanC8s regulate ADAM10 maturation and trafficking to the cell surface, and specific TspanC8-ADAM10 complexes provide cell- or substrate-specific ADAM10 targeting (Haining et al., 2012).

In cultured VSMCs, angiotensin II (AngII) increases ADAM17 mRNA expression, protein levels, and promoter activity. Also, AngII infusion in mice for 2 weeks increases ADAM17 in the aorta, heart and kidney vessels through hypoxia inducible factor 1α (HIF1α)-dependent transcriptional upregulation, leading to vascular malfunction and end-organ damage (Obama et al., 2015). MicroRNAs (miRs) are small single-stranded noncoding molecules that regulate gene expression, directly target mRNA at posttranscriptional level, and play a role in different pathological conditions. miR-634 is upregulated in blood of patients with anti-neutrophil cytoplasmic antibody-associated vasculitis, and miR-634 mimics induce a proinflammatory phenotype in monocyte-derived macrophages with enhanced expression/release of ADAM17 and interleukin 6 (IL-6) (Bertram et al., 2015).

Rhomboids are a conserved protein superfamily that binds membrane proteins and directs them to different cellular pathways. The iRhom1 and 2 have seven transmembrane domains and regulate ADAM17 enzymatic maturation and trafficking to cell surface and distinct substrates. In platelets, iRhom2 directs ADAM17 to promote the shedding of the von Willebrand factor (vWF) platelet receptor glycoprotein Ib (GPIb), leading to inhibition of vWF receptor function. Targeting platelet iRhom2 could activate ADAM17 and provide anti-thrombotic therapy without the side effects of activating ADAM17 in other cells (Matthews, Noy, Reyat, & Tomlinson, 2017).

ADAM17 regulates EGF receptor (EGFR) signaling by shedding and liberating EGFR ligands from their membrane anchor. ADAM17 deficiency reduces EGFR signaling, leading to skin and intestinal barrier defects. Like Egfr$^{-/-}$ mice, Adam17$^{-/-}$ mice die perinatally with open eyes. ADAM17-dependent EGFR ligand shedding requires its transmembrane domain but not its cytoplasmic tail, suggesting that ADAM17 is regulated by other integral membrane proteins. While iRhom2 controls the maturation and function of ADAM17 in myeloid cells, iRhom2$^{-/-}$ mice appear normal. On the other hand, iRhom1/2$^{-/-}$ double knockout (KO) mice resemble Adam17$^{-/-}$ and Egfr$^{-/-}$ mice in that they die perinatally with open eyes, misshapen heart valves, and growth plate defects. The iRhom1/2$^{-/-}$ tissues lack mature ADAM17 and show reduced EGFR phosphorylation. iRhom1 regulates ADAM17 maturation in the brain, except in microglia, where ADAM17 is controlled by iRhom2. Thus, during mouse development, iRhoms1/2 regulate ADAM17-dependent EGFR signaling, and targeting iRhoms1/2 may be useful in ADAM17/EGFR-related pathologies (Li et al., 2015).

ADAMs may differ in their activation process and its location. ADAM8 and 28 are activated in ECM. ADAM12 is stored as already active proteins, and transferred to the cell membrane when the cell is stimulated by cytokines (Sundberg et al., 2004), suggesting that removal of the pro-domain and proteolytic processing is not necessary for ADAM12 activation (Cao, Kang, Zhao, & Zolkiewska, 2002). Other ADAMs auto-catalytically remove their pro-domain for their transformation from inactive pro-protein to active enzyme (Schlomann et al., 2002).

The intracellular cytoplasmic tail and protein phosphorylation may contribute to ADAMs signal transmit and interaction with other proteins and receptors, but their role in ADAMs activation is unclear. For example, ADAM17 with truncated cytoplasmic tail can still function as a sheddase of TNFα, p75 TNFR and IL-1R-II. On the other hand, the ADAM17 transmembrane domain is essential for the shedding of these substrates (Reddy et al., 2000). Also, while phosphorylated Ser819 is an important reaction site during activation of ADAM17, mutation of this site did not suppress ADAM17 activity or cleavage of its substrates transforming growth factor-α (TGFα), TNFα or TNFα receptors, suggesting that the cytoplasmic tail is not responsible for ADAM17 sheddase activity (Reddy et al., 2000). However, the cytoplasmic tail of ADAM17 is linked to GPCR mediated EGFR signaling (Edwards et al., 2008), where Src causes stimulation of phosphatidylinositol 3-kinase (PI_3K) and activation of phosphoinositide-dependent kinase-1 (PDK1), which phosphorylates ADAM17

(Zhang et al., 2006). Also, agonist-induced phosphorylation of Thr735 of ADAM17 accounts for the transfer of ADAM17 from the endoplasmic reticulum to the cell surface, and in turn enhances cleavage of the TrkA neurotrophin receptor in cardiomyocytes (Soond, Everson, Riches, & Murphy, 2005).

Similar to ADAMs. ADAMTS activation involves cleavage of the N-terminal pro-domain next to the consensus sequence Arg-Xaa-(Arg/Lys)-Arg by the proprotein convertases furin and furin-like enzymes in the trans-Golgi or at the cell surface (Colige et al., 2005; Koo & Apte, 2010; Somerville, Longpre, et al., 2004). As metalloproteases, ADAMTS activity requires a neutral to slightly basic pH, Zn^{2+} and Ca^{2+} (Colige et al., 1995). Some ADAMTS may not require pro-domain cleavage for their activation. ADAMTS13 has an unusually short propeptide, and ADAMTS9 and 13 zymogens are active despite retention of the propeptide (Koo, Longpre, Somerville, Alexander, & Apte, 2007; Majerus, Zheng, Tuley, & Sadler, 2003). ADAMTS2 undergoes autocatalytic cleavage within the C-terminal end and the procollagen N-propeptidase domain (Bekhouche & Colige, 2015; Colige et al., 2005). Autocatalytic C-terminal cleavage and activation also occur with ADAMTS1, 4, 8, 9 and 12 (Porter et al., 2005), thus impacting their bio-disponibility, substrate recognition and activity (Bekhouche & Colige, 2015).

5. ADAMs targets, substrates, functions and mouse KO phenotype

ADAMs have multiple targets/substrates (Table 1). Similar to MMPs and SVMs, ADAMs were initially presumed as active proteases that cleave ECM substrates, but members of the ADAM family could be proteolytic or non-proteolytic. Proteolytic ADAMs including ADAM8, 9, 10 and 17 are active metalloproteases or sheddases that regulate proteolytic cleavage and ectodomain shedding of cell surface adhesion molecules, cytokines, chemokines and growth factors, resulting in the release of soluble proteins that exert agonistic or antagonistic effects. ADAM-mediated shedding could also affect a specific receptor, and in turn activate signaling pathways and cellular functions, or render the membrane protein or receptor inactive (van der Vorst et al., 2018). The ADAMs' M-domain, D-domain, and cysteine-rich C-domain with HVR are important for substrate recognition, proteolytic processing and protein degradation. During cell-cell and cell-matrix interactions, HVR guides proteolytically inactive ADAMs to recognize specific substrates, then the metalloproteinase M-domain conducts ADAM function as a proteolytic enzyme or sheddase. A specific factor may combine with the substrate before it can be recognized by HVR. Also, during inter-cellular interaction, an ADAM on one cell surface can liberate a ligand and activate a receptor on an adjacent cell surface. In contrast with proteolytic ADAMs, non-proteolytic ADAM11, 22 and 23 have no catalytic activity, and function as adhesion proteins or receptors (Hsia et al., 2019).

ADAMs have been implicated in multiple cellular processes including degradation of ECM proteins, cell adhesion and fusion, intracellular signaling, cell proliferation, migration and invasion, fertilization, neurogenesis, and inflammation (Pelisek et al., 2012). There are 22 ADAMs in humans (Klein & Bischoff, 2011), and 14 ADAMs including ADAM1, 2, 3, 6, 7, 18, 20, 21, 22, 28, 29, 30, 32 and 33 are mainly expressed in the testis, epididymis and uterus, and involved in embryo development. ADAM-induced shedding of membrane-associated growth factors also modulate key cell signaling pathways in cancer microenvironment. ADAM8, 9, 10, 12, 15, and 17 have a broader expression in human tissues particularly in the cardiovascular system, and may be involved in the pathogenesis of CVD, and therefore will be discussed in greater detail.

ADAM8 is highly expressed on immune cells, neutrophils, hematopoietic cells and breast cancer, ADAM8 is usually stored in granules and transported to the cell surface when the cell is stimulated by pro-inflammatory stimuli. L-selectin is a "homing receptor" for lymphocytes, and its shedding by ADAM8 is involved in regulation of neutrophil rolling and trans-endothelial extravasation. ADAM8 is implicated in inflammation, rheumatoid arthritis and asthma. The levels of ADAM8 are increased in the peri-infarct myocardium following MI and infiltration of inflammatory cells. ADAM8 also regulates ovulation and osteoclast differentiation (Vuohelainen et al., 2011). ADAM8$^{-/-}$ mice develop normally without a disease phenotype, but show suppressed reaction to autoimmune arthritis (Kelly et al., 2005).

ADAM9 (MDC9/meltrin-γ) is a widely expressed protease implicated in ectodomain cleavage of heparin-binding EGF-like growth factor (HB-EGF) and as an α-secretase for APP. During mouse development, *ADAM9* is ubiquitously expressed mainly in the mesenchyme, heart and brain. ADAM9 regulates myogenesis, formation of myotubes and myocardium development. However, *ADAM9*$^{-/-}$ mice develop normally, are viable and fertile with no major pathological phenotype or defects in muscle formation, and still show HB-EGF shedding and APP α-secretase products formation (Weskamp et al., 2002), suggesting that ADAM9 functions can be compensated by other ADAMs. Also, constitutive and stimulated ectodomain shedding of HB-EGF is comparable in embryonic fibroblasts from ADAM$9^{-/-}$ and WT mice, arguing against a role of ADAM9 in HB-EGF shedding in these cells. Also, the production of the APP α- and γ-secretase cleavage product 3-kDa peptide and of β- and γ-secretase cleavage product amyloid-β is not different in hippocampal neurons from *ADAM9*$^{-/-}$ and WT mice, arguing against a role as an α-secretase in mice (Weskamp et al., 2002). Angiotensin-I converting enzyme (ACE) is a zinc-dependent peptidase that regulates vasoactive peptide metabolism and a transmembrane protein that undergoes shedding primarily from endothelial cells (ECs) by proteinases to release catalytically active sACE. The MMP/ADAM inhibitor BB-94, tissue inhibitor of metalloproteinases (TIMP), and ADAM9 knockdown by siRNA block lipopolysaccharide (LPS)-induced ACE shedding from ECs, confirming a role of ADAM9 in ACE shedding (English, Corvol, & Murphy, 2012).

ADAM10 is a crucial α-secretase involved in ECM degradation, ectodomain shedding of cell surface substrates, adhesion molecules, chemokines and growth factor receptors (van der Vorst et al., 2015). ADAM10 is essential for embryonic development through cleavage of Notch proteins (Matthews, Noy, et al., 2017). By inducing Notch cleavage and controlling subsequent "regulated intramembrane proteolysis," ADAM10 releases cleaved intracellular domains which transfer to the nucleus and finetune gene transcription. ADAM10 regulation of Notch signaling is an important step in the embryonic development of the cardiovascular system (Cong & Jia, 2011; Howard & Glynn, 1995). Because of the crucial role of ADAM10 in biological processes, intramembrane proteolysis, Notch/Delta-like 4 (Dll4) signaling and APP processing, ADAM10 KO mice do not survive during early embryonic development, show multiple defects in the CNS and somites, and die of severe cardiovascular defects, similar to mice deficient in Notch/Dll4 signaling (Cong & Jia, 2011; Howard & Glynn, 1995). ADAM10 also regulate the Eph/ephrin pathway and plays a role in cancer, neurodegenerative diseases, Alzheimer and prion disease, bacterial infection, inflammation, heart attacks, stroke and asthma (Matthews, Szyroka, Collier, Noy, & Tomlinson, 2017).

ADAM12 participates in myogenesis and embryonic development (Yagami-Hiromasa et al., 1995). The two splice-variants ADAM12L and ADAM12S are proteolytically active, cleave membrane-bound proteins, and affect distant targets. ADAM12L promotes cardiomyocyte hypertrophy by inducing HB-EGF shedding and Notch signaling (Asakura et al., 2002;

Jorissen et al., 2010; Karkkainen, Rybnikova, Pelto-Huikko, & Huovila, 2000). ADAM12 also contributes to ectodomain shedding of EGFR ligands and EGFR transactivation (Tanaka et al., 2004), and may reduce inflammatory skin diseases and barrier defects. ADAM12$^{-/-}$ mice usually develop without functional deficiencies, although some studies found 30% mortality in ADAM12$^{-/-}$ pups within the first week (Kurisaki et al., 2003).

ADAM15 is linked to cell adhesion, cell-cell and cell-matrix interactions, inflammation, and shedding of cell surface molecules (Oksala et al., 2009), ADAM15 colocalizes with VE-cadherin. Accumulation of ADAM15 in cell-cell contacts is preceded by VE-cadherin-mediated EC adherens junction formation, supporting that ADAM15 is a component of adherens junctions that influence EC function (Ham, Levkau, Raines, & Herren, 2002). ADAM15 also cleaves epithelial cadherin (E-cadherin), thus compromising epithelial cell connections and tissue stability, and promoting inflammatory cell infiltration in different tissues (Sun, Wu, Lee, & Yuan, 2012). ADAM15 through cleaving E-cadherin, decreases EC stability, and promotes EC permeability and neutrophil trans-endothelial migration and vascular tissue infiltration (Sun et al., 2010). ADAM15 also promotes angiogenesis by inducing the expression of vascular endothelial growth factor (VEGF), VEGF receptor VEGFR1 and VEGFR2 (Xie et al., 2008). Recombinant human disintegrin domain of ADAM15 (rhddADAM15) inhibited proliferation/migration and induced partial G2/S arrest, apoptosis and caspases activity in Bel-7402 cells, and inhibited the growth and metastasis of Bel-7402 cell xenografts in zebrafish, suggesting inhibitory effects on tumor growth and metastasis that could be useful in cancer therapy (Hou et al., 2013). ADAM15$^{-/-}$ mice show no overt pathological phenotype, but display reduced neovascularization in a mouse model of retinopathy of prematurity, and reduced size of tumors resulting from implanted mouse melanoma cells (Horiuchi et al., 2003).

ADAM17 (TNFα converting enzyme, TACE) is expressed in most tissues, and is upregulated during inflammation and cancer. ADAM17 mediates ectodomain shedding of membrane-bound adhesion molecules, cytokines and their receptors (Black et al., 1997; Moss et al., 1997; Niu, Wang, & Li, 2015). ADAM17 is considered a first line of defense against infection and injury by releasing TNFα and promoting inflammation (Matthews, Noy, et al., 2017). ADAM17 also regulates the shedding of TNFα receptors, the growth factors TGFα, HB-EGF, VEGF, VEGFR2 and neuregulins (Blobel, 2005; Obama et al., 2015; Sommer et al., 2017). Shedding of membrane-anchored pro-TGFα (Peschon et al., 1998) and pro-HB-EGF

(Higashiyama & Nanba, 2005) to activate EGFR is among the critical functions of ADAM17 (Jackson et al., 2003; Lee et al., 2003; Sahul et al., 2011). ADAM17 is also involved in egg fertilization, embryonic development, angiogenesis and neurogenesis (Canault, Certel, Schatzberg, Wagner, & Hynes, 2010; Peschon et al., 1998). Mice with TACE$^{\Delta Zn/\Delta Zn}$ null mutation die at birth and show failure of eyelid fusion, hair and skin defects, abnormal lung development, and enlarged hearts with increased myocardial trabeculation, reduced cell compaction, larger cardiomyocyte size and increased cell proliferation. The heart of TACE$^{\Delta Zn/\Delta Zn}$ KO mouse shows reduced EGFR expression, attenuated cleavage of the receptor tyrosine-protein kinase ErbB4, and altered mitogen-activated protein kinase (MAPK) activity, supporting a role of TACE-mediated cell surface protein ectodomain shedding in cardiac development and modeling (Shi et al., 2003). ADAM17 KO mice embryos also show thickened and mis-shaped heart valves, similar to the mice lacking HB-EGF (Jackson et al., 2003; Lee et al., 2003; Sahul et al., 2011; Shi et al., 2003). Because ADAM17 regulates TNFα processing and TNFα levels are elevated in CVD, TNFα antagonists have been tested and have shown benefits in animal models of CVD (Sato et al., 2006; Sun et al., 2007). However, anti-TNFα treatment did not show much improvement in patients with late-stage heart failure (Anker & Coats, 2002; Coletta, Clark, Banarjee, & Cleland, 2002). Also, in contrast with the perinatal death of ADAM17 KO mice, TNFα-deficient mice develop normally and are viable and fertile, indicating that ADAM17 has other essential functions (Canault et al., 2010). Interestingly, TNFα processing is not completely inhibited in ADAM17 KO mice, as ADAM9 and 10 (Lunn et al., 1997; Rosendahl et al., 1997), and MMP17 (English et al., 2000) also promote TNFα shedding. In effect, ADAM17 could have a dual effect whereby it promotes inflammation by releasing soluble TNFα to activate TNFα receptor (TNFR), and at the same time cleaving TNFRI (p55) and TNFRII (p57) and reducing their sensitivity to TNFα (McClurg et al., 2015; Reddy et al., 2000; Weskamp et al., 2004; Zeinieh, Salehi, Rajkumar, & Barker, 2015).

While ADAM17 KO mice are not viable, conditional ADAM17 KO using novel gene targeting strategy generate mice with reduced ADAM17 levels in all tissues. The resulting ADAM17$^{ex/ex}$ mice are viable, show reduced shedding of ADAM17 cell surface substrates, and develop eye, heart, and skin defects due to failure of release of EGFR ligands and impaired EGFR signaling. Homozygous ADAM17$^{ex/ex}$ mice have normal intestine, but show increased susceptibility to inflammation in response to dextran sulfate sodium-induced colitis, likely due to impaired shedding of EGFR ligands and failure to activate EGFR and phosphorylate STAT3, leading to defective regeneration of epithelial cells and breakdown of the intestinal barrier. Thus, ADAM17 appears to regulate both the systemic release of the proinflammatory cytokine TNFα, and the EGFR-mediated regenerative activities during the immune response (Chalaris et al., 2010). ADAM17 also confers defense against skin infection and injury and maintains epidermal barrier function by proteolytic release of EGFR ligands (Li, Maretzky, et al., 2017). The skin barrier is formed by cross-linking activity of transglutaminases, and ADAM17/EGFR-driven PLCγ1 and PKC pathways promote transglutaminase-1 expression during terminal keratinocyte differentiation. Epidermal deficiency of ADAM17 in mice impedes transglutaminases activity and results in postnatal skin barrier defects (Wolf, Qian, Brooke, Kelsell, & Franzke, 2016). Of note, EGFR participates in CVD progression, and ADAM17 may promote atherosclerosis, cardiac hypertrophy, and cardiac and renal fibrosis through the release of EGFR ligands and activation of EGFR (Oikawa et al., 2014).

ADAM17 share aa sequence, crystal structure and function with ADAM10, and they both modulate vascular permeability by cleaving junctional adhesion molecule A (JAM-A) and VE-cadherin (Speck et al., 2015). Other ADAM17 substrates include syndecan-1 (Bertram et al., 2015), soluble intercellular adhesion molecule-1 (sICAM-1), soluble vascular cell adhesion molecule-1 (sVCAM-1), soluble IL-6 receptor (sIL-6R) and sTNFR1 (Rizza et al., 2015). Individuals with the single nucleotide polymorphism (SNP) rs2228145 of IL-6R (IL-6R Asp358Ala variant) show increased sIL-6R serum levels, reduced IL-6-induced C-reactive protein, and decreased risk for CAD likely due to increased ADAM10 and 17 mediated shedding of cell surface IL-6R Asp358Ala variant vs the common IL-6R variant (Garbers et al., 2014).

Angiotensin-converting enzyme-2 (ACE2) regulates heart function, and could act as a receptor for SARS-CoV spike protein. ACE2 is a type I transmembrane protein, with an extracellular N-terminal domain containing the active site and a short intracellular C-terminal tail. sACE2, lacking the transmembrane and cytosolic domains, could act as a decoy receptor for SARS-CoV spike protein preventing it from binding to the native ACE2 receptor (Xiang, Wang, Chen, & Chen, 2021). ADAM17 promotes ACE2 shedding, and ADAM17 siRNA reduces ACE2 shedding (Lambert et al., 2005).

Besides shedding of ADAM10, ADAM8 proteolytically releases the ADAM17 ectodomain. A study comparing the substrate spectrum of soluble ectodomains of ADAM10/17 (sADAM10/17) and their membrane-bound counterparts identified 134 protein cleavage events in total and 45 common substrates for sADAM10/17 within the secretome of murine cardiomyocytes. Further studies verified fibronectin, cystatin C, sN-cadherin, PCPE-1, and sAPP as direct substrates of sADAM10/17 (Scharfenberg et al., 2020).

6. ADAMTS targets, substrates, functions and mouse KO phenotype

In comparison with ADAMs, ADAMTS are secreted proteases and most of their targets/substrates are ECM proteins (Table 2) (Dubail & Apte, 2015; Mead & Apte, 2018). ADAMTS cleave proteoglycans including aggrecan, brevican, neurocan and versican, and degrade aggrecan and versican in blood vessels. ADAMTS also play a role in embryonic development, angiogenesis, coagulation, ECM proteolysis, and cartilage degradation, and ADAMTS KO mice show strong phenotypes in morphogenesis, mobility and reproduction.

ADAMTS1 (METH1) was originally cloned from a cancer cell line. ADAMTS1 is expressed in the yolk sac, placenta, heart, lung, liver, pancreas, spleen, kidney, brain, and limb bud of the developing mouse embryo and the tunica media of the aorta and pulmonary and hepatic vessels of adult mice (Thai & Iruela-Arispe, 2002). Osteotropic agents such as parathyroid hormone (PTH)-related protein (PTHrP), and prostaglandin PGE2 cause bone turnover partly via the cAMP/PKA pathway and rapid and transient increase in ADAMTS1 expression (Miles et al., 2000). ADAMTS1 deficient mice show morphological defects in the kidney, adrenal gland, heart and aorta, and different lymphocyte and myeloid cell population in the spleen and bone marrow (Rodriguez-Baena et al., 2018; Shindo et al., 2000). Almost 50% of newborn *Adamts1* null mice die likely due to a kidney malformation that becomes apparent at birth. Surviving female *Adamts1* null mice are subfertile, while males reproduce normally (Boerboom et al., 2011; Mittaz et al., 2005, 2004). LPS administration in mice induces *ADAMTS1* expression in the heart and kidney, suggesting a role in inflammation. In cultured fibroblast-like COS-7 cells treated with heparin, the mature form of ADAMTS1 is detected in the culture medium and associated with ECM. Deletion mutants of ADAMTS1 revealed that the spacer region and three thrombospondin 1 (TSP1) motifs in the C-terminal region are critical for interaction with ECM (Kuno & Matsushima, 1998).

Mutations in ADAMTS2, 3, 10, 13, 17 and 20 are linked to Mendelian disorders or birth defects (Mead & Apte, 2018). ADAMTS2, 3 and 14 are procollagen N-proteinases that play a role in procollagen processing and collagen fibrils formation, maturation and assembly (Bekhouche & Colige, 2015). ADAMTS2 heterozygous mice are normal at birth, but show progressively fragile skin, and adult males are sterile (Li et al., 2001).

ADAMTS3 is important for lymphangiogenesis and ADAMTS3 deficient mouse embryos do not survive past gestational day 15 due to lack of lymphangiogenesis and severe lymphedema (Janssen et al., 2016).

ADAMTS5 cleaves versican and plays a role in the development of heart valves. Adamts5$^{-/-}$ mice fed a high-fat diet show impaired cleavage of versican in the heart and increased diastolic posterior wall thickness and left ventricle volume, but with little effect on cardiac function (Hemmeryckx, Carai, & Roger Lijnen, 2019), making it important to further assess the effects of ADAMTS5 inhibition in obesity-related heart injury. ADAMTS5 is also implicated in osteoarthritis by degrading its cartilage substrate aggrecan (Mead & Apte, 2018).

vWF mediates platelet aggregation to sites of blood vessel injury, and its ultra-large multimer functions as a substrate that is proteolytically cleaved and regulated by ADAMTS13 (Petri et al., 2019).

ADAMTS15 is co-localized with hyaluronan in the developing heart and musculoskeletal system of the mouse embryo, and is expressed in the adult mouse colon and other systems with high versican processing capacity. In cultured HEK293T and COS-7 cells, ADAMTS15 is localized on cell surface where it undergoes propeptide processing and activation before cleaving V1 versican (Dancevic et al., 2013).

ADAMTS16 has been linked to blood pressure regulation, osteoarthritis, cancer, kidney function and testis development. Male homozygous Adamts16 deficient mice show cryptorchidism and sterility with small testes ~10% of controls, and seminiferous tubules that do not perform spermatogenesis, are gradually depleted of germ cells, show vacuoles, and do not contain sperms. Of note, male heterozygous Adamts16 mutants on C57BL/6N background show normal testis determination during fetal development and are fertile at 3 and 6 months, suggesting a recessive trait (Livermore et al., 2019). Adamts16 mutant rats also show renal abnormalities, suggesting that Adamts16 plays a role in maintaining normal functions of the male genitourinary system (Abdul-Majeed, Mell, Nauli, & Joe, 2014).

Heart valve defects are common disorders, making it important to determine their genetic underpinning. Studies have identified two consanguineous families, each family has two members affected with heart valve disease early in life, and whole-exome sequencing revealed homozygous alleles in *ADAMTS19* in the affected four individuals. Also, *Adamts19* KO mice show aortic valve dysfunction, supporting the role of *ADAMTS19* gene mutation in the human heart valve disorder (Wunnemann et al., 2020).

7. ADAMs and ADAMTS inhibitors

The "cysteine-switch" is a potent ADAM inhibitory mechanism, in which the cysteine residues in the pro-domain inhibit the protease activity (Lemjabbar & Basbaum, 2002; Ohtsu, Dempsey, & Eguchi, 2006). However, targeting the "cysteine-switch" in the metalloproteinase domain is not very specific due to structural similarity between ADAMs, ADAMTS and MMPs (Nyren-Erickson et al., 2013). TIMPs are endogenous four-member family with a broad inhibitory effect on most MMPs (Brew & Nagase, 2010), and relatively more specific inhibitory effects on ADAMs. TIMP-1 and -3 inhibit ADAM10, 12, 15 and 17 (Pelisek et al., 2012). In endotoxin-activated human macrophages, TIMP-3 inhibits ADAM17 only when it is bound to the cell surface, and the TIMP-3 cell surface levels are controlled by the endocytic receptor LRP1 (Schubert, Collins, Green, Nagase, & Troeberg, 2019). ADAM8, 9 and 19 are not inhibited by any TIMP (Amour et al., 2002; Chesneau et al., 2003). ADAM33 can be inhibited by TIMP-3 and -4, but not TIMP-1 (Zou et al., 2004).

TIMPs inhibit MMPs and ADAMs with different efficacies. The N-terminal domain of TIMPs accounts for inhibiting MMPs, while the N-terminus of TIMP-1 or -3 or that of TIMP-2 has little effect on ADAM10 or ADAM17, respectively. Also, while TIMP-3 has a solid inhibitory effect on the isolated catalytic domain of ADAM17, when the other domains are added or some parts of the domains such as cysteine-rich domain are modified, the TIMP-3 inhibitory effect is reduced (Blobel, 2005).

Most synthetic small molecule inhibitors also target the catalytic Zn^{2+} and have a broad inhibitory spectrum toward ADAMs and MMPs (Table 3). Zn^{2+} chelators 1,10-phenanthroline and hydroxamate are potent ADAMs inhibitors (Glassey & Civetta, 2004). INCB3619 is a potent inhibitor of ADAM10 and 17, but is a less potent against ADAM8, 9 and 33 (Fridman et al., 2007). TAPI-1, TAPI-2, and batimastat (BB-94) are potent inhibitors of ADAM17, but could affect MMPs. CGS27023,

Table 3 Endogenous and synthetic inhibitors of ADAMs and ADAMTS.

Inhibitor	Target	Reference
Endogenous:		
TIMP-1	ADAM10, 12, 15, 17	Pelisek et al. (2012), Rapti et al. (2008)
TIMP-2	ADAM17, 33 ADAMTS1	Kveiborg et al. (2010)
TIMP-3	ADAM10, 12, 15, 17, 28, 33 ADAMTS1, 2, 4, 5	Bekhouche and Colige (2015), Kashiwagi, Tortorella, Nagase, and Brew (2001), Pelisek et al. (2012), Rapti et al. (2008), Schubert et al. (2019), Wang, Ge, Lim, Nagase, and Greenspan (2006)
TIMP-4	ADAM17, 28, 33	Heijink et al. (2011)
α-2 macroglobulin	ADAMTS2, 4, 5	Bekhouche and Colige (2015), Tortorella et al. (2004), Wang et al. (2006)
Papilin	ADAMTS2	Kramerova et al. (2000)
Synthetic:		
Batimastat (BB-94)	ADAM8, 9, 17, MMPs	Heijink et al. (2011)
BK-1361 inhibitor peptide	ADAM8	Chen et al. (2016)
Calcium pentosan polysulfate	ADAMTS4, 5	Takizawa et al. (2008), Troeberg et al. (2008), Vistnes et al. (2014)
CGS27023	ADAM9, 10, 17	Qian et al. (2002)
Cis-1(S)2(R)-amino-2-indanol-based compounds	ADAMTS4, 5	Tortorella et al. (2009)
cyclo(RLsKDK) cyclic peptide	ADAM8	Yim et al. (2016)
Doxycycline	ADAMTS13, MMPs	Bartoli, Kang, et al. (2015)
FC143, FC387	ADAM8, 17	Schlomann et al. (2019)
GI254023	ADAM9, 10, 17, MMPs	Zhang et al. (2016)

Table 3 Endogenous and synthetic inhibitors of ADAMs and ADAMTS.—cont'd

Inhibitor	Target	Reference
Glycoconjugated arylsulfonamide	ADAMTS5	Santamaria et al. (2021)
GM6001	ADAM9, MMPs	Maretzky et al. (2017)
Granulin-epithelin precursor	ADAMTS7, 12	Guo et al. (2010), Kelwick, Desanlis, et al. (2015)
GW280264X	ADAM8, 9, 10, 17	Zhang et al. (2016)
INCB3619	ADAM8, 9, 10, 17, 33	Zhang et al. (2016)
KP457	ADAM10, 17	Zhang et al. (2016)
α-Lipolic acid	ADAM17	de Queiroz, Xia, Filipeanu, Braga, and Lazartigues (2015)
Marimastat	ADAM9, 17, MMPs	Maretzky et al. (2017), Parrish et al. (2018)
Propofol anesthetic	ADAM8	Yu, Shi, Wang, and Zhang (2019)
TAPI-1	ADAM17, MMPs	Moss and Rasmussen (2007)
TAPI-2	ADAM9, 17, other ADAMs, MMPs	Moss and Rasmussen (2007)

GW280264 and GI254023 exhibit specific inhibitory effect on ADAM9, 10 and 17 (Ludwig et al., 2005). Glycosylation of a substrate such as TNFα inhibited ADAM10 activity, but increased ADAM8 and 17 activities (Minond et al., 2012), and adopting the glycosylation strategy could allow targeting of a specific ADAM in CVD.

In Neuro2A cells, AngII increases ADAM17 expression and oxidative stress and these effects are attenuated by α-lipoic acid. Also, α-lipoic acid improves dysautonomia and baroreflex sensitivity, ameliorate HTN, and blunts the increase in ADAM17 and NADPH oxidase, and the decrease in ACE2 activity in the hypothalamus of deoxycorticosterone acetate (DOCA)-salt hypertensive mice. Thus, α-lipoic may preserve ACE2 compensatory activity by inhibiting ADAM17 and oxidative stress, resulting in amelioration of neurogenic HTN (de Queiroz et al., 2015).

Cilostazol is a phosphodiesterase inhibitor that inhibits VSMC proliferation by regulating ADAM17 expression. In cultured VSMCs, cilostazol inhibits IL-1α and IL-1β-induced ADAM17 expression likely through inhibition of MAPK kinase (MEK), extracellular signal-regulated protein kinase (ERK) phosphorylation and the ERK/NF-κB pathway (Takaguri, Morimoto, Imai, & Satoh, 2016).

ADAMTS family members have different susceptibilities to endogenous and synthetic inhibitors (Murphy, 2011; Santamaria et al., 2021; Santamaria & de Groot, 2019). As with other proteinases, α2-macroglobulin entrap ADAMTS2 after cleavage within its bait region (Bekhouche & Colige, 2015). ADAMTS1 is inhibited by TIMP-2 and 3, but not TIMP-1 and 4 (Rodriguez-Manzaneque et al., 2002). TIMP-3 inhibits ADAMTS2, 4 and 5 (Hashimoto, Aoki, Nakamura, Tanzawa, & Okada, 2001; Wang et al., 2006), and aggrecan and heparan sulfate promote the inhibition by interacting with TSR and spacer regions (Troeberg et al., 2009, 2014). Papilin inhibits ADAMTS2 by binding both the enzyme and its substrate (Kramerova et al., 2000). Calcium pentosan polysulfate interacts with the noncatalytic spacer domain of ADAMTS4 and the cysteine-rich domain of ADAMTS5, blocking activity against their natural substrate aggrecan (Troeberg et al., 2008). Granulin-epithelin precursor binds to the ancillary domains of ADAMTS7 and 12 and block the degradation of cartilage oligomeric matrix protein (COMP) substrate (Guo et al., 2010).

Many of the ADAMs and ADAMTS inhibitors have a broad spectrum and interact with other proteases such MMPs, and therefore their use has been limited to *in vitro* biochemical or cellar studies or in animal models *in vivo*. The development of new ADAMs and ADAMTS inhibitors with improved specificity would enhance their use in clinical applications.

8. ADAMs and ADAMTS in vascular processes and malfunction

ADAMs and ADAMTS play a role in several vascular processes including angiogenesis, VSMC proliferation and migration, intimal hyperplasia and neointima formation, vascular cell apoptosis, EC permeability, vascular inflammation, and tissue repair and wound healing (Fig. 3).

8.1 ADAMs and ADAMTS in angiogenesis

During sprouting angiogenesis, VEGF induces tip ECs to start sprouting and express delta-like 4 (Dll4), which activates Notch in the adjacent stalk cells

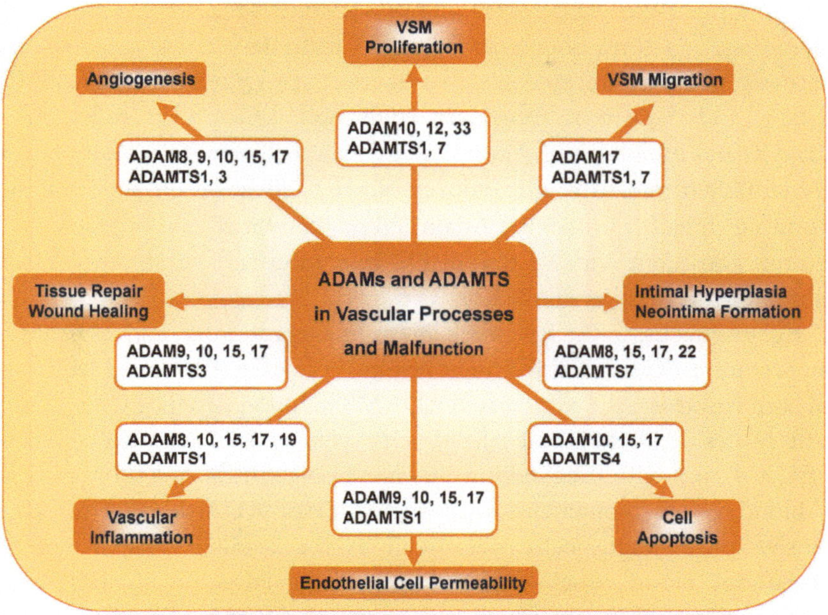

Fig. 3 Role of ADAMs and ADAMTS in vascular processes and malfunction.

and limit their sprouting. Notch signaling also regulates the level of VEGFR, and in turn affects the expression of the Notch ligand Dll4, thus creating an intercellular feedback loop (Jakobsson et al., 2010). VEGF also activates ADAMs, which promote Notch ectodomain shedding. Both ADAM10 and 17 are implicated in Notch-signaling, but they have different roles in angiogenesis. In mouse retinas, inhibition of ADAM10 induces, while inhibition of ADAM17 reduces, vascular sprouting. Retinal vessels analysis in ADAM17 hypomorphic mice (ADAM17$^{ex/ex}$) confirmed the requirement of ADAM17 in angiogenesis. ADAM17 overexpression decreased the expression of a naturally occurring inhibitor of angiogenesis Thrombospondin 1 (TSP1). Genetic and pharmacological ADAM17 blockade increased TSP1 expression in mouse retina. During ADAM17 inhibition, the TSP1 inhibitor LSKL restored VEGF-induced angiogenesis and EC tube formation. Thus, ADAM10 and 17 have opposite effects on sprouting angiogenesis that may be unrelated to Notch signaling and involve differentially expressed TSP1 (Caolo et al., 2015).

The density of preexisting collaterals varies widely and is a major determinant of severity of MI, stroke and PAD. VEGF affects collateral density in newborn and adult mice. In the mouse embryo, pial collaterals begin sprouting from existing cerebral arterioles. Global VEGF-A overexpressing mice (*Vegf*$^{hi/+}$) form more, and *Vegf*$^{lo/+}$ form fewer, collaterals during embryogenesis. Conditional global reduction of *Vegf* reduces collateral formation, and the effects remain in adulthood. EC-specific reduction of Adam10 and inhibition of γ-secretase increase collateral formation, consistent with their roles in VEGF-induced Notch1 activation and suppression of sprouting signals. EC-specific Adam17 knockdown reduces collateral formation, consistent with its role in EC migration and embryonic vascular stabilization (Lucitti et al., 2012).

EC loss occurs in the first week after spinal cord injury, and ADAMs are important for EC survival and angiogenesis. Adult C57Bl/6 mice with a spinal cord contusion show increased ADAM8 in blood vessels, ECs and spinal cord lysates. ADAM8 colocalized with platelet-EC adhesion molecule (PECAM) and with intravenously-injected isolectin B4 in a subpopulation of blood vessels, coincident with angiogenesis. ADAM8 and ADAM8-positive proliferating cells were seen at the leading end of isolectin B4-positive blood vessels, supporting a role of ADAM8 in proliferation and migration of ECs during angiogenesis following spinal cord injury (Mahoney, Benton, Maddie, Whittemore, & Hagg, 2009).

Proteolytic cleavage of VEGFR and the VEGF coreceptor neuropilin-1 are important factors in angiogenesis. Neuropilin-1 species that include the C-terminal and transmembrane domains but lack the ligand-binding A and B regions are constitutively expressed in ECs, upregulated by phorbol ester and Ca^{2+} ionophore, and reduced by ADAM9 knockdown using siRNA or by ADAM10 inhibitor. VEGF upregulates neuropilin-1 species in an ADAM9/ADAM10-dependent manner. Transfection of ECs with adenoviral constructs expressing neuropilin-1 C-terminal domain inhibited VEGF-induced EC motility and angiogenesis in aortic ring sprouting assays, suggesting a role of neuropilin-1 proteolysis by ADAM9 and 10 in modulating VEGF angiogenic signaling (Mehta et al., 2018).

ADAMTS1 has been linked to angiogenesis in gastric and lung cancer (Chen, Zhi, et al., 2013; Kilic et al., 2017; Tang et al., 2017). ADAMTS1 is abundant in rat embryonal epithelia of the intestines, nasal cavity, choroid plexus and skin, and is involved in the development of the heart, liver, adrenal glands, muscle, neuronal system and adipose tissue. At the time of birth, ADAMTS1 is reduced in most organs, but increases in the developing bone and skin. A 62 kDa ADAMTS1 fragment is detected in the heart, lung, intestines, kidneys and adrenal glands of the developing rat embryo and to a less extent in the corresponding adult rat organs. ADAMTS1 is found in principal cells of collecting ducts and renal medulla, ependymal cells of the ventricles, and some neurons. The distribution of ADAMTS1 in multiple organs during embryogenesis suggests a role in tissue remodeling and angiogenesis (Gunther et al., 2005).

ADAMTS3 cleaves pro-VEGF-C into active VEGF-C during embryonic lymphangiogenesis and placental angiogenesis (Janssen et al., 2016), and regulates VEGFR-3 signaling during lymphatic EC differentiation (Jeltsch et al., 2014). Loss of ADAMTS3 is linked to Hennekam lymphangiectasia-lymphedema syndrome (Brouillard et al., 2017).

On the other hand, recombinant ADAMTS2 (rADAMTS2) reduces EC proliferation and branching of capillary-like structures, and inhibits vessel formation in embryoid bodies (Dubail et al., 2010), partly through interaction of one of its C-terminal domains with nucleolin (Bekhouche & Colige, 2015; Dubail et al., 2010). Similarly, ADAMTS12 shows antiangiogenic effects independent of its enzymatic activity, as both the WT control form and mutated inactive form similarly inhibit EC sprouting in the aortic ring assay. These ADAMTS12 antiangiogenic properties could protect against tumor progression (El Hour et al., 2010). ADAMTS15 also reduces angiogenesis and liver cancer metastasis by modulating cell-ECM interactions (Kelwick, Wagstaff, et al., 2015).

8.2 ADAMs and ADAMTS in VSMC proliferation and migration

VSMC proliferation and migration are key events in atherosclerosis and intimal hyperplasia. In cultured human coronary VSMCs, the C-terminal fragment of the plasminogen activator urokinase (CTF-uPA) increases DNA synthesis, cell proliferation and EGFR phosphorylation/activation, and these effects are blocked by plasmin, EGFR inhibitors, TIMPs, and inhibitors of ADAM10, ADAM12 and HB-EGF (Duru et al., 2014). The N-terminal fragment of uPA (NTF-uPA) also promotes migration, EGFR phosphorylation/activation and HB-EGF release in human coronary VSMCs, and these effects are blocked by EGFR inhibitor AG1478, MMP and HB-EGF inhibitors, ADAM inhibitors TAPI-0 and TAPI-1, and ADAM9 and 10 siRNA. Thus, uPA induces domain-dependent VSMC proliferation through transactivation of EGFR by a plasmin-mediated, ADAM-induced and HB-EGF-dependent process, and EGFR and ADAM9, 10 or 12 could be potential targets to inhibit cell migration (Bakken, Protack, Roztocil, Nicholl, & Davies, 2009).

ADAM12 is an important mediator of VSMC proliferation in carotid artery lesions (Pelisek et al., 2012; Smiljanic et al., 2011).

In human airway SMCs, recombinant disintegrin domain of ADAM15 (ddADAM15), which contains an RGD integrin-binding motif, adhered to SMCs in a β1-integrin dependent manner. ddADAM15 inhibited platelet-derived growth factor (PDGF)-induced airway SMC migration, and this inhibition was reversed by β1-integrin antibody, supporting a role of ddADAM15 in inhibiting airway SMC adhesion and migration through interaction with β1-integrin (Lu et al., 2007).

ADAM17 is linked to VSMC hypertrophy and hyperplasia, possibly through activation of EGFR (Shen et al., 2017). AngII-induced HTN is suppressed in mice lacking ADAM17 in SMCs ($Adam17^{f/f}/Cre^{Sm22}$) during the first week of AngII infusion, but by the second week, HTN increases to levels observed in mice with intact ADAM17 ($Adam17^{f/f}$). $Adam17^{f/f}/Cre^{Sm22}$ mice also exhibit less cardiac hypertrophy and fibrosis and renal fibrosis at 2 weeks post-AngII, but this protection is reversed by the fourth week. EGFR activation is suppressed in $Adam17^{f/f/}Cre^{Sm22}$-AngII arteries. AngII-induced proliferation and migration, EGFR activation and Erk1/2 signaling were suppressed in VSMCs isolated from $Adam17^{f/f}/Cre^{Sm22}$. Thus, Adam17-deficiency suppresses AngII-induced VSMC remodeling, and transiently protect against AngII-mediated HTN and end-organ damage (Shen et al., 2017).

ADAM33, which is evolutionally related to ADAM15, has been suggested as a crucial factor in airway SMC proliferation and bronchial asthma pathology (Kim et al., 2017).

Plasma of CAD patients shows increased ADAMTS1 and decreased miR-362-3p. In human coronary VSMCs, PDGF-BB inhibits miR-365b-3p and upregulates ADAMTS1 expression. Overexpression of miR-365b-3p downregulates ADAMTS1 and attenuates PDGF-BB-induced VSMC proliferation/migration and G1/S cell cycle transition. miR-362-3p binds to ADAMTS1 3′-untranslated region and decreases its expression. Overexpression of ADAMTS1 reverses miR-362-3p-induced inhibition of VSMC proliferation/migration and, cell cycle. Thus, miR-362-3p inhibits VSMC proliferation/migration and attenuates atherosclerosis by targeting ADAMTS1 (Li, Liu, et al., 2017; Qu & Zhang, 2018).

ADAMTS7 could mediate VSMC migration and neointima formation (Wang, Zheng, et al., 2009). In rat model of carotid artery balloon-injury, luminal adenoviral delivery of ADAMTS7 aggravates intimal hyperplasia and increases proliferating cell nuclear antigen-positive cells in the intima and media. Perivascular ADAMTS7 siRNA reduces intimal thickening and VSMC replication. Cultured rat VSMCs show enhanced replication with ADAMTS7 overexpression and decreased proliferation with ADAMTS7 siRNA, supporting that ADAMTS7 promotes VSMC proliferation (Zhang et al., 2015). ADAMTS7 KO mice also show reduced risk of atherosclerosis likely due to loss of ADAMTS7-mediated VSM migration (Bauer et al., 2015).

8.3 ADAMs and ADAMTS in neointimal hyperplasia and vascular restenosis

Neointimal hyperplasia and vascular restenosis are major limitations of coronary angioplasty and involve abnormal proliferation/migration of VSMCs. In response to vascular injury, adventitia stem/progenitor cells (AdSPCs) migrate into the intima, where they differentiate into SMCs and participate in neointimal hyperplasia. Macrophage-derived MMP8 promotes SMC differentiation from AdSPCs, and contributes to injury-induced neointimal SMC hyperplasia by modulating TGF-β activity and ADAM10/Notch1 signaling (Yang et al., 2020). In support, the mouse carotid artery wire injury model shows fewer proliferating cells and smaller neointimal lesions in $ApoE^{-/-}MMP8^{-/-}$ mice. Also, MMP8 KO VSMCs and WT VSMCs treated with ADAM10 inhibitor GI254023X or transfected with ADAM10 siRNA show less proliferation/migration, and contain more pro-ADAM10 and less mature ADAM10, more N-cadherin and β-catenin in the plasma membrane, less β-catenin in the nucleus, and less cyclin D1. Treatment of MMP8 KO VSMCs with rADAM10 increases cell proliferation/migration and cyclin D1 expression. Immunohistochemistry show colocalization of ADAM10 with VSMCs and N-cadherin, and nuclear accumulation of β-catenin in the neointima of $ApoE^{-/-}MMP8^{+/+}$ mice, suggesting that MMP8 promotes VSMC proliferation/migration and neointima formation via an ADAM10, N-cadherin and β-catenin-mediated pathway (Xiao et al., 2014).

Methyl protodioscin reduces neointima formation in rat carotid artery balloon injury model, and inhibits growth and migration, arrests cell cycle at the G1 phase, and decreases ADAM15 expression in A7r5 VSMCs, suggesting a role of ADAM15 in neointima formation (Chung et al., 2016),

In rat carotid arteries after balloon angioplasty, neointimal cells are strongly positive for ADAM17. Intimal hyperplasia and proliferating cell nuclear antigen (PCNA)- and phospho-EGFR-positive cells are reduced in a dominant-negative ADAM17 adenovirus-treated carotid artery, and enhanced by WT ADAM17 adenovirus, supporting a role of ADAM17 in EGF activation and neointimal hyperplasia after vascular injury (Takaguri et al., 2011).

ADAM22 is upregulated in mouse carotid artery injury model and PDGF-BB-treated VSMCs. Wire injury induced neointima formation is ameliorated in ADAM22 heterozygous mice. VSMCs overexpressing ADAM22 show increased proliferation/migration and phenotypic switching, and these effects are reversed by ADAM22 siRNA or ERK inhibitors, suggesting a role of ERK phosphorylation in ADAM22-mediated neointima formation (Zhang, Jiang, et al., 2019).

ADAMTS7 accumulates in the neointima of rat carotid artery after balloon injury. Luminal delivery of ADAMTS7 adenovirus to carotid arteries exacerbates, while perivascular application of ADAMTS7 siRNA attenuates, intimal thickening. TNFα and PDGF-BB enhance ADAMTS7 expression in VSMCs. ADAMTS7 overexpression accelerates, and its siRNA knockdown retards VSMC migration. ADAMTS7 promotes degradation of cartilage oligomeric matrix protein (COMP) in injured vessels, and overexpression of COMP suppresses postinjury neointima formation and VSMC migration, suggesting that ADAMTS7 facilitates intimal hyperplasia by degrading COMP (Wang, Zheng, et al., 2009). Conversely, ADAMTS7 inhibits proliferation/migration in cultured ECs. In mouse carotid artery wire injury model, *Adamts7* KO promoted re-endothelialization and ameliorates neointima formation. ADAMTS7 degraded TSP1, and the inhibitory effect of ADAMTS7 on postinjury endothelium recovery was absent in $Tsp1^{-/-}$ mice. Thus ADAMTS7 inhibits re-endothelialization, delays EC repair and promotes TSP1 degradation and neointima formation, and could be a potential target in postinjury intimal hyperplasia and post-angioplasty restenosis (Kessler et al., 2015).

8.4 ADAMs and ADAMTS in vascular cell apoptosis

ADAM10, 15 and 17 play a role in vascular cell apoptosis (Fig. 3). ADAM10 cleaves N-cadherin and increases apoptosis in atherosclerotic lesions and the risk of vulnerable plaque (Schulz et al., 2008). Other studies suggest that ADAM10 promotes vascular cell survival, as ionizing radiation reduces ADAM10 expression and induces neurovascular cell senescence and death (McRobb et al., 2017). Recombinant human ADAM15 (rhADAM15) induces vascular apoptosis and inhibits tumor formation and angiogenesis (Hou et al., 2015). ADAM17 mediates vascular apoptosis and migratory invasion of liver cancer stem cells, making ADAM17 a promising target in cancer therapy (Jin et al., 2013; Wang, Li, et al., 2018). Deletion of Cdc42 increases ADAM17 activity, enhances VEGFR-2 shedding, and reduces vascular EC survival and angiogenesis, and ADAM17 inhibition reverses Cdc42 deletion-induced EC apoptosis (Jin et al., 2013).

Versican is a large proteoglycan required for development of the circulatory system and proper limb development (Timms & Maurice, 2020). ADAMTS4 degrades versican, induces VSMC apoptosis, and promotes inflammatory cell infiltration of blood vessels (Ren et al., 2017). Also, ADAMTS20 mutants have reduced versican proteolysis and impaired interdigit web regression, leading to soft tissue syndactyly. Versikine, the ADAMTS20-generated versican N-terminal bioactive proteolytic fragment, restores interdigit apoptosis in ADAMTS mutant webs, and may play an essential role in interdigital web regression (Nandadasa et al., 2021).

8.5 ADAMs and ADAMTS in endothelial permeability

VE-cadherin controls endothelial permeability, vascular integrity and leukocyte transmigration, and soluble VE-cadherin is elevated in atherosclerosis. In HUVECs, ADAM9 is localized at cell-cell junctions with VE-cadherin (English, Siviter, Hansen, & Murphy, 2017). Also, ADAM10 cleaves VE-cadherin ectodomain from HUVECs, and this cleavage is induced by Ca^{2+} influx or staurosporine, suggesting that it contributes to dissolution of adherens junctions during EC activation or apoptosis, respectively. ADAM10 contributes to thrombin-induced decrease of endothelial cell-cell adhesion and increased endothelial permeability. Also, ADAM10 siRNA inhibits T-cell transmigration in HUVECs (Schulz et al., 2008).

The renal glomeruli filter blood through fenestrated endothelium, glomerular basement membrane and podocyte foot processes. Glomeruli of mice lacking ADAM10 in ECs ($ADAM10^{\Delta EC}$) show increased vascular diameter and intussusceptive or splitting angiogenesis, suggesting a role of endothelial ADAM10 and Notch signaling in glomerular vessels development (Farber et al., 2018).

In bovine aortic ECs high shear stress modulates gene expression, promotes an anti-coagulant, anti-inflammatory, proliferative and promatrix remodeling, and upregulates the ECM processing factor ADAMTS1, metalloproteinase inhibitor TIMP-3, and the fibrinolysis factors tissue plasminogen activator (tPA) and urokinase plasminogen activator (uPA). Also, ADAMTS1 and uPA are increased in rabbit basilar arteries exposed to high flow after bilateral carotid artery ligation (Dolan, Sim, Meng, & Kolega, 2012).

Blood-brain barrier (BBB) defects and cerebrovascular dysfunction contribute to amyloid-β accumulation and Alzheimer disease. In APP and presenilin 1 (PS1) APPPS1 transgenic mice, ADAMTS13 deficiency leads to BBB breakdown, reduced vessel density, capillary perfusion and cerebral blood flow, impeded clearance of amyloid-β, increased brain plaque load and cerebral amyloid angiopathy, and further cognitive decline. Virus-induced expression of ADAMTS13 in APPPS1 mice attenuates BBB disruption, increases microvessels, capillary perfusion, cerebral blood flow and cerebral amyloid-β clearance, and improves cognitive performance, supporting that ADAMTS13 deficiency contributes to cerebrovascular dysfunction in Alzheimer disease (Cao et al., 2019).

8.6 ADAMs and ADAMTS in vascular inflammation

Cell-cell and cell-matrix interactions participate in leukocyte recruitment to inflammatory sites, and ADAMs adhesive and proteolytic activities contribute to the inflammatory process. In human macrophages, meprin-β promotes inflammation and increases the production of IL-1β, IL-6 and IL-18 through activation of ADAM10-ERK1/2 pathway and phosphorylation of NF-κB (Li, Fan, Tang, Li, & Yu, 2014).

ADAM15 through modulation of cell-cell and cell-ECM interactions and ectodomain shedding activities could mediate rheumatoid arthritis and other inflammatory disorders (Charrier-Hisamuddin et al., 2008).

ADAM17 regulates inflammation by shedding membrane-bound proteins, converting TNFα precursor to its mature form, and processing of TNFR1 and TNFR2 (Chemaly et al., 2017). Plasma ADAM17 and its substrate syndecan-1 are elevated in patients with anti-neutrophil cytoplasmic antibody-associated vasculitis (Bertram et al., 2015). TNFα and ADAM17 are also upregulated in endomyocardial biopsies from patients with myocarditis, and correlate positively with left ventricular volume and negatively with left ventricular systolic function, suggesting a role in myocarditis and cardiac dysfunction (Satoh et al., 2000).

Kawasaki disease is a childhood disease of systemic vasculitis and coronary artery lesions. ADAM17 cleaves TGF-β receptor type-1 and reduces TGF-β signaling. In the Han Chinese population three ADAM17 SNPs are associated with Kawasaki disease risk and coronary artery lesions likely through modulation of the TGF-β/SMAD3 pathway (Peng et al., 2016).

IL-1 induces ADAMTS1 expression in colon-26 cells, and injection of LPS in mice upregulates ADAMTS1 in the heart and kidney, supporting a role of ADAMTS1 in inflammation (Hirohata, Inagaki, & Ohtsuki, 2017; Kuno et al., 1997).

8.7 ADAMs and ADAMTS in tissue repair and wound healing

ADAM and ADAMTS show differential expression in wound healing tissues vs normal tissues. ADAM9, 10, 15 and 17 are highly expressed, and ADAMTS3 shows differential expression in healing wounds, suggesting potential roles in tissue repair (Hodgkinson et al., 2010).

ADAMTS5 could play a role in tissue repair and wound healing through regulation of versican proteolysis, pericellular matrix volume and dermal fibroblast-myofibroblast transition (Hattori et al., 2011). In a murine model of excisional wound healing, ADAMTS5 ablation was associated with impaired contraction and dermal collagen deposition, and accumulation of cell aggregates, fibroblastic cells and full-length aggrecan enriched pericellular matrix in the dermal layer. ADAMTS5 deficiency may block dermal repair through CD44-mediated aggrecan accumulation and changes in TGF-β1 signaling (Velasco et al., 2011)

9. ADAMs and ADAMTS in cardiovascular disease

ADAM8, 9, 10, 12, 13, 15, 17, 19 and 28, as well as ADAMTS1, 4 and 5 have been associated with different pathological conditions (Mochizuki & Okada, 2007). ADAM17 is involved in diabetes and inflammatory, immune and cardiovascular disorders (Chemaly et al., 2017; Palau, Pascual, Soler, & Riera, 2019). ADAMTS13 deficiency is linked to thrombotic microangiopathy (Akyol, Akyol, & Chen, 2016). ADAMs and ADAMTS have also been implicated in HTN, atherosclerosis, CAD, MI, heart failure, ischemic stroke, PAD and vascular aneurysm (Nyren-Erickson et al., 2013; Obama et al., 2015; Palau et al., 2019; Santamaria & de Groot, 2020) (Fig. 4).

9.1 ADAMs and ADAMTS in hypertension

Neurogenic, renal and vascular factors contribute to different forms of hypertension (HTN), and ADAMs and ADAMTS may be involved. Receptors-for-Advanced-Glycation-End-products (RAGE) activate inflammatory processes during cell stress. ADAM10 cleaves RAGE and releases sRAGE,

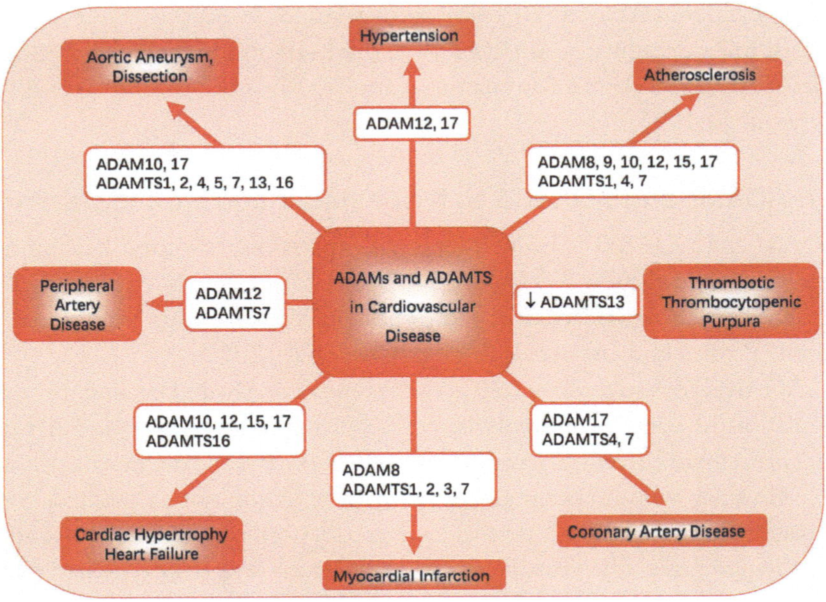

Fig. 4 Role of ADAMs and ADAMTS in cardiovascular disease.

which neutralizes RAGE ligands and reduces cardiovascular effects of increased sympathetic activity in HTN and diabetes (Raucci et al., 2008). Myocardial fibrosis and RAGE are increased, sRAGE is decreased, and ADAM10 myocardial and serum levels are elevated in obese spontaneously hypertensive rats (SHR), and these effects are reversed by renal denervation. Isoproterenol induces β1-adrenergic receptor-mediated RAGE expression in splenocytes and β2-adrenergic receptor-mediated suppression of ADAM10 activity and decreased sRAGE secretion from splenocytes and cardiac fibroblasts. Thus, sympathetic activity suppresses ADAM10 activity and sRAGE/RAGE balance, and sympathetic inhibition or renal denervation reverse these effects and prevent RAGE-induced cardiac damage in HTN and metabolic syndrome (Selejan et al., 2018).

ADAM12 has been implicated in HTN (Nyren-Erickson et al., 2013). GPCR agonists upregulate ADAM12 and other mediators to increase BP and cardiac hypertrophy (Berry, Bosonea, Wang, & Fernandez-Patron, 2013). Acute HTN induced by catecholamines, AngII or nitric oxide synthase inhibitor requires transcription of vascular MMP-7 and ADAM12. Myocardial ADAM12 is upregulated in mice with AngII-induced HTN and cardiac hypertrophy, and MMP-7 knockdown attenuates HTN,

ADAM12 overexpression and cardiac hypertrophy, making the MMP-7/ ADAM12 pathway a potential therapeutic target in HTN (Wang, Chow, et al., 2009).

ADAM17 is overexpressed in HTN (Obama et al., 2015; Palau et al., 2019). C57Bl/6 mice infused with AngII for 2 weeks show cardiac and vascular medial hypertrophy, perivascular fibrosis, increased vascular ADAM17, EGFR activation, and endoplasmic reticulum stress. These phenotypes are diminished in AngII-infused vascular ADAM17-deficient mice or C57Bl/6 mice treated with ADAM17 antibody independent of BP changes, suggesting a role of vascular ADAM17 in mediating AngII-induced cardiovascular remodeling via EGFR activation (Takayanagi et al., 2016). In other studies, AngII-infused mice show cardiac hypertrophy and fibrosis, and increased myocardial hypertrophy markers (α-actin, β-myosin heavy chain and brain natriuretic peptide), fibrosis markers (collagen types I and III and fibronectin), MMP-2 and ADAM12, and these effects are prevented by ADAM17 siRNA (Wang, Oka, et al., 2009). Also, loss of ADAM17 specifically in SMCs suppressed AngII-induced HTN, cardiac hypertrophy and fibrosis, and renal fibrosis (Shen et al., 2017). Thus, ADAM17, likely through transcriptional regulation of MMP-2 and ADAM12, may play a role in AngII-induced cardiac hypertrophy and fibrosis (Wang, Oka, et al., 2009).

Neurogenic HTN is characterized by increased sympathetic activity and drug resistance. Chronic activation of the brain renin angiotensin system (RAS) causes HTN by altering autonomic balance. ACE2 cleaves AngII to Ang(1-7) peptide, which counteracts the adverse effects of AngII. ACE2 activity is increased in the cerebrospinal fluid and correlates with systolic BP in patients with HTN. ADAM17 is also upregulated in the brain of patients with HTN as TNFα levels are increased in the cerebrospinal fluid. ADAM17 is also upregulated in neurons of DOCA-salt hypertensive mice, but not in mice lacking AngII receptor (AT_1R) in neurons. Thus, neuronal AT_1R, likely through increasing reactive oxygen species and ERK, causes ADAM17 activation, increased ADAM17-mediated ACE2 shedding, and reduced ACE2 compensatory activity in neurogenic HTN (Xu, Sriramula, et al., 2017).

ADAM17 is robustly expressed and promotes RAS activation in the brain. DOCA-salt increases BP, and cardiac and vascular sympathetic activity in WT mice, and these effects are reduced in mice lacking ADAM17 in glutamatergic neurons. Within the paraventricular nucleus, AngII-induced activation of kidney-related presympathetic glutamatergic neurons is reduced in ADAM17 knockdown mice, confirming the role of neuronal ADAM17 in increasing presympathetic neuronal activity and salt-sensitive HTN (Xu et al., 2019). In cultured cortical neurons, glutamate increases ADAM17 activity and reduces ACE2 activity, and these effects are reversed by blockers of oxidative stress, supporting a relationship between exaggerated glutamate stimulation, ADAM17-mediated impairment in ACE2 activity, oxidative stress and neurogenic HTN (Xu, Sriramula, & Lazartigues, 2018). Interestingly, α-lipoic acid reduces neurogenic HTN by blunting oxidative stress and the increase in ADAM17 (de Queiroz et al., 2015).

Neuronal ACE2 deletion reduces inhibitory inputs to presympathetic neurons involved in BP regulation. In primary neuron cultures, ACE2 is expressed on GABAergic neurons synapsing onto excitatory neurons within the hypothalamus. ADAM17 colocalizes with AT_1R on Sim1 neurons. ADAM17 knockdown in Sim1 neurons reduces *FosB* gene expression, increases vagal tone, and prevents the acute pressor response to centrally administered AngII. Sim1 neurons ADAM17 deficient mice show blunted BP and preserved ACE2 activity during DOCA salt-sensitive HTN, supporting contrasting effects of ACE2 and ADAM17 on neuronal excitability of presympathetic neurons within the paraventricular nucleus, and on neurogenic HTN (Mukerjee et al., 2019).

The renal RAS regulates salt and water excretion, plasma volume and BP. ADAM17 is highly expressed in distal renal tubules and in the diabetic kidney. In addition to shedding ACE2, ADAM17 promotes inflammation and fibrosis in chronic kidney disease (Palau et al., 2019).

HTN-in-pregnancy and preeclampsia (PE) affect 5–8% of pregnancies in the United States. Maternal serum level of sADAM12, a marker of fetal aneuploidy and growth, is altered in PE. In the first-trimester, serum sADAM12 level is reduced in women who developed PE and further reduced in those delivering prior to 35 weeks. Combining sADAM12 with pregnancy-associated plasma protein A (PAPP-A) results in a further 1% increase in detecting women who developed PE. Combining sADAM12 with uterine artery Doppler Pulsatility Index increases PE detection rate to 66%. In the second trimester at 22–24 weeks, serum sADAM12 levels are increased in women developing PE (Spencer, Cowans, & Stamatopoulou, 2008). Other studies have shown that in normal pregnant women ADAM12 levels increase with fetal crown rump length, decrease with maternal weight, are higher in African-American than white women, and show an association with PAPP-A levels. ADAM12 levels are reduced in pregnant women with small for gestational age neonates, and are not markedly different in PE pregnancies, gestational HTN, or spontaneous preterm delivery (Poon, Chelemen, Granvillano, Pandeva, & Nicolaides, 2008). Also, studies examining the efficiency of ADAM12, PAPP-A, uterine artery Doppler and maternal characteristics in predicting PE in the first-trimester showed that ADAM12 serum levels were lower in women who developed PE than those who did not. ADAM12, PAPP-A, or uterine artery Doppler pulsatility indices each individually in combination with maternal characteristics identified ~50% of women who developed PE. Combining these first-trimester parameters did not improve their predictive efficiency (Goetzinger et al., 2013). Other studies showed an association between decreased first trimester ADAM12s levels and gestational HTN, but combined ADAM12s and placental protein 13 (PP13) measurements did not further predict PE, gestational HTN and small for gestational age fetuses (Deurloo et al., 2013), making it important to more thoroughly examine the role of ADAM12 in PE.

α-Klotho is an anti-aging protein produced by the kidney, brain and placenta. Because of mRNA splicing, α-klotho is present as both a full-length membrane-bound form and a truncated circulating soluble protein. Membrane-bound α-klotho is an obligate co-receptor for fibroblast growth factor 23 (FGF23) and its action on FGF receptor (FGFR). ADAM17 causes proteolytic shedding of α-Klotho from the cell membrane, a process that could affect kidney function and the course of chronic kidney disease (Perna et al., 2017). Maternal plasma levels of α-Klotho are elevated in PE, and patients with the highest levels have less placental accelerated villous maturation. α-Klotho, ADAM17 and FGFR are expressed in syncytiotrophoblasts and cytotrophoblasts. Between 32 and 40 weeks gestation, placental levels of α-Klotho, ADAM17 and FGFR are decreased in normal pregnant, but not PE women, suggesting their involvement in PE (Loichinger, Towner, Thompson, Ahn, & Bryant-Greenwood, 2016).

Pulmonary arterial HTN (PAH) is characterized by pulmonary vascular remodeling, SMC proliferation, endothelial dysfunction, and excess ECM. Collagen accumulation plays a role in hypoxic pulmonary HTN, and baicalin prevents bleomycin-induced pulmonary fibrosis. ADAMTS1 degrades ECM substrates associated with vascular remodeling. In rats exposed to hypoxia for 4 weeks, baicalin treatment reduced pulmonary arterial pressure, increased ADAMTS1 expression, attenuated pulmonary artery remodeling, and decreased synthesis of type I collagen (Liu et al., 2015).

In old mice, AngII infusion for 3 days is associated with HTN, kidney damage and increased ADAMTS7 mRNA expression and protein levels, suggesting that ADAMTS7 may contribute to AngII-mediated early inflammatory kidney damage and age-related HTN (Gao et al., 2013).

ADAMTS8 is upregulated in pulmonary artery SMCs (PASMCs) and the lung of mice with hypoxia-induced PAH. Hypoxia-induced PAH is attenuated in SMC-specific ADAMTS8 KO (ADAMTS8$^{\Delta SM22}$) mice. ADAMTS8 overexpression increases PASMC proliferation and downregulates AMP-activated protein kinase (AMPK), while ADAMTS8 deletion causes decreased PASMC proliferation and AMPK upregulation. ADAMTS8 deletion reduces mitochondrial fragmentation in hypoxic conditions. rADAMTS8 induces endothelial dysfunction and MMP activation. Cardiomyocyte-specific ADAMTS8 KO (ADAMTS8$^{\Delta\alpha MHC}$) mice show ameliorated right ventricle failure in response to chronic hypoxia, enhanced angiogenesis and reduced right ventricle ischemia and fibrosis. Mebendazole reduces ADAMTS8 expression and PAH-PASMC proliferation, and ameliorates HTN and right ventricular failure in PAH models, suggesting that ADAMTS8 could be a potential therapeutic target in PAH (Omura et al., 2019).

Non-cirrhotic intrahepatic portal HTN (NCIPH) is characterized by thrombotic microangiopathy of the portal venous system. Plasma vWF/ADAMTS13 balance is altered in NCIPH. Initial sequencing of ADAMTS13 CUB domain revealed one NCIPH patient with a rare missense variant at position c.3829C >T (rs14045669) associated with severe ADAMTS13 deficiency, high vWF, and other missense variants in ADAMTS13, vWF and complement genes. The patient liver biopsy revealed globules of ADAMTS13 in stellate cells. Missense variants in ADAMTS13, vWF and complement genes, and decreased ADAMTS13 activity may play a role in NCIPH (Goel et al., 2017).

ADAMTS16 has been linked to systolic and diastolic BP in the Quebec Family Study. Multiple variants including an Ala to Pro variant in codon 90 (rs2086310) of human ADAMTS16 have been associated with resting systolic BP. Also, a BP quantitative trait locus on rat chromosome 1 was isolated in a short congenic segment spanning 804.6 kb, and contained two genes, LOC306664 and LOC306665. LOC306664 is predicted to translate into Adamts16. Similar to human ADAMTS16, the rat Adamts16 transcript was detected in multiple tissues including the kidney. Also, several genes related to BP were differentially expressed between congenic and Dahl Salt-sensitive (S) rat, and in kidney cell lines with or without Adamts16 knockdown (Joe et al., 2009). Systolic BP is lower and aortic pulse wave velocity and vascular media thickness are less in homozygous Adamts16 mutant rats than S rats. The mechanosensory cilia of ECs are longer and glomerular capillaries show splitting, thickening and longer survival rate in Adamts16 mutant than S rats, suggesting a link between Adamts16, the vascular system and BP regulation (Gopalakrishnan et al., 2012).

9.2 ADAMs and ADAMTS in atherosclerosis

Atherosclerosis is characterized by accumulation of lipoproteins and inflammatory cytokines, and formation of lipid-rich plaques on the arterial inner walls. Macrophages play a role in all stages of atherosclerosis including foam cell formation, ROS production, inflammation, and plaque stability. Apoptosis in the fibrous cap, which is rich in VSMCs and macrophages, and its subsequent weakening and erosion affect plaque stability (Musumeci et al., 2014). In the unstable plaque, perturbed ECs secrete vWF, which interacts with platelet GPIbα and enables platelet adherence to the damaged endothelium. Following plaque rupture, vWF and platelets contact subendothelial collagen, which further supports platelet aggregation, leading to thrombus formation and ischemic events (Howes, Knauper, Malcor, & Farndale, 2020).

ADAM8 is implicated in inflammatory processes, atherosclerosis and MI by regulating immune cell response. In patients undergoing coronary artery bypass graft (CABG), serum levels of sADAM8 are correlated with sCXCL16 levels. ADAM8 expression is increased in left internal thoracic (mammary) arterial graft from coronary bypass patients, suggesting an association with atherosclerosis and CAD. ADAM8 is also upregulated in ECs, circulating neutrophils and in macrophages of high fat diet-fed $ApoE^{-/-}$ and $Ldlr^{-/-}$ mice models of atherosclerosis and mouse model of coronary artery ligation and MI, Human mononuclear cells and neutrophils, and cultured human umbilical artery ECs and arterial SMCs under basal and inflammatory conditions show correlation of ADAM8 with the vascular disease markers ICAM-1, VCAM-1, TNFα, IL-6 and CCL-2 (Schick et al., 2019). ADAM8 deficient mouse macrophages show reduced inflammatory mediators. Although whole-body or hematopoietic-specific ADAM8 deficiency does not influence atherosclerotic lesion size and plaque development in mice, ADAM8 expression is increased in vulnerable atherosclerotic lesions and might still distinguish between stable and unstable lesions (Theodorou et al., 2017).

In atherosclerotic plaques from patients undergoing carotid endarterectomy, ADAM8, 9, 10, 12, 15 and 17 are expressed in both early and advanced lesions, with the highest expression for ADAM15 then ADAM8. ADAM10 and 12 are upregulated in unstable plaques, suggesting their contribution to atherosclerosis progression (Pelisek et al., 2012). ADAM9, 15, and 17 are upregulated and co-localize with CD68-positive cells of monocytic origin in advanced human atherosclerotic lesions from carotid, aortic and femoral territories. Cells expressing ADAMs co-localize with SMCs in the carotid territory, and with CD31-positive ECs in femoral territory, supporting vascular bed-specific ADAM distribution (Oksala et al., 2009). ADAM9 and 15 and αvβ3 and α5β1 integrins are upregulated and colocalized in human atherosclerotic arteries. PDGF increases ADAM9 and 15 and αvβ3 and α5β1 in human VSMCs. ADAM9 and 15 could regulate integrin-ECM interactions and αvβ3 and α5β1 promotion of SMC proliferation/migration during neointima progression (Al-Fakhri et al., 2003).

ADAM10, 15 and 17 regulate inflammatory cell recruitment and macrophage activity by cleaving TNFα, TNFR1, TNFR2 and the scavenger receptor CD163, and promote neovessel formation and atherosclerosis by shedding of VEGFR2 and the angiopoietin growth factor receptor Tie-2 (van der Vorst, Keijbeck, de Winther, & Donners, 2012). In low density lipoprotein receptor *Ldlr*$^{-/-}$ mice on atherogenic diet, myeloid Adam10 deficiency increases plaque collagen content. Adam10-deficient macrophages show impaired MMP-2, 9 and 13 expression/activity, reduced migration toward monocyte chemoattractant protein-1 (MCP-1) and transmigration through collagen, increased anti-inflammatory IL-10, and reduced release of TNFα, IL-12 and nitric oxide in response to LPS, suggesting a role of myeloid ADAM10 in leukocyte recruitment, cytokine production, ECM degradation, and plaque progression/stability (van der Vorst et al., 2015). Atherosclerotic plaques and THP-1 macrophage-derived foam cells show upregulated ADAM10 and downregulated cyclin-dependent kinase inhibitor 2B antisense RNA-1 (CDKN2B-AS1). CDKN2B-AS1 overexpression or ADAM10 silencing reduces lipid accumulation and increases cholesterol efflux. Nuclear CDKN2B-AS1 may bind DNA methyltransferase, increase methylation of ADAM10 promoter, and inhibit ADAM10 transcription, leading to suppressed atherosclerotic inflammatory response and increased cholesterol efflux (Li et al., 2019). Atherosclerotic plaques from internal carotid artery of symptomatic patients show increased caspase-3 and ADAM10, and decreased N-cadherin in the fibrous cap, suggesting a role of apoptotic events triggered by ADAM10-induced N-cadherin cleavage in plaque vulnerability (Musumeci et al., 2014). VEGF upregulates ADAM10 in ECs, induces

ADAM10-mediated cleavage of VE-cadherin, increases vascular permeability and facilitates EC migration, while ADAM10 inhibition reduces EC migration, supporting a role of ADAM10 in atherosclerosis, neovascularization and VEGF-induced EC migration (Donners et al., 2010).

Endothelium injury is an initiating event in atherosclerosis, and ADAM15 regulates endothelial permeability. In $ApoE^{-/-}$ mice, ADAM15 ablation decreases aortic atherosclerotic lesion size, plaque macrophage infiltration and SMC accumulation. EC-derived ADAM15 causes endothelium barrier dysfunction, dissociation of endothelial adherens junctions VE-cadherin/γ-catenin and monocyte transmigration across mouse aortic ECs and HUVECs (Sun et al., 2012). Platelet adhesion to immobilized rADAM15 and ADAM15-overexpressing HUVECs is enhanced under both static and high shear rate conditions, and is reduced by blocking GPIIb-IIIa using neutralizing anti-$\alpha_{IIb}\beta_3$ antibody. sADAM15 binds to activated GPIIb-IIIa. Platelets adherent to ADAM15 attract more platelets under high shear rates indicating platelet-ADAM15 interactions during thrombus formation. Endothelial ADAM15, through GPIIb-IIIa binding, may promote platelet adhesion and activation and thrombus formation, making ADAM15 a potential target for antithrombotic therapies (Langer, May, Bultmann, & Gawaz, 2005).

ADAM17 is upregulated in atherosclerosis (Obama et al., 2015; Palau et al., 2019). In advanced atherosclerosis, vulnerable plaques show defective efferocytosis and reduced removal of apoptotic cells by phagocytic cells. In macrophages, AngII decreases surface expression of Mer tyrosine kinase (MerTK) through ADAM17-mediated shedding of sMerTK, leading to efferocytosis suppression. AngII-activated ADAM17 requires ROS and p38 MAPK phosphorylation. AT_1R blockers suppress ROS production, and ROS scavengers prevent p38 MAPK phosphorylation. Mutant $MERTK^{\Delta 483-488}$ resists AngII-induced shedding and efferocytosis suppression. Thus AngII-activated AT_1R/ROS/MAPK/ADAM17 pathway and MerTK shedding in macrophages leads to defective efferocytosis and atherosclerosis progression (Zhang, Wang, et al., 2019). Among patients from the Vascular Diabetes study the risk for nonfatal MI, nonfatal strokes, peripheral artery procedures and cardiovascular death is increased in individuals with high ADAM17 circulating substrates sICAM-1, sVCAM-1, sIL-6R and sTNFR1. ADAM17 score increased the prediction accuracy of the Framingham Recurring-Coronary-Heart-Disease-Score, and improved the discrimination and correct reclassification of events and non-events, supporting potential usefulness of measuring ADAM17 activity in predicting cardiovascular events in individuals with atherosclerosis (Rizza et al., 2015). Fish oil exerts anti-atherogenic effects by decreasing ADAM10 and 17 activity. In *Ldlr*$^{-/-}$ mice fed a high fat diet, fish oil decreased early atherosclerotic lesions, and reduced circulating EC adhesion molecules JAM-A, ICAM-1 and VE-cadherin, indicating decreased ADAM activity in ECs. The reduced release of adhesion molecules from ECs should improve endothelial barrier function and prevent intimal lipoprotein insudation and macrophage accumulation (Speck et al., 2015). Some studies suggest an opposite role of ADAM17 in atherosclerosis. Adam17 deficient mice (Adam17$^{ex/ex}$) crossed onto Ldlr$^{-/-}$, develop larger atherosclerotic lesions with more macrophages and SMCs than control Adam17$^{wt/wt}$.Ldlr$^{-/-}$ mice. Reduced Adam17-mediated shedding leads to increased membrane-resident TNFα and TNFR2 activation. Cultured Adam17-deficient macrophages and SMCs show proatherosclerotic potential, increased proliferation, reduced apoptosis, and increased adhesion to ECs, and these effects are prevented by Tnfr2 siRNA. Thus, ADAM17 may exert atheroprotective effects mediated by cleaving membrane-bound TNFα and TNFR2, and preventing over-activation of TNFR2 (Nicolaou et al., 2017).

Oxidized low-density lipoprotein (ox-LDL)-induced oxidative stress and apoptosis play a role in atherosclerosis partly through ADAM22 activation. In macrophages, ox-LDL suppresses miR-221-3p expression, transfection of miR-221-3p mimic or silencing ADAM22 reduces, and a miR-221-3p inhibitor increases ox-LDL-induced foam cell formation and cell apoptosis. Thus, miR-221-3p may inhibit ox-LDL-induced foam cell formation and apoptosis by targeting ADAM22 (Zhuang et al., 2019).

ADAM33 is upregulated in atheromas' SMCs and inflammatory cells. ADAM33 gene variants are associated with the extent of atherosclerosis in patients with CAD. ADAM33 neutralizing antibody increases SMC migration through a reconstituted basement membrane, suggesting an inhibitory effect of ADAM33 on SMC migration that could affect the course of atherosclerosis (Holloway et al., 2010).

ADAMTS members also participate in atherosclerosis (Santamaria & de Groot, 2020). ADAMTS1, 4, 5 and 13 are expressed in carotid plaques, especially in SMCs and macrophages, with higher expression of ADAMTS1, little increase in ADAMTS4 and 5, and reduced TIMP-1 in unstable vs stable plaques (Pelisek et al., 2017). Also, while ADAMTS4 or 5 immunoreactive areas are similar, ADAMTS1 immunoreactive area is greater and overlap with those positive for CD68 and versican cleavage products in coronary atherectomy specimens from patients with acute MI vs stable angina, supporting a role of ADMATS1 in the fibrous cap weakening and plaque instability (Lee et al., 2011). Shear stress on ECs promotes atherogenesis, fibrous cap thinning and rupture. Pericytes in the sub-endothelial space have vasoprotective effects, but are subjected to shear stress when EC integrity is disrupted. In cultured ECs and pericytes subjected to high shear stress ECs upregulate ADAMTS1 while pericytes upregulate the ADAMTS1 inhibitor TIMP-3, and ECM proteins are differentially expressed in ECs and pericytes co-cultures. Thus during atherosclerosis development, pericytes sense direct flow and counter-regulate EC ADAMTS1 by protective TIMP-3 expression to prevent ECM degradation and maintain vascular stability (Schrimpf et al., 2017). ADAMTS1, 4 and 5 are upregulated during differentiation of monocytes into macrophages. TGF-β induced ADAMTS1 and 5 and downregulated ADAMTS4. IFN-γ suppressed ADAMTS1 expression. TL-1A or IL-17A alone did not affect ADAMTS1, 4 and 5 expression, but induced their expression synergistically when present together, suggesting differential cytokine-induced regulation of ADAMTS proteases in macrophages which would affect atherosclerotic lesion progression and plaque stability (Ashlin, Kwan, & Ramji, 2013).

ADAMTS1 is upregulated in atherosclerotic plaques and in proliferating/migrating aortic SMCs. ADAMTS1 cleaves versican and other proteoglycans purified from cultured human aortic SMCs. Also, the carotid artery no-flow mouse model shows increased intimal hyperplasia in ADAMTS1 transgenic/ApoE$^{-/-}$ vs ApoE$^{-/-}$ mice, supporting that ADAMTS1 promotes atherogenesis by cleaving versican and facilitating SMC migration (Jonsson-Rylander et al., 2005). In THP-1 macrophages, lauric fatty acid reduces PI_3K and JNK activity and downregulates ADAMTS1, and these effects are reversed by JNK1 siRNA, suggesting that lauric acid stabilizes atherosclerotic plaques and prevents thrombosis by interfering with PI_3K/JNK pathways and ADAMTS1 expression (Ong, Wong, Tengku-Muhammad, Choo, & Chew, 2019).

ADAMTS4 regulates versican turnover in the arterial wall. In patients undergoing carotid endarterectomy, ADAMTS4 expression in the atherosclerotic plaques and its serum level are higher, versican levels are lower, and symptomatic cerebral ischemic events are higher in the vulnerable than stable group, suggesting that ADAMTS4 is an independent risk factor and a potential biomarker for plaque vulnerability (Dong et al., 2018). ADAMTS4 is expressed in macrophages of atherosclerotic lesions, and TGF-β likely through Smads, p38 MAPK and c-Jun pathways downregulates ADAMTS4 in human macrophages and in turn promotes anti-atherogenic and plaque stabilization actions (Salter et al., 2011). In ApoE$^{-/-}$ mice fed high-fat diet, ADAMTS4 expression is increased in plaques as atherosclerosis progresses. ApoE$^{-/-}$Adamts4$^{-/-}$ showed reduced plaque burden, vulnerability index, lipid content and macrophages, more stable plaques, increased SMCs, collagen deposition and fibrotic cap thickness, and altered plasma inflammatory cytokines, further supporting a role of ADAMTS4 in atherosclerosis progression and plaque instability (Chen, Bui, et al., 2013; Kumar et al., 2016).

Biglycan and versican are important lipoprotein-binding proteoglycans. ADAMTS5 releases versican and aggrecan fragments, biglycan and link protein from the aortic wall. ADAMTS5 is reduced while biglycan and versican are increased in atherosclerotic aortas of ApoE$^{-/-}$ mice. Aortas of ADAMTS5-deficient mice show no detectable versican fragments and increased biglycan levels, highlighting the role of ADAMTS5 in degrading vascular proteoglycans reducing their LDL binding ability, and releasing LDL from aortic lesions, thus reducing lipoprotein retention in atherosclerosis (Didangelos, Mayr, Monaco, & Mayr, 2012). ADAMTS5 also degrade the ECM protein matrilin-2. Calcified human aortic valves show reduced ADAMTS5 and increased matrilin-2 and α-smooth muscle actin (α-SMA). Treatment of normal valvular interstitial cells with soluble matrilin-2 increases α-SMA, and these effects are enhanced by ADAMTS5 knockdown. α-SMA knockdown reduces, while α-SMA overexpression increases pro-osteogenic factors and calcium deposits in valvular interstitial cells. Thus, ADAMTS5 deficiency and matrilin-2 accumulation in valvular interstitial cells promote myofibroblastic transition and pro-osteogenic activity, which may contribute to calcific aortic valve disease (Li, Song, et al., 2017).

Large-scale genome-wide association studies (GWAS) have identified SNPs in ADAMTS7 gene with associations to CAD. ADAMTS7 levels were higher in carotid plaques from patients with cerebrovascular symptoms than asymptomatic patients, and correlated with intense CD68-staining and high lipid content and low SMC and collagen content, which are characteristics of a vulnerable plaque. ADAMTS7 levels above median were associated with increased risk for postoperative cardiovascular events, supporting an association of ADAMTS7 with a vulnerable plaque phenotype in human carotid lesions (Bengtsson et al., 2017). COMP is a matricellular protein expressed in cartilage and VSMCs, and maintains VSMC contractile phenotype. COMP is also secreted by platelets and reduces hemostasis and thrombosis. COMP mediates its effects through COMP binding proteins such as integrin $\alpha_7\beta_1$, integrin β_3, thrombin, and bone morphogenetic protein 2.

COMP deficient mice show increased VSMC migration, atherosclerosis and dilated cardiomyopathy. ADAMTS7 degrades COMP, and ADAMTS7 expression correlates with atherosclerosis and vascular calcification in both human GWAS and animal models (Fu & Kong, 2017). In rat carotid artery balloon injury model, ADAMTS7 is accumulated in the neointima mainly in SMCs. Adenovirus-induced ADAMTS7 overexpression increases VSMC proliferation/migration and neointima thickening, and ADAMTS7 siRNA produces opposite effects. Thus, ADAMTS7 facilitates VSMC migration by degrading COMP, and may be a target in atherosclerosis and postangioplasty restenosis (Wang, Wang, & Kong, 2010).

ADAMTS4 and 8 are expressed in macrophage-rich areas of human atherosclerotic carotid plaques and coronary unstable plaques. ADAMTS4 is upregulated in atherosclerotic aortas of $Ldlr^{-/-}ApoB^{100/100}$ mice. ADAMTS4 and 8 are induced during monocyte to macrophage differentiation, and IFN-γ and TNFα enhance ADAMTS4 and 8 expression in macrophages, supporting a role of ADAMTS4 and 8 in the regulation of macrophage-rich areas of atherosclerotic plaques (Wagsater et al., 2008). Also, cardiovascular risk score is increased and show positive correlation with ADAMTS4 and 9 levels in patients with primary hyperparathyroidism and atherosclerosis (Karakose et al., 2018).

ADAMTS13 is released by hepatic stellate cells and ECs, and modulates early atherosclerosis through proteolytic cleavage of ultra-large vWF multimers. vWF is synthesized by ECs and megakaryocytes. Endothelium-derived vWF contributes to atherosclerosis by promoting platelet adhesion and vascular inflammation, whereas platelet-derived vWF, even in the absence of ADAMTS13, is not sufficient to promote atherosclerosis (Doddapattar et al., 2018). Low plasma ADAMTS13 activity is associated with cardiovascular events, MI and stroke. ADAMTS13 co-localizes with vWF in coronary thrombi from patients with acute MI. ADAMTS13 cleaves vWF and reduces inflammation, plaque formation and thrombosis during early atherosclerosis in mice. In kidney podocytes, simvastatin increases while IL-6 decreases ADAMTS13 expression, and simvastatin reverses IL-6 induced inhibition of ADAMTS13 expression, which contributes to its anti-atherosclerotic and anti-thrombotic properties (Shen, Lu, Dong, Ma, & Ruan, 2013). In $ApoE^{-/-}$ and $Adamts13^{-/-}ApoE^{-/-}$ mice fed a high-fat diet, plasma cholesterol levels are similar, but $Adamts13^{-/-}ApoE^{-/-}$ mice show more atherosclerotic lesions in the aorta, increased ratio of plasma high- to low-molecular-weight vWF multimers, reduced leukocyte rolling velocities, and increased number of leukocyte rolling and macrophage infiltration into the atherosclerotic lesions (Jin et al., 2012). Also, an antibody to ADAMTS13 disintegrin domain augments the average surface covered by platelet adhesion and the long axes of platelet thrombi, reduces the ability of plasma ADAMTS13 to cleave ultra-large vWF multimers in type I collagen-coated flow chamber, and augments thrombus formation on injured neointima of rabbit femoral artery, supporting a role of ADAMTS13 in attenuating thrombus growth on injured arteries (Moriguchi-Goto et al., 2009).

9.3 ADAMTS13 deficiency and thrombotic thrombocytopenic purpura (TTP)

vWF is a multimeric hemostatic plasma glycoprotein that acts as a bridging molecule at sites of vascular injury for normal platelet adhesion, and platelet aggregation during high shear. Plasma ADAMTS13 recognizes and cleaves ultra-large vWF multimer into smaller less coagulant forms, and thereby counterbalances its platelet adhesion and prothrombogenic effects (Zheng, 2015). ADAMTS13-mediated proteolysis is determined by rheological shear stress-induced conformational changes in vWF that unfold the A2 domain cleavage site, and its own conformational activation. ADAMTS13 circulates in a closed conformation maintained by a CUB-spacer domain binding, and is conformationally activated on demand through interaction with vWF (South et al., 2014). The ADAMTS13 cysteine-rich and spacer domain exosites bring the enzyme and substrate into proximity to each other, then binding of ADAMTS13 disintegrin domain to vWF allosterically activates the adjacent metalloprotease domain to facilitate proteolysis, such that vWF functions as both a substrate and activating cofactor for ADAMTS13 (Petri et al., 2019). ADAMTS13 cleaves vWF at the Tyr1605-Met1606 (P1-P1′) bond in vWF A2 domain (Xiang, de Groot, Crawley, & Lane, 2011). Truncated ADAMTS13 variants suggest the importance of the disintegrin domain for enzyme activity. Targeted mutagenesis of nonconserved regions in the disintegrin domain identified three ADAMTS13 mutants (R349A, L350G, V352G) with reduced proteolytic activity toward vWF115 (vWF residues 1554–1668). These residues form a predicted exposed exosite on the disintegrin domain ~26 Å from the active site. Kinetic analysis of vWF115 carrying the D1614A mutation suggested that Arg349 in ADAMTS13 disintegrin domain interacts directly with Asp1614 in vWF A2. This interaction positions the scissile bond within the active site of ADAMTS13 and in turn determines the cleavage parameters (K_m and k_{cat}), while the binding affinity

(K_d) of ADAMTS13 for vWF is determined by the spacer domain (de Groot, Bardhan, Ramroop, Lane, & Crawley, 2009).

ADAMTS13 deficiency (inherited or acquired) increases ultra-large vWF multimers and leads to platelet clumping and a microvascular thrombotic disorder termed thrombotic thrombocytopenic purpura (TTP, Moschcowitz disease). Mutations in *ADAMTS13* gene cause chronic relapsing TTP, and ADAMTS13 autoantibodies cause sporadic TTP (Zheng, Majerus, & Sadler, 2002). TTP is characterized by severe thrombocytopenia, microangiopathic hemolytic anemia and ischemic damage in the brain, heart and kidneys. In the microvasculature high shear environment, hyperreactive ultra-large vWF strings remain uncleaved after EC secretion and anchorage, bind to platelets, cause platelet aggregation and form microthrombi, leading to the clinical manifestations of TTP.

Congenital TTP (Upshaw-Schulman syndrome) is a rare autosomal recessive thrombomicroangiopathy caused by inherited ADAMTS13 deficiency. Data from the United Kingdom over 15 years showed 73 cases diagnosed with congenital TTP and confirmed by genetic analysis, with presentation peaks in childhood (age ~3.5 years) and adulthood, typically related to pregnancy (age ~31 years). Genetic mutations differed by age of onset with prespacer mutations more likely associated with childhood onset (Alwan et al., 2019). Congenital TTP results from homozygous or compound heterozygous mutations in ADAMTS13, whereas acquired TTP is an autoimmune disorder caused by circulating ADAMTS13 autoantibodies. TTP is diagnosed by a combination of symptoms, severe deficiency in plasma ADAMTS13 activity, and detection of ADAMTS13 antibodies (Crawley & Scully, 2013), with some cases showing open ADAMTS13 conformation and exposed cryptic epitope in the spacer domain (Roose et al., 2018).

Current treatment of acute TTP includes plasma exchange to provide functional ADAMTS13 and remove inhibitory antibodies. In patients with congenital TTP in the United Kingdom, fresh-frozen plasma and factor VIII concentrate were used, and 88% of patients showed normal blood counts and symptoms resolution. The 3-weekly regimen of fresh-frozen plasma was insufficient for 70% of patients, and weekly or fortnightly infusions were required. Stroke incidence was reduced with prophylactic therapy, but long-term the risk of end-organ damage was seen in 75% of patients with late diagnosis of congenital TTP (Alwan et al., 2019). Immunosuppressive drugs such as corticosteroids and rituximab (RTX) supplement plasma exchange (PEX) therapy in patients with acquired

TTP (Kremer Hovinga et al., 2017). Following PEX/RTX therapy, patients remain in remission for extended periods, with continuing reduction in ADAMTS13 antibodies (Becerra et al., 2015). Anti-CD20, rADAMTS13, hyperreactive ADAMTS13 variant and anti-vWF therapy are under development (Crawley & Scully, 2013). Prophylactic ADAMTS13 replacement may decrease the risk of end-organ damage and ischemic stroke (Alwan et al., 2019). In patients with severe congenital ADAMTS13 deficiency and plasma activity <6% rADAMTS13 (BAX 930) increased vWF cleavage products and reduced vWF multimeric size, and was well tolerated with no serious adverse events or detection of anti-ADAMTS13 antibodies (Scully et al., 2017).

Acute MI may occur secondary to TTP. A report described an 80-year-old male with acute MI, who was treated by percutaneous coronary intervention, but then developed thrombocytopenia, acute kidney injury and hemolytic anemia. Acquired TTP was diagnosed based on decreased ADAMTS13 levels and the presence of ADAMTS13 autoantibodies, and the patient eventually died of multiorgan failure despite repeated plasma exchanges and immunosuppressive therapies with corticosteroid and RTX, thus alerting that TTP could be an underlying cause of acute MI (Takimoto et al., 2016).

TTP can also present in pregnancy with typical microangiopathy and thrombocytopenia, and risk of *in utero* fetal loss. ADAMTS13 activity <10% is consistent with late-onset congenital TTP or acquired TTP; the former will require plasma therapy and the latter immunosuppression (Scully, 2016).

ADAMTS13$^{-/-}$ mice receiving rh-ultra-large vWF multimers show TTP-like features, thrombocytopenia, schistocytosis (increased fragmented red blood cells), decreased hematocrit, elevated serum lactate dehydrogenase, platelet aggregation in the ventricles and myocardial necrosis, and rhADAMTS13 reduces the incidence and severity of TTP in ADAMTS13$^{-/-}$ mice (Schiviz et al., 2012).

Of note, complete ADAMTS13 deficiency does not lead to continuous microangiopathy, Plasminogen binds to vWF A1 domain. In the absence of ADAMTS13, plasminogen activation by uPA or streptokinase causes rapid degradation of platelet-vWF complexes on ECs. Plasminogen activation and plasma levels of plasmin-α2-antiplasmin complexes increase with the extent of thrombocytopenia in acute TTP, independent of ADAMTS13 activity. Also, streptokinase shows benefits in Adamts13$^{-/-}$ mouse model of TTP. Thus, plasminogen activation on ECs may be a natural backup for

ADAMTS13 to degrade platelet-vWF complexes, and thrombolytic agents may bypass ADAMTS13 autoantibodies and have benefits in microangiopathies (Tersteeg et al., 2014).

Bleeding events are frequent complications of left ventricular assist device, due to shear stress-induced unfolding of large vWF multimers and its accelerated proteolysis by ADAMTS13 (Proudfoot, Davidson, & Strueber, 2017). Blood of patients with a left ventricular assist device shows reduced large vWF multimers and increased 10/11 vWF degradation fragments. Also, in normal human blood exposed to supraphysiologic shear stress in a laboratory vortexer ADAMTS13 cleaves large vWF multimers and generates 11/11 vWF degradation fragments, suggesting that ADAMTS13 could be targeted to reduce vWF degradation and bleeding complications of left ventricular assist device (Bartoli, Restle, Zhang, Acker, & Atluri, 2015).

9.4 ADAMs and ADAMTS in coronary artery disease

Coronary artery disease (CAD) results from blockage of the coronary arteries by plaque buildup. In HUVECs, IL-6 and sIL-6R induce inflammation, increase glycoprotein130 and decrease soluble glycoprotein130 levels, and these effects are reversed by estradiol treatment. Estradiol-through activation of estrogen α/β receptor and increased release of ADAM10 and 17 could alter the inflammatory pathways and the course of inflammation in atherosclerosis and CAD (Zhou, Dai, Cui, & Li, 2020).

Decreased endothelial ADAM10 activity is linked to dysregulated Notch signaling and defective coronary arterial cell differentiation. Endothelium-specific ADAM10 deficient mice ($ADAM10^{\Delta EC}$) show reduced coronary endothelial EGFR signaling, enlarged hearts, abnormal myocardial compaction, and immature endothelium markers, implicating ADAM10/Notch signaling in coronary arterial cell specification and heart development, and suggesting a role of endothelial ADAM10 in EGFR signaling and the regenerative capacity and maturation of the coronary vasculature (Farber et al., 2019).

Circulating ADAM17 substrates sICAM-1, sVCAM-1, sIL-6R and sTNFR1 have been linked to recurring cardiovascular events in patients with atherosclerosis, making ADAM17 an attractive biomarker and therapeutic target in CAD (Rizza et al., 2015). ADAM17 also regulate angiogenesis and myocardial cell repair post-MI in patients with CAD (Fan et al., 2015; van der Vorst et al., 2012).

ADAMTS aggrecanases regulate vascular proteoglycans and ECM remodeling during in-stent restenosis. Immunostaining shows more aggrecan and its fragments in human stented coronary arteries at the contacts of the stent struts with the artery, in human arteries than veins, and on grafting a vein into the arterial circulation, suggesting aggrecan contribution to vascular plasticity. In pig coronary arteries implanted with overstretched drug-eluting stents, the neointima shows increases in calcification proteins, and the media shows changes in inflammatory and thrombotic factors, followed by changes in ECM proteins. By day 28 post-implantation, basement membrane proteins are less in drug-eluting than bare-metal stents, and aggrecan is increased with a shift from ADAMTS1 and 5 to ADAMTS4 gene expression, implicating aggrecan and aggrecanases in the vascular injury response after stenting. Mice lacking ADAMTS5 show aggrecan accumulation and dilation of thoracic aorta, supporting a role of aggrecanases in vascular remodeling (Suna et al., 2018).

Plasma ADAMTS4 level is increased in acute coronary syndromes, and further elevated with progression from stable angina to unstable angina, to non-ST-segment elevation MI (NSTEMI), to ST-segment elevation MI (STEMI), and serial measurements of plasma ADAMTS4 may be a marker of plaque destabilization in acute coronary syndromes (Zha et al., 2010). Also, in patients undergoing elective coronary angiography, ADAMTS4 levels are higher in patients with than without CAD, are increased with the number of diseased vessels, are associated with the severity of stenosis score, are correlated with the presence/severity of CAD, and are lower in statin-treated than non-treated patients, suggesting that serum ADAMTS4 levels may be an independent predictor of CAD (Chen, Yang, Zha, & Cui, 2011).

In patients with stable obstructive CAD, plasma ADAMTS7 levels are positively correlated with the Syntax score CAD severity tertiles (low, moderate, high), and are greater in the high than the low Syntax score group. Event-free survival rate is less in the high than low plasma ADAMTS7 group, supporting that ADAMTS7 contributes to severity of CAD (Yu et al., 2016). ADAMTS7 accumulates in VSMCs in coronary atherosclerotic plaques. In a population-based study, an inverse association was observed between atherosclerosis prevalence and rs3825807, a non-synonymous SNP (A to G) leading to a Ser-to-Pro substitution in ADAMTS7 pro-domain. The rs3825807 variant-mediated protection from atherosclerosis and CAD may involve reduced ADAMTS7 maturation and its prodomain cleavage, decreased cleavage of thrombospondin-5, and reduced VSMC migration (Pu et al., 2013). CABG is a beneficial approach in CAD, but is prone to vein graft restenosis. Upregulation of ADAMTS7 contributes to neointima formation and graft restenosis by promoting VSMC proliferation/migration and inhibiting EC proliferation/migration. Aberrant miR-423 levels in plasma of CAD patients prior to and following CABG suggest that it may affect vein graft patency. Dual-luciferase reporter gene assay indicates that miR-423 interacts with ADAMTS7. Overexpression of miR-423 suppresses ADAMTS7, decreases proliferation/migration of human umbilical vein SMCs, increases proliferation/migration of HUVECs, enhances re-endothelialization and decreases neointima formation in a rat vein graft model, suggesting that upregulation of miR-423 and downregulation of ADAMTS7 could reduce autologous vein graft restenosis in patients undergoing CABG (Ren et al., 2020). Rat model of carotid artery balloon injury show neointima formation and increased Adamts7 expression. *Adamts7*-deficient mice show reduced neointima formation following vascular injury, supporting that ADAMTS7 could be a target for intervention in CAD (Muller, Kessler, Schunkert, Erdmann, & Tennstedt, 2016).

Studies examined the association of genetic variants of ADAMTS13 (P475S, Q448E, rs2073932, P618A, A900V, S903L, rs652600, rs4962153) and vWF (V1565L, Y1584C), as well as ADAMTS13 activity, vWF antigen and vWF activity with CAD risk in Thai CAD and non-CAD patients. None of ADAMTS13 polymorphisms or haplotypes was associated with ADAMTS13 activity. vWF V1565L polymorphism was associated with increased ADAMTS13 activity, and the QAGA or H4 haplotype of ADAMTS13 gene had an independent protective effect on CAD (Lasom et al., 2017).

9.5 ADAMs and ADAMTS in myocardial infarction

Genotyping of samples from the Finnish cardiovascular study showed increased MI risk and higher sADAM8 serum levels for carriers of the rs2995300 C allele and rs2275725 A allele, suggesting a prognostic potential of ADAM8 in MI (Raitoharju et al., 2011). In rats undergoing cardiac transplantation after cardiac arrest to induce I/R injury and rats undergoing left anterior coronary artery ligation to cause MI, edematous intramyocardial artery nuclei and periadventitial inflammation were more prominent in MI than I/R injury and control rats. In MI rats, ADAM8 expression was increased and localized to the vicinity of the infarcted area and to remote intramyocardial arteries (Vuohelainen et al., 2011).

In Wistar rats subjected to MI by ligation of left anterior descending coronary artery, ADAM15 expression initially increases then gradually decreases. ADAM15 is localized at cardiac myocytes in the border area of MI and at macrophages in the border and infarcted areas, suggesting a role in the inflammatory response and cardiac remodeling associated with MI (Li, Du, Jiang, & Tian, 2009).

Compared with sham-controls, Wistar rats with ligated coronary artery show MI, worse systolic function, greater left ventricular weight index, increased ADAM17 expression, upregulated TNFα, and decreased TIMP-3. In MI rats, ADAM17 expression correlates positively with increased left ventricular end-diastolic and end-systolic diameters and negatively with left ventricular ejection fraction, suggesting a link between ADAM17 expression, increased TNFα, and post-MI cardiac remodeling (Zheng, Zhao, Yang, Wang, & Zhang, 2016). Other studies suggest a protective role of ADAM17 in ischemic cardiomyopathy. Cardiomyocyte-specific ADAM17 knockdown mice ($ADAM17^{flox/flox/\alpha\text{-}MHC\text{-}Cre}$) are more vulnerable to coronary artery ligation-induced MI than control mice ($ADAM17^{flox/flox}$), and show unfavorable survival, higher rates of cardiac rupture, more severe ventricular dilation and decreased ejection fraction, and the infarcted areas show reduced myocardial vascular density, lectin perfusion, CD31 staining, NF-κB activity and VEGFR2 expression. Thus ADAM17 may promote post-MI recovery by regulating VEGFR2 transcription and angiogenesis, and limiting left ventricular dysfunction (Fan et al., 2015).

ADAMTS1 shows diffuse distribution in the myocardium of individuals who died of MI or trauma. The MI group show no ADAMTS1 staining around fibrotic areas, and slight ADAMTS1 staining and similar localization of fragmented versican in coagulative and necrotic zones (Pehlivan et al., 2016). In rat MI model, ADAMTS1 is upregulated in the endothelium and myocardium of infarcted heart 3h post-MI, making it one of the early genes expressed in the ischemic heart (Nakamura et al., 2004).

In patients with STEMI and NSTEMI, plasma ADAMTS7 levels are higher in patients with left ventricular ejection fraction (LVEF) $\leq$35% than those with LVEF >35%, correlate positively with brain natriuretic peptide, left ventricular mass index, and left ventricular end-diastolic and end-systolic diameters, and correlate negatively with the 6-min walk test of aerobic capacity and endurance, suggesting a role of ADAMTS7 in ventricular remodeling after acute MI (Wu et al., 2015).

Culprit atherosclerotic plaques from patients with acute MI show a smaller area for smooth muscle α-actin, and a greater area for the EC marker CD31 or macrophage marker CD68 than plaques from patients with stable angina. Also, the immunoreactive areas for ADAMTS2, 3, and 13 overlap with CD31 or CD68, and are larger in acute MI (Lee et al., 2012). On the other hand, the Glasgow MI Study showed no correlation between ADAMTS13 and vWF levels in MI cases. ADAMTS13 levels correlated positively with serum cholesterol and triglycerides and body mass index, and negatively with high-density lipoprotein-cholesterol. vWF levels correlated with age, fibrinogen and C-reactive protein. vWF correlated positively and ADAMTS13 correlated negatively with risk of MI (Crawley, Lane, Woodward, Rumley, & Lowe, 2008). Another study showed elevated vWF activity and vWF antigen and decreased ADAMTS13 activity following percutaneous coronary intervention in STEMI patients with intramyocardial hemorrhage vs those without intramyocardial hemorrhage. However, vWF and ADAMTS13 activities were not correlated with infarct size. Also, intracoronary administration of rADAMTS13 did not decrease infarct size or intramyocardial hemorrhage in a porcine model of myocardial I/R, suggesting that vWF/ADAMTS13 imbalance may not be the cause of no reflow (Eerenberg et al., 2016). Nevertheless, vWF/ADAMTS13 imbalance should be monitored in patients with MI. A study reported an old male patient who was receiving the purinergic P2Y12 receptor antagonist ticagrelor for STEMI, and presented with severe thrombocytopenia, anemia, renal and liver dysfunction, heart failure and fever. Blood samples showed schistocytosis and low ADAMTS13 activity, consistent with TTP. Cessation of ticagrelor and plasma exchange improved the patient condition, but re-administration of ticagrelor aggravated TTP and led to the patient's death, highlighting the risk of purinergic receptor antagonist-induced low ADAMTS13 and TTP in patients with MI (Wang, Zhang, et al., 2018).

9.6 ADAMs and ADAMTS in cardiac hypertrophy and heart failure

Patients with dilated cardiomyopathy show increased myocardial ADAM10 and 15 expression and integrin-β1D cleavage. ADAM10 expression correlates with chamber dilatation and systolic dysfunction. Hemodynamic unloading reduced ADAM10 and 12 and increased integrin-β1D expression. ADAM12 and integrin-β1D are increased in hypertrophic obstructive cardiomyopathy, and ADAM17 is increased in dilated cardiomyopathy and hypertrophic obstructive cardiomyopathy, suggesting different roles of ADAMs in myocardial structural remodeling and integrin shedding (Fedak et al., 2006).

Cardiac ADAM12 levels are increased in a mouse model of heart failure induced by aorta-to-vena cava shunt (Mishra, Tyagi, Sen, Givvimani, & Tyagi, 2010), and hydrogen sulfide (H_2S) donors ameliorate heart failure by decreasing ADAM12 (Donnarumma, Trivedi, & Lefer, 2017; Mishra et al., 2010; Salloum, 2015). In cardiomyocytes, GPCR agonists cause hypertrophy and HB-EGF shedding through metalloproteinase and EGFR transactivation. Also, the ADAM12 inhibitor KB-R7785 blocks HB-EGF shedding and ameliorates cardiac hypertrophy in mouse transaortic constriction model (Asakura et al., 2002). In mice with transverse aortic constriction, atorvastatin causes reduction of heart/body weight, decreased left ventricular end-diastolic pressure, increased fractional shortening, downregulation of ADAM12, ADAM17 and HB-EGF, and reduced EGFR and ERK activity. In neonatal rat cardiomyocytes, atorvastatin inhibits phenylephrine-induced protein synthesis, EGFR phosphorylation and ERK activity (Liao et al., 2008). However, 4 weeks after transaortic constriction ADAM12 KO mice show advanced cardiac hypertrophy, higher mortality rates, and more cardiac fibrosis and collagen-related gene expression in failing hearts than WT mice. ADAM12 deficient mice also show enhanced focal adhesion- and fibrosis-related signaling pathways, increased integrin β1 and TGF-β receptor I and III, and phosphorylation of focal adhesion kinase, Akt, mammalian target of rapamycin, ERK, and Smad2/3 in the heart, resulting in cardiac dysfunction (Nakamura et al., 2020). These discrepant findings make it important to further examine the role of ADAM12 in heart failure.

ADAM17 and TNFα levels are higher in mononuclear cells from patients with severe congestive heart failure (CHF) than mild CHF patients and controls (Satoh, Iwasaka, et al., 2004). The peroxisome proliferator-activated receptor-α (PPAR-α) agonist fenofibrate reduces heart/body weight, left ventricular wall thickness and ADAM17 expression In aortic constriction-induced hypertensive rats, and reduces AngII-induced hypertrophy and ADAM17 expression in cardiomyocytes, suggesting that PPAR-α agonists ameliorate cardiac hypertrophy by downregulating ADAM17 (Zeng, Lu, Yan, & Zou, 2018). ACE2 cleaves AngII to Ang-(1-7) and protects against cardiac hypertrophy, while ADAM17 cleaves ACE2 and contributes to AngII-induced heart damage. In AngII-infused mice Dickkopf-3 overexpression is associated with less cardiac hypertrophy and fibrosis, decreased expression of the hypertrophic genes atrial natriuretic peptide and β-myosin heavy chain and the fibrotic genes collagen I and III, reduced ADAM17 phosphorylation, and increased ACE2 expression and AngII degradation (Zhai, Xu, et al., 2018). Rats with aortic coarctation-induced myocardial hypertrophy show increased nicotinamide adenine dinucleotide phosphate oxidase 4 (Nox4) and ADAM17. Nox4 and ROS mediate AngII-induced hypertrophy of cardiac myocytes partly through upregulation of ADAM17 and increased release of mature HB-EGF, and ADAM17 siRNA decreases phospho-EGFR/EGFR ratio and EGFR activation in hypertrophic cardiomyocytes (Zeng et al., 2013). However, in mice with cardiac pressure-overload induced by transverse aortic constriction, cardiomyocyte-specific ADAM17 knockdown mice (ADAM17$^{f/f}$/Cre) show enhanced myocardial hypertrophy, fibrosis, left ventricular dilation, and systolic dysfunction, and greater upregulation of integrin β1 and activation of the focal adhesion kinase pathway vs mice with intact ADAM17 (ADAM17$^{f/f}$). ADAM17 knockdown does not affect AngII infusion-induced myocardial hypertrophy, which does not require integrin β1-mediated pathway. ADAM17 knockdown also enhances hypertrophy induced by cyclic mechanical stretching in neonatal rat cardiomyocytes. Thus, ADAM17 could be cardioprotective in pressure overload but not agonist-induced cardiac hypertrophy likely through cleavage of cardiac integrin β1 (Fan et al., 2016).

ADAM22 expression is increased in patients with hypertrophic cardiomyopathy. In mice with transaortic constriction, cardiac-specific ADAM22 KO deteriorates, while ADAM22 overexpression mitigates, cardiac hypertrophy. Cardiac-specific ADAM22 KO is associated with enhanced Akt activity in transaortic constriction-induced mice and AngII-stimulated neonatal rat cardiomyocytes, and Akt inhibitors attenuate transaortic constriction-induced cardiac hypertrophy, suggesting that ADAM22 reduces Akt activity and cardiac hypertrophy (Ren et al., 2018).

ADAM23 expression is decreased in failing human heart and hypertrophic mouse heart. Cardiac-specific ADAM23 KO mice show increased cardiac hypertrophy, fibrosis, and dysfunction, and mice overexpressing ADAM23 in the heart show reduced pressure overload-induced cardiac hypertrophy. Similar findings are observed in AngII-induced neonatal rat cardiomyocyte hypertrophy. The focal adhesion kinase inhibitor PF-562271 reverses the detrimental effects in ADAM23 KO mice subjected to aortic banding, supporting that ADAM23 protects against cardiac hypertrophy through inhibition of the focal adhesion kinase-Akt signaling pathway (Xiang et al., 2018).

ADAMTS2 is upregulated in failing human heart and hypertrophic mouse heart. GPCR agonists induce cardiac hypertrophy, and *Adamts2* gene could drive isoproterenol-induced cardiac hypertrophy in mice (Rau et al., 2017). Other studies suggest that ADAMTS2 cleaves the N-propeptides from procollagens type I, II, III and V, thus allowing the formation and assembly of collagen fibrils (Bekhouche & Colige, 2015). Mice lacking ADAMTS2 show increased pressure overload-induced cardiac hypertrophy, because their collagen fibrils have inadequate mechanical strength to counteract pressure overload, while mice with cardiac-specific overexpression of ADAMTS2 show alleviated cardiac hypertrophy. Also, loss or gain of function experiments in neonatal rat cardiomyocytes show that ADAMTS2 decreases AngII-induced cardiomyocyte hypertrophy. Blocking the phosphoinositide 3-kinase (PI_3K)/Akt pathway ameliorates the hypertrophic response to the loss of ADAMTS2, supporting that ADAMTS2 attenuates cardiac hypertrophy through inhibition of PI_3K/Akt signaling (Wang et al., 2017).

Myocardial ADAMTS1, 4 and 8, and versican and aggrecan levels are increased in rat aortic banding model, and TNFα and IL-1β increase ADAMTS4 and versican in neonatal cardiomyocytes. Pentosan polysulfate was used to inhibit ADAMTS4 and was found to improve left ventricular systolic function and fractional shortening after aortic banding, and reduce extracellular versican fragments, supporting a role of increased versicanase activity in hypertrophic cardiomyopathy, and that ADAMTS4 inhibition could improve systolic function in heart failure (Vistnes et al., 2014).

In mice with pressure overload hypertrophic cardiomyopathy, treatment with rhADAMTS13 is associated with less endothelium-associated vWF, platelet aggregates and profibrotic TGF-β1 levels, preservation of cardiac function and less fibrotic remodeling (Witsch et al., 2018).

9.7 ADAMs and ADAMTS in ischemic stroke

Ischemic stroke is linked to Alzheimer's disease and increased amyloid-β and APP. ADAM10 is upregulated in patients with atherosclerotic cerebral infarction carrying the rs653765 C > T mutation (Li et al., 2013). In neuronal SH-SY5Y cells, exposure to hypoxia decreases ADAM10 levels and reduces APP processing by the neuroprotective ADAM10 α-secretase pathway (Webster, Green, Settle, Peers, & Vaughan, 2004).

The frequencies of ADAM17 SNPs rs11684747, rs11689958, rs12692386, rs55790676 and rs1524668 or ADAM17 haplotypes do not differ between ischemic stroke patients and healthy subjects. However, ADAM17-rs1524668 A > G polymorphism shows higher ADAM17 expression and an association with the partial anterior circulation infarcts subtype of ischemic stroke (Li et al., 2014). ADAM17-induced ectodomain shedding of platelet GPIbα is important in hemostasis and thrombosis. Patients with acute atherosclerotic ischemic stroke show increased plasma glycocalicin and ADAM17 levels and decreased platelet GPIbα, suggesting ADAM17 as a risk factor for acute ischemic stroke, and GPIbα expression as a measure for stroke severity (Ling et al., 2013).

ADAMTS1, 4, 5 and 9 proteoglycanases play a role in ECM turnover in the CNS and their expression is dysregulated in cerebral ischemic stroke and acute spinal cord injury (Lemarchant et al., 2013). Studies of ADAMTS1 gene polymorphism suggest that the frequencies of the rs402007 GC + CC genotype and the C allele are different and may represent susceptibility factors in ischemic stroke patients vs controls (Lyu et al., 2015). Rat models of focal cerebral ischemia induced by transient middle cerebral artery occlusion show increased ADAMTS1 and 4, IL-1β, IL-1 receptor antagonist and TNFα in the occluded hemisphere. Also, in human astrocytes, TNFα upregulates ADAMTS4, suggesting that TNFα-induced ADAMTS1 and 4 facilitate ECM breakdown, inflammatory cell infiltration and brain injury following stroke (Cross et al., 2006). Other studies confirmed an increase in ADAMTS4 expression in the ischemic brain hemisphere of stroke patients and mice models of cerebral ischemia. However, in primary microglia or astrocytes, pretreatment with rhADAMTS4 decreased while transfection with ADAMTS4 siRNA increased LPS-induced production of NO and the inflammatory cytokines MCP-1, TNFα, IL-1β and MMP-9. In a mouse model of neuroinflammation induced by middle cerebral artery occlusion, ADAMTS4 decreased astrogliosis and macrophage infiltration, and increased microglia expressing arginase-1, a marker of reduced inflammation, and IL-10 production in the peri-ischemic area, suggesting ADAMTS4 anti-inflammatory and neuro-regenerative effects that could be useful in ischemic stroke and traumatic brain or spinal cord injury (Lemarchant et al., 2016).

Studies of SNPs of ADAMTS13 gene showed an association of rs2285467 with stroke. Also, ADAMTS13 mRNA is elevated in blood cells of systemic lupus erythematosus patients with history of stroke (Lopez De Padilla et al., 2013). In a prospective study, patients with ADAMTS13 activity in the lowest quartile had a higher risk of ischemic stroke than those in the highest quartile. Adding ADAMTS13 to the predictive model improved the accuracy of risk prediction of ischemic stroke (Sonneveld et al., 2015).

Patients with cerebral infarction also show higher vWF antigen, and lower ADAMTS13, vWF collagen binding activity/vWF antigen and ADAMTS13/vWF antigen, supporting that increased vWF levels and reduced ADAMTS13 activity may contribute to the pathogenesis of cerebral infarction (Qu et al., 2016). vWF/ADAMTS13 imbalance is also a risk factor of neonatal thrombosis, pediatric stroke and secondary microangiopathies (Katneni, Ibla, Hunt, Schiller, & Kimchi-Sarfaty, 2019). In pediatric patients with ischemic stroke, 22% of patients showed decreased ADAMTS13 levels (Lambers et al., 2013). Also, among pediatric stroke patients 241 variants (SNPs or insertions/deletions) in the ADAMTS13 gene have been identified, 10 SNPs were associated with pediatric stroke, and rs2285489 and rs28793911 were associated with ADAMTS13 levels. A protective haplotype H1.1. was associated with increased ADAMTS13 levels, supporting a link between decreased ADAMTS13 levels and stroke susceptibility (Stoll et al., 2016).

Inherited TTP may present with ischemic stroke in adults. A young male with recurrent strokes, who relapsed despite anticoagulant therapy showed plasma ADAMTS13 activity <5% with no anti-ADAMTS13 IgG, and sequencing of the ADAMTS13 gene led to the diagnosis of Upschaw-Schulman syndrome. The patient received fresh frozen plasma every 2 weeks, and 1 year after diagnosis was free of neurological symptoms (Beauvais et al., 2019). ADAMTS13 may promote brain angiogenesis, neovascularization and ischemic brain repair. Studies in patients undergoing endovascular treatment of ischemic stroke showed that low ADAMTS13 activity and missing of statin therapy were independently associated with poor clinical outcome to recanalization therapies (Schuppner et al., 2018). While thrombolysis with tissue plasminogen activator (tPA) is effective in acute ischemic stroke, ADAMTS13 by virtue of cleaving vWF could be an alternative therapy if tPA is not available or in tPA resistant thrombi (Chen, Cheng, Zhang, & Wu, 2019). Notably, in acute ischemic stroke cases with arterial occlusion, patients who achieved intravenous tPA-induced recanalization had higher baseline ADAMTS13 activity compared to futile recanalization in patients treated with mechanical thrombectomy. Absence of early ischemic signs and ADAMTS13 activity >75% were independent predictors of recanalization, and reduced ADAMTS13 level was an independent predictor of futile recanalization (Bustamante et al., 2018).

In mouse model of ischemic stroke, *Adamts13*$^{-/-}$ mice show reduced neovascularization, brain capillary perfusion, pericyte and SMC coverage on microvessels and expression of tight junction proteins, and accelerated BBB breakdown and extravascular deposits of serum proteins in the peri-infarct cortex, as well as decreased angiopoietin-2 and galectin-3 in brain microvessels, and these effects were reversed in vWF deficient mice, by treatment with anti-vWF antibody, or by adenovirus-mediated overexpression of angiopoietin-2 or galectin-3 (Xu, Cao, et al., 2017). Also, in mouse model of focal cerebral ischemia, vWF deficiency reduced infarct volume, while ADAMTS13 deficiency resulted in larger infarctions. Infusion of rhADAMTS13 in WT mice reduced infarct volume, increased neovascularization and vascular repair, and improved functional outcome, supporting potential benefits of ADAMTS13 in ischemic stroke (Zhao et al., 2009). Although tPA is approved for treatment of acute ischemic stroke, it increases the risk of cerebral hemorrhage. In normal mice, rADAMTS13 blocked tPA- and vWF-induced BBB permeability. In mouse stroke model, intravenous tPA exacerbated BBB disruption and cerebral hemorrhage. rADAMTS13 attenuated these effects through inhibition of tPA-mediated Akt phosphorylation, RhoA activation and upregulation of VEGF, and rvWF reversed the antihemorrhagic effect of rADAMTS13 (Wang et al., 2013). Also, in a mouse model of cerebral hemorrhage induced by intracerebral infusion of autologous blood, rADAMTS13 reduced chemokines and cytokines levels, neutrophil recruitment, myeloperoxidase activity and microglia activation. rADAMTS13 also reduced ICAM-1 levels and MMP-9 activity, attenuated BBB disruption, cerebral edema and hemorrhagic lesion volume, increased pericyte coverage of brain microvessels, and improved neurological functions. Also, in brain ECs, rADAMTS13 decreased LPS-induced IL-6 expression, and rvWF reversed this effect, supporting potential benefits of rADAMTS13 against inflammation and BBB dysfunction following intracerebral hemorrhage (Cai et al., 2015).

ADAMTS18 secretion by ECs enhances platelet fragmentation and thrombus dissolution. A C-terminal 385-aa fragment of ADAMTS18 induces platelet fragmentation and destroys platelet aggregates induced *ex vivo* by ADP or collagen and fibrinogen. Also, the C-terminal ADAMTS18 fragment with a glutathione S-transferase tag (named rADAMTS-351) promotes platelet fragmentation (Dang et al., 2012), facilitates platelet thrombus dissolution, and protects against $FeCI_3$-induced carotid artery thrombosis and cerebral infarction in a mouse model of ischemic stroke (Li et al., 2009). In support, anti-ADAMTS18 antibody shortens the tail vein bleeding time (Li, Nardi, et al., 2009). Also, *Adamts18*$^{-/-}$ *mice* display accelerated $FeCl_3$-induced carotid artery thrombosis and aggravated postischemic cerebral infarction, due to lack of ADAMTS18-mediated-platelet fragmentation (Dang et al., 2018).

9.8 ADAMs and ADAMTS in ischemia-reperfusion injury

I/R injury causes structural and functional changes in the heart, liver, kidney and brain. I/R injury interferes with blood flow restoration to ischemic myocardium, and causes oxidative stress and apoptosis. In mouse models of I/R injury, all-trans retinoic acid promotes anti-apoptotic effects, improves cardiac function, decreases the infarcted area, ROS production and phosphorylation of MAPKs p38, JNK and ERK, increases ADAM10 expression and RAGE cleavage, and decreases RAGE, and the cardiac protective effects are not observed in RAGE KO mice (Zhu et al., 2015).

In isolated rabbit heart, ischemic preconditioning (induced by two cycles of 5 min ischemia/5 min reperfusion) or pretreatment with AngII reduced infarction size (induced by 30 min ischemia/2 h reperfusion), increased TNFα release into the coronary effluent, and augmented tyrosine phosphorylation of target proteins running at ~60 and 90 kDa in gel electrophoresis of cardiac tissue samples, and these effects were abolished by the tyrosine kinase inhibitor genistein or ADAM17 inhibitor KB-R7785. Pretreatment with TNFα decreased infarct size and induced tyrosine phosphorylation of 60 kDa protein, suggesting that ADAM17 regulates TNFα shedding, and promotes ischemic preconditioning through a tyrosine kinase pathway (Ichikawa et al., 2004).

The endothelial glycocalyx could be damaged during hypoxia, I/R injury, stress-related sympathoadrenal activation, and inflammation. In HUVECs, epinephrine or epinephrine + hydrogen peroxide (H_2O_2) increased ADAM17 and MMP-9 activity, glycocalyx degradation and shedding of syndecan-1, hyaluronic acid and TNFα, and these effects were prevented by the serine protease inhibitor tranexamic acid or MMP inhibitor doxycycline, supporting the clinical practice of early tranexamic acid treatment in severely injured patients (Diebel, Martin, Liberati, & Diebel, 2018).

Hepatic I/R injury could cause serious liver damage and affect the outcome of liver surgery or transplantation. TNFα and its receptors play a role in the inflammatory response after hepatic I/R injury. ADAM17 levels are low in normal rat liver. Rats subjected to hepatic I/R show increases in ADAM17 expression and upregulation of TNFα, TNFR1 and IL-6. ADAM17 inhibition by TIMP-3 decreased circulating TNFα and alanine transferase and improved hepatic I/R injuries (Tang, Loss, Carmody, & Cohen, 2006).

In rats subjected to bilateral renal I/R injury, renal VEGF and VEGFR1 (flt-1) were reduced, plasma soluble flt-1 was elevated, and the expression of

ADAMTS1, which inhibits VEGF, was increased in proximal tubules. ADAMTS1-mediated inhibition of the VEGF pathway during early renal I/R injury may reduce renal microvascular density and lead to chronic renal damage (Basile, Fredrich, Chelladurai, Leonard, & Parrish, 2008).

ADAMTS13 deficiency causes thrombotic microangiopathy and multi-organ damage during I/R of the heart, liver, kidney and brain. In mice with MI produced by transient ligation of left anterior descending coronary artery, mortality and infarct size was in ADAMTS13$^{-/-}$ > WT > WT + ADAMTS13 mice, and microvascular reflow in the risk area was in ADAMTS13$^{-/-}$ < WT < WT + ADAMTS13 mice. Platelet glycoprotein GPIbα and vWF imaging signals were higher in the postischemic risk area of ADAMTS13$^{-/-}$ than WT mice, and were abolished in WT mice treated with ADAMTS13. (Ozawa et al., 2018).

Children with biliary cirrhosis due to congenital biliary atresia sometimes show thrombotic microangiopathy and decreased ADAMTS13 activity. In these children, disappearance of clinical TTP after liver transplantation confirms that hepatic stellate cells are major sources of plasma ADAMTS13. Also, acute rejection in liver transplant recipients and patients who underwent hepatectomy for liver tumors often show decreased ADAMTS13 levels and the presence of ultra-large vWF, and the ADAMTS13/vWF imbalance in the hepatic sinusoids may represent a localized TTP-like microcirculatory disturbance leading to liver damage following liver surgery (Ko et al., 2015). Studies supported an association between plasma ADAMTS13 activity, vWF antigen and ultra-large vWF multimers, and adverse events in liver transplant recipients, and measurements of ADAMTS13 and vWF could be good indicators of graft dysfunction in the early stage after liver transplantation (Ko et al., 2006). In mice with hepatic I/R injury, vWF KO mice showed improved hepatic blood flow, and reduced alanine aminotransferase levels, hepatocellular necrosis and neutrophil infiltration of vessel wall. Also, in WT mice, treatment with rhADAMTS13, improved alanine aminotransferase levels and hepatic blood flow and decreased neutrophil infiltration and hepatic I/R injury (Urisono et al., 2018).

Mice with bilateral renal I/R injury show increased plasma vWF and decreased ADAMTS13 levels, and treatment with rhADAMTS13 recovers renal function, reduces tubular cell apoptosis, renal inflammation, p38/ERK phosphorylation and cyclooxygenase-2 expression, and improves eNOS phosphorylation, afferent arteriolar dilation and microvascular endothelial function (Zhou et al., 2019).

During brain I/R, vWF multimer promotes platelet aggregation and microvascular plugging. ADAMTS13 cleaves vWF multimer, and ADAMTS13 deficiency amplifies post-ischemic cerebral hypoperfusion. In mouse model of middle cerebral artery occlusion and reperfusion, ADAMTS13$^{-/-}$ mice show larger brain infarcts and less regional cerebral blood flow, suggesting protective effects of ADAMTS13 against brain I/R injury by reducing vWF-mediated microvascular plugging (Fujioka et al., 2012).

9.9 ADAMs and ADAMTS in peripheral artery disease

Peripheral artery disease (PAD) presents as intermittent claudication and critical limb ischemia. ADAM12 may modify the severity of PAD possibly through preserving endothelial and skeletal muscle cells (Okeke & Dokun, 2018). In mice with experimental PAD, *ADAM12* showed less expression in Balb/c mice which exhibited poor outcomes than in C57Bl/6 mice which had favorable outcomes. ADAM12 overexpression improved outcomes in Balb/c mice, and ADAM12 knockdown worsened outcomes in C57Bl/6 mice. Also, ADAM12 expression modulated EC proliferation and survival through activation of tyrosine-protein kinase receptor (Tie-2) (Dokun et al., 2015).

ADAMTS7 mRNA levels are elevated in peripheral blood mononuclear cells of Turkish patients with PAD. The frequency of rs1994016 and rs3825807 SNPs was not different in PAD patients vs controls, but in PAD patients ADAMTS7 mRNA levels were increased in the CC genotype of rs1994016 and TT genotype of rs3825807, suggesting a role of ADAMTS7 in PAD (Bayoglu et al., 2018).

PAD patients that experienced cardiovascular events may not show statistically higher vWF levels and vWF/ADAMTS13 ratio than PAD controls, but in patients with complete bimonthly data a trend toward an increase in vWF/ADAMTS13 was observed, supporting the value of measuring vWF/ADAMTS13 ratio in monitoring PAD patients for ischemic cardiovascular events (Green et al., 2017).

9.10 ADAMs and ADAMTS in vascular aneurysm

Abdominal aortic aneurysm (AAA) involves ECM degradation and aortic wall inflammation. ADAM9 promotes inflammation, macrophage infiltration and cell apoptosis and is overexpressed in murine models of AAA and in AngII treated human aortic ECs and SMCs. Expression of miR-126 was decreased and inversely correlated with ADAM9 expression in AngII-treated ECs and SMCs. Also, miR-126 decreased ADAM9 gene expression, inflammatory cytokines and aneurysm formation, and improved cell survival in murine AAA, supporting that ADAM9 plays a role in AAA, and that miR-126 controls AAA development by modulating ADAM9 expression (Shen et al., 2020).

Dilation of the ascending aorta involves ECM modifications and inflammation, and acute aortic dissection involves progressive degeneration of the aortic media. In patients undergoing aortic repair, B-cells in the entire aortic wall and intimal plasma cells were more abundant, and ADAM8 and 15 expression in the aortic media was greater in aortic dissection than aortic dilation. Also, two of the patients with aortic dilation and increased ADAM8 and 15 developed aortic dissection (Levula et al., 2011). However, a causal relationship between ADAM8 and 15 and aortic dissection needs to be further tested.

ADAM10 and 17 have been linked to AAA (Folkesson et al., 2015). TNFα and ADAM17 mRNA is greater in the transition zone between non-dilated aorta and proximal aspect of AAA than the mid-portion of AAA, and in AAA than control infrarenal aorta. TNFα mRNA expression correlated with ADAM17 mRNA, and both TNFα and ADAM17 were localized in CD68 macrophages in the media and adventitia of the transition zone of AAA (Satoh, Nakamura, et al., 2004). In WT mice treated with AngII and the lysyl oxidase inhibitor β-aminopropionitrile, 52.4% of mice died from aortic rupture, and the surviving mice showed increased ADAM17 expression in the AAA lesions. In contrast, all mice lacking ADAM17 in SMCs survived and showed reduced aortic diameter, and no aortic EGFR activation, IL-6 induction, endoplasmic reticulum/oxidative stress or ECM deposition. Treatment of WT mice with ADAM17 antibody prevented AAA formation, suggesting that decreasing SMC ADAM17 could prevent AAA formation by suppressing EGFR activation (Kawai et al., 2017). Ursolic acid decreased AAA incidence, alleviated degradation of elastin fibers and inflammation, and decreased MMP2, MMP9, ADAM17 and phospho-STAT3 (signal transducer and activator of transcription 3) in AngII-infused ApoE$^{-/-}$ mice and in AngII- and TNFα-treated VSMCs, suggesting that ursolic acid ameliorates AAA by inhibiting ADAM17 and phospho-STAT3 expression (Zhai, Guo, et al., 2018). ADAM17 is increased in tunica media and intima of thoracic aortic aneurysm (TAA). In experimental elastase-induced TAA, mice lacking ADAM17 in SMCs ($Adam17^{f/f}/Sm22^{Cre/+}$) or ECs ($Adam17^{f/f}/Tie2^{Cre/+}$) showed decreased TAA dilation. ADAM17 deficiency in SMCs prevented the contractile-to-synthetic phenotypic switching, perivascular fibrosis, inflammation and adverse aortic remodeling. Loss of ADAM17 in ECs protected the intimal barrier integrity and preserved the adherens junction (VE-cadherin) and tight junctions (JAM-A and claudin). ADAM17 inhibitor PF-548 prevented TAA progression, supporting a role of ADAM17 in aortic SMC remodeling, impaired EC barrier integrity and TAA progression (Shen, Hu, Fedak, Oudit, & Kassiri, 2018).

ADAMTS1, 5, and 16 are increased in AAA, TAA and acute aortic dissection (Gao et al., 2016; Gunes et al., 2016). Also, while ADAMTS1, 4, 5, 6, 8, 9, 10, 13 and 17 mRNA may show a decrease, ADAMTS1 protein levels are elevated in SMCs and macrophages of AAA (Vorkapic et al., 2017). ADAMTS1 is also elevated in blood of acute aortic dissection patients. Aged AngII-infused mouse model of acute aortic dissection shows upregulation of ADAMTS1 in aortic media, macrophages and neutrophils, and increased degradation of versican (Gao et al., 2016). Other studies have shown decreased ADAMTS1 and elevated inducible NOS2 levels in the aorta of patients with Marfan syndrome. *Adamts1*-deficient mice show TAA and dissection and elevated aortic NO and NOS2 levels similar to mouse model of Marfan syndrome, and Nos2 inactivation protected both types of mice from aortic dilation and medial degeneration, suggesting a role for the ADAMTS1-NOS2 axis in TAA and dissection, and potential benefits of NOS2 inhibitors (Oller et al., 2017).

ADAMTS2 gene variant rs11750568 has been associated with cerebral aneurysm and pediatric stroke (Arning et al., 2012, 2016). Also, ADAMTS4 is increased in aortic SMCs from patients with sporadic ascending TAA and dissection. In mice with sporadic aortic aneurysm and dissection induced by high-fat diet and AngII infusion, ADAMTS4 deficiency reduced aortic diameter, aneurysm formation, dissection and rupture. Also, *Adamts4*$^{-/-}$ aortas showed less elastic fiber destruction, versican degradation, macrophage infiltration and SMC apoptosis (Ren et al., 2017).

ADAMTS5-mediated aggrecan cleavage is important during development of the aorta. Adamts5$^{-/-}$Smad2$^{+/-}$ and Adamts5$^{-/-}$ mice exhibit aortic anomalies and accumulation of aggrecan at the onset of elastogenesis. Aggrecan accumulation could promote the generation of DIPEN and FFGVG aggrecan neoepitope by local MMPs. In support, Adamts5$^{-/-}$ aortas show aggrecan neo-DIPEN and neo-FFGVG fragments in the aortic adventitia, and increased aggrecan neo-FFGVG in the aortic media concomitant with SMC loss (Dupuis et al., 2019). In AngII-induced aortic dilation model, mice lacking ADAMTS5 catalytic domain (Adamts5$^{\Delta cat}$) show attenuated BP, increased ascending aorta dilation and versican, and decreased versican cleavage products (versikine) and LDL-related protein 1. Silencing LDL-related protein 1 expression in human aortic SMCs reduced ADAMTS5 expression and versikine production, suggesting a role of ADAMTS5 in TAA, partly through regulation of versican metabolism (Fava et al., 2018).

ADAMTS7 degrades COMP, and ADAMTS7 mRNA expression is increased and COMP protein level is decreased in human aortic aneurysm (Qin, Cao, Li, Chen, & Chen, 2017). Whether the observed ADAMTS increased expression and its degradation of COMP are causally linked to atherosclerosis and aortic aneurysm need to be further tested.

While genetic ADAMTS13 variants rs2301612 and rs2285489 have been associated with the risk of cerebral aneurysm, ADAMTS12 variant rs1364044, and ADAMTS13 variants rs739469 and rs4962153 may be protective against cerebral aneurysm (Arning et al., 2016).

9.11 ADAMs and ADAMTS in venous thromboembolism

Studies investigating the relationship between plasma levels of ADAMTS13 and vWF antigen and venous thromboembolism (VTE) showed that the median ADAMTS13 level was reduced and the mean vWF antigen level was elevated in VTE. Whether lower ADAMTS13 levels and higher vWF antigen levels cause VTE or are related to another pathology remain to be examined (Karakaya, Tombak, Serin, & Tiftik, 2016).

9.12 ADAMs and ADAMTS in obesity and diabetes-related vascular disease

Obesity and diabetes are major risks for CVD particularly in aging individuals. Obesity is associated with impaired endothelium-dependent dilation in coronary arterioles from aging patients undergoing open heart surgery and from aged mice. Transplantation of adipose tissue from aged obese mice increased serum TNFα levels, and impaired coronary artery dilation in young recipient mice. In aging patients and mice, obesity was associated with activation of endothelial ADAM17, partly due to its decreased inhibition by caveolin-1 resulting from reduced caveolin-1 expression with age. In bioassay cascade experiments, ADAM17-induced TNFα shedding in the upstream adipose tissue arteries of older obese patients reduced dilation in the downstream coronary arterioles. Thus, aging- and obesity-related reduction in caveolin-1 increases endothelial ADAM17 activity and TNFα release in adipose tissue, leading to coronary microvascular dysfunction (Dou et al., 2017).

ADAM28 is upregulated in the liver of mice with metabolic syndrome. ADAM28 KO or its downregulation by siRNA is associated with reduced body weight and liver TNFα, and increased insulin sensitivity/glucose tolerance and high density lipoprotein cholesterol in diet-induced obese mouse, supporting a role of ADAM28 in metabolic syndrome and high fat-induced obesity (Herat et al., 2017).

Increased prevalence of obesity has been linked to non-alcoholic steatohepatitis. Studies in mice on a high fat diet have suggested that ADAMTS5 may enhance visceral/gonadal adipose tissue expansion and promote liver pathology (Bauters, Scroyen, Deprez-Poulain, & Lijnen, 2016). In a high-fat diet induced obesity mouse model, ADAMTS5$^{-/-}$ mice showed lower liver weight and less steatohepatitis and fibrosis than wild-type mice, suggesting that ADAMTS5 deficiency preserves liver integrity in mice with diet-induced obesity, and that targeting ADAMTS5 could reduce obesity-related steatohepatitis (Bauters, Spincemaille, et al., 2016).

ADAMTS13 gene polymorphisms and the frequencies of QE genotype and E allele carrier of ADAMTS13 Q448E, AG genotype and G allele carrier of ADAMTS13 rs2073932, and AA genotype of ADAMTS13 rs652600 are higher in diabetic individuals than controls. E allele and AA genotype of Q448E and rs652600 are associated with multi-vessel coronary stenosis, and the E and G allele of Q448E and rs2073932 are associated with high CAD severity score, suggesting contribution of ADAMTS13 polymorphisms to atherosclerotic coronary stenosis in diabetes (Lasom et al., 2018). WT mice with streptozotocin-induced diabetes show low plasma ADAMTS13 activity and high vWF levels. *Adamts13*$^{-/-}$ diabetic mice show impaired renal function, and increased albuminuria, urea, intrarenal thrombosis, plasminogen activator inhibitor-1, vWF, fibrin(ogen), and ECM deposition, and these effects are reversed by deletion of vWF, supporting that vWF/ADAMTS13 imbalance contributes to thrombotic angiopathy, intrarenal thrombosis and diabetic nephropathy (Dhanesha et al., 2017).

Visceral adiposity poses greater risk than subcutaneous adiposity for diabetes and CVD. In mice, *Adamts18* mRNA expression is abundant in visceral (gonadal) white adipose tissue during early development after birth. *Adamts18*$^{-/-}$ mice show increased body fat, larger adipocyte size in visceral white adipose tissue, early metabolic syndrome, hyperlipidemia and HTN, suggesting a role of ADAMTS18 in the regulation of visceral white adipose tissue and metabolic disorders (Zhu et al., 2018).

10. Conclusion

ADAMs play a role in the shedding of various membrane-bound proteins, and regulate numerous biological processes by cleaving different cytokines, growth factors and their receptions. ADAMs are also associated with different vascular processes, vascular malfunction and CVD. ADAM10 and 17 are promising biomarkers and therapeutic targets in HTN and atherosclerosis, ADAMTS family members also contribute to various biological processes and may be involved in vascular malfunction and CVD. Decreased levels of ADAMTS13 have been related to the TTP, and modulation of its activity could be useful in treatment of thrombotic microangiopathies. TIMPs are endogenous inhibitors of specific ADAMs and ADAMTS. Synthetic ADAM and ADAMTS inhibitors have also been developed, but with varying specificity and selectivity. Further research into the potential substrates, targets and functions of ADAMs and ADAMTS should help develop specific modulators with potential use in the management of CVD.

Acknowledgments

This work was supported by BRI Fund to Sustain Research Excellence from Brigham Research Institute, and grants from National Heart, Lung, and Blood Institute (HL111775, R56HL147889, and R01HL147889-A1). Dr. HaiFeng Yang was a visiting scholar from Department of Neurosurgery, Union Hospital, Tongji Medical College, Huazhong University of Science and Technology, Wuhan, Hubei, China. We thank Yael Day, Clara Frothingham, Annie Heuer, Jedidiah Kim, Cameron Muniz, and Vijay Sherring for their assistance in reviewing and editing the manuscript.

Conflict of interest

The authors state there are no conflicts of interest.

References

Abbaszade, I., Liu, R. Q., Yang, F., Rosenfeld, S. A., Ross, O. H., Link, J. R., et al. (1999). Cloning and characterization of ADAMTS11, an aggrecanase from the ADAMTS family. *The Journal of Biological Chemistry*, *274*(33), 23443–23450.

Abdul-Majeed, S., Mell, B., Nauli, S. M., & Joe, B. (2014). Cryptorchidism and infertility in rats with targeted disruption of the Adamts16 locus. *PLoS ONE*, *9*(7), e100967.

Adams, J. C., & Lawler, J. (2011). The thrombospondins. *Cold Spring Harbor Perspectives in Biology*, *3*(10), a009712.

Akyol, O., Akyol, S., & Chen, C. H. (2016). Update on ADAMTS13 and VWF in cardiovascular and hematological disorders. *Clinica Chimica Acta*, *463*, 109–118.

Al-Fakhri, N., Wilhelm, J., Hahn, M., Heidt, M., Hehrlein, F. W., Endisch, A. M., et al. (2003). Increased expression of disintegrin-metalloproteinases ADAM-15 and ADAM-9 following upregulation of integrins alpha5beta1 and alphavbeta3 in atherosclerosis. *Journal of Cellular Biochemistry*, *89*(4), 808–823.

Alwan, F., Vendramin, C., Liesner, R., Clark, A., Lester, W., Dutt, T., et al. (2019). Characterization and treatment of congenital thrombotic thrombocytopenic purpura. *Blood*, *133*(15), 1644–1651.

Amour, A., Knight, C. G., English, W. R., Webster, A., Slocombe, P. M., Knauper, V., et al. (2002). The enzymatic activity of ADAM8 and ADAM9 is not regulated by TIMPs. *FEBS Letters*, *524*(1–3), 154–158.

Anders, A., Gilbert, S., Garten, W., Postina, R., & Fahrenholz, F. (2001). Regulation of the alpha-secretase ADAM10 by its prodomain and proprotein convertases. *The FASEB Journal*, *15*(10), 1837–1839.

Anker, S. D., & Coats, A. J. (2002). How to RECOVER from RENAISSANCE? The significance of the results of RECOVER, RENAISSANCE, RENEWAL and ATTACH. *International Journal of Cardiology*, *86*(2–3), 123–130.

Arning, A., Hiersche, M., Witten, A., Kurlemann, G., Kurnik, K., Manner, D., et al. (2012). A genome-wide association study identifies a gene network of ADAMTS genes in the predisposition to pediatric stroke. *Blood*, *120*(26), 5231–5236.

Arning, A., Jeibmann, A., Kohnemann, S., Brokinkel, B., Ewelt, C., Berger, K., et al. (2016). ADAMTS genes and the risk of cerebral aneurysm. *Journal of Neurosurgery*, *125*(2), 269–274.

Asakura, M., Kitakaze, M., Takashima, S., Liao, Y., Ishikura, F., Yoshinaka, T., et al. (2002). Cardiac hypertrophy is inhibited by antagonism of ADAM12 processing of HB-EGF: Metalloproteinase inhibitors as a new therapy. *Nature Medicine*, *8*(1), 35–40.

Ashlin, T. G., Kwan, A. P., & Ramji, D. P. (2013). Regulation of ADAMTS-1, -4 and -5 expression in human macrophages: Differential regulation by key cytokines implicated in atherosclerosis and novel synergism between TL1A and IL-17. *Cytokine*, *64*(1), 234–242.

Ataca, D., Aouad, P., Constantin, C., Laszlo, C., Beleut, M., Shamseddin, M., et al. (2020). The secreted protease Adamts18 links hormone action to activation of the mammary stem cell niche. *Nature Communications*, *11*(1), 1571.

Bai, X. H., Wang, D. W., Luan, Y., Yu, X. P., & Liu, C. J. (2009). Regulation of chondrocyte differentiation by ADAMTS-12 metalloproteinase depends on its enzymatic activity. *Cellular and Molecular Life Sciences*, *66*(4), 667–680.

Bakken, A. M., Protack, C. D., Roztocil, E., Nicholl, S. M., & Davies, M. G. (2009). Cell migration in response to the amino-terminal fragment of urokinase requires epidermal growth factor receptor activation through an ADAM-mediated mechanism. *Journal of Vascular Surgery*, *49*(5), 1296–1303.

Bartoli, C. R., Kang, J., Restle, D. J., Zhang, D. M., Shabahang, C., Acker, M. A., et al. (2015). Inhibition of ADAMTS-13 by doxycycline reduces von Willebrand factor degradation during supraphysiological shear stress: Therapeutic implications for left ventricular assist device-associated bleeding. *JACC: Heart Failure*, *3*(11), 860–869.

Bartoli, C. R., Restle, D. J., Zhang, D. M., Acker, M. A., & Atluri, P. (2015). Pathologic von Willebrand factor degradation with a left ventricular assist device occurs via two distinct mechanisms: Mechanical demolition and enzymatic cleavage. *The Journal of Thoracic and Cardiovascular Surgery*, *149*(1), 281–289.

Basile, D. P., Fredrich, K., Chelladurai, B., Leonard, E. C., & Parrish, A. R. (2008). Renal ischemia reperfusion inhibits VEGF expression and induces ADAMTS-1, a novel VEGF inhibitor. *American Journal of Physiology. Renal Physiology*, *294*(4), F928–F936.

Bauer, R. C., Tohyama, J., Cui, J., Cheng, L., Yang, J., Zhang, X., et al. (2015). Knockout of Adamts7, a novel coronary artery disease locus in humans, reduces atherosclerosis in mice. *Circulation, 131*(13), 1202–1213.

Bauters, D., Scroyen, I., Deprez-Poulain, R., & Lijnen, H. R. (2016). ADAMTS5 promotes murine adipogenesis and visceral adipose tissue expansion. *Thrombosis and Haemostasis, 116*(4), 694–704.

Bauters, D., Spincemaille, P., Geys, L., Cassiman, D., Vermeersch, P., Bedossa, P., et al. (2016). ADAMTS5 deficiency protects against non-alcoholic steatohepatitis in obesity. *Liver International, 36*(12), 1848–1859.

Bayoglu, B., Arslan, C., Tel, C., Ulutin, T., Dirican, A., Deser, S. B., et al. (2018). Genetic variants rs1994016 and rs3825807 in ADAMTS7 affect its mRNA expression in atherosclerotic occlusive peripheral arterial disease. *Journal of Clinical Laboratory Analysis, 32*(1), e22174.

Beauvais, D., Venditti, L., Chassin, O., Joly, B., Ameri, A., Boisseau, P., et al. (2019). Inherited thrombotic thrombocytopenic purpura revealed by recurrent strokes in a male adult: Case report and literature review. *Journal of Stroke and Cerebrovascular Diseases, 28*(6), 1537–1539.

Becerra, E., Scully, M. A., Leandro, M. J., Heelas, E. O., Westwood, J. P., De La Torre, I., et al. (2015). Effect of rituximab on B cell phenotype and serum B cell-activating factor levels in patients with thrombotic thrombocytopenic purpura. *Clinical and Experimental Immunology, 179*(3), 414–425.

Bekhouche, M., & Colige, A. (2015). The procollagen N-proteinases ADAMTS2, 3 and 14 in pathophysiology. *Matrix Biology, 44–46*, 46–53.

Bengtsson, E., Hultman, K., Duner, P., Asciutto, G., Almgren, P., Orho-Melander, M., et al. (2017). ADAMTS-7 is associated with a high-risk plaque phenotype in human atherosclerosis. *Scientific Reports*, 7(1), 3753.

Berry, E., Bosonea, A. M., Wang, X., & Fernandez-Patron, C. (2013). Insights into the activity, differential expression, mutual regulation, and functions of matrix metalloproteinases and a disintegrin and metalloproteinases in hypertension and cardiac disease. *Journal of Vascular Research, 50*(1), 52–68.

Bertram, A., Lovric, S., Engel, A., Beese, M., Wyss, K., Hertel, B., et al. (2015). Circulating ADAM17 level reflects disease activity in proteinase-3 ANCA-associated vasculitis. *Journal of the American Society of Nephrology, 26*(11), 2860–2870.

Black, R. A., Rauch, C. T., Kozlosky, C. J., Peschon, J. J., Slack, J. L., Wolfson, M. F., et al. (1997). A metalloproteinase disintegrin that releases tumour-necrosis factor-alpha from cells. *Nature, 385*(6618), 729–733.

Blobel, C. P. (1997). Metalloprotease-disintegrins: Links to cell adhesion and cleavage of TNF alpha and Notch. *Cell, 90*(4), 589–592.

Blobel, C. P. (2005). ADAMs: Key components in EGFR signalling and development. *Nature Reviews. Molecular Cell Biology, 6*(1), 32–43.

Blobel, C. P., & White, J. M. (1992). Structure, function and evolutionary relationship of proteins containing a disintegrin domain. *Current Opinion in Cell Biology, 4*(5), 760–765.

Bode, W., Gomis-Ruth, F. X., & Stockler, W. (1993). Astacins, serralysins, snake venom and matrix metalloproteinases exhibit identical zinc-binding environments (HEXXHXX GXXH and Met-turn) and topologies and should be grouped into a common family, the 'metzincins'. *FEBS Letters, 331*(1–2), 134–140.

Boerboom, D., Lafond, J. F., Zheng, X., Lapointe, E., Mittaz, L., Boyer, A., et al. (2011). Partially redundant functions of Adamts1 and Adamts4 in the perinatal development of the renal medulla. *Developmental Dynamics, 240*(7), 1806–1814.

Brew, K., & Nagase, H. (2010). The tissue inhibitors of metalloproteinases (TIMPs): An ancient family with structural and functional diversity. *Biochimica et Biophysica Acta, 1803*(1), 55–71.

Brouillard, P., Dupont, L., Helaers, R., Coulie, R., Tiller, G. E., Peeden, J., et al. (2017). Loss of ADAMTS3 activity causes Hennekam lymphangiectasia-lymphedema syndrome 3. *Human Molecular Genetics, 26*(21), 4095–4104.

Bustamante, A., Ning, M., Garcia-Berrocoso, T., Penalba, A., Boada, C., Simats, A., et al. (2018). Usefulness of ADAMTS13 to predict response to recanalization therapies in acute ischemic stroke. *Neurology, 90*(12), e995–e1004.

Cai, P., Luo, H., Xu, H., Zhu, X., Xu, W., Dai, Y., et al. (2015). Recombinant ADAMTS 13 attenuates brain injury after intracerebral hemorrhage. *Stroke, 46*(9), 2647–2653.

Cal, S., Obaya, A. J., Llamazares, M., Garabaya, C., Quesada, V., & Lopez-Otin, C. (2002). Cloning, expression analysis, and structural characterization of seven novel human ADAMTSs, a family of metalloproteinases with disintegrin and thrombospondin-1 domains. *Gene, 283*(1–2), 49–62.

Canault, M., Certel, K., Schatzberg, D., Wagner, D. D., & Hynes, R. O. (2010). The lack of ADAM17 activity during embryonic development causes hemorrhage and impairs vessel formation. *PLoS ONE, 5*(10), e13433.

Cao, Y., Kang, Q., Zhao, Z., & Zolkiewska, A. (2002). Intracellular processing of metalloprotease disintegrin ADAM12. *The Journal of Biological Chemistry, 277*(29), 26403–26411.

Cao, Y., Xu, H., Zhu, Y., Shi, M. J., Wei, L., Zhang, J., et al. (2019). ADAMTS13 maintains cerebrovascular integrity to ameliorate Alzheimer-like pathology. *PLoS Biology, 17*(6), e3000313.

Caolo, V., Swennen, G., Chalaris, A., Wagenaar, A., Verbruggen, S., Rose-John, S., et al. (2015). ADAM10 and ADAM17 have opposite roles during sprouting angiogenesis. *Angiogenesis, 18*(1), 13–22.

Chalaris, A., Adam, N., Sina, C., Rosenstiel, P., Lehmann-Koch, J., Schirmacher, P., et al. (2010). Critical role of the disintegrin metalloprotease ADAM17 for intestinal inflammation and regeneration in mice. *The Journal of Experimental Medicine, 207*(8), 1617–1624.

Charrier-Hisamuddin, L., Laboisse, C. L., & Merlin, D. (2008). ADAM-15: A metalloprotease that mediates inflammation. *The FASEB Journal, 22*(3), 641–653.

Chemaly, M., McGilligan, V., Gibson, M., Clauss, M., Watterson, S., Alexander, H. D., et al. (2017). Role of tumour necrosis factor alpha converting enzyme (TACE/ADAM17) and associated proteins in coronary artery disease and cardiac events. *Archives of Cardiovascular Diseases, 110*(12), 700–711.

Chen, J., Deng, L., Dreymuller, D., Jiang, X., Long, J., Duan, Y., et al. (2016). A novel peptide ADAM8 inhibitor attenuates bronchial hyperresponsiveness and Th2 cytokine mediated inflammation of murine asthmatic models. *Scientific Reports, 6*, 30451.

Chen, J., Zhi, Y., Chang, X., Zhang, S., & Dai, D. (2013). Expression of ADAMTS1 and its correlation with angiogenesis in primary gastric cancer and lymph node metastasis. *Digestive Diseases and Sciences, 58*(2), 405–413.

Chen, L., Yang, L., Zha, Y., & Cui, L. (2011). Association of serum a disintegrin and metalloproteinase with thrombospodin motif 4 levels with the presence and severity of coronary artery disease. *Coronary Artery Disease, 22*(8), 570–576.

Chen, X., Cheng, X., Zhang, S., & Wu, D. (2019). ADAMTS13: An emerging target in stroke therapy. *Frontiers in Neurology, 10*, 772.

Chen, Y. C., Bui, A. V., Diesch, J., Manasseh, R., Hausding, C., Rivera, J., et al. (2013). A novel mouse model of atherosclerotic plaque instability for drug testing and mechanistic/therapeutic discoveries using gene and microRNA expression profiling. *Circulation Research, 113*(3), 252–265.

Chesneau, V., Becherer, J. D., Zheng, Y., Erdjument-Bromage, H., Tempst, P., & Blobel, C. P. (2003). Catalytic properties of ADAM19. *The Journal of Biological Chemistry, 278*(25), 22331–22340.

Cho, C. (2012). Testicular and epididymal ADAMs: Expression and function during fertilization. *Nature Reviews. Urology*, *9*(10), 550–560.

Chung, Y. L., Pan, C. H., Wang, C. C., Hsu, K. C., Sheu, M. J., Chen, H. F., et al. (2016). Methyl protodioscin, a steroidal saponin, inhibits neointima formation in vitro and in vivo. *Journal of Natural Products*, *79*(6), 1635–1644.

Coletta, A. P., Clark, A. L., Banarjee, P., & Cleland, J. G. (2002). Clinical trials update: Renewal (renaissance and recover) and attach. *European Journal of Heart Failure*, *4*(4), 559–561.

Colige, A., Beschin, A., Samyn, B., Goebels, Y., Van Beeumen, J., Nusgens, B. V., et al. (1995). Characterization and partial amino acid sequencing of a 107-kDa procollagen I N-proteinase purified by affinity chromatography on immobilized type XIV collagen. *The Journal of Biological Chemistry*, *270*(28), 16724–16730.

Colige, A., Li, S. W., Sieron, A. L., Nusgens, B. V., Prockop, D. J., & Lapiere, C. M. (1997). cDNA cloning and expression of bovine procollagen I N-proteinase: A new member of the superfamily of zinc-metalloproteinases with binding sites for cells and other matrix components. *Proceedings of the National Academy of Sciences of the United States of America*, *94*(6), 2374–2379.

Colige, A., Ruggiero, F., Vandenberghe, I., Dubail, J., Kesteloot, F., Van Beeumen, J., et al. (2005). Domains and maturation processes that regulate the activity of ADAMTS-2, a metalloproteinase cleaving the aminopropeptide of fibrillar procollagens types I-III and V. *The Journal of Biological Chemistry*, *280*(41), 34397–34408.

Cong, L., & Jia, J. (2011). Promoter polymorphisms which regulate ADAM9 transcription are protective against sporadic Alzheimer's disease. *Neurobiology of Aging*, *32*(1), 54–62.

Crawley, J. T., Lane, D. A., Woodward, M., Rumley, A., & Lowe, G. D. (2008). Evidence that high von Willebrand factor and low ADAMTS-13 levels independently increase the risk of a non-fatal heart attack. *Journal of Thrombosis and Haemostasis*, *6*(4), 583–588.

Crawley, J. T., & Scully, M. A. (2013). Thrombotic thrombocytopenic purpura: Basic pathophysiology and therapeutic strategies. *Hematology. American Society of Hematology. Education Program*, *2013*, 292–299.

Cross, A. K., Haddock, G., Stock, C. J., Allan, S., Surr, J., Bunning, R. A., et al. (2006). ADAMTS-1 and -4 are up-regulated following transient middle cerebral artery occlusion in the rat and their expression is modulated by TNF in cultured astrocytes. *Brain Research*, *1088*(1), 19–30.

Dancevic, C. M., Fraser, F. W., Smith, A. D., Stupka, N., Ward, A. C., & McCulloch, D. R. (2013). Biosynthesis and expression of a disintegrin-like and metalloproteinase domain with thrombospondin-1 repeats-15: A novel versican-cleaving proteoglycanase. *The Journal of Biological Chemistry*, *288*(52), 37267–37276.

Dang, S., Bu, D., Lu, T., Wang, Z., Liu, J., & Zhang, W. (2018). Adamts18 deficiency increases arterial thrombus formation associated with vascular defects in mice. *Biochemical and Biophysical Research Communications*, *496*(4), 1362–1368.

Dang, S., Hong, T., Bu, D., Tang, J., Fan, J., & Zhang, W. (2012). Optimized refolding and characterization of active C-terminal ADAMTS-18 fragment from inclusion bodies of Escherichia coli. *Protein Expression and Purification*, *82*(1), 32–36.

de Groot, R., Bardhan, A., Ramroop, N., Lane, D. A., & Crawley, J. T. (2009). Essential role of the disintegrin-like domain in ADAMTS13 function. *Blood*, *113*(22), 5609–5616.

de Queiroz, T. M., Xia, H., Filipeanu, C. M., Braga, V. A., & Lazartigues, E. (2015). alpha-Lipoic acid reduces neurogenic hypertension by blunting oxidative stress-mediated increase in ADAM17. *American Journal of Physiology. Heart and Circulatory Physiology*, *309*(5), H926–H934.

Desanlis, I., Felstead, H. L., Edwards, D. R., & Wheeler, G. N. (2018). ADAMTS9, a member of the ADAMTS family, in Xenopus development. *Gene Expression Patterns*, *29*, 72–81.

Deurloo, K. L., Linskens, I. H., Heymans, M. W., Heijboer, A. C., Blankenstein, M. A., & van Vugt, J. M. (2013). ADAM12s and PP13 as first trimester screening markers for adverse pregnancy outcome. *Clinical Chemistry and Laboratory Medicine*, *51*(6), 1279–1284.

Dhanesha, N., Doddapattar, P., Chorawala, M. R., Nayak, M. K., Kokame, K., Staber, J. M., et al. (2017). ADAMTS13 retards progression of diabetic nephropathy by inhibiting intrarenal thrombosis in mice. *Arteriosclerosis, Thrombosis, and Vascular Biology*, *37*(7), 1332–1338.

Didangelos, A., Mayr, U., Monaco, C., & Mayr, M. (2012). Novel role of ADAMTS-5 protein in proteoglycan turnover and lipoprotein retention in atherosclerosis. *The Journal of Biological Chemistry*, *287*(23), 19341–19345.

Diebel, M. E., Martin, J. V., Liberati, D. M., & Diebel, L. N. (2018). The temporal response and mechanism of action of tranexamic acid in endothelial glycocalyx degradation. *Journal of Trauma and Acute Care Surgery*, *84*(1), 75–80.

Doddapattar, P., Dhanesha, N., Chorawala, M. R., Tinsman, C., Jain, M., Nayak, M. K., et al. (2018). Endothelial cell-derived Von Willebrand factor, but not platelet-derived, promotes atherosclerosis in apolipoprotein E-deficient mice. *Arteriosclerosis, Thrombosis, and Vascular Biology*, *38*(3), 520–528.

Dokun, A. O., Chen, L., Okutsu, M., Farber, C. R., Hazarika, S., Jones, W. S., et al. (2015). ADAM12: A genetic modifier of preclinical peripheral arterial disease. *American Journal of Physiology. Heart and Circulatory Physiology*, *309*(5), H790–H803.

Dolan, J. M., Sim, F. J., Meng, H., & Kolega, J. (2012). Endothelial cells express a unique transcriptional profile under very high wall shear stress known to induce expansive arterial remodeling. *American Journal of Physiology. Cell Physiology*, *302*(8), C1109–C1118.

Dong, H., Du, T., Premaratne, S., Zhao, C. X., Tian, Q., Li, Y., et al. (2018). Relationship between ADAMTS4 and carotid atherosclerotic plaque vulnerability in humans. *Journal of Vascular Surgery*, *67*(4), 1120–1126.

Donnarumma, E., Trivedi, R. K., & Lefer, D. J. (2017). Protective actions of H2S in acute myocardial infarction and heart failure. *Comprehensive Physiology*, 7(2), 583–602.

Donners, M. M., Wolfs, I. M., Olieslagers, S., Mohammadi-Motahhari, Z., Tchaikovski, V., Heeneman, S., et al. (2010). A disintegrin and metalloprotease 10 is a novel mediator of vascular endothelial growth factor-induced endothelial cell function in angiogenesis and is associated with atherosclerosis. *Arteriosclerosis, Thrombosis, and Vascular Biology*, *30*(11), 2188–2195.

Dou, H., Feher, A., Davila, A. C., Romero, M. J., Patel, V. S., Kamath, V. M., et al. (2017). Role of adipose tissue endothelial ADAM17 in age-related coronary microvascular dysfunction. *Arteriosclerosis, Thrombosis, and Vascular Biology*, *37*(6), 1180–1193.

Dubail, J., & Apte, S. S. (2015). Insights on ADAMTS proteases and ADAMTS-like proteins from mammalian genetics. *Matrix Biology*, *44–46*, 24–37.

Dubail, J., Kesteloot, F., Deroanne, C., Motte, P., Lambert, V., Rakic, J. M., et al. (2010). ADAMTS-2 functions as anti-angiogenic and anti-tumoral molecule independently of its catalytic activity. *Cellular and Molecular Life Sciences*, *67*(24), 4213–4232.

Dupuis, L. E., Nelson, E. L., Hozik, B., Porto, S. C., Rogers-DeCotes, A., Fosang, A., et al. (2019). Adamts5(-/-) mice exhibit altered aggrecan proteolytic profiles that correlate with ascending aortic anomalies. *Arteriosclerosis, Thrombosis, and Vascular Biology*, *39*(10), 2067–2081.

Duru, E. A., Fu, Y., & Davies, M. G. (2014). Protease-mediated human smooth muscle cell proliferation by urokinase requires epidermal growth factor receptor transactivation by triple membrane signaling. *The Journal of Surgical Research*, *192*(2), 254–262.

Edwards, D. R., Handsley, M. M., & Pennington, C. J. (2008). The ADAM metalloproteinases. *Molecular Aspects of Medicine*, *29*(5), 258–289.

Eerenberg, E. S., Teunissen, P. F., van den Born, B. J., Meijers, J. C., Hollander, M. R., Jansen, M., et al. (2016). The role of ADAMTS13 in acute myocardial infarction: Cause or consequence? *Cardiovascular Research*, *111*(3), 194–203.

El Hour, M., Moncada-Pazos, A., Blacher, S., Masset, A., Cal, S., Berndt, S., et al. (2010). Higher sensitivity of Adamts12-deficient mice to tumor growth and angiogenesis. *Oncogene*, *29*(20), 3025–3032.

English, W. R., Corvol, P., & Murphy, G. (2012). LPS activates ADAM9 dependent shedding of ACE from endothelial cells. *Biochemical and Biophysical Research Communications*, *421*(1), 70–75.

English, W. R., Puente, X. S., Freije, J. M., Knauper, V., Amour, A., Merryweather, A., et al. (2000). Membrane type 4 matrix metalloproteinase (MMP17) has tumor necrosis factor-alpha convertase activity but does not activate pro-MMP2. *The Journal of Biological Chemistry*, *275*(19), 14046–14055.

English, W. R., Siviter, R. J., Hansen, M., & Murphy, G. (2017). ADAM9 is present at endothelial cell–cell junctions and regulates monocyte–endothelial transmigration. *Biochemical and Biophysical Research Communications*, *493*(2), 1057–1062.

Fan, D., Takawale, A., Shen, M., Samokhvalov, V., Basu, R., Patel, V., et al. (2016). A disintegrin and metalloprotease-17 regulates pressure overload-induced myocardial hypertrophy and dysfunction through proteolytic processing of integrin beta1. *Hypertension*, *68*(4), 937–948.

Fan, D., Takawale, A., Shen, M., Wang, W., Wang, X., Basu, R., et al. (2015). Cardiomyocyte a disintegrin and metalloproteinase 17 (ADAM17) Is essential in post-myocardial infarction repair by regulating angiogenesis. *Circulation. Heart Failure*, *8*(5), 970–979.

Farber, G., Hurtado, R., Loh, S., Monette, S., Mtui, J., Kopan, R., et al. (2018). Glomerular endothelial cell maturation depends on ADAM10, a key regulator of Notch signaling. *Angiogenesis*, *21*(2), 335–347.

Farber, G., Parks, M. M., Lustgarten Guahmich, N., Zhang, Y., Monette, S., Blanchard, S. C., et al. (2019). ADAM10 controls the differentiation of the coronary arterial endothelium. *Angiogenesis*, *22*(2), 237–250.

Fava, M., Barallobre-Barreiro, J., Mayr, U., Lu, R., Didangelos, A., Baig, F., et al. (2018). Role of ADAMTS-5 in aortic dilatation and extracellular matrix remodeling. *Arteriosclerosis, Thrombosis, and Vascular Biology*, *38*(7), 1537–1548.

Fedak, P. W., Moravec, C. S., McCarthy, P. M., Altamentova, S. M., Wong, A. P., Skrtic, M., et al. (2006). Altered expression of disintegrin metalloproteinases and their inhibitor in human dilated cardiomyopathy. *Circulation*, *113*(2), 238–245.

Fernandes, R. J., Hirohata, S., Engle, J. M., Colige, A., Cohn, D. H., Eyre, D. R., et al. (2001). Procollagen II amino propeptide processing by ADAMTS-3. Insights on dermatosparaxis. *The Journal of Biological Chemistry*, *276*(34), 31502–31509.

Folkesson, M., Li, C., Frebelius, S., Swedenborg, J., Wagsater, D., Williams, K. J., et al. (2015). Proteolytically active ADAM10 and ADAM17 carried on membrane microvesicles in human abdominal aortic aneurysms. *Thrombosis and Haemostasis*, *114*(6), 1165–1174.

Fridman, J. S., Caulder, E., Hansbury, M., Liu, X., Yang, G., Wang, Q., et al. (2007). Selective inhibition of ADAM metalloproteases as a novel approach for modulating ErbB pathways in cancer. *Clinical Cancer Research*, *13*(6), 1892–1902.

Fu, Y., & Kong, W. (2017). Cartilage oligomeric matrix protein: Matricellular and matricrine signaling in cardiovascular homeostasis and disease. *Current Vascular Pharmacology*, *15*(3), 186–196.

Fujioka, M., Nakano, T., Hayakawa, K., Irie, K., Akitake, Y., Sakamoto, Y., et al. (2012). ADAMTS13 gene deletion enhances plasma high-mobility group box1 elevation and neuroinflammation in brain ischemia-reperfusion injury. *Neurological Sciences*, *33*(5), 1107–1115.

Gao, Y., Wu, W., Yu, C., Zhong, F., Li, G., Kong, W., et al. (2016). A disintegrin and metalloproteinase with thrombospondin motif 1 (ADAMTS1) expression increases in acute aortic dissection. *Science China. Life Sciences*, *59*(1), 59–67.

Gao, Y. X., Yu, C. A., Lu, J. H., Gao, H. M., Li, G., Kong, W., et al. (2013). ADAMTS-7 expression increases in the early stage of angiotensin II-induced renal injury in elderly mice. *Kidney & Blood Pressure Research*, *38*(1), 121–131.

Garbers, C., Monhasery, N., Aparicio-Siegmund, S., Lokau, J., Baran, P., Nowell, M. A., et al. (2014). The interleukin-6 receptor Asp358Ala single nucleotide polymorphism rs2228145 confers increased proteolytic conversion rates by ADAM proteases. *Biochimica et Biophysica Acta*, *1842*(9), 1485–1494.

Georgiadis, K. E., Hirohata, S., Seldin, M. F., & Apte, S. S. (1999). ADAM-TS8, a novel metalloprotease of the ADAM-TS family located on mouse chromosome 9 and human chromosome 11. *Genomics*, *62*(2), 312–315.

Glassey, B., & Civetta, A. (2004). Positive selection at reproductive ADAM genes with potential intercellular binding activity. *Molecular Biology and Evolution*, *21*(5), 851–859.

Goel, A., Raghupathy, V., Amirtharaj, G. J., Chapla, A., Venkatraman, A., Ramakrishna, B., et al. (2017). ADAMTS13 missense variants associated with defective activity and secretion of ADAMTS13 in a patient with non-cirrhotic portal hypertension. *Indian Journal of Gastroenterology*, *36*(5), 380–389.

Goertsches, R., Comabella, M., Navarro, A., Perkal, H., & Montalban, X. (2005). Genetic association between polymorphisms in the ADAMTS14 gene and multiple sclerosis. *Journal of Neuroimmunology*, *164*(1–2), 140–147.

Goetzinger, K. R., Zhong, Y., Cahill, A. G., Odibo, L., Macones, G. A., & Odibo, A. O. (2013). Efficiency of first-trimester uterine artery Doppler, a-disintegrin and metalloprotease 12, pregnancy-associated plasma protein a, and maternal characteristics in the prediction of preeclampsia. *Journal of Ultrasound in Medicine*, *32*(9), 1593–1600.

Gopalakrishnan, K., Kumarasamy, S., Abdul-Majeed, S., Kalinoski, A. L., Morgan, E. E., Gohara, A. F., et al. (2012). Targeted disruption of Adamts16 gene in a rat genetic model of hypertension. *Proceedings of the National Academy of Sciences of the United States of America*, *109*(50), 20555–20559.

Gould, R. J., Polokoff, M. A., Friedman, P. A., Huang, T. F., Holt, J. C., Cook, J. J., et al. (1990). Disintegrins: A family of integrin inhibitory proteins from viper venoms. *Proceedings of the Society for Experimental Biology and Medicine*, *195*(2), 168–171.

Green, D., Tian, L., Greenland, P., Liu, K., Kibbe, M., Tracy, R., et al. (2017). Association of the von Willebrand factor-ADAMTS13 ratio with incident cardiovascular events in patients with peripheral arterial disease. *Clinical and Applied Thrombosis/Hemostasis*, *23*(7), 807–813.

Gunes, M. F., Akpinar, M. B., Comertoglu, I., Akyol, S., Demircelik, B., Gurel, O. M., et al. (2016). The investigation of a disintegrin and metalloproteinase with thrombospondin motifs (ADAMTS) 1, 5 and 16 in thoracic aortic aneurysms and dissections. *Clinical Laboratory*, *62*(3), 425–433.

Gunther, W., Skaftnesmo, K. O., Arnold, H., Bjerkvig, R., & Terzis, A. J. (2005). Distribution patterns of the anti-angiogenic protein ADAMTS-1 during rat development. *Acta Histochemica*, *107*(2), 121–131.

Guo, F., Lai, Y., Tian, Q., Lin, E. A., Kong, L., & Liu, C. (2010). Granulin-epithelin precursor binds directly to ADAMTS-7 and ADAMTS-12 and inhibits their degradation of cartilage oligomeric matrix protein. *Arthritis and Rheumatism*, *62*(7), 2023–2036.

Haining, E. J., Yang, J., Bailey, R. L., Khan, K., Collier, R., Tsai, S., et al. (2012). The TspanC8 subgroup of tetraspanins interacts with A disintegrin and metalloprotease 10 (ADAM10) and regulates its maturation and cell surface expression. *The Journal of Biological Chemistry*, *287*(47), 39753–39765.

Ham, C., Levkau, B., Raines, E. W., & Herren, B. (2002). ADAM15 is an adherens junction molecule whose surface expression can be driven by VE-cadherin. *Experimental Cell Research*, *279*(2), 239–247.

Hanby, H. A., & Zheng, X. L. (2013). Biochemistry and physiological functions of ADAMTS7 metalloprotease. *Advances in Biochemistry*, *1*(3). https://doi.org/10.11648/j.ab.20130103.11.

Hartmann, D., de Strooper, B., Serneels, L., Craessaerts, K., Herreman, A., Annaert, W., et al. (2002). The disintegrin/metalloprotease ADAM 10 is essential for Notch signalling but not for alpha-secretase activity in fibroblasts. *Human Molecular Genetics*, *11*(21), 2615–2624.

Hashimoto, G., Aoki, T., Nakamura, H., Tanzawa, K., & Okada, Y. (2001). Inhibition of ADAMTS4 (aggrecanase-1) by tissue inhibitors of metalloproteinases (TIMP-1, 2, 3 and 4). *FEBS Letters*, *494*(3), 192–195.

Hattori, N., Carrino, D. A., Lauer, M. E., Vasanji, A., Wylie, J. D., Nelson, C. M., et al. (2011). Pericellular versican regulates the fibroblast-myofibroblast transition: A role for ADAMTS5 protease-mediated proteolysis. *The Journal of Biological Chemistry*, *286*(39), 34298–34310.

Heijink, I. H., Brandenburg, S. M., Noordhoek, J. A., Slebos, D. J., Postma, D. S., & van Oosterhout, A. J. (2011). Role of aberrant metalloproteinase activity in the pro-inflammatory phenotype of bronchial epithelium in COPD. *Respiratory Research*, *12*, 110.

Hemmeryckx, B., Carai, P., & Roger Lijnen, H. (2019). ADAMTS5 deficiency in mice does not affect cardiac function. *Cell Biology International*, *43*(6), 593–604.

Herat, L., Rudnicka, C., Okada, Y., Mochizuki, S., Schlaich, M., & Matthews, V. (2017). The metalloproteinase ADAM28 promotes metabolic dysfunction in mice. *International Journal of Molecular Sciences*, *18*(4), 884.

Higashiyama, S., & Nanba, D. (2005). ADAM-mediated ectodomain shedding of HB-EGF in receptor cross-talk. *Biochimica et Biophysica Acta*, *1751*(1), 110–117.

Hirohata, S., Inagaki, J., & Ohtsuki, T. (2017). Diverse functions of a disintegrin and metalloproteinase with thrombospondin motif-1. *Yakugaku Zasshi*, *137*(7), 811–814.

Hodgkinson, L. M., Wang, L., Duncan, G., Edwards, D. R., & Wormstone, I. M. (2010). ADAM and ADAMTS gene expression in native and wound healing human lens epithelial cells. *Molecular Vision*, *16*, 2765–2776.

Holloway, J. W., Laxton, R. C., Rose-Zerilli, M. J., Holloway, J. A., Andrews, A. L., Riaz, Z., et al. (2010). ADAM33 expression in atherosclerotic lesions and relationship of ADAM33 gene variation with atherosclerosis. *Atherosclerosis*, *211*(1), 224–230.

Horiuchi, K., Weskamp, G., Lum, L., Hammes, H. P., Cai, H., Brodie, T. A., et al. (2003). Potential role for ADAM15 in pathological neovascularization in mice. *Molecular and Cellular Biology*, *23*(16), 5614–5624.

Horiuchi, K., Zhou, H. M., Kelly, K., Manova, K., & Blobel, C. P. (2005). Evaluation of the contributions of ADAMs 9, 12, 15, 17, and 19 to heart development and ectodomain shedding of neuregulins beta1 and beta2. *Developmental Biology*, *283*(2), 459–471.

Hou, Y., Chu, M., Cai, Y., Lei, J., Chen, Y., Zhu, R., et al. (2015). Antitumor and anti-angiogenic activity of the recombinant human disintegrin domain of A disintegrin and metalloproteinase 15. *Molecular Medicine Reports*, *12*(2), 2360–2366.

Hou, Y., Chu, M., Du, F. F., Lei, J. Y., Chen, Y., Zhu, R. Y., et al. (2013). Recombinant disintegrin domain of ADAM15 inhibits the proliferation and migration of Bel-7402 cells. *Biochemical and Biophysical Research Communications*, *435*(4), 640–645.

Howard, L., & Glynn, P. (1995). Membrane-associated metalloproteinase recognized by characteristic cleavage of myelin basic protein: Assay and isolation. *Methods in Enzymology*, *248*, 388–395.

Howes, J. M., Knauper, V., Malcor, J. D., & Farndale, R. W. (2020). Cleavage by MMP-13 renders VWF unable to bind to collagen but increases its platelet reactivity. *Journal of Thrombosis and Haemostasis*, *18*(4), 942–954.

Hsia, H. E., Tushaus, J., Brummer, T., Zheng, Y., Scilabra, S. D., & Lichtenthaler, S. F. (2019). Functions of 'A disintegrin and metalloproteases (ADAMs)' in the mammalian nervous system. *Cellular and Molecular Life Sciences*, *76*(16), 3055–3081.

Hubmacher, D., & Apte, S. S. (2015). ADAMTS proteins as modulators of microfibril formation and function. *Matrix Biology*, *47*, 34–43.

Hurskainen, T. L., Hirohata, S., Seldin, M. F., & Apte, S. S. (1999). ADAM-TS5, ADAM-TS6, and ADAM-TS7, novel members of a new family of zinc metalloproteases. General features and genomic distribution of the ADAM-TS family. *The Journal of Biological Chemistry*, *274*(36), 25555–25563.

Iba, K., Albrechtsen, R., Gilpin, B., Frohlich, C., Loechel, F., Zolkiewska, A., et al. (2000). The cysteine-rich domain of human ADAM 12 supports cell adhesion through syndecans and triggers signaling events that lead to beta1 integrin-dependent cell spreading. *The Journal of Cell Biology*, *149*(5), 1143–1156.

Ichikawa, Y., Miura, T., Nakano, A., Miki, T., Nakamura, Y., Tsuchihashi, K., et al. (2004). The role of ADAM protease in the tyrosine kinase-mediated trigger mechanism of ischemic preconditioning. *Cardiovascular Research*, *62*(1), 167–175.

Jackson, L. F., Qiu, T. H., Sunnarborg, S. W., Chang, A., Zhang, C., Patterson, C., et al. (2003). Defective valvulogenesis in HB-EGF and TACE-null mice is associated with aberrant BMP signaling. *The EMBO Journal*, *22*(11), 2704–2716.

Jakobsson, L., Franco, C. A., Bentley, K., Collins, R. T., Ponsioen, B., Aspalter, I. M., et al. (2010). Endothelial cells dynamically compete for the tip cell position during angiogenic sprouting. *Nature Cell Biology*, *12*(10), 943–953.

Janssen, L., Dupont, L., Bekhouche, M., Noel, A., Leduc, C., Voz, M., et al. (2016). ADAMTS3 activity is mandatory for embryonic lymphangiogenesis and regulates placental angiogenesis. *Angiogenesis*, *19*(1), 53–65.

Jeltsch, M., Jha, S. K., Tvorogov, D., Anisimov, A., Leppanen, V. M., Holopainen, T., et al. (2014). CCBE1 enhances lymphangiogenesis via A disintegrin and metalloprotease with thrombospondin motifs-3-mediated vascular endothelial growth factor-C activation. *Circulation*, *129*(19), 1962–1971.

Jha, S. K., Rauniyar, K., Karpanen, T., Leppanen, V. M., Brouillard, P., Vikkula, M., et al. (2017). Efficient activation of the lymphangiogenic growth factor VEGF-C requires the C-terminal domain of VEGF-C and the N-terminal domain of CCBE1. *Scientific Reports*, 7(1), 4916.

Jin, S. Y., Tohyama, J., Bauer, R. C., Cao, N. N., Rader, D. J., & Zheng, X. L. (2012). Genetic ablation of Adamts13 gene dramatically accelerates the formation of early atherosclerosis in a murine model. *Arteriosclerosis, Thrombosis, and Vascular Biology*, *32*(8), 1817–1823.

Jin, Y., Liu, Y., Lin, Q., Li, J., Druso, J. E., Antonyak, M. A., et al. (2013). Deletion of Cdc42 enhances ADAM17-mediated vascular endothelial growth factor receptor 2 shedding and impairs vascular endothelial cell survival and vasculogenesis. *Molecular and Cellular Biology*, *33*(21), 4181–4197.

Joe, B., Saad, Y., Dhindaw, S., Lee, N. H., Frank, B. C., Achinike, O. H., et al. (2009). Positional identification of variants of Adamts16 linked to inherited hypertension. *Human Molecular Genetics*, *18*(15), 2825–2838.

Jonsson-Rylander, A. C., Nilsson, T., Fritsche-Danielson, R., Hammarstrom, A., Behrendt, M., Andersson, J. O., et al. (2005). Role of ADAMTS-1 in atherosclerosis: Remodeling of carotid artery, immunohistochemistry, and proteolysis of versican. *Arteriosclerosis, Thrombosis, and Vascular Biology*, *25*(1), 180–185.

Jorissen, E., Prox, J., Bernreuther, C., Weber, S., Schwanbeck, R., Serneels, L., et al. (2010). The disintegrin/metalloproteinase ADAM10 is essential for the establishment of the brain cortex. *The Journal of Neuroscience*, *30*(14), 4833–4844.

Karakaya, B., Tombak, A., Serin, M. S., & Tiftik, N. (2016). Change in plasma a disintegrin and metalloprotease with thrombospondin type-1 repeats-13 and von Willebrand factor levels in venous thromboembolic patients. *Hematology*, *21*(5), 295–299.

Karakose, M., Caliskan, M., Arslan, M. S., Demirci, T., Karakose, S., Tutal, E., et al. (2018). Association of ADAMTS4 and ADAMTS9 levels with cardiovascular risk in patients with primary hyperparathyroidism. *Endocrine Research*, *43*(1), 15–20.

Karkkainen, I., Rybnikova, E., Pelto-Huikko, M., & Huovila, A. P. (2000). Metalloprotease-disintegrin (ADAM) genes are widely and differentially expressed in the adult CNS. *Molecular and Cellular Neurosciences*, *15*(6), 547–560.

Karoulias, S. Z., Taye, N., Stanley, S., & Hubmacher, D. (2020). The ADAMTS/fibrillin connection: Insights into the biological functions of ADAMTS10 and ADAMTS17 and their respective sister proteases. *Biomolecules*, *10*(4), 596.

Kashiwagi, M., Tortorella, M., Nagase, H., & Brew, K. (2001). TIMP-3 is a potent inhibitor of aggrecanase 1 (ADAM-TS4) and aggrecanase 2 (ADAM-TS5). *The Journal of Biological Chemistry*, *276*(16), 12501–12504.

Katneni, U. K., Ibla, J. C., Hunt, R., Schiller, T., & Kimchi-Sarfaty, C. (2019). von Willebrand factor/ADAMTS-13 interactions at birth: Implications for thrombosis in the neonatal period. *Journal of Thrombosis and Haemostasis*, *17*(3), 429–440.

Kawai, T., Takayanagi, T., Forrester, S. J., Preston, K. J., Obama, T., Tsuji, T., et al. (2017). Vascular ADAM17 (a disintegrin and metalloproteinase domain 17) is required for angiotensin II/beta-aminopropionitrile-induced abdominal aortic aneurysm. *Hypertension*, *70*(5), 959–963.

Kelly, K., Hutchinson, G., Nebenius-Oosthuizen, D., Smith, A. J., Bartsch, J. W., Horiuchi, K., et al. (2005). Metalloprotease-disintegrin ADAM8: Expression analysis and targeted deletion in mice. *Developmental Dynamics*, *232*(1), 221–231.

Kelwick, R., Desanlis, I., Wheeler, G. N., & Edwards, D. R. (2015). The ADAMTS (a disintegrin and metalloproteinase with thrombospondin motifs) family. *Genome Biology*, *16*, 113.

Kelwick, R., Wagstaff, L., Decock, J., Roghi, C., Cooley, L. S., Robinson, S. D., et al. (2015). Metalloproteinase-dependent and -independent processes contribute to inhibition of breast cancer cell migration, angiogenesis and liver metastasis by a disintegrin and metalloproteinase with thrombospondin motifs-15. *International Journal of Cancer*, *136*(4), E14–E26.

Kessler, T., Zhang, L., Liu, Z., Yin, X., Huang, Y., Wang, Y., et al. (2015). ADAMTS-7 inhibits re-endothelialization of injured arteries and promotes vascular remodeling through cleavage of thrombospondin-1. *Circulation*, *131*(13), 1191–1201.

Kilic, M. O., Aynekin, B., Kara, A., Icen, D., & Demircan, K. (2017). Differentially regulated ADAMTS1, 8, and 18 in gastric adenocarcinoma. *Bratislavské Lekárske Listy*, *118*(2), 71–76.

Kim, S. H., Pei, Q. M., Jiang, P., Yang, M., Qian, X. J., & Liu, J. B. (2017). Effect of active vitamin D3 on VEGF-induced ADAM33 expression and proliferation in human airway smooth muscle cells: Implications for asthma treatment. *Respiratory Research*, *18*(1), 7.

Klein, T., & Bischoff, R. (2011). Active metalloproteases of the A disintegrin and metalloprotease (ADAM) family: Biological function and structure. *Journal of Proteome Research*, *10*(1), 17–33.

Ko, S., Chisuwa, H., Matsumoto, M., Fujimura, Y., Okano, E., & Nakajima, Y. (2015). Relevance of ADAMTS13 to liver transplantation and surgery. *World Journal of Hepatology*, 7(13), 1772–1781.

Ko, S., Okano, E., Kanehiro, H., Matsumoto, M., Ishizashi, H., Uemura, M., et al. (2006). Plasma ADAMTS13 activity may predict early adverse events in living donor liver transplantation: Observations in 3 cases. *Liver Transplantation, 12*(5), 859–869.

Koo, B. H., & Apte, S. S. (2010). Cell-surface processing of the metalloprotease pro-ADAMTS9 is influenced by the chaperone GRP94/gp96. *The Journal of Biological Chemistry, 285*(1), 197–205.

Koo, B. H., Coe, D. M., Dixon, L. J., Somerville, R. P., Nelson, C. M., Wang, L. W., et al. (2010). ADAMTS9 is a cell-autonomously acting, anti-angiogenic metalloprotease expressed by microvascular endothelial cells. *The American Journal of Pathology, 176*(3), 1494–1504.

Koo, B. H., Longpre, J. M., Somerville, R. P., Alexander, J. P., Leduc, R., & Apte, S. S. (2007). Regulation of ADAMTS9 secretion and enzymatic activity by its propeptide. *The Journal of Biological Chemistry, 282*(22), 16146–16154.

Kramerova, I. A., Kawaguchi, N., Fessler, L. I., Nelson, R. E., Chen, Y., Kramerov, A. A., et al. (2000). Papilin in development; a pericellular protein with a homology to the ADAMTS metalloproteinases. *Development, 127*(24), 5475–5485.

Kremer Hovinga, J. A., Coppo, P., Lammle, B., Moake, J. L., Miyata, T., & Vanhoorelbeke, K. (2017). Thrombotic thrombocytopenic purpura. *Nature Reviews. Disease Primers, 3*, 17020.

Kumar, S., Chen, M., Li, Y., Wong, F. H., Thiam, C. W., Hossain, M. Z., et al. (2016). Loss of ADAMTS4 reduces high fat diet-induced atherosclerosis and enhances plaque stability in ApoE(-/-) mice. *Scientific Reports, 6*, 31130.

Kuno, K., Kanada, N., Nakashima, E., Fujiki, F., Ichimura, F., & Matsushima, K. (1997). Molecular cloning of a gene encoding a new type of metalloproteinase-disintegrin family protein with thrombospondin motifs as an inflammation associated gene. *The Journal of Biological Chemistry, 272*(1), 556–562.

Kuno, K., & Matsushima, K. (1998). ADAMTS-1 protein anchors at the extracellular matrix through the thrombospondin type I motifs and its spacing region. *The Journal of Biological Chemistry, 273*(22), 13912–13917.

Kurisaki, T., Masuda, A., Osumi, N., Nabeshima, Y., & Fujisawa-Sehara, A. (1998). Spatially- and temporally-restricted expression of meltrin alpha (ADAM12) and beta (ADAM19) in mouse embryo. *Mechanisms of Development, 73*(2), 211–215.

Kurisaki, T., Masuda, A., Sudo, K., Sakagami, J., Higashiyama, S., Matsuda, Y., et al. (2003). Phenotypic analysis of Meltrin alpha (ADAM12)-deficient mice: Involvement of Meltrin alpha in adipogenesis and myogenesis. *Molecular and Cellular Biology, 23*(1), 55–61.

Kurohara, K., Komatsu, K., Kurisaki, T., Masuda, A., Irie, N., Asano, M., et al. (2004). Essential roles of Meltrin beta (ADAM19) in heart development. *Developmental Biology, 267*(1), 14–28.

Kutz, W. E., Wang, L. W., Bader, H. L., Majors, A. K., Iwata, K., Traboulsi, E. I., et al. (2011). ADAMTS10 protein interacts with fibrillin-1 and promotes its deposition in extracellular matrix of cultured fibroblasts. *The Journal of Biological Chemistry, 286*(19), 17156–17167.

Kveiborg, M., Jacobsen, J., Lee, M. H., Nagase, H., Wewer, U. M., & Murphy, G. (2010). Selective inhibition of ADAM12 catalytic activity through engineering of tissue inhibitor of metalloproteinase 2 (TIMP-2). *The Biochemical Journal, 430*(1), 79–86.

Lambers, M., Goldenberg, N. A., Kenet, G., Kirkham, F. J., Manner, D., Bernard, T., et al. (2013). Role of reduced ADAMTS13 in arterial ischemic stroke: A pediatric cohort study. *Annals of Neurology, 73*(1), 58–64.

Lambert, D. W., Yarski, M., Warner, F. J., Thornhill, P., Parkin, E. T., Smith, A. I., et al. (2005). Tumor necrosis factor-alpha convertase (ADAM17) mediates regulated ectodomain shedding of the severe-acute respiratory syndrome-coronavirus

(SARS-CoV) receptor, angiotensin-converting enzyme-2 (ACE2). *The Journal of Biological Chemistry*, *280*(34), 30113–30119.

Langer, H., May, A. E., Bultmann, A., & Gawaz, M. (2005). ADAM 15 is an adhesion receptor for platelet GPIIb-IIIa and induces platelet activation. *Thrombosis and Haemostasis*, *94*(3), 555–561.

Lasom, S., Komanasin, N., Settasatian, N., Settasatian, C., Kukongviriyapan, U., & Intharapetch, P. (2018). Association of a disintegrin and metalloproteinase with a thrombospondin type 1 motif member 13 polymorphisms with severity of coronary stenosis in type 2 diabetes mellitus. *Journal of Research in Medical Sciences : The Official Journal of Isfahan University of Medical Sciences*, *23*, 59.

Lasom, S., Komanasin, N., Settasatian, N., Settasatian, C., Kukongviriyapan, U., Intharapetch, P., et al. (2017). Protective effect of a disintegrin and metalloproteinase with a thrombospondin type 1 motif, member 13 haplotype on coronary artery disease. *Blood Coagulation & Fibrinolysis*, *28*(4), 286–294.

Le Goff, C., & Cormier-Daire, V. (2009). Genetic and molecular aspects of acromelic dysplasia. *Pediatric Endocrinology Reviews*, *6*(3), 418–423.

Le, H. T., Atif, J., Mara, D. L., Castellana, B., Treissman, J., Baltayeva, J., et al. (2018). ADAM8 localizes to extravillous trophoblasts within the maternal-fetal interface and potentiates trophoblast cell line migration through a beta1 integrin-mediated mechanism. *Molecular Human Reproduction*, *24*(10), 495–509.

Lee, C. W., Hwang, I., Park, C. S., Lee, H., Park, D. W., Kang, S. J., et al. (2011). Comparison of ADAMTS-1, -4 and -5 expression in culprit plaques between acute myocardial infarction and stable angina. *Journal of Clinical Pathology*, *64*(5), 399–404.

Lee, C. W., Hwang, I., Park, C. S., Lee, H., Park, D. W., Kang, S. J., et al. (2012). Expression of ADAMTS-2, -3, -13, and -14 in culprit coronary lesions in patients with acute myocardial infarction or stable angina. *Journal of Thrombosis and Thrombolysis*, *33*(4), 362–370.

Lee, D. C., Sunnarborg, S. W., Hinkle, C. L., Myers, T. J., Stevenson, M. Y., Russell, W. E., et al. (2003). TACE/ADAM17 processing of EGFR ligands indicates a role as a physiological convertase. *Annals of the New York Academy of Sciences*, *995*, 22–38.

Lemarchant, S., Dunghana, H., Pomeshchik, Y., Leinonen, H., Kolosowska, N., Korhonen, P., et al. (2016). Anti-inflammatory effects of ADAMTS-4 in a mouse model of ischemic stroke. *Glia*, *64*(9), 1492–1507.

Lemarchant, S., Pruvost, M., Montaner, J., Emery, E., Vivien, D., Kanninen, K., et al. (2013). ADAMTS proteoglycanases in the physiological and pathological central nervous system. *Journal of Neuroinflammation*, *10*, 133.

Lemjabbar, H., & Basbaum, C. (2002). Platelet-activating factor receptor and ADAM10 mediate responses to Staphylococcus aureus in epithelial cells. *Nature Medicine*, *8*(1), 41–46.

Letronne, F., Laumet, G., Ayral, A. M., Chapuis, J., Demiautte, F., Laga, M., et al. (2016). ADAM30 downregulates APP-linked defects through cathepsin D activation in Alzheimer's disease. *eBioMedicine*, *9*, 278–292.

Levula, M., Paavonen, T., Valo, T., Pelto-Huikko, M., Laaksonen, R., Kahonen, M., et al. (2011). A disintegrin and metalloprotease -8 and -15 and susceptibility for ascending aortic dissection. *Scandinavian Journal of Clinical and Laboratory Investigation*, *71*(6), 515–522.

Li, F., Song, R., Ao, L., Reece, T. B., Cleveland, J. C., Jr., Dong, N., et al. (2017). ADAMTS5 deficiency in calcified aortic valves is associated with elevated pro-osteogenic activity in valvular interstitial cells. *Arteriosclerosis, Thrombosis, and Vascular Biology*, *37*(7), 1339–1351.

Li, H., Han, S., Sun, Q., Yao, Y., Li, S., Yuan, C., et al. (2019). Long non-coding RNA CDKN2B-AS1 reduces inflammatory response and promotes cholesterol efflux in atherosclerosis by inhibiting ADAM10 expression. *Aging (Albany NY)*, *11*(6), 1695–1715.

Li, J. K., Du, W. J., Jiang, S. L., & Tian, H. (2009). Expression of ADAM-15 in rat myocardial infarction. *International Journal of Experimental Pathology*, *90*(3), 347–354.

Li, M., Liu, Q., Lei, J., Wang, X., Chen, X., & Ding, Y. (2017). MiR-362-3p inhibits the proliferation and migration of vascular smooth muscle cells in atherosclerosis by targeting ADAMTS1. *Biochemical and Biophysical Research Communications*, *493*(1), 270–276.

Li, S. W., Arita, M., Fertala, A., Bao, Y., Kopen, G. C., Langsjo, T. K., et al. (2001). Transgenic mice with inactive alleles for procollagen N-proteinase (ADAMTS-2) develop fragile skin and male sterility. *The Biochemical Journal*, *355*(Pt. 2), 271–278.

Li, X., Maretzky, T., Perez-Aguilar, J. M., Monette, S., Weskamp, G., Le Gall, S., et al. (2017). Structural modeling defines transmembrane residues in ADAM17 that are crucial for Rhbdf2-ADAM17-dependent proteolysis. *Journal of Cell Science*, *130*(5), 868–878.

Li, X., Maretzky, T., Weskamp, G., Monette, S., Qing, X., Issuree, P. D., et al. (2015). iRhoms 1 and 2 are essential upstream regulators of ADAM17-dependent EGFR signaling. *Proceedings of the National Academy of Sciences of the United States of America*, *112*(19), 6080–6085.

Li, Y., Cui, L. L., Li, Q. Q., Ma, G. D., Cai, Y. J., Chen, Y. Y., et al. (2014). Association between ADAM17 promoter polymorphisms and ischemic stroke in a Chinese population. *Journal of Atherosclerosis and Thrombosis*, *21*(8), 878–893.

Li, Y., Liao, F., Yin, X. J., Cui, L. L., Ma, G. D., Nong, X. X., et al. (2013). An association study on ADAM10 promoter polymorphisms and atherosclerotic cerebral infarction in a Chinese population. *CNS Neuroscience & Therapeutics*, *19*(10), 785–794.

Li, Y. J., Fan, Y. H., Tang, J., Li, J. B., & Yu, C. H. (2014). Meprin-beta regulates production of pro-inflammatory factors via a disintegrin and metalloproteinase-10 (ADAM-10) dependent pathway in macrophages. *International Immunopharmacology*, *18*(1), 77–84.

Li, Z., Nardi, M. A., Li, Y. S., Zhang, W., Pan, R., Dang, S., et al. (2009). C-terminal ADAMTS-18 fragment induces oxidative platelet fragmentation, dissolves platelet aggregates, and protects against carotid artery occlusion and cerebral stroke. *Blood*, *113*(24), 6051–6060.

Liao, Y., Zhao, H., Ogai, A., Kato, H., Asakura, M., Kim, J., et al. (2008). Atorvastatin slows the progression of cardiac remodeling in mice with pressure overload and inhibits epidermal growth factor receptor activation. *Hypertension Research*, *31*(2), 335–344.

Ling, J. Y., Shen, L., Liu, Q., Xue, S., Ma, W., Wu, H., et al. (2013). Changes in platelet GPIbalpha and ADAM17 during the acute stage of atherosclerotic ischemic stroke among Chinese. *Journal of Huazhong University of Science and Technology. Medical Sciences*, *33*(3), 438–442.

Liu, P., Yan, S., Chen, M., Chen, A., Yao, D., Xu, X., et al. (2015). Effects of baicalin on collagen Iota and collagen IotaIotaIota expression in pulmonary arteries of rats with hypoxic pulmonary hypertension. *International Journal of Molecular Medicine*, *35*(4), 901–908.

Livermore, C., Warr, N., Chalon, N., Siggers, P., Mianne, J., Codner, G., et al. (2019). Male mice lacking ADAMTS-16 are fertile but exhibit testes of reduced weight. *Scientific Reports*, *9*(1), 17195.

Llamazares, M., Cal, S., Quesada, V., & Lopez-Otin, C. (2003). Identification and characterization of ADAMTS-20 defines a novel subfamily of metalloproteinases-disintegrins with multiple thrombospondin-1 repeats and a unique GON domain. *The Journal of Biological Chemistry*, *278*(15), 13382–13389.

Loichinger, M. H., Towner, D., Thompson, K. S., Ahn, H. J., & Bryant-Greenwood, G. D. (2016). Systemic and placental alpha-klotho: Effects of preeclampsia in the last trimester of gestation. *Placenta*, *41*, 53–61.

Lopez De Padilla, C. M., Hein, M. S., Crowson, C. S., Choo, C. S., Green, A. B., Petri, M., et al. (2013). Increased expression of ADAMTS13 mRNA correlates with ischemic cerebrovascular disease in systemic lupus erythematosus patients. *SAGE Open Medicine*, *1*, 2050312113514404.

Lopez, J. A., & Dong, J. F. (2004). Cleavage of von Willebrand factor by ADAMTS-13 on endothelial cells. *Seminars in Hematology*, *41*(1), 15–23.
Lu, D., Xie, S., Sukkar, M. B., Lu, X., Scully, M. F., & Chung, K. F. (2007). Inhibition of airway smooth muscle adhesion and migration by the disintegrin domain of ADAM-15. *American Journal of Respiratory Cell and Molecular Biology*, *37*(4), 494–500.
Lucitti, J. L., Mackey, J. K., Morrison, J. C., Haigh, J. J., Adams, R. H., & Faber, J. E. (2012). Formation of the collateral circulation is regulated by vascular endothelial growth factor-A and a disintegrin and metalloprotease family members 10 and 17. *Circulation Research*, *111*(12), 1539–1550.
Ludwig, A., Hundhausen, C., Lambert, M. H., Broadway, N., Andrews, R. C., Bickett, D. M., et al. (2005). Metalloproteinase inhibitors for the disintegrin-like metalloproteinases ADAM10 and ADAM17 that differentially block constitutive and phorbol ester-inducible shedding of cell surface molecules. *Combinatorial Chemistry & High Throughput Screening*, *8*(2), 161–171.
Lunn, C. A., Fan, X., Dalie, B., Miller, K., Zavodny, P. J., Narula, S. K., et al. (1997). Purification of ADAM 10 from bovine spleen as a TNFalpha convertase. *FEBS Letters*, *400*(3), 333–335.
Lyu, C., Chen, Y., Zhu, M., Jin, X., Liu, P., Zheng, Z., et al. (2015). Association of ADAMTS-1 gene polymorphisms with ischemic stroke caused by large artery atherosclerosis. *Zhonghua Yi Xue Yi Chuan Xue Za Zhi*, *32*(6), 844–848.
Mahoney, E. T., Benton, R. L., Maddie, M. A., Whittemore, S. R., & Hagg, T. (2009). ADAM8 is selectively up-regulated in endothelial cells and is associated with angiogenesis after spinal cord injury in adult mice. *The Journal of Comparative Neurology*, *512*(2), 243–255.
Majerus, E. M., Zheng, X., Tuley, E. A., & Sadler, J. E. (2003). Cleavage of the ADAMTS13 propeptide is not required for protease activity. *The Journal of Biological Chemistry*, *278*(47), 46643–46648.
Maretzky, T., Swendeman, S., Mogollon, E., Weskamp, G., Sahin, U., Reiss, K., et al. (2017). Characterization of the catalytic properties of the membrane-anchored metalloproteinase ADAM9 in cell-based assays. *The Biochemical Journal*, *474*(9), 1467–1479.
Matthews, A. L., Noy, P. J., Reyat, J. S., & Tomlinson, M. G. (2017). Regulation of A disintegrin and metalloproteinase (ADAM) family sheddases ADAM10 and ADAM17: The emerging role of tetraspanins and rhomboids. *Platelets*, *28*(4), 333–341.
Matthews, A. L., Szyroka, J., Collier, R., Noy, P. J., & Tomlinson, M. G. (2017). Scissor sisters: Regulation of ADAM10 by the TspanC8 tetraspanins. *Biochemical Society Transactions*, *45*(3), 719–730.
McClurg, U. L., Danjo, K., King, H. O., Scott, G. B., Robinson, P. A., & Crabtree, J. E. (2015). Epithelial cell ADAM17 activation by Helicobacter pylori: Role of ADAM17 C-terminus and Threonine-735 phosphorylation. *Microbes and Infection*, *17*(3), 205–214.
McRobb, L. S., McKay, M. J., Gamble, J. R., Grace, M., Moutrie, V., Santos, E. D., et al. (2017). Ionizing radiation reduces ADAM10 expression in brain microvascular endothelial cells undergoing stress-induced senescence. *Aging (Albany NY)*, *9*(4), 1248–1268.
Mead, T. J., & Apte, S. S. (2018). ADAMTS proteins in human disorders. *Matrix Biology*, *71-72*, 225–239.
Mehta, V., Fields, L., Evans, I. M., Yamaji, M., Pellet-Many, C., Jones, T., et al. (2018). VEGF (vascular endothelial growth factor) induces NRP1 (neuropilin-1) cleavage via ADAMs (a disintegrin and metalloproteinase) 9 and 10 to generate novel carboxy-terminal NRP1 fragments that regulate angiogenic signaling. *Arteriosclerosis, Thrombosis, and Vascular Biology*, *38*(8), 1845–1858.
Miles, R. R., Sluka, J. P., Halladay, D. L., Santerre, R. F., Hale, L. V., Bloem, L., et al. (2000). ADAMTS-1: A cellular disintegrin and metalloprotease with thrombospondin motifs is a target for parathyroid hormone in bone. *Endocrinology*, *141*(12), 4533–4542.

Minond, D., Cudic, M., Bionda, N., Giulianotti, M., Maida, L., Houghten, R. A., et al. (2012). Discovery of novel inhibitors of a disintegrin and metalloprotease 17 (ADAM17) using glycosylated and non-glycosylated substrates. *The Journal of Biological Chemistry*, *287*(43), 36473–36487.

Mishra, P. K., Tyagi, N., Sen, U., Givvimani, S., & Tyagi, S. C. (2010). H2S ameliorates oxidative and proteolytic stresses and protects the heart against adverse remodeling in chronic heart failure. *American Journal of Physiology. Heart and Circulatory Physiology*, *298*(2), H451–H456.

Mittaz, L., Ricardo, S., Martinez, G., Kola, I., Kelly, D. J., Little, M. H., et al. (2005). Neonatal calyceal dilation and renal fibrosis resulting from loss of Adamts-1 in mouse kidney is due to a developmental dysgenesis. *Nephrology, Dialysis, Transplantation*, *20*(2), 419–423.

Mittaz, L., Russell, D. L., Wilson, T., Brasted, M., Tkalcevic, J., Salamonsen, L. A., et al. (2004). Adamts-1 is essential for the development and function of the urogenital system. *Biology of Reproduction*, *70*(4), 1096–1105.

Moake, J. L. (2004). von Willebrand factor, ADAMTS-13, and thrombotic thrombocytopenic purpura. *Seminars in Hematology*, *41*(1), 4–14.

Mochizuki, S., & Okada, Y. (2007). ADAMs in cancer cell proliferation and progression. *Cancer Science*, *98*(5), 621–628.

Moriguchi-Goto, S., Yamashita, A., Tamura, N., Soejima, K., Takahashi, M., Nakagaki, T., et al. (2009). ADAMTS-13 attenuates thrombus formation on type I collagen surface and disrupted plaques under flow conditions. *Atherosclerosis*, *203*(2), 409–416.

Moss, M. L., Jin, S. L., Milla, M. E., Bickett, D. M., Burkhart, W., Carter, H. L., et al. (1997). Cloning of a disintegrin metalloproteinase that processes precursor tumour-necrosis factor-alpha. *Nature*, *385*(6618), 733–736.

Moss, M. L., & Rasmussen, F. H. (2007). Fluorescent substrates for the proteinases ADAM17, ADAM10, ADAM8, and ADAM12 useful for high-throughput inhibitor screening. *Analytical Biochemistry*, *366*(2), 144–148.

Mukerjee, S., Gao, H., Xu, J., Sato, R., Zsombok, A., & Lazartigues, E. (2019). ACE2 and ADAM17 interaction regulates the activity of presympathetic neurons. *Hypertension*, *74*(5), 1181–1191.

Muller, M., Kessler, T., Schunkert, H., Erdmann, J., & Tennstedt, S. (2016). Classification of ADAMTS binding sites: The first step toward selective ADAMTS7 inhibitors. *Biochemical and Biophysical Research Communications*, *471*(3), 380–385.

Murphy, G. (2011). Tissue inhibitors of metalloproteinases. *Genome Biology*, *12*(11), 233.

Musumeci, G., Coleman, R., Imbesi, R., Magro, G., Parenti, R., Szychlinska, M. A., et al. (2014). ADAM-10 could mediate cleavage of N-cadherin promoting apoptosis in human atherosclerotic lesions leading to vulnerable plaque: A morphological and immunohistochemical study. *Acta Histochemica*, *116*(7), 1148–1158.

Nakamura, K., Hirohata, S., Murakami, T., Miyoshi, T., Demircan, K., Oohashi, T., et al. (2004). Dynamic induction of ADAMTS1 gene in the early phase of acute myocardial infarction. *Journal of Biochemistry*, *136*(4), 439–446.

Nakamura, Y., Kita, S., Tanaka, Y., Fukuda, S., Obata, Y., Okita, T., et al. (2020). A disintegrin and metalloproteinase 12 prevents heart failure by regulating cardiac hypertrophy and fibrosis. *American Journal of Physiology. Heart and Circulatory Physiology*, *318*(2), H238–H251.

Nandadasa, S., Burin des Roziers, C., Koch, C., Tran-Lundmark, K., Dours-Zimmermann, M. T., Zimmermann, D. R., et al. (2021). A new mouse mutant with cleavage-resistant versican and isoform-specific versican mutants demonstrate that proteolysis at the Glu(441)-Ala(442) peptide bond in the V1 isoform is essential for interdigital web regression. *Matrix Biology Plus*, *10*, 100064.

Nicolaou, A., Zhao, Z., Northoff, B. H., Sass, K., Herbst, A., Kohlmaier, A., et al. (2017). Adam17 deficiency promotes atherosclerosis by enhanced TNFR2 signaling in mice. *Arteriosclerosis, Thrombosis, and Vascular Biology*, *37*(2), 247–257.

Niu, A., Wang, B., & Li, Y. P. (2015). TNFalpha shedding in mechanically stressed cardiomyocytes is mediated by Src activation of TACE. *Journal of Cellular Biochemistry*, *116*(4), 559–565.

Nyren-Erickson, E. K., Jones, J. M., Srivastava, D. K., & Mallik, S. (2013). A disintegrin and metalloproteinase-12 (ADAM12): Function, roles in disease progression, and clinical implications. *Biochimica et Biophysica Acta*, *1830*(10), 4445–4455.

Obama, T., Takayanagi, T., Kobayashi, T., Bourne, A. M., Elliott, K. J., Charbonneau, M., et al. (2015). Vascular induction of a disintegrin and metalloprotease 17 by angiotensin II through hypoxia inducible factor 1alpha. *American Journal of Hypertension*, *28*(1), 10–14.

Ogino, H., Hisanaga, A., Kohno, T., Kondo, Y., Okumura, K., Kamei, T., et al. (2017). Secreted metalloproteinase ADAMTS-3 inactivates reelin. *The Journal of Neuroscience*, *37*(12), 3181–3191.

Ohtsu, H., Dempsey, P. J., & Eguchi, S. (2006). ADAMs as mediators of EGF receptor transactivation by G protein-coupled receptors. *American Journal of Physiology. Cell Physiology*, *291*(1), C1–10.

Oikawa, H., Maesawa, C., Tatemichi, Y., Nishinari, Y., Nishiya, M., Mizugai, H., et al. (2014). A disintegrin and metalloproteinase 17 (ADAM17) mediates epidermal growth factor receptor transactivation by angiotensin II on hepatic stellate cells. *Life Sciences*, *97*(2), 137–144.

Okeke, E., & Dokun, A. O. (2018). Role of genetics in peripheral arterial disease outcomes; significance of limb-salvage quantitative locus-1 genes. *Experimental Biology and Medicine (Maywood, N.J.)*, *243*(2), 190–197.

Oksala, N., Levula, M., Airla, N., Pelto-Huikko, M., Ortiz, R. M., Jarvinen, O., et al. (2009). ADAM-9, ADAM-15, and ADAM-17 are upregulated in macrophages in advanced human atherosclerotic plaques in aorta and carotid and femoral arteries—Tampere vascular study. *Annals of Medicine*, *41*(4), 279–290.

Oller, J., Mendez-Barbero, N., Ruiz, E. J., Villahoz, S., Renard, M., Canelas, L. I., et al. (2017). Nitric oxide mediates aortic disease in mice deficient in the metalloprotease Adamts1 and in a mouse model of Marfan syndrome. *Nature Medicine*, *23*(2), 200–212.

Omura, J., Satoh, K., Kikuchi, N., Satoh, T., Kurosawa, R., Nogi, M., et al. (2019). ADAMTS8 promotes the development of pulmonary arterial hypertension and right ventricular failure: A possible novel therapeutic target. *Circulation Research*, *125*(10), 884–906.

Ong, M. H., Wong, H. K., Tengku-Muhammad, T. S., Choo, Q. C., & Chew, C. H. (2019). Pro-atherogenic proteoglycanase ADAMTS-1 is down-regulated by lauric acid through PI3K and JNK signaling pathways in THP-1 derived macrophages. *Molecular Biology Reports*, *46*(3), 2631–2641.

Ozawa, K., Packwood, W., Varlamov, O., Qi, Y., Xie, A., Wu, M. D., et al. (2018). Molecular imaging of VWF (von Willebrand factor) and platelet adhesion in postischemic impaired microvascular reflow. *Circulation. Cardiovascular Imaging*, *11*(11), e007913.

Palau, V., Pascual, J., Soler, M. J., & Riera, M. (2019). Role of ADAM17 in kidney disease. *American Journal of Physiology. Renal Physiology*, *317*(2), F333–F342.

Parrish, D. C., Francis Stuart, S. D., Olivas, A., Wang, L., Nykjaer, A., Ripplinger, C. M., et al. (2018). Transient denervation of viable myocardium after myocardial infarction does not alter arrhythmia susceptibility. *American Journal of Physiology. Heart and Circulatory Physiology*, *314*(3), H415–H423.

Pehlivan, S., Gurses, M. S., Ural, M. N., Akyol, S., Eren, F., Turkmen Inanir, N., et al. (2016). The role of ADAMTS1 and Versican in human myocardial infarction: A postmortem study. *Laboratoriums Medizin*, *47*(3), 205–212.

Pelisek, J., Deutsch, L., Ansel, A., Pongratz, J., Stadlbauer, T., Gebhard, H., et al. (2017). Expression of a metalloproteinase family of ADAMTS in human vulnerable carotid lesions. *Journal of Cardiovascular Medicine (Hagerstown, Md.)*, *18*(1), 10–18.

Pelisek, J., Pongratz, J., Deutsch, L., Reeps, C., Stadlbauer, T., & Eckstein, H. H. (2012). Expression and cellular localization of metalloproteases ADAMs in high graded carotid artery lesions. *Scandinavian Journal of Clinical and Laboratory Investigation*, *72*(8), 648–656.

Peng, Q., Deng, Y., Yang, X., Leng, X., Yang, Y., & Liu, H. (2016). Genetic variants of ADAM17 are implicated in the pathological process of Kawasaki disease and secondary coronary artery lesions via the TGF-beta/SMAD3 signaling pathway. *European Journal of Pediatrics*, *175*(5), 705–713.

Perna, A. F., Pizza, A., Di Nunzio, A., Bellantone, R., Raffaelli, M., Cicchella, T., et al. (2017). ADAM17, a new player in the pathogenesis of chronic kidney disease-mineral and bone disorder. *Journal of Renal Nutrition*, *27*(6), 453–457.

Peschon, J. J., Slack, J. L., Reddy, P., Stocking, K. L., Sunnarborg, S. W., Lee, D. C., et al. (1998). An essential role for ectodomain shedding in mammalian development. *Science*, *282*(5392), 1281–1284.

Petri, A., Kim, H. J., Xu, Y., de Groot, R., Li, C., Vandenbulcke, A., et al. (2019). Crystal structure and substrate-induced activation of ADAMTS13. *Nature Communications*, *10*(1), 3781.

Polverino, F., Rojas-Quintero, J., Wang, X., Petersen, H., Zhang, L., Gai, X., et al. (2018). A disintegrin and metalloproteinase domain-8: A novel protective proteinase in chronic obstructive pulmonary disease. *American Journal of Respiratory and Critical Care Medicine*, *198*(10), 1254–1267.

Poon, L. C., Chelemen, T., Granvillano, O., Pandeva, I., & Nicolaides, K. H. (2008). First-trimester maternal serum a disintegrin and metalloprotease 12 (ADAM12) and adverse pregnancy outcome. *Obstetrics and Gynecology*, *112*(5), 1082–1090.

Poonpet, T., Honsawek, S., Tammachote, N., Kanitnate, S., & Tammachote, R. (2013). ADAMTS14 gene polymorphism associated with knee osteoarthritis in Thai women. *Genetics and Molecular Research*, *12*(4), 5301–5309.

Porter, S., Clark, I. M., Kevorkian, L., & Edwards, D. R. (2005). The ADAMTS metalloproteinases. *The Biochemical Journal*, *386*(Pt. 1), 15–27.

Prins, B. P., Mead, T. J., Brody, J. A., Sveinbjornsson, G., Ntalla, I., Bihlmeyer, N. A., et al. (2018). Exome-chip meta-analysis identifies novel loci associated with cardiac conduction, including ADAMTS6. *Genome Biology*, *19*(1), 87.

Proudfoot, A. G., Davidson, S. J., & Strueber, M. (2017). von Willebrand factor disruption and continuous-flow circulatory devices. *The Journal of Heart and Lung Transplantation*, *36*(11), 1155–1163.

Pu, X., Xiao, Q., Kiechl, S., Chan, K., Ng, F. L., Gor, S., et al. (2013). ADAMTS7 cleavage and vascular smooth muscle cell migration is affected by a coronary-artery-disease-associated variant. *American Journal of Human Genetics*, *92*(3), 366–374.

Qi, B., Newcomer, R. G., & Sang, Q. X. (2009). ADAM19/adamalysin 19 structure, function, and role as a putative target in tumors and inflammatory diseases. *Current Pharmaceutical Design*, *15*(20), 2336–2348.

Qian, L. W., Mizumoto, K., Urashima, T., Nagai, E., Maehara, N., Sato, N., et al. (2002). Radiation-induced increase in invasive potential of human pancreatic cancer cells and its blockade by a matrix metalloproteinase inhibitor, CGS27023. *Clinical Cancer Research*, *8*(4), 1223–1227.

Qin, W., Cao, Y., Li, L., Chen, W., & Chen, X. (2017). Upregulation of ADAMTS7 and downregulation of COMP are associated with aortic aneurysm. *Molecular Medicine Reports*, *16*(4), 5459–5463.

Qu, L., Jiang, M., Qiu, W., Lu, S., Zhao, Y., Xia, L., et al. (2016). Assessment of the diagnostic value of plasma levels, activities, and their ratios of von Willebrand factor and ADAMTS13 in patients with cerebral infarction. *Clinical and Applied Thrombosis/Hemostasis*, *22*(3), 252–259.

Qu, Y., & Zhang, N. (2018). miR-365b-3p inhibits the cell proliferation and migration of human coronary artery smooth muscle cells by directly targeting ADAMTS1 in coronary atherosclerosis. *Experimental and Therapeutic Medicine*, *16*(5), 4239–4245.

Raitoharju, E., Seppala, I., Levula, M., Kuukasjarvi, P., Laurikka, J., Nikus, K., et al. (2011). Common variation in the ADAM8 gene affects serum sADAM8 concentrations and the risk of myocardial infarction in two independent cohorts. *Atherosclerosis*, *218*(1), 127–133.

Ramdas, V., McBride, M., Denby, L., & Baker, A. H. (2013). Canonical transforming growth factor-beta signaling regulates disintegrin metalloprotease expression in experimental renal fibrosis via miR-29. *The American Journal of Pathology*, *183*(6), 1885–1896.

Rapti, M., Atkinson, S. J., Lee, M. H., Trim, A., Moss, M., & Murphy, G. (2008). The isolated N-terminal domains of TIMP-1 and TIMP-3 are insufficient for ADAM10 inhibition. *The Biochemical Journal*, *411*(2), 433–439.

Rau, C. D., Romay, M. C., Tuteryan, M., Wang, J. J., Santolini, M., Ren, S., et al. (2017). Systems genetics approach identifies gene pathways and Adamts2 as drivers of isoproterenol-induced cardiac hypertrophy and cardiomyopathy in mice. *Cell Systems*, *4*(1), 121–128 e124.

Raucci, A., Cugusi, S., Antonelli, A., Barabino, S. M., Monti, L., Bierhaus, A., et al. (2008). A soluble form of the receptor for advanced glycation endproducts (RAGE) is produced by proteolytic cleavage of the membrane-bound form by the sheddase a disintegrin and metalloprotease 10 (ADAM10). *The FASEB Journal*, *22*(10), 3716–3727.

Reddy, P., Slack, J. L., Davis, R., Cerretti, D. P., Kozlosky, C. J., Blanton, R. A., et al. (2000). Functional analysis of the domain structure of tumor necrosis factor-alpha converting enzyme. *The Journal of Biological Chemistry*, *275*(19), 14608–14614.

Ren, L., Wu, C., Yang, K., Chen, S., Ye, P., Wu, J., et al. (2018). A disintegrin and metalloprotease-22 attenuates hypertrophic remodeling in mice through inhibition of the protein kinase B signaling pathway. *Journal of the American Heart Association*, 7(2), e005696.

Ren, P., Hughes, M., Krishnamoorthy, S., Zou, S., Zhang, L., Wu, D., et al. (2017). Critical role of ADAMTS-4 in the development of sporadic aortic aneurysm and dissection in mice. *Scientific Reports*, 7(1), 12351.

Ren, W., Liang, L., Li, Y., Wei, F. Y., Mu, N., Zhang, L., et al. (2020). Upregulation of miR423 improves autologous vein graft restenosis via targeting ADAMTS7. *International Journal of Molecular Medicine*, *45*(2), 532–542.

Reyat, J. S., Chimen, M., Noy, P. J., Szyroka, J., Rainger, G. E., & Tomlinson, M. G. (2017). ADAM10-interacting tetraspanins Tspan5 and Tspan17 regulate VE-cadherin expression and promote T lymphocyte transmigration. *Journal of Immunology*, *199*(2), 666–676.

Rizza, S., Copetti, M., Cardellini, M., Menghini, R., Pecchioli, C., Luzi, A., et al. (2015). A score including ADAM17 substrates correlates to recurring cardiovascular event in subjects with atherosclerosis. *Atherosclerosis*, *239*(2), 459–464.

Rodriguez-Baena, F. J., Redondo-Garcia, S., Peris-Torres, C., Martino-Echarri, E., Fernandez-Rodriguez, R., Plaza-Calonge, M. D. C., et al. (2018). ADAMTS1 protease is required for a balanced immune cell repertoire and tumour inflammatory response. *Scientific Reports*, *8*(1), 13103.

Rodriguez-Lopez, J., Pombo-Suarez, M., Loughlin, J., Tsezou, A., Blanco, F. J., Meulenbelt, I., et al. (2009). Association of a nsSNP in ADAMTS14 to some osteoarthritis phenotypes. *Osteoarthritis and Cartilage*, *17*(3), 321–327.

Rodriguez-Manzaneque, J. C., Westling, J., Thai, S. N., Luque, A., Knauper, V., Murphy, G., et al. (2002). ADAMTS1 cleaves aggrecan at multiple sites and is differentially inhibited by metalloproteinase inhibitors. *Biochemical and Biophysical Research Communications*, *293*(1), 501–508.

Roose, E., Vidarsson, G., Kangro, K., Verhagen, O., Mancini, I., Desender, L., et al. (2018). Anti-ADAMTS13 autoantibodies against cryptic epitopes in immune-mediated thrombotic thrombocytopenic purpura. *Thrombosis and Haemostasis*, *118*(10), 1729–1742.

Rosendahl, M. S., Ko, S. C., Long, D. L., Brewer, M. T., Rosenzweig, B., Hedl, E., et al. (1997). Identification and characterization of a pro-tumor necrosis factor-alpha--processing enzyme from the ADAM family of zinc metalloproteases. *The Journal of Biological Chemistry*, *272*(39), 24588–24593.

Roychaudhuri, R., Hergrueter, A. H., Polverino, F., Laucho-Contreras, M. E., Gupta, K., Borregaard, N., et al. (2014). ADAM9 is a novel product of polymorphonuclear neutrophils: Regulation of expression and contributions to extracellular matrix protein degradation during acute lung injury. *Journal of Immunology*, *193*(5), 2469–2482.

Saha, N., Robev, D., Himanen, J. P., & Nikolov, D. B. (2019). ADAM proteases: Emerging role and targeting of the non-catalytic domains. *Cancer Letters*, *467*, 50–57.

Sahin, U., Weskamp, G., Kelly, K., Zhou, H. M., Higashiyama, S., Peschon, J., et al. (2004). Distinct roles for ADAM10 and ADAM17 in ectodomain shedding of six EGFR ligands. *The Journal of Cell Biology*, *164*(5), 769–779.

Sahul, Z. H., Mukherjee, R., Song, J., McAteer, J., Stroud, R. E., Dione, D. P., et al. (2011). Targeted imaging of the spatial and temporal variation of matrix metalloproteinase activity in a porcine model of postinfarct remodeling: Relationship to myocardial dysfunction. *Circulation. Cardiovascular Imaging*, *4*(4), 381–391.

Salloum, F. N. (2015). Hydrogen sulfide and cardioprotection—Mechanistic insights and clinical translatability. *Pharmacology & Therapeutics*, *152*, 11–17.

Salter, R. C., Arnaoutakis, K., Michael, D. R., Singh, N. N., Ashlin, T. G., Buckley, M. L., et al. (2011). The expression of a disintegrin and metalloproteinase with thrombospondin motifs 4 in human macrophages is inhibited by the anti-atherogenic cytokine transforming growth factor-beta and requires Smads, p38 mitogen-activated protein kinase and c-Jun. *The International Journal of Biochemistry & Cell Biology*, *43*(5), 805–811.

Santamaria, S., Cuffaro, D., Nuti, E., Ciccone, L., Tuccinardi, T., Liva, F., et al. (2021). Exosite inhibition of ADAMTS-5 by a glycoconjugated arylsulfonamide. *Scientific Reports*, *11*(1), 949.

Santamaria, S., & de Groot, R. (2019). Monoclonal antibodies against metzincin targets. *British Journal of Pharmacology*, *176*(1), 52–66.

Santamaria, S., & de Groot, R. (2020). ADAMTS proteases in cardiovascular physiology and disease. *Open Biology*, *10*(12), 200333.

Sarila, G., Bao, T., Abeydeera, S. A., Li, R., Mell, B., Joe, B., et al. (2020). Interplay between collagenase and undescended testes in Adamts16 knockout rats. *Journal of Pediatric Surgery*, *55*(9), 1952–1958.

Sato, T., Suzuki, H., Shibata, M., Kusuyama, T., Omori, Y., Soda, T., et al. (2006). Tumor-necrosis-factor-alpha-gene-deficient mice have improved cardiac function through reduction of intercellular adhesion molecule-1 in myocardial infarction. *Circulation Journal*, *70*(12), 1635–1642.

Satoh, H., Nakamura, M., Satoh, M., Nakajima, T., Izumoto, H., Maesawa, C., et al. (2004). Expression and localization of tumour necrosis factor-alpha and its converting enzyme in human abdominal aortic aneurysm. *Clinical Science (London, England)*, *106*(3), 301–306.

Satoh, M., Iwasaka, J., Nakamura, M., Akatsu, T., Shimoda, Y., & Hiramori, K. (2004). Increased expression of tumor necrosis factor-alpha converting enzyme and tumor necrosis factor-alpha in peripheral blood mononuclear cells in patients with advanced congestive heart failure. *European Journal of Heart Failure*, *6*(7), 869–875.

Satoh, M., Nakamura, M., Satoh, H., Saitoh, H., Segawa, I., & Hiramori, K. (2000). Expression of tumor necrosis factor-alpha-converting enzyme and tumor necrosis factor-alpha in human myocarditis. *Journal of the American College of Cardiology*, *36*(4), 1288–1294.

Scharfenberg, F., Helbig, A., Sammel, M., Benzel, J., Schlomann, U., Peters, F., et al. (2020). Degradome of soluble ADAM10 and ADAM17 metalloproteases. *Cellular and Molecular Life Sciences*, 77(2), 331–350.

Schick, D., Babendreyer, A., Wozniak, J., Awan, T., Noels, H., Liehn, E., et al. (2019). Elevated expression of the metalloproteinase ADAM8 associates with vascular diseases in mice and humans. *Atherosclerosis*, *286*, 163–171.

Schiviz, A., Wuersch, K., Piskernik, C., Dietrich, B., Hoellriegl, W., Rottensteiner, H., et al. (2012). A new mouse model mimicking thrombotic thrombocytopenic purpura: Correction of symptoms by recombinant human ADAMTS13. *Blood*, *119*(25), 6128–6135.

Schlomann, U., Dorzweiler, K., Nuti, E., Tuccinardi, T., Rossello, A., & Bartsch, J. W. (2019). Metalloprotease inhibitor profiles of human ADAM8 in vitro and in cell-based assays. *Biological Chemistry*, *400*(6), 801–810.

Schlomann, U., Wildeboer, D., Webster, A., Antropova, O., Zeuschner, D., Knight, C. G., et al. (2002). The metalloprotease disintegrin ADAM8. Processing by autocatalysis is required for proteolytic activity and cell adhesion. *The Journal of Biological Chemistry*, *277*(50), 48210–48219.

Schouten, L. R., Helmerhorst, H. J., Wagenaar, G. T., Haltenhof, T., Lutter, R., Roelofs, J. J., et al. (2016). Age-dependent changes in the pulmonary renin-angiotensin system are associated with severity of lung injury in a model of acute lung injury in rats. *Critical Care Medicine*, *44*(12), e1226–e1235.

Schrimpf, C., Koppen, T., Duffield, J. S., Boer, U., David, S., Ziegler, W., et al. (2017). TIMP3 is regulated by pericytes upon shear stress detection leading to a modified endothelial cell response. *European Journal of Vascular and Endovascular Surgery*, *54*(4), 524–533.

Schubert, K., Collins, L. E., Green, P., Nagase, H., & Troeberg, L. (2019). LRP1 controls TNF release via the TIMP-3/ADAM17 axis in endotoxin-activated macrophages. *Journal of Immunology*, *202*(5), 1501–1509.

Schulz, B., Pruessmeyer, J., Maretzky, T., Ludwig, A., Blobel, C. P., Saftig, P., et al. (2008). ADAM10 regulates endothelial permeability and T-Cell transmigration by proteolysis of vascular endothelial cadherin. *Circulation Research*, *102*(10), 1192–1201.

Schuppner, R., Dirks, M., Grosse, G. M., Bockmann, M., Goetz, F., Pasedag, T., et al. (2018). ADAMTS-13 activity predicts outcome in acute ischaemic stroke patients undergoing endovascular treatment. *Thrombosis and Haemostasis*, *118*(4), 758–767.

Scully, M. (2016). Thrombotic thrombocytopenic purpura and atypical hemolytic uremic syndrome microangiopathy in pregnancy. *Seminars in Thrombosis and Hemostasis*, *42*(7), 774–779.

Scully, M., Knobl, P., Kentouche, K., Rice, L., Windyga, J., Schneppenheim, R., et al. (2017). Recombinant ADAMTS-13: First-in-human pharmacokinetics and safety in congenital thrombotic thrombocytopenic purpura. *Blood*, *130*(19), 2055–2063.

Seals, D. F., & Courtneidge, S. A. (2003). The ADAMs family of metalloproteases: Multidomain proteins with multiple functions. *Genes & Development*, *17*(1), 7–30.

Selejan, S. R., Linz, D., Tatu, A. M., Hohl, M., Speer, T., Ewen, S., et al. (2018). Sympathoadrenergic suppression improves heart function by upregulating the ratio of sRAGE/RAGE in hypertension with metabolic syndrome. *Journal of Molecular and Cellular Cardiology*, *122*, 34–46.

Shen, G., Sun, Q., Yao, Y., Li, S., Liu, G., Yuan, C., et al. (2020). Role of ADAM9 and miR-126 in the development of abdominal aortic aneurysm. *Atherosclerosis*, *297*, 47–54.

Shen, L., Lu, G., Dong, N., Ma, Z., & Ruan, C. (2013). Simvastatin increases ADAMTS13 expression in podocytes. *Thrombosis Research*, *132*(1), 94–99.

Shen, M., Hu, M., Fedak, P. W. M., Oudit, G. Y., & Kassiri, Z. (2018). Cell-specific functions of ADAM17 regulate the progression of thoracic aortic aneurysm. *Circulation Research*, *123*(3), 372–388.

Shen, M., Morton, J., Davidge, S. T., & Kassiri, Z. (2017). Loss of smooth muscle cell disintegrin and metalloproteinase 17 transiently suppresses angiotensin II-induced hypertension and end-organ damage. *Journal of Molecular and Cellular Cardiology*, *103*, 11–21.

Shi, W., Chen, H., Sun, J., Buckley, S., Zhao, J., Anderson, K. D., et al. (2003). TACE is required for fetal murine cardiac development and modeling. *Developmental Biology*, *261*(2), 371–380.

Shindo, T., Kurihara, H., Kuno, K., Yokoyama, H., Wada, T., Kurihara, Y., et al. (2000). ADAMTS-1: A metalloproteinase-disintegrin essential for normal growth, fertility, and organ morphology and function. *The Journal of Clinical Investigation*, *105*(10), 1345–1352.

Smiljanic, K., Dobutovic, B., Obradovic, M., Nikolic, D., Marche, P., & Isenovic, E. R. (2011). Involvement of the ADAM 12 in thrombin-induced rat's VSMCs proliferation. *Current Medicinal Chemistry*, *18*(22), 3382–3386.

Smith, K. M., Gaultier, A., Cousin, H., Alfandari, D., White, J. M., & DeSimone, D. W. (2002). The cysteine-rich domain regulates ADAM protease function in vivo. *The Journal of Cell Biology*, *159*(5), 893–902.

Somerville, R. P., Jungers, K. A., & Apte, S. S. (2004). Discovery and characterization of a novel, widely expressed metalloprotease, ADAMTS10, and its proteolytic activation. *The Journal of Biological Chemistry*, *279*(49), 51208–51217.

Somerville, R. P., Longpre, J. M., Apel, E. D., Lewis, R. M., Wang, L. W., Sanes, J. R., et al. (2004). ADAMTS7B, the full-length product of the ADAMTS7 gene, is a chondroitin sulfate proteoglycan containing a mucin domain. *The Journal of Biological Chemistry*, *279*(34), 35159–35175.

Somerville, R. P., Longpre, J. M., Jungers, K. A., Engle, J. M., Ross, M., Evanko, S., et al. (2003). Characterization of ADAMTS-9 and ADAMTS-20 as a distinct ADAMTS subfamily related to Caenorhabditis elegans GON-1. *The Journal of Biological Chemistry*, *278*(11), 9503–9513.

Sommer, A., Duppe, M., Baumecker, L., Kordowski, F., Buch, J., Chico, J. F., et al. (2017). Extracellular sphingomyelinase activity impairs TNF-alpha-induced endothelial cell death via ADAM17 activation and TNF receptor 1 shedding. *Oncotarget*, *8*(42), 72584–72596.

Sonneveld, M. A., de Maat, M. P., Portegies, M. L., Kavousi, M., Hofman, A., Turecek, P. L., et al. (2015). Low ADAMTS13 activity is associated with an increased risk of ischemic stroke. *Blood*, *126*(25), 2739–2746.

Soond, S. M., Everson, B., Riches, D. W., & Murphy, G. (2005). ERK-mediated phosphorylation of Thr735 in TNFalpha-converting enzyme and its potential role in TACE protein trafficking. *Journal of Cell Science*, *118*(Pt. 11), 2371–2380.

South, K., Luken, B. M., Crawley, J. T., Phillips, R., Thomas, M., Collins, R. F., et al. (2014). Conformational activation of ADAMTS13. *Proceedings of the National Academy of Sciences of the United States of America*, *111*(52), 18578–18583.

Speck, N., Brandsch, C., Schmidt, N., Yazdekhasti, N., Hirche, F., Lucius, R., et al. (2015). The antiatherogenic effect of fish oil in male mice is associated with a diminished release of endothelial ADAM17 and ADAM10 substrates. *The Journal of Nutrition*, *145*(6), 1218–1226.

Spencer, K., Cowans, N. J., & Stamatopoulou, A. (2008). ADAM12s in maternal serum as a potential marker of pre-eclampsia. *Prenatal Diagnosis*, *28*(3), 212–216.

Srinivasan, S., Romagnoli, M., Bohm, A., & Sonenshein, G. E. (2014). N-glycosylation regulates ADAM8 processing and activation. *The Journal of Biological Chemistry*, *289*(48), 33676–33688.

Stoll, M., Ruhle, F., Witten, A., Barysenka, A., Arning, A., Strauss, C., et al. (2016). Rare variants in the ADAMTS13 Von Willebrand factor-binding domain contribute to pediatric stroke. *Circulation. Cardiovascular Genetics*, *9*(4), 357–367.

Stone, A. L., Kroeger, M., & Sang, Q. X. (1999). Structure-function analysis of the ADAM family of disintegrin-like and metalloproteinase-containing proteins (review). *Journal of Protein Chemistry*, *18*(4), 447–465.

Sun, C., Wu, M. H., Guo, M., Day, M. L., Lee, E. S., & Yuan, S. Y. (2010). ADAM15 regulates endothelial permeability and neutrophil migration via Src/ERK1/2 signalling. *Cardiovascular Research*, *87*(2), 348–355.

Sun, C., Wu, M. H., Lee, E. S., & Yuan, S. Y. (2012). A disintegrin and metalloproteinase 15 contributes to atherosclerosis by mediating endothelial barrier dysfunction via Src family kinase activity. *Arteriosclerosis, Thrombosis, and Vascular Biology*, *32*(10), 2444–2451.

Sun, M., Chen, M., Dawood, F., Zurawska, U., Li, J. Y., Parker, T., et al. (2007). Tumor necrosis factor-alpha mediates cardiac remodeling and ventricular dysfunction after pressure overload state. *Circulation*, *115*(11), 1398–1407.

Suna, G., Wojakowski, W., Lynch, M., Barallobre-Barreiro, J., Yin, X., Mayr, U., et al. (2018). Extracellular matrix proteomics reveals interplay of aggrecan and aggrecanases in vascular remodeling of stented coronary arteries. *Circulation*, *137*(2), 166–183.

Sundberg, C., Thodeti, C. K., Kveiborg, M., Larsson, C., Parker, P., Albrechtsen, R., et al. (2004). Regulation of ADAM12 cell-surface expression by protein kinase C epsilon. *The Journal of Biological Chemistry*, *279*(49), 51601–51611.

Takaguri, A., Kimura, K., Hinoki, A., Bourne, A. M., Autieri, M. V., & Eguchi, S. (2011). A disintegrin and metalloprotease 17 mediates neointimal hyperplasia in vasculature. *Hypertension*, *57*(4), 841–845.

Takaguri, A., Morimoto, M., Imai, S., & Satoh, K. (2016). Cilostazol inhibits interleukin-1-induced ADAM17 expression through cAMP independent signaling in vascular smooth muscle cells. *Cell Biology International*, *40*(3), 269–276.

Takahashi, E., Sagane, K., Oki, T., Yamazaki, K., Nagasu, T., & Kuromitsu, J. (2006). Deficits in spatial learning and motor coordination in ADAM11-deficient mice. *BMC Neuroscience*, 7, 19.

Takawale, A., Sakamuri, S. S., & Kassiri, Z. (2015). Extracellular matrix communication and turnover in cardiac physiology and pathology. *Comprehensive Physiology*, *5*(2), 687–719.

Takayanagi, T., Forrester, S. J., Kawai, T., Obama, T., Tsuji, T., Elliott, K. J., et al. (2016). Vascular ADAM17 as a novel therapeutic target in mediating cardiovascular hypertrophy and perivascular fibrosis induced by angiotensin II. *Hypertension*, *68*(4), 949–955.

Takeda, S. (2016). ADAM and ADAMTS family proteins and snake venom metalloproteinases: A structural overview. *Toxins (Basel)*, *8*(5).

Takeda, S., Igarashi, T., Mori, H., & Araki, S. (2006). Crystal structures of VAP1 reveal ADAMs' MDC domain architecture and its unique C-shaped scaffold. *The EMBO Journal*, *25*(11), 2388–2396.

Takimoto, T., Nakao, M., Nakajo, T., Chinen, Y., Kuroda, J., & Taniwaki, M. (2016). Acute myocardial infarction as the initial thrombotic event of thrombotic thrombocytopenic purpura. *Blood Coagulation & Fibrinolysis*, *27*(8), 948–951.

Takizawa, M., Yatabe, T., Okada, A., Chijiiwa, M., Mochizuki, S., Ghosh, P., et al. (2008). Calcium pentosan polysulfate directly inhibits enzymatic activity of ADAMTS4 (aggrecanase-1) in osteoarthritic chondrocytes. *FEBS Letters*, *582*(19), 2945–2949.

Tanaka, M., Nanba, D., Mori, S., Shiba, F., Ishiguro, H., Yoshino, K., et al. (2004). ADAM binding protein Eve-1 is required for ectodomain shedding of epidermal growth factor receptor ligands. *The Journal of Biological Chemistry, 279*(40), 41950–41959.

Tang, J. H., Zhang, H. M., Zhang, Z. H., & Zhang, X. L. (2017). Effect of tetramethylpyrazine combined with cisplatin on VEGF, KLF4 and ADAMTS1 in Lewis lung cancer mice. *Asian Pacific Journal of Tropical Medicine, 10*(8), 813–818.

Tang, Z. Y., Loss, G., Carmody, I., & Cohen, A. J. (2006). TIMP-3 ameliorates hepatic ischemia/reperfusion injury through inhibition of tumor necrosis factor-alpha-converting enzyme activity in rats. *Transplantation, 82*(11), 1518–1523.

Tersteeg, C., de Maat, S., De Meyer, S. F., Smeets, M. W., Barendrecht, A. D., Roest, M., et al. (2014). Plasmin cleavage of von Willebrand factor as an emergency bypass for ADAMTS13 deficiency in thrombotic microangiopathy. *Circulation, 129*(12), 1320–1331.

Thai, S. N., & Iruela-Arispe, M. L. (2002). Expression of ADAMTS1 during murine development. *Mechanisms of Development, 115*(1–2), 181–185.

Theodorou, K., van der Vorst, E. P. C., Gijbels, M. J., Wolfs, I. M. J., Jeurissen, M., Theelen, T. L., et al. (2017). Whole body and hematopoietic ADAM8 deficiency does not influence advanced atherosclerotic lesion development, despite its association with human plaque progression. *Scientific Reports*, 7(1), 11670.

Timms, K. P., & Maurice, S. B. (2020). Context-dependent bioactivity of versican fragments. *Glycobiology, 30*(6), 365–373.

Toba, H., de Castro Bras, L. E., Baicu, C. F., Zile, M. R., Lindsey, M. L., & Bradshaw, A. D. (2016). Increased ADAMTS1 mediates SPARC-dependent collagen deposition in the aging myocardium. *American Journal of Physiology. Endocrinology and Metabolism, 310*(11), E1027–E1035.

Torabi, F., Bogle, O. A., Estanyol, J. M., Oliva, R., & Miller, D. (2017). Zona pellucida-binding protein 2 (ZPBP2) and several proteins containing BX7B motifs in human sperm may have hyaluronic acid binding or recognition properties. *Molecular Human Reproduction, 23*(12), 803–816.

Tortorella, M. D., Arner, E. C., Hills, R., Easton, A., Korte-Sarfaty, J., Fok, K., et al. (2004). Alpha2-macroglobulin is a novel substrate for ADAMTS-4 and ADAMTS-5 and represents an endogenous inhibitor of these enzymes. *The Journal of Biological Chemistry, 279*(17), 17554–17561.

Tortorella, M. D., Tomasselli, A. G., Mathis, K. J., Schnute, M. E., Woodard, S. S., Munie, G., et al. (2009). Structural and inhibition analysis reveals the mechanism of selectivity of a series of aggrecanase inhibitors. *The Journal of Biological Chemistry, 284*(36), 24185–24191.

Troeberg, L., Fushimi, K., Khokha, R., Emonard, H., Ghosh, P., & Nagase, H. (2008). Calcium pentosan polysulfate is a multifaceted exosite inhibitor of aggrecanases. *The FASEB Journal, 22*(10), 3515–3524.

Troeberg, L., Fushimi, K., Scilabra, S. D., Nakamura, H., Dive, V., Thogersen, I. B., et al. (2009). The C-terminal domains of ADAMTS-4 and ADAMTS-5 promote association with N-TIMP-3. *Matrix Biology, 28*(8), 463–469.

Troeberg, L., Lazenbatt, C., Anower, E. K. M. F., Freeman, C., Federov, O., Habuchi, H., et al. (2014). Sulfated glycosaminoglycans control the extracellular trafficking and the activity of the metalloprotease inhibitor TIMP-3. *Chemistry & Biology, 21*(10), 1300–1309.

Urisono, Y., Sakata, A., Matsui, H., Kasuda, S., Ono, S., Yoshimoto, K., et al. (2018). Von Willebrand factor aggravates hepatic ischemia-reperfusion injury by promoting neutrophil recruitment in mice. *Thrombosis and Haemostasis, 118*(4), 700–708.

van der Vorst, E. P., Jeurissen, M., Wolfs, I. M., Keijbeck, A., Theodorou, K., Wijnands, E., et al. (2015). Myeloid A disintegrin and metalloproteinase domain 10 deficiency modulates atherosclerotic plaque composition by shifting the balance from inflammation toward fibrosis. *The American Journal of Pathology, 185*(4), 1145–1155.

van der Vorst, E. P., Keijbeck, A. A., de Winther, M. P., & Donners, M. M. (2012). A disintegrin and metalloproteases: Molecular scissors in angiogenesis, inflammation and atherosclerosis. *Atherosclerosis, 224*(2), 302–308.

van der Vorst, E. P. C., Weber, C., & Donners, M. (2018). A disintegrin and metalloproteases (ADAMs) in cardiovascular, metabolic and inflammatory diseases: Aspects for theranostic approaches. *Thrombosis and Haemostasis, 118*(7), 1167–1175.

Van Wart, H. E., & Birkedal-Hansen, H. (1990). The cysteine switch: A principle of regulation of metalloproteinase activity with potential applicability to the entire matrix metalloproteinase gene family. *Proceedings of the National Academy of Sciences of the United States of America, 87*(14), 5578–5582.

Vazquez, F., Hastings, G., Ortega, M. A., Lane, T. F., Oikemus, S., Lombardo, M., et al. (1999). METH-1, a human ortholog of ADAMTS-1, and METH-2 are members of a new family of proteins with angio-inhibitory activity. *The Journal of Biological Chemistry, 274*(33), 23349–23357.

Velasco, J., Li, J., DiPietro, L., Stepp, M. A., Sandy, J. D., & Plaas, A. (2011). Adamts5 deletion blocks murine dermal repair through CD44-mediated aggrecan accumulation and modulation of transforming growth factor beta1 (TGFbeta1) signaling. *The Journal of Biological Chemistry, 286*(29), 26016–26027.

Vistnes, M., Aronsen, J. M., Lunde, I. G., Sjaastad, I., Carlson, C. R., & Christensen, G. (2014). Pentosan polysulfate decreases myocardial expression of the extracellular matrix enzyme ADAMTS4 and improves cardiac function in vivo in rats subjected to pressure overload by aortic banding. *PLoS ONE, 9*(3), e89621.

Vorkapic, E., Folkesson, M., Magnell, K., Bohlooly, Y. M., Lanne, T., & Wagsater, D. (2017). ADAMTS-1 in abdominal aortic aneurysm. *PLoS ONE, 12*(6), e0178729.

Vuohelainen, V., Raitoharju, E., Levula, M., Lehtimaki, T., Pelto-Huikko, M., Honkanen, T., et al. (2011). Myocardial infarction induces early increased remote ADAM8 expression of rat hearts after cardiac arrest. *Scandinavian Journal of Clinical and Laboratory Investigation, 71*(7), 553–562.

Wagsater, D., Bjork, H., Zhu, C., Bjorkegren, J., Valen, G., Hamsten, A., et al. (2008). ADAMTS-4 and -8 are inflammatory regulated enzymes expressed in macrophage-rich areas of human atherosclerotic plaques. *Atherosclerosis, 196*(2), 514–522.

Wang, L., Fan, W., Cai, P., Fan, M., Zhu, X., Dai, Y., et al. (2013). Recombinant ADAMTS13 reduces tissue plasminogen activator-induced hemorrhage after stroke in mice. *Annals of Neurology, 73*(2), 189–198.

Wang, L., Hoggard, J. A., Korleski, E. D., Long, G. V., Ree, B. C., Hensley, K., et al. (2018). Multiple non-catalytic ADAMs are novel integrin alpha4 ligands. *Molecular and Cellular Biochemistry, 442*(1–2), 29–38.

Wang, L., Wang, X., & Kong, W. (2010). ADAMTS-7, a novel proteolytic culprit in vascular remodeling. *Sheng Li Xue Bao, 62*(4), 285–294.

Wang, L., Zheng, J., Bai, X., Liu, B., Liu, C. J., Xu, Q., et al. (2009). ADAMTS-7 mediates vascular smooth muscle cell migration and neointima formation in balloon-injured rat arteries. *Circulation Research, 104*(5), 688–698.

Wang, R., Li, Y., Tsung, A., Huang, H., Du, Q., Yang, M., et al. (2018). iNOS promotes CD24(+)CD133(+) liver cancer stem cell phenotype through a TACE/ADAM17-dependent Notch signaling pathway. *Proceedings of the National Academy of Sciences of the United States of America, 115*(43), E10127–E10136.

Wang, W. M., Ge, G., Lim, N. H., Nagase, H., & Greenspan, D. S. (2006). TIMP-3 inhibits the procollagen N-proteinase ADAMTS-2. *The Biochemical Journal, 398*(3), 515–519.

Wang, X., Chen, W., Zhang, J., Khan, A., Li, L., Huang, F., et al. (2017). Critical role of ADAMTS2 (a disintegrin and metalloproteinase with thrombospondin motifs 2) in cardiac hypertrophy induced by pressure overload. *Hypertension, 69*(6), 1060–1069.

Wang, X., Chow, F. L., Oka, T., Hao, L., Lopez-Campistrous, A., Kelly, S., et al. (2009). Matrix metalloproteinase-7 and ADAM-12 (a disintegrin and metalloproteinase-12) define a signaling axis in agonist-induced hypertension and cardiac hypertrophy. *Circulation, 119*(18), 2480–2489.

Wang, X., Oka, T., Chow, F. L., Cooper, S. B., Odenbach, J., Lopaschuk, G. D., et al. (2009). Tumor necrosis factor-alpha-converting enzyme is a key regulator of agonist-induced cardiac hypertrophy and fibrosis. *Hypertension, 54*(3), 575–582.

Wang, X., Zhang, S., Li, L., Hua, J., Zhu, L., & Zhang, G. (2018). Ticagrelor-induced thrombotic thrombocytopenic purpura: A case report and review of the literature. *Medicine (Baltimore), 97*(26), e11206.

Webster, N. J., Green, K. N., Settle, V. J., Peers, C., & Vaughan, P. F. (2004). Altered processing of the amyloid precursor protein and decreased expression of ADAM 10 by chronic hypoxia in SH-SY5Y: No role for the stress-activated JNK and p38 signalling pathways. *Brain Research. Molecular Brain Research, 130*(1–2), 161–169.

Weskamp, G., Cai, H., Brodie, T. A., Higashyama, S., Manova, K., Ludwig, T., et al. (2002). Mice lacking the metalloprotease-disintegrin MDC9 (ADAM9) have no evident major abnormalities during development or adult life. *Molecular and Cellular Biology, 22*(5), 1537–1544.

Weskamp, G., Schlondorff, J., Lum, L., Becherer, J. D., Kim, T. W., Saftig, P., et al. (2004). Evidence for a critical role of the tumor necrosis factor alpha convertase (TACE) in ectodomain shedding of the p75 neurotrophin receptor (p75NTR). *The Journal of Biological Chemistry, 279*(6), 4241–4249.

Wichert, R., Scharfenberg, F., Colmorgen, C., Koudelka, T., Schwarz, J., Wetzel, S., et al. (2019). Meprin beta induces activities of A disintegrin and metalloproteinases 9, 10, and 17 by specific prodomain cleavage. *The FASEB Journal, 33*(11), 11925–11940.

Witsch, T., Martinod, K., Sorvillo, N., Portier, I., De Meyer, S. F., & Wagner, D. D. (2018). Recombinant human ADAMTS13 treatment improves myocardial remodeling and functionality after pressure overload injury in mice. *Journal of the American Heart Association, 7*(3), e007004.

Wolf, C., Qian, Y., Brooke, M. A., Kelsell, D. P., & Franzke, C. W. (2016). ADAM17/EGFR axis promotes transglutaminase-dependent skin barrier formation through phospholipase C gamma1 and protein kinase C pathways. *Scientific Reports, 6*, 39780.

Wolf, Z. T., Brand, H. A., Shaffer, J. R., Leslie, E. J., Arzi, B., Willet, C. E., et al. (2015). Genome-wide association studies in dogs and humans identify ADAMTS20 as a risk variant for cleft lip and palate. *PLoS Genetics, 11*(3), e1005059.

Wu, W., Zhou, Y., Li, Y., Li, J., Ke, Y., Wang, Y., et al. (2015). Association between plasma ADAMTS-7 levels and ventricular remodeling in patients with acute myocardial infarction. *European Journal of Medical Research, 20*, 27.

Wunnemann, F., Ta-Shma, A., Preuss, C., Leclerc, S., van Vliet, P. P., Oneglia, A., et al. (2020). Loss of ADAMTS19 causes progressive non-syndromic heart valve disease. *Nature Genetics, 52*(1), 40–47.

Xiang, M., Luo, H., Wu, J., Ren, L., Ding, X., Wu, C., et al. (2018). ADAM23 in cardiomyocyte inhibits cardiac hypertrophy by targeting FAK–AKT signaling. *Journal of the American Heart Association, 7*(18), e008604.

Xiang, Y., de Groot, R., Crawley, J. T., & Lane, D. A. (2011). Mechanism of von Willebrand factor scissile bond cleavage by a disintegrin and metalloproteinase with a thrombospondin type 1 motif, member 13 (ADAMTS13). *Proceedings of the National Academy of Sciences of the United States of America, 108*(28), 11602–11607.

Xiang, Y., Wang, M., Chen, H., & Chen, L. (2021). Potential therapeutic approaches for the early entry of SARS-CoV-2 by interrupting the interaction between the spike protein on SARS-CoV-2 and angiotensin-converting enzyme 2 (ACE2). *Biochemical Pharmacology, 192*, 114724.

Xiao, Q., Zhang, F., Grassia, G., Hu, Y., Zhang, Z., Xing, Q., et al. (2014). Matrix metalloproteinase-8 promotes vascular smooth muscle cell proliferation and neointima formation. *Arteriosclerosis, Thrombosis, and Vascular Biology*, *34*(1), 90–98.

Xie, B., Shen, J., Dong, A., Swaim, M., Hackett, S. F., Wyder, L., et al. (2008). An Adam15 amplification loop promotes vascular endothelial growth factor-induced ocular neovascularization. *The FASEB Journal*, *22*(8), 2775–2783.

Xu, H., Cao, Y., Yang, X., Cai, P., Kang, L., Zhu, X., et al. (2017). ADAMTS13 controls vascular remodeling by modifying VWF reactivity during stroke recovery. *Blood*, *130*(1), 11–22.

Xu, J., Molinas, A. J. R., Mukerjee, S., Morgan, D. A., Rahmouni, K., Zsombok, A., et al. (2019). Activation of ADAM17 (a disintegrin and metalloprotease 17) on glutamatergic neurons selectively promotes sympathoexcitation. *Hypertension*, *73*(6), 1266–1274.

Xu, J., Sriramula, S., & Lazartigues, E. (2018). Excessive glutamate stimulation impairs ACE2 activity through ADAM17-mediated shedding in cultured cortical neurons. *Cellular and Molecular Neurobiology*, *38*(6), 1235–1243.

Xu, J., Sriramula, S., Xia, H., Moreno-Walton, L., Culicchia, F., Domenig, O., et al. (2017). Clinical relevance and role of neuronal AT1 receptors in ADAM17-mediated ACE2 shedding in neurogenic hypertension. *Circulation Research*, *121*(1), 43–55.

Yagami-Hiromasa, T., Sato, T., Kurisaki, T., Kamijo, K., Nabeshima, Y., & Fujisawa-Sehara, A. (1995). A metalloprotease-disintegrin participating in myoblast fusion. *Nature*, *377*(6550), 652–656.

Yang, F., Chen, Q., Yang, M., Maguire, E. M., Yu, X., He, S., et al. (2020). Macrophage-derived MMP-8 determines smooth muscle cell differentiation from adventitia stem/progenitor cells and promotes neointima hyperplasia. *Cardiovascular Research*, *116*(1), 211–225.

Yao, Y., Hu, C., Song, Q., Li, Y., Da, X., Yu, Y., et al. (2020). ADAMTS16 activates latent TGF-beta, accentuating fibrosis and dysfunction of the pressure-overloaded heart. *Cardiovascular Research*, *116*(5), 956–969.

Yim, V., Noisier, A. F. M., Hung, K. Y., Bartsch, J. W., Schlomann, U., & Brimble, M. A. (2016). Synthesis and biological evaluation of analogues of the potent ADAM8 inhibitor cyclo(RLsKDK) for the treatment of inflammatory diseases and cancer metastasis. *Bioorganic & Medicinal Chemistry*, *24*(18), 4032–4037.

Yu, J., Zhou, B., Yu, H., Han, J., Cui, M., Zhang, F., et al. (2016). Association between plasma ADAMTS-7 levels and severity of disease in patients with stable obstructive coronary artery disease. *Medicine (Baltimore)*, *95*(48), e5523.

Yu, X., Shi, J., Wang, X., & Zhang, F. (2019). Propofol affects the growth and metastasis of pancreatic cancer via ADAM8. *Pharmacological Reports*, *72*(2), 418–426.

Zeinieh, M., Salehi, A., Rajkumar, V., & Barker, P. A. (2015). p75NTR-dependent Rac1 activation requires receptor cleavage and activation of an NRAGE and NEDD9 signaling cascade. *Journal of Cell Science*, *128*(3), 447–459.

Zeng, S. Y., Chen, X., Chen, S. R., Li, Q., Wang, Y. H., Zou, J., et al. (2013). Upregulation of Nox4 promotes angiotensin II-induced epidermal growth factor receptor activation and subsequent cardiac hypertrophy by increasing ADAM17 expression. *The Canadian Journal of Cardiology*, *29*(10), 1310–1319.

Zeng, S. Y., Lu, H. Q., Yan, Q. J., & Zou, J. (2018). A reduction in ADAM17 expression is involved in the protective effect of the PPAR-alpha activator fenofibrate on pressure overload-induced cardiac hypertrophy. *PPAR Research*, *2018*, 7916953.

Zha, Y., Chen, Y., Xu, F., Li, T., Zhao, C., & Cui, L. (2010). ADAMTS4 level in patients with stable coronary artery disease and acute coronary syndromes. *Biomedicine & Pharmacotherapy*, *64*(3), 160–164.

Zhai, C. G., Xu, Y. Y., Tie, Y. Y., Zhang, Y., Chen, W. Q., Ji, X. P., et al. (2018). DKK3 overexpression attenuates cardiac hypertrophy and fibrosis in an angiotensin-perfused

animal model by regulating the ADAM17/ACE2 and GSK-3beta/beta-catenin pathways. *Journal of Molecular and Cellular Cardiology*, *114*, 243–252.
Zhai, M., Guo, J., Ma, H., Shi, W., Jou, D., Yan, D., et al. (2018). Ursolic acid prevents angiotensin II-induced abdominal aortic aneurysm in apolipoprotein E-knockout mice. *Atherosclerosis*, *271*, 128–135.
Zhang, C., Tian, L., Chi, C., Wu, X., Yang, X., Han, M., et al. (2010). Adam10 is essential for early embryonic cardiovascular development. *Developmental Dynamics*, *239*(10), 2594–2602.
Zhang, L., Yu, F., Wang, L., Zheng, J., Du, Y., Huang, Y., et al. (2015). ADAMTS-7 promotes vascular smooth muscle cells proliferation in vitro and in vivo. *Science China. Life Sciences*, *58*(7), 674–681.
Zhang, P., Shen, M., Fernandez-Patron, C., & Kassiri, Z. (2016). ADAMs family and relatives in cardiovascular physiology and pathology. *Journal of Molecular and Cellular Cardiology*, *93*, 186–199.
Zhang, Q., Thomas, S. M., Lui, V. W., Xi, S., Siegfried, J. M., Fan, H., et al. (2006). Phosphorylation of TNF-alpha converting enzyme by gastrin-releasing peptide induces amphiregulin release and EGF receptor activation. *Proceedings of the National Academy of Sciences of the United States of America*, *103*(18), 6901–6906.
Zhang, S. M., Jiang, L., Zhao, X., Liu, J. F., Liang, B., Liu, C., et al. (2019). A disintegrin and metalloprotease 22 accelerates neointima formation by activating ERK signaling. *Atherosclerosis*, *283*, 92–99.
Zhang, Y., Wang, Y., Zhou, D., Zhang, L. S., Deng, F. X., Shu, S., et al. (2019). Angiotensin II deteriorates advanced atherosclerosis by promoting MerTK cleavage and impairing efferocytosis through the AT1R/ROS/p38 MAPK/ADAM17 pathway. *American Journal of Physiology. Cell Physiology*, *317*(4), C776–C787.
Zhao, B. Q., Chauhan, A. K., Canault, M., Patten, I. S., Yang, J. J., Dockal, M., et al. (2009). von Willebrand factor-cleaving protease ADAMTS13 reduces ischemic brain injury in experimental stroke. *Blood*, *114*(15), 3329–3334.
Zheng, D. Y., Zhao, J., Yang, J. M., Wang, M., & Zhang, X. T. (2016). Enhanced ADAM17 expression is associated with cardiac remodeling in rats with acute myocardial infarction. *Life Sciences*, *151*, 61–69.
Zheng, X., Chung, D., Takayama, T. K., Majerus, E. M., Sadler, J. E., & Fujikawa, K. (2001). Structure of von Willebrand factor-cleaving protease (ADAMTS13), a metalloprotease involved in thrombotic thrombocytopenic purpura. *The Journal of Biological Chemistry*, *276*(44), 41059–41063.
Zheng, X., Majerus, E. M., & Sadler, J. E. (2002). ADAMTS13 and TTP. *Current Opinion in Hematology*, *9*(5), 389–394.
Zheng, X. L. (2015). ADAMTS13 and von Willebrand factor in thrombotic thrombocytopenic purpura. *Annual Review of Medicine*, *66*, 211–225.
Zhou, H. M., Weskamp, G., Chesneau, V., Sahin, U., Vortkamp, A., Horiuchi, K., et al. (2004). Essential role for ADAM19 in cardiovascular morphogenesis. *Molecular and Cellular Biology*, *24*(1), 96–104.
Zhou, M., Dai, W., Cui, Y., & Li, Y. (2020). Estrogen downregulates gp130 expression in HUVECs by regulating ADAM10 and ADAM17 via the estrogen receptor. *Biochemical and Biophysical Research Communications*, *523*(3), 753–758.
Zhou, S., Jiang, S., Guo, J., Xu, N., Wang, Q., Zhang, G., et al. (2019). ADAMTS13 protects mice against renal ischemia-reperfusion injury by reducing inflammation and improving endothelial function. *American Journal of Physiology. Renal Physiology*, *316*(1), F134–F145.
Zhu, R., Cheng, M., Lu, T., Yang, N., Ye, S., Pan, Y. H., et al. (2018). A disintegrin and metalloproteinase with thrombospondin motifs 18 deficiency leads to visceral adiposity

and associated metabolic syndrome in mice. *The American Journal of Pathology, 188*(2), 461–473.

Zhu, Z., Zhu, J., Zhao, X., Yang, K., Lu, L., Zhang, F., et al. (2015). All-trans retinoic acid ameliorates myocardial ischemia/reperfusion injury by reducing cardiomyocyte apoptosis. *PLoS ONE, 10*(7), e0133414.

Zhuang, X., Li, R., Maimaitijiang, A., Liu, R., Yan, F., Hu, H., et al. (2019). miR-221-3p inhibits oxidized low-density lipoprotein induced oxidative stress and apoptosis via targeting a disintegrin and metalloprotease-22. *Journal of Cellular Biochemistry, 120*(4), 6304–6314.

Zou, J., Zhu, F., Liu, J., Wang, W., Zhang, R., Garlisi, C. G., et al. (2004). Catalytic activity of human ADAM33. *The Journal of Biological Chemistry, 279*(11), 9818–9830.

CHAPTER NINE

Beyond hypertension: Diastolic dysfunction associated with cancer treatment in the era of cardio-oncology

Giorgio Minotti[a,*], Pierantonio Menna[b], Massimiliano Camilli[c], Emanuela Salvatorelli[a], and Roberto Levi[d]

[a]Department of Medicine, Campus Bio-Medico University and Fondazione Policlinico, Rome, Italy
[b]Department of Health Sciences, Campus Bio-Medico University and Fondazione Policlinico, Rome, Italy
[c]Department of Cardiovascular Medicine, Fondazione Policlinico Universitario A. Gemelli IRCCS, Rome
[d]Department of Pharmacology, Weill Cornell Medicine, New York, NY, United States
[*]Corresponding author: e-mail address: g.minotti@unicampus.it

Contents

Abstract

Cancer patients are at an increased risk of cardiovascular events. Both old-generation cytostatics/cytotoxics and new-generation "targeted" drugs can in fact damage cardiomyocytes, endothelial cells of veins and arteries, specialized cells of the conduction system, pericardium, and valves. A new discipline, cardio-oncology, has therefore developed with the aim of protecting cancer patients from cardiovascular events, while also providing them with the best possible oncologic treatment. Anthracyclines have long

Advances in Pharmacology, Volume 94
ISSN 1054-3589
https://doi.org/10.1016/bs.apha.2022.02.002

been known to elicit cardiotoxicity that, depending on treatment- or patient-related factors, may progress with a variable velocity toward cardiomyopathy and systolic heart failure. However, early compromise of diastolic function may precede systolic dysfunction, and a progression of early diastolic dysfunction to diastolic rather than systolic heart failure has been documented in long-term cancer survivors. This chapter first describes general notions about hypertension in the cancer patient and then moves on reviewing the pathophysiology and clinical trajectories of diastolic dysfunction, and the molecular mechanisms of anthracycline-induced diastolic dysfunction. Diastolic dysfunction can in fact be caused and/or aggravated by hypertension. Pharmacologic foundations and therapeutic opportunities to prevent or treat diastolic dysfunction before it progresses toward heart failure are also reviewed, with a special emphasis on the mechanisms of action of drugs that raised hopes to treat diastolic dysfunction in the general population (sacubitril/valsartan, guanylyl cyclase activators, phosphodiesterase inhibitors, ranolazine, inhibitors of type-2 sodium-glucose-inked transporter). Cardio-oncologists will be confronted with the risk:benefit ratio of using these drugs in the cancer patient.

Abbreviations

ACEi	angiotensin converting enzyme inhibitor
ARB	angiotensin receptor blocker
BCR-ABL	breakpoint cluster region-Abelson gene tyrosine kinase
BNP	B-type natriuretic peptide
cGMP	cyclic guanosine monophosphate
CV	cardiovascular
DD	diastolic dysfunction
GC	guanylyl cyclase
HF	heart failure
HFmrEF	heart failure with mildly reduced ejection fraction
HFpEF	heart failure with preserved ejection fraction
HFrEF	heart failure with reduced ejection fraction
LV	left ventricle
LVEF	left ventricular ejection fraction
NCX	sodium-calcium exchanger
NO	nitric oxide
NYHA	New York Heart Association
Nt-proBNP	aminoterminal fragment of B-type natriuretic peptide prohormone
PDE	phosphodiesterase
PKG	protein kinase G
RAAS	renin-angiotensin-aldosterone-system
ROS	reactive oxygen species
SERCA	sarco-endoplasmic reticulum Ca^{2+}/Mg^{2+} ATPase
SGLT2(i)	sodium-glucose linked transporter 2 (inhibitor)
S/V	sacubitril/valsartan

1. Introduction

Cancer patients have long been known to be plagued by cardiovascular (CV) events, some of which are directly related to the growth and spreading of malignancy, as is the case of thromboembolism. But other events are more directly related to the drugs that oncologists and hematologists prescribe to treat cancer. Cancer drug-induced CV events may sometime be life-threatening. This is the historical lesson from antitumor antibiotics, primarily anthracyclines, notorious for causing systolic dysfunction and heart failure (HF) upon chronic administration (Minotti, Menna, Salvatorelli, Cairo, & Gianni, 2004).

As our understanding of cancer biology has improved over the years, many new drugs have been developed that make the pharmacologic portfolium of oncologists and hematologists remarkably wider and more versatile to design an effective cancer treatment. Regrettably, however, no single player in the CV system (myocardium, conduction system, valves, pericardium, arteries, veins) can be said to escape the risk of untoward effects of new drugs such as antibodies, small inhibitors of growth factors or receptor-associated tyrosine kinases, hormones, proteasome inhibitors, immune check point inhibitors, or chimeric antigen receptor-engineered T cells. Yet, all such drugs and therapies were intended to hit tumor-specific moieties or pathways, while having little or no effect on the cardiovascular system and other healthy tissues (Zamorano et al., 2020).

The unexpected outbreak of CV toxicities of "targeted" drugs and therapies illustrates the complexity of cancer growth and dissemination, and shows that mechanism(s) of action of new drugs should be considered in a multidimensional context, where selectivity cannot be given for granted. On a different note, the remarkable improvements in tumor curability or chronicization that the new drugs introduce, often in combination with anthracyclines or other "old" chemotherapeutics, call for a judicious risk: benefit assessment of therapeutic decisions. This is where cardio-oncology comes into a play.

Cardio-oncology is a relatively new discipline that harmonizes the expertise of oncologists, hematologists, radiation therapists, cardiologists and other care givers (such as nurses or rehabilitation experts), to jointly assess the risk:benefit of antitumor therapies and identify the best possible modalities of cardiac protection and surveillance with a patient-tailored approach (Ewer, Carver, & Minotti, 2019). The main goal of cardio-oncology is in fact to provide any given patient with the best possible cancer treatment in the face of risk of cardiovascular sequelae. It is no surprise that Pubmed entries reading "cancer drugs and cardiovascular toxicities" have been surpassed and eventually replaced by an exponential growth of entries that read "cardio-oncology." This denotes how the conceptual framework of cardio-oncology moved the scientific community from anedoctically reporting on the CV toxicity from a given drug to deciphering the foundations and clinical readouts of the complex interplay that exists between that drug, patient's characteristics, and opportunities for devising optimal cancer treatment while also mitigating CV risk (Fig. 1).

With certain drugs, like the anthracyclines, refinements of dose density and intensity have limited the risk of CV events over the weeks or months in which these drugs are administered to treat a tumor; yet, the risk of delayed events has not been abated. Childhood cancer survivors may develop heart failure (HF) anytime over the years, sometime decades after the last anthracycline administration (Camilli, Del Buono, Crea, & Minotti, 2020; Howard et al., 2019). Adult patients too may develop HF some 5 to 10 years after cancer treatment (Pinder et al., 2007). The hiatus between patient exposure to anthracyclines and clinical manifestations of CV toxicity probably recapitulates a continuum that begins with the first anthracycline infusion and proceeds through a slow dissipation of cardiac defense and repair mechanisms (Benjamin & Minotti, 2021). Cardio-oncologists should be committed to identify subclinical cardiotoxicity as early as possible, so that progression of asymptomatic reversible damage to irreversible deterioration of cardiac function can be halted or delayed by appropriate medications.

Other drugs, like antileukemic BCR-ABL inhibitors, are administered chronically until the disease relapses. In the latter scenario the hiatus from

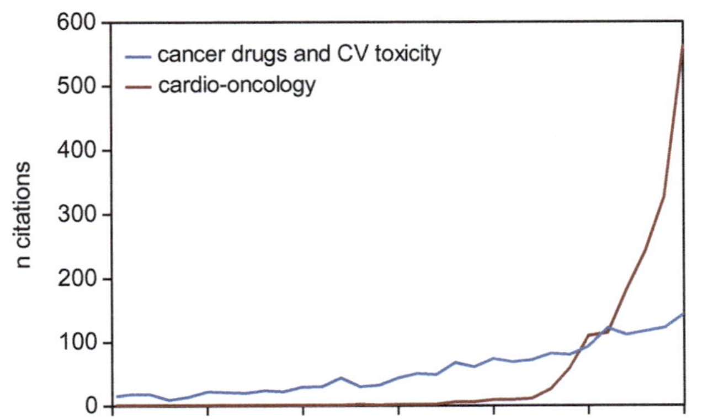

Fig. 1 Number of Pubmed entries reading "Cancer drugs and cardiovascular (CV) toxicity" or "Cardio-Oncology." *Pubmed, September 2021.*

the first dose of the drug and the clinical manifestations of CV toxicity may be shorter, and given that patients often switch from an inhibitor to another to prevent resistance or mitigate noncardiovascular side effects, it may not always be possible to understand which particular drug caused the early damage, and which other drug caused subclinical toxicity progress toward clinical symptoms (Breccia et al., 2017). Needless to say, however, both the anthracycline scenario and the Bcr-Abl inhibitors scenario are heavily influenced by competing CV risk factors that predispose to early damage or accelerate the transition from subclinical toxicity to clinical symptoms. Hypertension is one of such factors (Cohen, Geara, Hogan, & Townsend, 2019).

Pre-existing hypertension increases CV toxicity of cancer drugs (Zamorano et al., 2020) while many cancer drugs, particularly inhibitors of angiogenesis, alkylators and proteasome inhibitors, can both induce hypertension in previously normotensive patients or exacerbate pre-existing hypertension. Also adjuvant treatments, like abdominal or head-neck radiation therapy, pain relievers and bone marrow growth factors, can cause hypertension during cancer treatment (Cohen et al., 2019). With the new cancer drugs, including the angiogenesis inhibitors, on-off interception of growth factors or inhibition of receptor-associated tyrosine kinases make hypertension transient and clinically manageable, so that cancer treatment does not always need to be interrupted or can safely be resumed following event resolution (Ewer et al., 2014). Other drugs introduce long-standing pharmacologic signatures and thus expose the cancer patient to a life-long risk of hypertension. Studies of survivors of testicular cancer treated with cisplatin show that this drug accumulates in endothelial cells over the years, laying the foundations for persistent vasoconstriction to occur (Vaughn, Palmer, Carver, Jacobs, & Mohler, 2008). Regrettably, however, there is a paucity of high quality data on the impact of antihypertensive therapy on CV risk in the cancer patient (Cohen et al., 2019), and concerns about vasodilators interfering with the oncologic efficacy of angiogenesis inhibitors have been reported (Cohen et al., 2019; Salvatorelli et al., 2015).

Hypertension can thus occur both during and after cancer treatment. Hypertension is one of the chronic medical conditions that accumulate in adult cancer survivors (Jiang et al., 2021) and its prevalence in childhood cancer survivors may be as high as $\geq$70% by age 50 years (Gibson et al., 2017). Cause-and-effect relations between one cancer drug and delayed hypertension are not always as obvious as we described for cisplatin. In many cases hypertension is just one component of complex metabolic syndromes characterized by obesity, diabetes, and dislipidemia, with each comorbidity possibly representing an independent risk factor for hypertension. Cisplatin exposure itself is associated with risk of metabolic syndrome in survivors (Zaid et al., 2018). Regardless of such complexity, hypertension exposes cancer survivors to an accelerated course of CV toxicity of cancer drugs.

In this chapter we will go beyond hypertension to discuss the pharmacologic foundations and pharmacotherapy of asymptomatic anthracycline-induced diastolic dysfunction (DD), currently considered as one of the earliest manifestations of a long process that eventually manifests as systolic dysfunction and HF. There was a multifaceted rationale for moving from hypertension to DD: (i) hypertension is a well established risk factor for DD; (ii), hypertension can accelerate DD progression toward HF; (iii), early DD identifies patients that carry an increased CV risk and may thus merit careful monitoring and treatment of hypertension; (iv), the pharmacology of anthracycline-related early cardiotoxicity is one of the most popular themes of modern cardio-oncology. Given the complex pathobiologic scenario, and the paucity of successful medications for DD, anthracycline-related DD will be contextualized in the settings of what we know in terms of etiology and therapeutic chances for the general population.

2. Diastolic versus systolic dysfunction

Anthracyclines carry a three- to five-fold greater risk for cardiotoxicity than other cancer drugs (Smith et al., 2010), with cardiotoxicity usually being defined as systolic dysfunction that progresses toward HF with reduced left ventricular ejection fraction (HFrEF, sometime referred to as systolic heart failure).

The most important determinant of anthracycline-related systolic dysfunction and HF risk is the cumulative dose of anthracycline. There is a dose range over which HF risk is low or nearly undetectable by standard cardiologic assessments, but there is a threshold dose beyond which HF risk increases exponentially. With doxorubicin the inflection point occurs at 240 mg/m^2, which represents the cumulative dose most commonly adopted in contemporary oncology regimens for treatment of early breast cancer. A cumulative dose of 400 mg/m^2 associates with a rather well established 5% risk of HF (Swain, Whaley, & Ewer, 2003) (Fig. 2).

The exponential relation between dose and risk suggests that at low doses there is a balance between the damage anthracyclines can inflict and the defense or repair mechanisms that cardiomyocytes can put in place, while

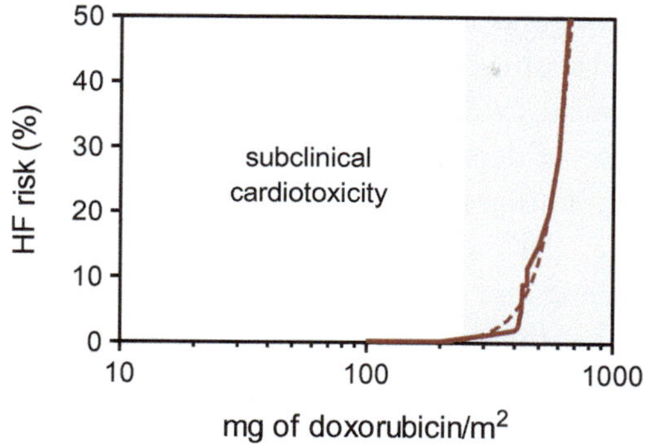

Fig. 2 Risk-versus dose relations for anthracycline-related heart failure (HF). The dashed curve represent absolute risk values as determined by experts at MD Anderson Cancer Center, Houston TX. The solid curve is a best-fit exponential representation of clinical data. Subclinical cardiotoxicity occurs over dose ranges <400 mg/m^2 *Based on Swain, S. M., Whaley, F. S., & Ewer, M. S. (2003). Congestive heart failure in patients treated with doxorubicin: A retrospective analysis of three trials.* Cancer, 97, *2869–2879.*

at higher doses damage accumulates in excess of the detoxifying capacity of cardiomyocytes.

This having been said, when does HF occur? The threshold at 400 mg/m^2 clearly introduces a risk of on-treatment HF if the transition from low to high anthracycline doses occurs within a therapeutic continuum (i.e., the patient is treated with anthracyclines until tumor response occurs or unacceptable hematologic or non-hematologic toxicities occur). On-treatment HF may nonetheless ensue when the transition from low to high anthracycline doses occurs discontinuously (i.e. the patient receives a first course of low-dose anthracycline and then receives additional anthracycline courses when tumor relapse or metastatization occurs, and the oncologist believes there is a potential benefit from rechallenging the patient with an anthracycline). In contemporary oncology, however, relatively few patients are continuously exposed to anthracycline doses that reach and eventually exceed the threshold of ≥400 mg/m^2, and relatively few patients receive separate anthracycline courses that would amount to lifetime doses of ≥400 mg/m^2. The vast majority of patients usually receive ≤300 mg/m^2, with concerns about HF discouraging second- or third-line rechallenges with anthracyclines.

A significant percentage of patients treated with "low" anthracycline doses may nonetheless develop HF after the oncologic treatment. Absent post-treatment injuries such as irradiation of cardiac area, sequential exposure to other oncologic treatments, or developing comorbidities that predispose to HF (such as hypertension, diabetes, overweight and others), the hiatus between anthracycline exposure and HF symptoms illuminates the role of subclinical cardiotoxicity induced by low-dose anthracycline and the importance of detecting, monitoring or treating it before it progresses toward HF. This is where asymptomatic DD may come into focus.

Left ventricular (LV) diastolic function plays an important role in determining LV filling and thus, stroke volume. Diastolic function is characterized by LV relaxation, chamber stiffness and early diastolic recoil (Kass, Bronzwaer, & Paulus, 2004; Zile & Gaasch, 1990). Abnormal diastolic function has been recognized in many cardiovascular diseases and is associated with worse outcomes, including total mortality and hospitalization due to HF (Borlaug & Kass, 2006).

The Frank-Starling mechanism, defined as the heart capability to translate an increased LV filling pressure into an increased cardiac output, is central to the pathophysiology of DD. When the Frank-Starling mechanism decompensates, such that an increased LV filling pressure is no longer coupled with an increased output, or the latter only increases when filling pressures are abnormally elevated, a well-known clinical syndrome occurs that is called heart failure with preserved ejection fraction (HFpEF, sometime referred to as diastolic heart failure) (Abbate et al., 2015). HFpEF shows some unique characteristics that make it different from HFrEF. Definitions and main features of these two pathophysiological entities are summarized in Table 1.

In brief, HFpEF (also referred to as diastolic failure) is characterized primarily by cardiomyocyte concentric hypertrophy, fibrosis, and inflammation, all leading to a LV wall that is thickened and unable to relax but maintains stroke efficiency; in contrast, HFrEF (systolic heart failure) is characterized primarily by a significant loss of cardiomyocytes with eccentric hypertrophy, leading to LV wall thinning, chamber dilation and loss of stroke efficiency. Also, ion homeostasis is differentially perturbed in HFrEF vis-à-vis HFpEF, with the latter showing calcium dysregulation that will require considerations when discussing pharmacologic interventions in patients with cancer-treatment related DD.

HFrEF and HFpEF also show distinct risk factors and predisposing comorbidities, but for the aims of our analyses in cardio-oncology settings, it is worth noting that they also share common predisposing factors such as hypertension, diabetes or obesity (Fig. 3). Again, this will need to be considered when the trajectory from early DD to overt systolic dysfunction and HFrEF will be discussed.

Table 1 General similarities and differences between HFrEF and HFpEF.

	HFrEF	HFpEF	
		Symptoms and/or signs of HF	
Definition	Symptoms and/or signs of HF (LVEF ≤40%)	LVEF ≥50%	Simmonds, Cuijpers, Heymans, and Jones (2020)
		Objective evidence of cardiac structural and/or functional abnormalities consistent with the presence of LV diastolic dysfunction/raised LV filling pressures, including raised natriuretic peptides	
Sex prevalence	Male	Female	Krumholz, Larson, and Levy (1993)
Cardiac hypertrophy	Eccentric	Concentric	Penn (2008); Zile et al. (2011)
Cardiomyocyte cell death	Present	Absent	Brouwers et al. (2013)
Cardiac fibrosis	↑ Perivascular fibrosis	↑↑ Perivascular fibrosis	Dai, Aoki, Fukumoto, and Shimokawa (2012)
			Roy et al. (2018)
	Interstitial fibrosis	Interstitial fibrosis	Kasner et al. (2011)
	Replacement fibrosis		
	Fibrotic signaling: ↑ Serum TGFβ1	Fibrotic signaling: ↑↑ Serum TGFβ1	Aoki et al. (2011)
			Forte, Furtado, and Rosenthal (2018)
	↓ MCP-1	↑ MCP-1	Bielecka-Dabrowa et al. (2016)
			Collier et al. (2011)

Continued

Table 1 General similarities and differences between HFrEF and HFpEF.—cont'd

	HFrEF	HFpEF	
Ion homeostasis disorders	↑ $[Na+]_i$	↑ $[Ca^{2+}]_i$	Pieske et al. (2002) Schwinger et al. (1999)
Systemic and cardiac inflammation	Secondary to cardiomyocyte damage and death (infections, toxins or ischemia)	Induced by extra-cardiac metabolic and inflammatory risk factors	Chen and Nunez (2010) Paulus and Tschöpe (2013) Pollack, Kontorovich, Fuster, and Dec (2015)

MCP-1, monocyte chemoattractant protein 1; TGFβ1, transforming growth factor beta 1.
Concept summary from Simmonds, S. J., Cuijpers, I., Heymans, S., & Jones, E. A. V. (2020). Cellular and molecular differences between HFpEF and HFreEF: A step ahead in an improved pathological understanding. *Cell, 9*, 242. doi:10.3390/cells9010242.

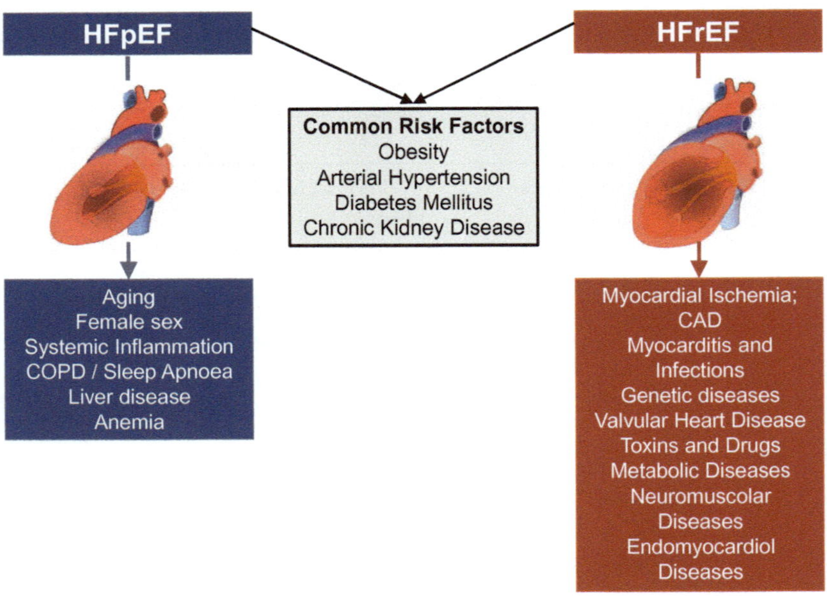

Fig. 3 Common and distinctive risk factors for HFpEF and HFrEF. *Based on Ho, J. E., Lyass, A., Lee, D. S., Vasan, R. S., Kannel, W. B., Larson, M. G., et al. (2013). Predictors of new-onset heart failure: Differences in preserved versus reduced ejection fraction.*

3. Anthracyclines and the mechanisms of diastolic dysfunction

Microvascular dysfunction and inappropriate interactions of Ca^{2+} with myofilaments during diastole are relevant causes of DD (Mohammed et al., 2015). As for Ca^{2+} disorders, much attention has been focused on inadequate sarcolemmal Ca^{2+} removal not compensated by an increased re-uptake of Ca^{2+} in sarcoplasmic reticulum. Ca^{2+} removal from cardiomyocytes is in fact largely mediated by the sarcolemmal Na^+/Ca^{2+} exchanger (NCX), a transporter protein that is governed in its function by the trans-sarcolemmal Na^+ gradient (Bers, Barry, & Intracellular, 2003). When $[Na^+]_i$ increases through e.g., a hyperactive late sodium current (I_{Na}-late current), the Na^+ gradient dissipates and the ability of NCX to extrude Ca^{2+} from within the cell to the extracellular space diminishes. In HFrEF inappropriate sources of elevated $[Ca^{2+}]_i$ have been located also to invaginations of the sarcolemmal membrane called t-tubules, which appear structurally disorganized in terms of reduced density and loss of a uniform striated pattern, as well as functionally altered in terms of delayed and desynchronized Ca^{2+} transients (Guo, Zhang, Wei, Chen, & Song, 2013). In the settings of HFpEF, however, t-tubule density actually increases as these structures proliferate during cellular hypertrophy, and rates of Ca^{2+} release remain in normality ranges (Frisk et al., 2021). As for microvascular dysfunction, much of the evidence was built on experimental observations that comorbidities known to predispose the general population to DD, like e.g., diabetes and obesity, are fingerprinted by systemic inflammation, which eventually perturbs the cardiac endothelial nitric oxide (NO) pathway (Paulus & Tschöpe, 2013).

Fig. 3—Cont'd *Circulation. Heart Failure, 6*, 279–286; Jeong, E. M., & Dudley, S. C., Jr. (2015). Diastolic dysfunction. *Circulation Journal, 79*, 470–477; Krumholz, H. M., Larson, M., & Levy, D. (1993). Sex differences in cardiac adaptation to isolated systolic hypertension. *The American Journal of Cardiology, 72*, 310–313; Lee, D. S., Gona, P., Vasan, R. S., Larson, M. G., Benjamin, E. J., Wang, T. J., et al. (2009). Relation of disease pathogenesis and risk factors to heart failure with preserved or reduced ejection fraction: Insights from the Framingham heart study of the National Heart, Lung, and Blood Institute. *Circulation, 119*, 3070–3077. Ergatoudes, C., Schaufelberger, M., Andersson, B., Pivodic, A., Dahlstrom, U., & Fu, M. (2019). Non-cardiac comorbidities and mortality in patients with heart failure with reduced vs. preserved ejection fraction: A study using the Swedish Heart Failure Registry. *Clinical Research in Cardiology, 108*, 1025–1033.

Mechanisms of Ca^{2+} disorders and microvasculature dysfunction, as described for experimental models tailored to reproduce conditions in the general population, should nonetheless be scrutinized with caution before translatability to oncologic settings is considered. Elevated myocardial Ca^{2+} levels were unequivocally demonstrated in HFpEF associated with arterial hypertension, but a triggering role of excess Na^{+} influx was not supported by experimental evidence (Runte et al., 2017). Impaired diastolic Ca^{2+} removal was demonstrated in experimental models of diabetic HfpEF, but not in ischemic and hypertensive disease models (Frisk et al., 2021). These findings should be taken to conclude that mechanisms of Ca^{2+} disorders in HFpEF are most likely etiology-dependent. On a different note, evidence for one mechanism of Ca^{2+} dysregulation or another cannot be used to generalize on the mechanisms occurring during the early phases of DD. HFpEF is the end-stage manifestation of a long trajectory where one mechanism of disease may be replaced by another over time, and compensatory mechanisms may occur that correct for one malfunction but not others.

Cancer treatment-related DD is often seen in normal-weight and non-diabetic patients, hence the inflammatory constellation that causes HFpEF in diabetic or obese patients cannot be invoked *bona fide* to explain asymptomatic DD from low anthracycline doses as those described in Fig. 2. Cause-and-effect relations between cardiac anthracycline exposure and DD must therefore be searched among mechanisms of damage that anthracyclines may inflict on cardiomyocyte directly and independent of coexisting morbidities. Anthracyclines, whether directly or through the action of hydroxymetabolites, aglyconic derivatives or reactive oxygen species, can in fact inhibit NCX (Olson & Mushlin, 1990), downregulate the expression and impair the Ca^{2+} sequestering activity of sarcoplasmic reticulum Ca^{2+}-ATPase (SERCA), while also inhibiting the expression of satellite Ca^{2+} regulators such as phospholamban and calsequestrin (Jeyaseelan et al., 1997; Jeyaseelan, Poizat, Wu, & Kedes, 1997). Anthracyclines can also dissipate mitochondrial membrane potential and impair mitochondrial Ca^{2+} storage in favor of passive Ca^{2+} efflux (Sokolove, 1994). As a deleterious readout of such multiple mechanisms of Ca^{2+} dysregulation, anthracyclines promote calcium-dependent protease degradation of titin, a giant myofilament that, by spanning the half sarcomere from M-line to Z-line, functions as a sort of entropic spring, i.e., it provides both the restoring force that the sarcomere needs to recover its resting length in diastole and the passive force that the sarcomere needs to initiate the systole (Peng, Chen, Lim, & Sawyer, 2005). Titin degradation impacts on diastolic relaxation and paves the road to DD.

Anthracyclines can also cause endothelial dysfunction via unique mechanisms. Anthracyclines can in fact bind to the reductase domain of

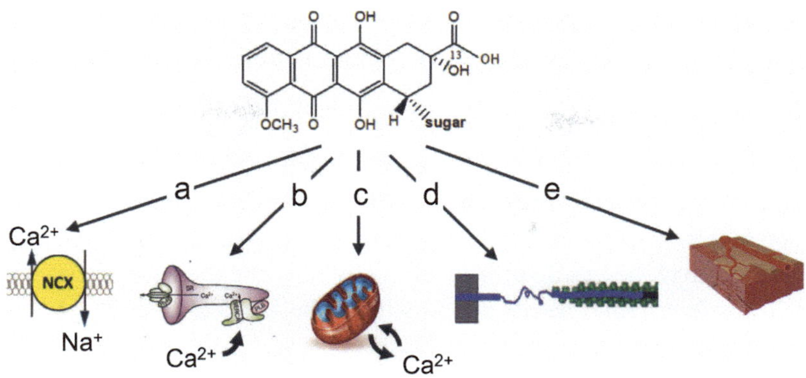

Fig. 4 Anthracycline targets likely involved in DD pathophysiology. Anthracyclines, here represented by doxorubicin chemical structure, can dysregulate Ca^{2+} homeostasis by inhibiting NCX (A), which mediates cellular Ca^{2+} extrusion, or Ca^{2+}-Mg^{2+} ATPase (SERCA) (B), which mediates Ca^{2+} re-uptake in sarcoplasmic reticulum. Anthracyclines depolarize mitochondria (C), altering an equilibrium of Ca^{2+} storage with Ca^{2+} efflux, and promote Ca^{2+} dependent protease degradation of the giant myofilament protein, titin (D, blu filament), which is important for diastolic relaxation. Anthracyclines can also target endothelial cells (E), causing microvascular dysfunction.

NO synthase, inhibiting NO production and downstream vasodilating effects. Moreover, anthracyclines can induce NO synthase to switch from producing NO to producing superoxide anion (Vásquez-Vivar et al., 1997), favoring the conversion of residual NO to peroxynitrite, a potent vasoconstrictor agent (Luu et al., 2018). Biochemical evidence of anthracycline-related perturbances of NO biosynthesis has been documented in women treated with doxorubicin for breast cancer (Finkelman et al., 2017).

Targets of anthracyclines, likely related to DD pathophysiology, are sketched in Fig. 4.

4. Anthracyclines and pathophysiologic trajectories of diastolic dysfunction

The literature counts 14 longitudinal studies of cancer treatment-related DD (Mincu et al., 2021). All of them describe patients treated with cumulative doses of doxorubicin or its closely related analogue, epirubicin, but in 6 of them the anthracycline dose was slightly ($\sim$300 mg/m^2) or significantly ($\geq$400 mg/m^2) beyond the inflection point of the curve that describes the transition from subclinical to clinical cardiotoxicity (see Fig. 2). Moreover, and more importantly, as many as 11 studies included patients with one or more CV risk factors that predispose to DD.

Considerations about anthracycline dose and CV risk factors complicate an interpretation of these studies and make it difficult to disentangle the role that low-dose anthracycline in itself may have on perturbing players and mechanisms of diastolic relaxation, eventually causing asymptomatic DD as an early manifestation of cardiotoxicity. Of the two studies of comorbid-free patients treated with $\leq 300\,mg/m^2$, one demonstrated indices of DD in virtually all patients examined at 2-years follow-up (Nagy, Cserép, Tolnay, Nagykálnai, & Forster, 2008), while the other showed that 19% of patients could be diagnosed with grade I DD as early as one week after the last chemotherapy cycle (Calabrese et al., 2018). Grade I DD (also referred to as impaired relaxation) is the mildest manifestation of DD, and hence, its very early detection in low-risk patients shows that cardiotoxicity begins with the first anthracycline infusion. Accordingly, inter-treatment echocardiographic evaluations showed that indices of transmitral flow began to decline after one or two chemotherapy cycles (Menna et al., 2018).

Having previously described the mechanisms of anthracycline-induced DD, and having now described how early DD can occur and be detected in low-risk cancer patients, questions should be asked about DD progressing to symptomatic cardiac events and what type of such events the survivor could anticipate experiencing. Here, it remains controversial whether DD represents the cause of a cardiotoxicity cascade that, with a variable velocity, proceeds to HFrEF. Regardless of how DD was measured in one or another study, the likelihood of DD progressing to HFrEF depends on a constellation of factors. Sequential exposure to other potentially cardiotoxic agents is an important factor, as demonstrated for breast cancer patients treated with regimens that include anthracyclines followed by the anti ErbB2 monoclonal antibody, trastuzumab (Klein et al., 2019). Post-anthracycline left chest irradiation is another factor to consider, given that radiation therapy is an independent risk factor for DD with a preserved LVEF (Cao et al., 2015; Saiki et al., 2017) and imaging studies show early microvascular dysfunction in irradiated cardiac areas (Song et al., 2017). Developing comorbidities play a remarkable important role. As we already mentioned both pediatric and adult cancer survivors are in fact at an increased risk of hypertension, diabetes or obesity, often aggravated by unfavorable lifestyles like limited physical activity or smoking. When taken in aggregate, all such factors may well compound a cardiac tissue that is inherently more vulnerable due to the presence of an early DD.

The process leading from early DD to HFrEF can therefore be contextualized as a multiple hit mechanism, where DD is the first hit and sequential treatments or developing comorbidities represent secondary hits (Menna, Salvatorelli, & Minotti, 2008; Thavendiranathan & Nolan, 2017).

How long this process will take may depend on further variables such as patient risk awareness, perception of symptoms, and appropriate attendance to cardiologic visits. Recent analyses of survivors of 20 adult cancer types confirm that this process may easily take decades (Strongman et al., 2019).

HFrEF is not the only negative outcome of an uncontrolled progression of early asymptomatic DD. Long term survivors of childhood cancer may show worsening DD, and grade II or III patterns can be documented that prelude to restrictive rather than dilated cardiomyopathy (Armstrong et al., 2015). In these subjects the risk of HFpEF may eventually increase and prevail over HFrEF. Other childhood cancer survivors may experience a different cardiomyopathy phenotype that is initially characterized by an HFrEF-like syndrome (systolic dysfunction with reduced ventricular wall thickness), which then evolves toward another phenotype characterized by a fall in ventricular dimension and mass, and by an increased wall thickness not caused by hypertrophy but secondary to decreasing chamber size. This process takes 15 or more years and generates a "small for age" heart (Grinch Syndrome) (Lipshultz et al., 2014). Thus, cardiotoxicity transitions from an early dilated cardiomyopathy to a restrictive cardiomyopathy that is similar to, but not fully identical with HFrEF.

The broad spectrum of late events possibly associated with early DD is summarized in Fig. 5 along with the essential components of the multiple-hits hypothesis of cardiotoxicity. Opportunities for pharmacologic interventions against DD should therefore be considered.

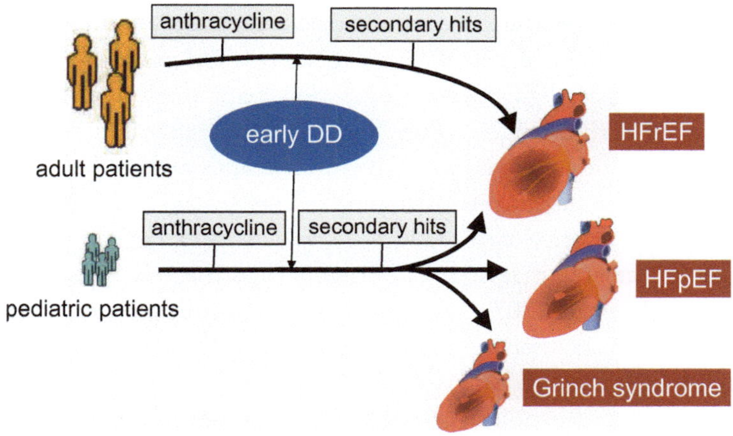

Fig. 5 Pathways of DD progression to late cardiac events in adult and pediatric cancer patients. Early DD, induced by anthracyclines and aggravated by secondary hits (sequential treatments, developing comorbidities), may eventually progress to HFrEF (adult patients) or HFrEF, HFpEF or small-for-age heart (Grinch syndrome) (pediatric patients).

5. General considerations on anthracycline cardiotoxicity prevention

There is a lack of guidelines for preventing anthracycline-related cardiotoxicity. Statements from the European Society of Cardiology (Zamorano et al., 2016) and the European Society for Medical Oncology (Curigliano et al., 2020), or expert groups (Zamorano et al., 2020) have resulted in common-sense recommendations, such as identifying and controlling pre-existing CV risk factors, and initiating cardioprotective treatments with inhibitors of renin-angiotensin-aldosterone-system (RAAS), and/or β-blockers, in patients with pre-existing HF or significant systolic dysfunction or elevated troponin as a biochemical index of cardiomyocyte necrosis. Statins are recommended for patients with coronary artery disease. According to the American Society of Clinical Oncology, data on the efficacy and safety of primary prevention with CV drugs in otherwise low-risk patients are of insufficient evidence for recommending their use on a routine basis, although *ad interim* analyses of most recent studies maintain that angiotensin converting enzyme inhibitors (ACEi) and/or β-blockers should be considered to prevent subclinical systolic dysfunction in low-risk breast cancer patients (Livi et al., 2021).

According to the American Society of Clinical Oncology dexrazoxane remains the only valuable option to prevent anthracycline cardiotoxicity (Armenian et al., 2017), but dexrazoxane is a very misfortunate drug that merits a number of considerations. Dexrazoxane is a bis-ketopiperazine that hydrolyzes intracellularly to become a diacid-diamide with iron chelating properties (Minotti et al., 2004). Iron chelation then prevents or mitigates free radical reactions that have extensively been implicated to mediate anthracycline cardiotoxicity. The "iron and free radical hypothesis" of cardiotoxicity is nonetheless limited by uncertainties such as the lack of efficacy of clinical interventions with antioxidants (Ladas et al., 2004), or an inconsistent occurrence of free radical-dependent mitochondriopathy across anthracycline analogs that cause comparable clinical levels of cardiotoxicity (Lebrecht & Walker, 2007). On the other hand, cardioprotective effects of dexrazoxane are themselves only partly understood. New drugs that were designed to chelate and redox-inactivate iron even more effectively than dexrazoxane, were unable to provide equal or better cardiac protection (Menna et al., 2012). Dexrazoxane might well prevent cardiotoxicity by other mechanisms; for example, dexrazoxane diminishes DNA double-strand breaks that occur following formation of complexes between anthracyclines and the β isoform of topoisomerase II which is constitutively expressed in cardiomyocytes (Yeh et al., 2019).

Absent dexrazoxane, DNA double strand breaks would be followed by altered mitochondrial biogenesis, mitochondrial dysfunction leading to ROS formation, and p53 relayed apoptosis (Yeh et al., 2019). Once disregraded as a causative mechanism of anthracycline cardiotoxicity, historically attributed to necrosis and replacement fibrosis, apoptosis is now considered a hallmark of it. Numerous studies have convincingly shown that anthracyclines may cause cardiomyocyte apoptosis via the mitochondrial intrinsic pathway (Minotti et al., 2004; Shi, Abdelwahid, & Wei, 2011) and investigational agents hold promise for preventing cardiomyocyte apoptosis by blocking proapoptoxic factors like e.g., Bax (Amgalan et al., 2020). Cardiac inflammation is another newly identified mechanism of anthracycline cardiotoxicity and C1q/tumor necrosis factor-related protein-3 overexpression may serve a mechanism to prevent both apoptosis and inflammation (Yuan et al., 2018). At this point in time, however, dexrazoxane would remain the only approved agent to prevent apoptosis in anthracycline-treated patients.

Regardless of uncertainties and doubts about its mechanism of cardioprotection, clinical use of dexrazoxane has been limited by just one unconfirmed report that it could interfere with anthracycline activity (Swain et al., 1997). More recently, dexrazoxane has also been plagued by unconfirmed concerns that it could increase the incidence of secondary malignancies in cancer survivors (Tebbi et al., 2007). Because of all such unfortunate circumstances, dexrazoxane label was revised and re-revised by regulatory agencies over the years, and despite compelling evidence of its efficacy and safety, also in terms of no interference with anthracycline activity, clinical use of dexrazoxane has been confined to, and recommended for, pediatric and adult patients candidate to high dose anthracycline regimens (Armenian et al., 2017; Kopp et al., 2019). For patients treated with $\leq 250\,mg/m^2$ dexrazoxane should be considered off label. Similar prescription limitations apply to liposomal anthracycline formulations or prolonged infusions schemes that significantly limit cardiac exposure to anthracyclines and convincingly limit cardiotoxicity in many patients, but are formally approved in only limited clinical settings (Minotti et al., 2004; Salvatorelli, Menna, Chello, Covino, & Minotti, 2017).

6. Pharmacologic interventions on cancer treatment-related diastolic dysfunction: Lessons from natriuretic peptide

6.1 Pathophysiology and role of B-type natriuretic peptide in diastolic dysfunction

In light of the disappointing considerations on the prevention of anthracycline-dependent cardiotoxicity, pharmacologic interventions on DD are limited to using conventional CV drugs; regrettably, however, DD is a difficult-to-treat condition, and very few drugs hold promise for successfully curing DD. Before addressing the risk:benefit of possible therapeutic strategies, the role and mechanisms of action of the endogenous cardiac relaxant agent, B-type natriuretic peptide (BNP), must be discussed. Understanding the role of BNP in the general and oncologic population might in fact help understanding which drug or classes drugs would be of some benefit to treat DD.

Under conditions of hemodynamic stress, varying from ventricular dilation to hypertrophy and diastolic wall tension, cardiomyocytes release a prohormone that is cleaved to BNP by circulating endoproteases (Braunwald, 2008). BNP release is associated with the formation of the amino-terminal fragment of the BNP prohormone, Nt-proBNP, which is hemodynamically inactive, but endowed with a longer half-life (120 vs 20 min). Inasmuch as BNP and Nt-proBNP are formed in a 1:1 ratio, the longer-lived Nt-proBNP is particularly suitable for improving BNP detection and prognostic value in a variety of cardiovascular diseases (Masson et al., 2006; Omland et al., 2007).

BNP acts as an hormone that modulates a number of cardiovascular functions: (i) it increases glomerular filtration rate and natriuresis in the kidney; (ii) it inhibits the activity of the sympathetic nervous system, eventually inhibiting also renin release from the kidney and thus, the consequent formation of angiotensin II and aldosterone, and (iii) it induces dilation and prevents fibrogenesis in arteries. Due to such conspicuous hemodynamic effects, BNP opposes the pathophysiology of HF, and circulating levels of BNP increase in both chronic and acutely decompensated HF. BNP also acts as an autocrine agent that modulates cardiac functions and structure. In fact, BNP causes cardiac relaxant effects (positive lusitropy) and diminishes hypertrophy and fibrosis, thus opposing pathophysiologic causes of DD such as myocardial stiffness and hypertrophic-fibrotic remodeling.

How does BNP behave as an endogenous lusitropic agent? Similar to other natriuretic peptides of atrial or endothelial origin, BNP binds to receptors associated with particulate guanylyl cyclase and cGMP production within cardiomyocytes. cGMP then activates protein kinase G (PKG) that phosphorylates titin, and by so doing, reduces cardiomyocyte passive tension in diastole (Bishu et al., 2011; Michel et al., 2020). BNP is less effective in phosphorylating other relaxation-coupled proteins such as troponin or phospholamban (Moltzau et al., 2014), but interestingly enough it mobilizes C-type endothelial natriuretic peptide, which is more effective in phosphorylating both proteins (Hillock et al., 2008). It is in keeping with these mechanisms that defects in receptor-driven cGMP formation were documented in patients with severe DD (van Heerebeek et al., 2012).

There is, however, another important ramification of the BNP-PKG signaling cascade, this being the inhibition of type 3 PDE, followed by cAMP accumulation, cAMP/protein kinase-induced Ca^{2+} increase, and catecholamine exocytosis from cardiac sympathetic nerve endings (Chan, Seyedi, Takano, & Levi, 2012). Catecholamine activation of β1 or β2 receptors would then induce positive lusitropy among other cardiac effects (Molenaar et al., 2007). An unsuspected role for BNP in upregulating catecholamine exocytosis, and hence cardiac sympathetic tone, was demonstrated by investigators who scrutinized potential reasons why infusional therapy with recombinant human BNP (nesiritide) lacked protective efficacy in patients with acutely decompensated HF (O'Connor et al., 2011). Cardiac sympathetic overdrive, possibly associated with e.g., tachyarrhythmias, would well explain such a lack of protective efficacy. In fact, protective effects were observed when excess cardiac exposure to BNP was avoided by switching from intravenous to subcutaneous administration, and a β1 blocker was given to all patients to blunt sympathetic overdrive (Thireau et al., 2014). Whether endogenous pathophysiologic levels of BNP upregulate cardiac sympathetic tone remains to be firmly established. Sympathetic overdrive would be an intuitively undesired effect if BNP had to be regarded as an endogenous curative agent for DD.

In addition to inducing cardiac relaxant effects, BNP can also influence heart rate (HR). Catecholamine exocytosis might well induce positive chronotropism but receptor-mediated mechanisms might be involved as well. BNP binding to the A subtype of natriuretic peptide receptors can in fact increase electrical conduction velocity both within the sinoatrial node and from the node toward surrounding cardiomyocytes (Azer, Hua, Krishnaswamy, & Rose, 2014). Again, these effects seem to be mediated by cGMP formation and cGMP activation of L-type Ca^{2+} sinoatrial currents (Springer et al., 2012).

In the settings of cancer patients, lusitropic and chronotropic effects of BNP elevations were demonstrated in the pilot prospective study of the incidence of early DD in comorbid-free patients evaluated at one week after chemotherapy (Calabrese et al., 2018; Menna et al., 2018). That study looked at two pre-specified events: grade I DD at echocardiography and BNP above the upper limit of normal, with the latter showing cardiac adaptation to anthracycline-induced impairment of myocardial relaxation. The two events occurred in a total of 29 of 80 patients and proved to be mutually exclusive, with just one patient showing both DD and BNP above the upper limit of normal (Fig. 6).

These results suggested that BNP could in fact induce positive lusitropic effects, which counteracted anthracycline impairment of myocardial relaxation and prevented grade I DD before this could be detected by echocardiography. While responding to BNP elevations by maintaining normal indices of myocardial relaxation, the same patients developed inappropriate tachycardia that was at least in part secondary to chemotherapy-related anemia and activation autonomic reflexes from carotid body (Lahiri et al., 2006); however, clinically measured HR exceeded that calculated on the basis of hemoglobin loss and increased when BNP levels were above the upper limit of normal. The net difference between measured and theoretical HR was due to the positive chronotropism of high BNP levels (Menna et al., 2018). A conceptual summary of how BNP effects on contractility or sinoatrial node activity relieved DD, but caused tachycardia, is shown in Fig. 7.

The effects of an endogenously increased BNP on mitigating DD risk, while also increasing HR, were reminiscent of the possible balance between beneficial and detrimental effects that limited a protective efficacy of intravenous nesiritide in patients with acutely decompensated HF; however, the chronotropic effect induced by an endogenously elevated BNP was of a limited magnitude and clinically manageable, and no tachyarrhythmia was observed in these patients. These findings therefore lend support to the notion that DD could be treated by an appropriate modulation of endogenous BNP or its second messenger, cGMP.

6.2 BNP and cGMP to treat DD: Current status and perspectives

In pre-clinical models of DD, pharmacologic inhibition of RAAS with ACEi or angiotensin II receptor blockers (ARBs) was generally shown

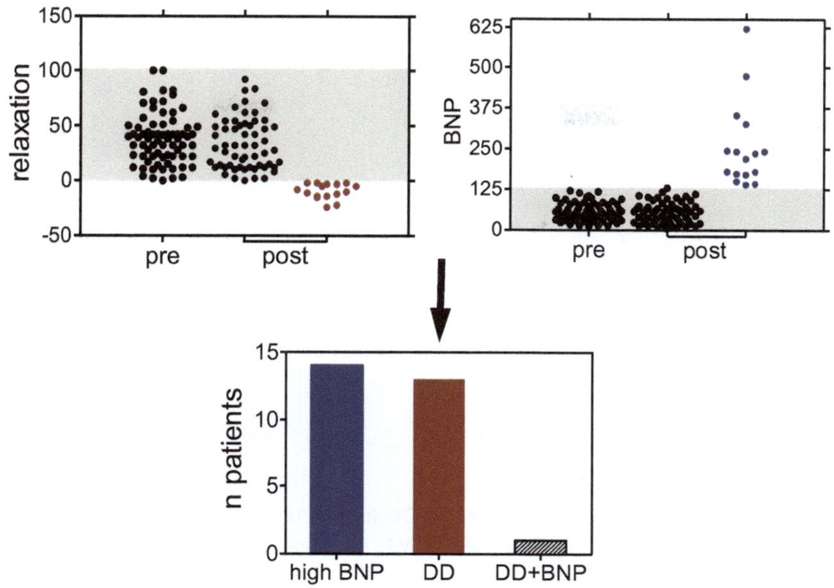

Fig. 6 Grade I DD and BNP elevations are mutually exclusive consequences of anthracycline-based chemotherapy. The upper panels show that all patients presented at chemotherapy with relaxation values within the age-adjusted range of normality (left panel, shaded area) and BNP values below the upper limit of normal (right panel, shaded area). At the end of chemotherapy some patients presented with low-for-age relaxation values (left panel, red symbols), while others presented with BNP values above the upper limit of normal (right panel, blue symbols). The bottom panel shows that DD and high BNP were mutually exclusive, only one patient presenting with both DD and high BNP. Relaxation was measured by transmitral flow (mean ratio of peak early filling (E wave) to late diastolic filling (A wave), E/A ratio). BNP was measured as Nt-proBNP (pg/mL). *Based on Calabrese, V., Menna, P., Annibali, O., Armento, G., Carpino, A., Cerchiara, E., et al. (2018). Early diastolic dysfunction after cancer chemotherapy: Primary endpoint results of a multicenter cardio-oncology study.* Chemotherapy, 63, *55–63; Menna, P., Calabrese, V., Armento, G., Annibali, O., Greco, C., Salvatorelli, E., et al. (2018). Pharmacology of cardio-oncology: Chronotropic and lusitropic effects of B-type natriuretic peptide in cancer patients with early diastolic dysfunction induced by anthracycline or nonanthracycline chemotherapy.* The Journal of Pharmacology and Experimental Therapeutics, 366, *158–168.*

to be of some efficacy, but clinical trials performed in patients with HFpEF have long failed to demonstrate mortality benefits. The CHARM Preserved trial (Effects of candesartan in patients with chronic heart failure and preserved left-ventricular ejection fraction) (Emdin, Callender, Cao, McMurray, & Rahimi, 2015) was one of the few trials to show benefit from an ARB in patients with an LVEF $\geq$40%, at least in terms of reduced

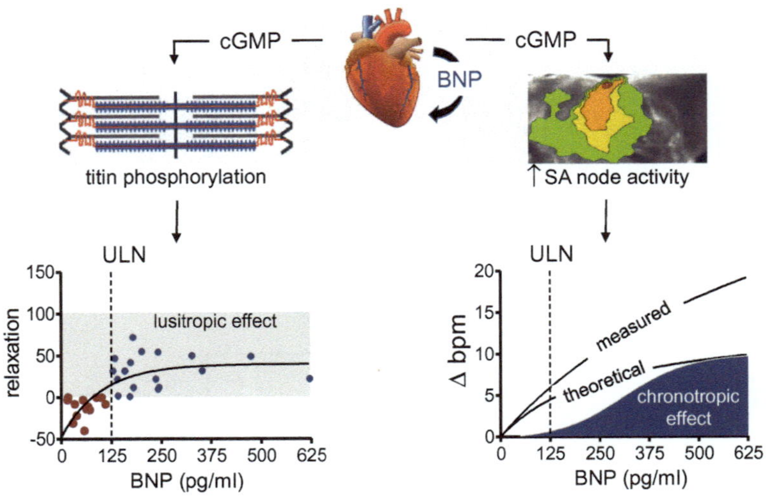

Fig. 7 Autocrine effects of BNP to relieve DD and increase HR. Cardiac-released BNP elicits autocrine effects, mediated by cGMP, that are important in patients with chemotherapy-related DD. Left panels show that by targeting and phosphorylating titin, BNP causes lusitropic effects. Patients with BNP below the upper limit of normal (ULN) will therefore present at post-chemotherapy assessment with grade I DD (red symbols), while patients with BNP above the upper limit of normal present with relaxation values within the age-adjusted range of normality (blue symbols in shaded area). Right panels show that BNP increases conduction velocity in the sinoatrial (SA) node and toward surrounding myocardium, increasing HR in excess of the tachycardia promoted by chemotherapy-induced hemoglobin loss. Relaxation and BNP were measured as described in the legend to Fig. 6. *Adapted from Azer, J., Hua, R., Krishnaswamy, P. S., & Rose, R. A. (2014). Effects of natriuretic peptides on electrical conduction in the sinoatrial node and atrial myocardium of the heart.* The Journal of Physiology, 592, *1025–1045; Calabrese, V., Menna, P., Annibali, O., Armento, G., Carpino, A., Cerchiara, E., et al. (2018). Early diastolic dysfunction after cancer chemotherapy: Primary endpoint results of a multicenter cardio-oncology study.* Chemotherapy, 63, *55–63; Menna, P., Calabrese, V., Armento, G., Annibali, O., Greco, C., Salvatorelli, E., et al. (2018). Pharmacology of cardio-oncology: Chronotropic and lusitropic effects of B-type natriuretic peptide in cancer patients with early diastolic dysfunction induced by anthracycline or non-anthracycline chemotherapy.* The Journal of Pharmacology and Experimental Therapeutics, 366, *158-168.*

hospitalization for decompensated HF. Things have changed since the pharmacological treatment of HF was transformed by the advent of sacubitril/valsartan (S/V).

Sacubitril/valsartan (S/V) is the first-in-class agent of a new family of drugs called angiotensin receptor/neprilysin inhibitors (ARNI). Sacubitril/valsartan is a combination product in which the role of sacubitril is to inhibit neprilysin, a protease involved in degrading natriuretic peptides. Sacubitril therefore prolongs the half-life of BNP and makes its beneficial effects extend over time. Because neprilysin degrades angiotensin II as well, valsartan is needed to blunt untoward effects of the accumulating angiotensin II. Thus, whereas sacubitril cannot be used as a single agent, its combination with valsartan ensures that beneficial effects of BNP are accompanied by beneficial effects of RAAS inhibition. In the pivotal Prospective comparison of ARNI with ACEi to Determine Impact on Global Mortality and morbidity in Heart Failure trial (PARADIGM-HF), randomizing patients with an LVEF of ≤40% to receive S/V or enalapril, S/V did prove significantly superior to enalapril in reducing the risks of death and hospitalization for HF, which was a long-waited improvement in HFrEF treatment (McMurray et al., 2014). Interestingly, S/V had earlier been shown to be of potential efficacy also in the settings of HFpEF. The phase II study PARAMOUNT-HF (Prospective comparison of ARNI with ARB on Management Of heart failUre with preserved ejection fracTion) had in fact reported that S/V was superior to valsartan in reducing Nt-proBNP levels, left atrial size and severity of functional status in patients with an LVEF of >45%. This was an obvious demonstration of how effectively an extended half-life of BNP could relieve cardiac stress and prevent further production of BNP prohormone (Solomon et al., 2012).

Given that PARADIGM-HF and PARAMOUNT-HF trials had been so successful in their respective settings, the PARAGON-HF trial (Angiotensin Receptor Neprilysin Inhibition in Heart Failure With Preserved Ejection Fraction) was designed by mirroring the same patient characteristics and protocol procedures as those of PARAMOUNT-HF with the intuitive exception that only patients with an LVEF of 45% or higher met the inclusion criteria. In this study, the primary endpoint of reduced total HF hospitalizations or cardiovascular death was barely missed by S/V ($P=0.059$), although other parameters, such as quality of life and New York Heart Association (NYHA) functional class, were improved in the S/V group as compared to the valsartan group (Solomon et al., 2019). Despite such neutral outcome, sacubitril/valsartan is now approved for both HFrEF and HFpEF, and Heart Failure guidelines now read a class IIb C recommendation for using S/V not only in patients with HFrEF (LVEF < 40%), but also in patients with HF symptoms and LVEF somewhere between 41% and 49% (McDonagh et al., 2021).

A point of criticism should now be brought on stage. The 2016 ESC heart failure guidelines would define an HF with LVEF of 40–49% as heart failure with midrange ejection fraction (Ponikowski et al., 2016). As correctly pointed out (Savarese, Stolfo, Sinagra, & Lund, 2021), heart failure with midrange ejection fraction remains largely unexplored compared with HFrEF (LVEF < 40%) and HFpEF (LVEF ≥ 50%). The prevalence of heart failure with midrange ejection fraction is much lower than that of HFpEF, and clinical and prognostic characteristics are somehow intermediate between HFrEF and HFpEF in some respects, while being more similar to HFrEF in others. Heart failure with midrange ejection fraction should probably be better defined as HF with mildly reduced ejection fraction (HFmrEF) (Savarese et al., 2021). These considerations are way more than semantic, but allude to the fact that HFpEF is such an unmet medical need that any drug with a measurable activity in patients with LVEF >40% is regarded as a new promising agent to treat authentic HFpEF. This was the case for S/V.

In oncologic settings there are reports showing the efficacy of S/V in rats with anthracycline-induced systolic dysfunction (Boutagy et al., 2020), as well as clinical studies showing S/V efficacy in patients with anthracycline-induced HFrEF (Camilli et al., 2020; Martín-Garcia et al., 2020). The PRADA II trial has been designed and is currently ongoing to probe the efficacy of S/V in primary prevention of anthracycline-induced systolic dysfunction in breast cancer patients (Mecinaj et al., 2021). There also are preclinical reports suggesting that S/V might afford cardioprotection independently of its CV effects, e.g., by counteracting anthracycline-induced expression and phosphorylation of the fission protein dynamin-related protein 1, which fragmentates the mitochondrial network and its perinuclear clustering (Xia et al., 2017). In spite of such growing evidence for S/V efficacy in the settings of systolic dysfunction and HF, studies that specifically look at early DD are lacking at this point in time. The road to such studies seems nonetheless to have been paved.

Augmentation of cGMP levels is another promising strategy to treat DD. Neutral result of trials of cGMP augmentation by means of sildenafil inhibition of PDE 5 (to prevent decomposition of cGMP to GMP) (Redfield et al., 2013), NO donors (to promote activation of soluble guanylyl cyclase) (Greene et al., 2013), or direct activators of soluble guanylyl cyclase, like vericiguat (Armstrong et al., 2020; Pieske et al., 2017), should not be interpreted to dismiss the validity of manipulating cGMP levels. These studies looked at the efficacy of one strategy or the other on improving CV performance of patients with HFpEF, but again HFpEF is the end stage disease of a long pathophysiologic trajectory, where multiple players come into a play at different times and with a different role in promoting early DD progression from grade I (asymptomatic impaired relaxation) to grade >II stages (symptomatic restrictive patterns). HFpEF is too late a stage of disease for interventions to be always as efficacious as one would anticipate from laboratory findings or conceptual design.

Things should be narrowed, and the efficacy of cGMP manipulations should be explored in the early phases of DD. Encouraging results were in fact obtained when pharmacological maneuvres around cGMP looked at improvements of early DD. Chronic subcutaneous BNP, as a strategy to increase cGMP via the receptor-associated particulate guanylyl cyclase, improved echocardiographic indices of diastolic function in patients with subclinical DD (McKie et al., 2011). Concomitant administration of BNP and tadalafil, as a strategy to increase cGMP while also inhibiting PDE 5 to prevent cGMP decomposition to GMP, improved diastolic indices in patients with grade II DD (Wan et al., 2021). Given that tadalafil alone was ineffective, these results hint that, with increasing DD severity from Grade I to Grade II, combination therapies would be more effective than single agent interventions.

Whereas the opportunities offered by cGMP as a therapeutic target for DD treatment call for confirmation in clinical oncologic settings, there are preclinical data to suggest that cGMP manipulations might be considered for primary prevention as well, i.e., for preventing the very early pathophysiologic steps and manifestations of DD. For example, tadalafil prevented DD in a juvenile mouse model of anthracycline cardiotoxicity (Nagiub, Filippone, Durrant, Das, & Kukreja, 2017). These results should be weighed against previous concerns about the etiology-dependence of DD development in animal models and the highly variable responses to pharmacological agents that one may observe in one model or another (Frisk et al., 2021). This having been acknowledged, the effects of tadalafil on a juvenile diabetic model of DD should be prospectively considered as a conceptual basis for halting the year-long trajectory that goes from childhood or adolescent cancer treatment to late manifestations such as HFrEF, HFpEF or Grinch syndrome, especially if one appreciates that childhood cancer survivors carry an increased risk of diabetes and other metabolic disturbances (Novetsky Friedman, Tonorezos, & Cohen, 2019).

On the side of PDEs that degrade cGMP downstream of particulate guanylyl cyclase, the novel PDE 9 inhibitor, CRD-733, was shown to improve HF induced by transverse aortic constriction. CRD-733 could in fact ameliorate LV hypertrophy, LV dysfunction, left atrial dilation, and pulmonary edema (Richards et al., 2021). These results, while being of greater relevance to HFrEF than HFpEF at this point in time, show that the cGMP arena can accommodate many potential new drugs of interest, raising hopes that some of them could eventually prove useful in the settings of HFpEF and particularly of early DD (van Heerebeek & Paulus, 2016). Indeed, DD should be treated as soon as a clinical diagnosis is made after cancer treatment. Equally interesting is that CRD-733 caused remarkable increases in plasma cGMP, which might be used to monitor treatment efficacy and design dose-finding studies in early clinical trials (Richards et al., 2021).

The role of cGMP and opportunities for therapeutic interventions are sketched in Fig. 8.

6.3 cGMP-independent lusitropic agents: Ranolazine

Means for inducing positive lusitropy in patients with myocardial stiffness and DD, whether occurring in the general population, or in cancer patients

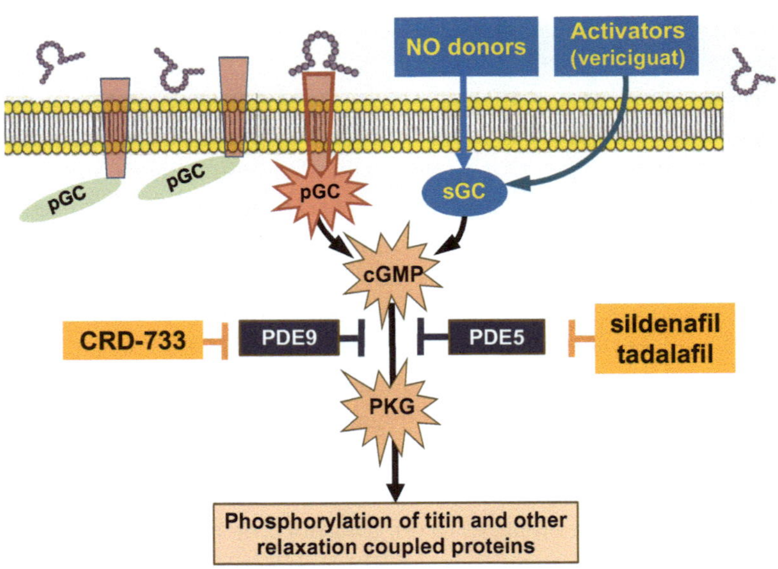

Fig. 8 Cardiac effects of cGMP modulation and relevance to DD. Schematic representation of how BNP binding to its receptors activates particulate guanylyl cyclase (pGC) to generate cGMP that then phosphorylates titin and other relaxation-coupled proteins. Similar effects could derive from activation of soluble guanylyl cyclase (sGC) by NO donors or sensitizing agents (e.g., vericiguat). This framework accommodates therapeutic interventions with drugs that further increase cGMP levels by inhibiting PDE5 or PDE9. PDE, phosphodiesterase; PKG, protein kinase G. *Concepts from van Heerebeek, L., & Paulus, W. J. (2016). Understanding heart failure with preserved ejection fraction: Where are we today?* Netherlands Heart Journal, 24, *227–236.*

treated with cardiotoxic drugs, may extend beyond the BNP-cGMP cascade. The ranolazine story has been particularly instructive in this setting.

Ranolazine is an orally available piperazine derivative approved by the Food and Drug Administration as first-line or top-on-therapy agent for chronic angina patients who are not adequately controlled by other drugs (β blockers, ACEi, ARB, calcium channel blockers) or show intolerance to them. In Europe, ranolazine was granted approval as top-on-therapy agent only. Once believed to afford anti-ischemic effects by inhibiting fatty acid oxidation, and thus shifting metabolism toward energy-building glucose oxidation (McCormack, Barr, Wolff, & Lopaschuk, 1996), ranolazine was subsequently shown to act primarily by inhibiting I_{Na}-late current (Belardinelli, Shryock, & Fraser, 2006; Hale, Shryock, Belardinelli, Sweeney, & Kloner, 2008). There is compelling evidence of delayed or incomplete inactivation of I_{Na}-late current in the repolarizing ischemic LV, likely caused by accumulating reactive oxygen species and ischemic metabolites. Hyperactive I_{Na}-late current forces NCX to operate in a reverse mode to extrude excess Na^+ in exchange with Ca^{2+} entry. Cardiomyocyte are thus exposed to inappropriate Ca^{2+} activation of myofilaments in diastole, which increases wall tension and reduces coronary conductance (Hale et al., 2008).

By inhibiting I_{Na}-late current ranolazine relieves Ca^{2+}-dependent diastolic stiffness and coronary arteries compression, eventually improving blood flow and oxygen supply. On a different note, ranolazine lacks effects on HR or blood pressure (Rousseau, Pouleur, Cocco, & Wolff, 2005; Venkataraman, Belardinelli, Blackburn, Heo, & Iskandrian, 2009), and can thus be viewed as a pure positive lusitropic agent. Moreover, and interestingly, ranolazine may cause pleiotropic effects that extend beyond inhibition of I_{Na}-late current but still result in positive lusitropic effects. For example, studies of oxidative stress-prone deoxycorticosterone acetate-salt hypertensive mouse models showed that ranolazine relieved echocardiographic indices of severe DD through direct effects on improving myofilament-Ca^{2+} interactions and cross-bridge kinetics (Lovelock et al., 2012).

Because of such convincing evidence that antianginal effects of ranolazine were in fact due to its positive lusitropic effects, ranolazine attracted attention as a potential new agent to treat DD and HFpEF (Stone, 2008). Limited studies with an intravenous formulation showed that ranolazine improved diastolic function in patients with long QT syndrome 3, caused by SCN5A gene mutations that slow inactivation of $I_{Na,Late}$ (Moss et al., 2008), or in patients with worsening DD due to a previous transmural myocardial infarction (Hayashida, van Eyll, Rousseau, & Pouleur, 1994). Relatively less convincing were the results of RALI-DHF (RAnoLazIne for the Treatment of Diastolic Heart Failure) trial, a small proof-of-concept study of the potential efficacy of ranolazine in patients with HFpEF. This study revealed that intravenous ranolazine improved some hemodynamic parameters (left ventricular end diastolic pressure, pulmonary capillary wedge pressure), but lacked effects on relaxation indices and did not reduce BNP levels that were significantly increased at patient study entry (Maier et al., 2013). Equally disappointing were the results of a small study of ranolazine in patients with DD secondary to moderate or severe aortic stenosis. In the latter study ranolazine caused a borderline significant increase in total exercise duration, but lacked effects on imaging indices of diastolic atrial relaxation (Singh, Steadman, Khan, Reggiardo, & McCann, 2016). Finally, based on preclinical evidence for ranolazine reversing electrophysiological and mechanical abnormalities of cardiomyocytes from patients with hypertrophic cardiomyopathy (Coppini et al., 2013), a clinical study of ranolazine efficacy in this setting showed that ranolazine lacked measurable effects on exercise performance, BNP levels and DD as compared to placebo (Olivotto et al., 2018).

Negative evidence for the efficacy of ranolazine in the settings of DD and HFpEF should be weighed against unanimous consensus on its positive lusitropic effects in patients with chronic angina. It may perhaps be appropriate considering that one size does not fit all. Clinical phenotypes of cardiomyopathy in chronic angina and DD are remarkably different. DD often develops in response to primary morbidities (diabetes, hypertension, infarction, etc.) that are too heterogeneous for a cohesive picture to be obtained. And again, DD is such a difficult condition to treat that the efficacy of potentially valuable drugs should be probed in early stages of DD rather than high-grade DD or end-stage HFpEF.

These reasonings formed the basis to probe ranolazine in cancer patients diagnosed with the mildest manifestation of DD (grade I) as early as one week after completing chemotherapy (Minotti, 2013). Having previously considered that BNP could compensate for DD, the study also recruited patients with persistent elevations of BNP at the end of chemotherapy. There were mechanistic reasonings to explore ranolazine efficacy in these settings. By continuously generating reactive oxygen species, anthracyclines may well cause metabolic hypoxia that activates I_{Na}-late current, similar to what ischemia does in patients with chronic angina; moreover, and accordingly, ranolazine was effective in relieving diastolic dysfunction in a rat model of doxorubicin cardiotoxicity (Cappetta et al., 2017). Finally, pleiotropic effects of ranolazine, as discussed earlier, might further contribute to counteract negative effects of anthracyclines on diastolic function. Attrition in patient recruitment made this clinical study a sort of an exploratory minitrial in which only 24 comorbid-free patients with post-chemotherapy DD or BNP elevations were randomized 1:1 to ranolazine or common cardiovascular drugs (β-blockers, ACEi, diuretics, or combinations of them). Although remarkably limited in its sample size, the study did provide some proof-of-concept opportunities: (i) it probed the efficacy of ranolazine against DD that was attributable to just one causative factor (chemotherapy), excluding biases from competing CV risk factors; (ii) it evaluated ranolazine vis-à-vis CV drugs after a short 5-weeks treatment, giving a chance to evaluate if ranolazine relieved DD as quickly as it improved myocardial relaxation and coronary blood flow in perfusion imaging studies of patients with chronic angina (Venkataraman et al., 2009); and (iii) inasmuch as CV drugs were anticipated to cause hemodynamic effects like e.g., hypotension, it gave a chance to confirm that ranolazine lacked such effects even in frail and often hemodynamically unstable oncologic patients.

Results showed that all patients randomized to ranolazine recovered from grade I DD or BNP elevations while 3 of 12 patients randomized to common CV drugs failed treatment. Moreover, ranolazine normalized echocardiographic indices of diastolic function or BNP levels without lowering systolic blood pressure, while patients treated with CV drugs experienced significant decreases of both systolic and diastolic pressure (Minotti et al., 2019). Limitations in sample size clearly precluded further considerations around ranolazine as a candidate off-label agent to cure cancer treatment-related early DD or prevent it from progressing toward advanced stages. Yet, some differential effects of ranolazine in patients with or without BNP elevations were of a noticeable interest.

In patients with grade I DD and normal BNP levels at the end of chemotherapy, changes of HR were well within the pathophysiologic range predicted by cancer treatment-induced bone marrow toxicity and hemoglobin loss. Following 5-week ranolazine, diastolic function normalized and HR decreased in a manner consistent with the returning of hemoglobin to pre-chemotherapy levels (Fig. 9). These findings showed that in presence of normal BNP levels, DD was relieved by ranolazine, while HR was governed only by autonomic reflexes driven by increases or decreases of hemoglobin levels.

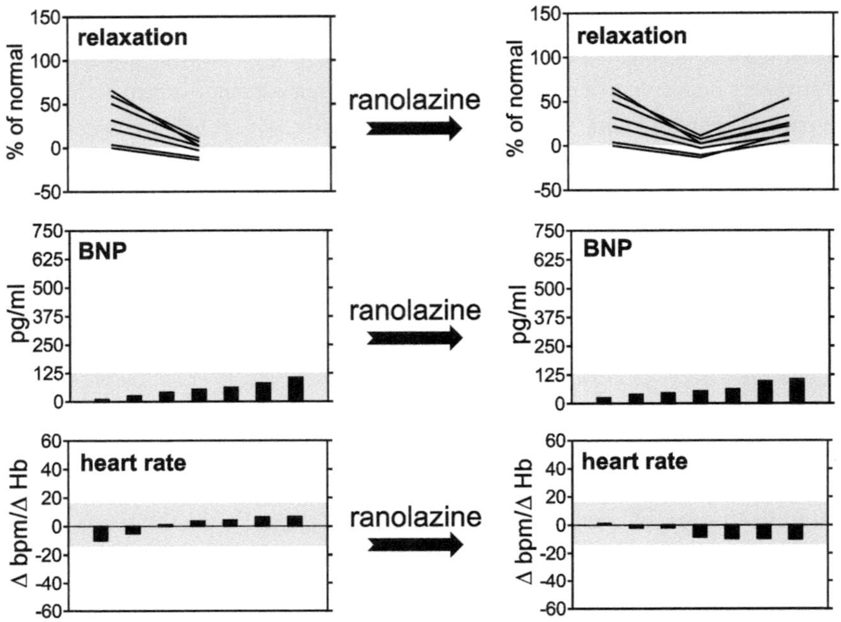

Fig. 9 Effects of ranolazine in cancer patients with chemotherapy-induced DD and normal BNP levels. In patients with post-chemotherapy grade I DD (impaired relaxation) and normal BNP levels, ranolazine improved diastolic function without affecting HR. Grey areas indicate normal ranges of relaxation, BNP levels, and hemoglobin-adjusted increases or decreases of beats per minute after chemotherapy or ranolazine. Relaxation and BNP were measured as described in the legend to Fig. 6. *Concept summary from Minotti, G., Menna, P., Calabrese, V., Greco, C., Armento, G., Annibali, O., et al. (2019). Pharmacology of ranolazine versus common cardiovascular drugs in patients with early diastolic dysfunction induced by anthracyclines or nonanthracycline chemotherapeutics: A phase 2b minitrial.* The Journal of Pharmacology and Experimental Therapeutics, 370, *197–205.*

Different results occurred when patients with normal diastolic function and high BNP levels were considered. In the latter patients, chemotherapy caused HR to increase in excess of hemoglobin loss, which was well explained by the positive chronotropic effect of high BNP, while five-week ranolazine blunted BNP levels and made HR decrease below the range predicted by normalization of hemoglobin levels (Fig. 10). Since ranolazine *per se* lacks negative chronotropic effects, the latter findings showed that in patients in whom DD was corrected by BNP lusitropy, ranolazine was able to mitigate the diastolic distress that stimulated BNP elevations and, by so doing, diminished both BNP levels and the accompanying chronotropic effects.

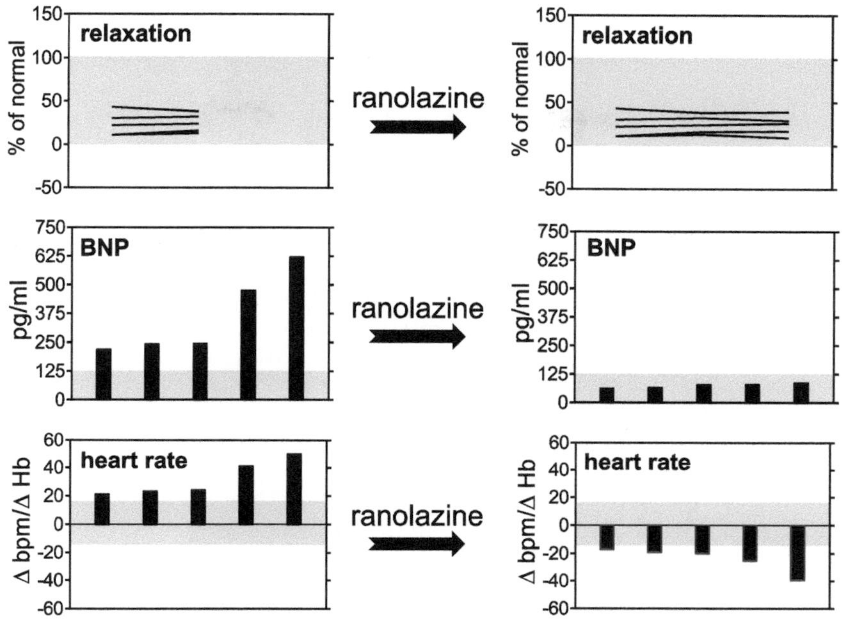

Fig. 10 Effects of ranolazine in cancer patients with post-chemotherapy normal diastolic function and high BNP levels. In patients with post-chemotherapy normal diastolic function and high BNP levels, HR increased in excess of hemoglodin-predicted changes. Ranolazine blunted BNP levels and made HR decrease in excess of hemoglobin-predicted changes. Grey areas indicate normal ranges of relaxation, BNP levels, and hemoglobin-adjusted increases or decreases of beats per minute after chemotherapy or ranolazine. Relaxation and BNP were measured as described in the legend to Fig. 6. *Concept summary from Minotti, G., Menna, P., Calabrese, V., Greco, C., Armento, G., Annibali, O., et al. (2019). Pharmacology of ranolazine versus common cardiovascular drugs in patients with early diastolic dysfunction induced by anthracyclines or non-anthracycline chemotherapeutics: A phase 2b minitrial.* The Journal of Pharmacology and Experimental Therapeutics, 370, *197–205.*

Face-to-face comparisons of patients with DD and normal BNP vs patients with normal diastolic function and high BNP thus recapitulate beneficial effects of ranolazine on improving myocardial relaxation or relieving compensatory elevations of BNP as an endogenous lusitropic and chronotropic agent. The effects of ranolazine were strongly reminiscent of those observed in patients randomized to ranolazine for treatment of non-ST-segment elevation acute coronary syndrome. After patients' stratification by BNP levels, it turned out that ranolazine efficacy on cardiovascular death, myocardial infarction, and recurrent ischemia was significantly higher in patients with high BNP levels than in patients with low BNP levels (Morrow et al., 2010).

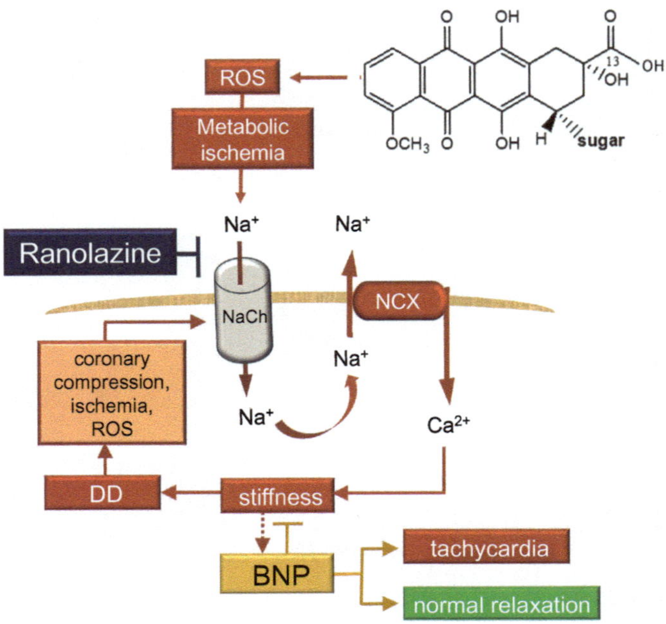

Fig. 11 Ranolazine breaks vicious cycles downstream of anthracycline activation of I_{Na}-late current. Schematic representation of how anthracyclines (here represented by the chemical structure of doxorubicin) would activate I_{Na}-late current, causing downstream Ca^{2+}-dependent myocardial stiffness, DD, and perpetuation of activation of I_{Na}-late current. In some patients stiffnesss would stimulate BNP production that in turn mitigates stiffness while also inducing inappropriate tachycardia. Ranolazine-induced inhibition of I_{Na}-late current would be of benefit to interrupt vicious cycles. NaCh, sodium channel forming subunit of I_{Na}-late current; ROS, reactive oxygen species. *Concept summary from Minotti, G. (2013). Pharmacology at work for cardio-oncology: Ranolazine to treat early cardiotoxicity induced by antitumor drugs.* The Journal of Pharmacology and Experimental Therapeutics, 346, *343–349; Minotti, G., Menna, P., Calabrese, V., Greco, C., Armento, G., Annibali, O., et al. (2019). Pharmacology of ranolazine versus common cardiovascular drugs in patients with early diastolic dysfunction induced by anthracyclines or nonanthracycline chemotherapeutics: A phase 2b minitrial.* The Journal of Pharmacology and Experimental Therapeutics, 370, *197–205.*

While waiting for larger confirmatory studies, ranolazine merits consideration in cardio-oncologic settings. Tentative vicious cycles linking anthracyclines to I_{Na}-late current and ranolazine are sketched in Fig. 11.

7. Novel potential pharmacologic opportunities

Whereas successful treatment of DD remains an unmet medical need, new drugs hold promise for providing unanticipated benefit in this setting.

Inhibitors of sodium-dependent glucose cotransporter 2 (or sodium-glucose linked transporter 2 inhibitors, SGLT2i) warrant attention.

SGLT2i were developed to improve glycemic control in patients with type 2 diabetes. They act by inhibiting glucose reabsorption in the proximal convoluted tubule of the kidney, thus causing glycosuria, natriuresis, body mass reduction and blood pressure lowering. Interestingly, however, cardiovascular outcome trials of patients with diabetes showed that SGLT2i could also diminish rates of hospitalization for HF (Cowie & Fisher, 2020). This was a game-changing result as SGLT2i were the first glucose-lowering drug class to show a measurable benefit in this setting as compared to neutral or harmful effects of other antidiabetic drugs. Several studies primarily designed to evaluate HF outcomes, then showed that SGLT2i reduced CV death or hospitalization rates also in patients without diabetes, including subgroups treated with sacubitril/valsartan (Camilli et al., 2021).

Given that normal or diseased heart seems to not express SGLT2 (Uthman et al., 2018), results of clinical trials have triggered basic research efforts to decipher how SGLT2i could positively influence the failing heart either directly or indirectly. Studies of a neurogenic hypertensive mouse model first revealed that a cross talk exists between kidney SGLT2 expression or activity and the sympathetic nervous system; in fact, chemical denervation reduced SGLT2 expression, while SGLT2 inhibition by dapaglifozin reduced kidney levels of noradrenaline (Herat et al., 2020).

These findings anticipated a possible role for SGLT2i in mitigating vicious neurohumoral reflexes that govern HF and make it progress toward end stage; however, many other SGLT2i effects have been provisionally characterized at a cellular level that could explain CV effects. Studies of empagliflozin, dapagliflozin and canagliflozin on various cardiac cell types have shown that SGLT2i reduce $[Na^{+}]_{I}$ (possibly by inhibiting the plasma membrane Na^{+}/H^{+} exchanger) and free $[Ca^{2+}]_{I}$ (possibly by improving Ca^{2+} accumulation in mitochondria) (Uthman et al., 2018). SGLT2i improved ATP content and cell viability after hypoxia/reoxygenation stress in cardiomyocytes and endothelial cells, showed antifibrotic effects and induced anti-inflammatory effects capable of mitigating metabolic syndrome in HF patients (Uthman et al., 2018). On molecular grounds, such beneficial effects of SGLT2i may at least in part be mediated by downregulation of NADPH oxidases, suppression of TGF-β related pathways, stimulation of gluconeogenesis and ketogenesis coupled with an alleviation of oxidative stress, and blunting of inflammatory cytokines (Gager et al., 2021). In a rat model of salt-induced hypertensive DD dapagliflozin did not only improve echocardiographic indices of myocardial stiffness but also reversed endothelial dysfunction and mitigated fibrogenesis, particularly in coronary vessels (Cappetta et al., 2020). In a randomized trial of patients with type 2 diabetes, known to be at risk for both HFrEF and HFpEF, dapagliflozin significantly reduced left ventricular mass compared with placebo, an effect that proved to be independent of baseline mass, blood pressure, weight, and systolic blood pressure-lowering effects of dapaglifozin. Moreover, and consistent with anti-dismetabolic and anti-inflammatory effects, dapaglifozin reduced visceral and subcutaneous adipose tissue as well as insulin resistance and high-sensitivity C-reactive protein levels (Brown et al., 2020).

In the recently completed EMPEROR-Preserved Trial, empaglifozin produced early and long-lasting reduction in the risk and severity of a broad range of worsening HF events in patients with New York Heart Association class II-IV HFpEF, defined as LVEF between 40% and 49% (Packer et al., 2021). This study highlighted empaglifozin as a valuable drug to treat HFmrEF, similar to the evidence that brought S/V to receive regulatory approval in the same setting. A much smaller but equally important study of diabetic patients with acute coronary syndrome, and lacking HF symptoms and with LVEF >50%, showed that early commencement of empaglifozin halted hypertrophy progression and improved numerous echocardiographic indices of DD (Lan et al., 2021). Considering that intermittent administration of oxygen-consuming drugs like anthracyclines can in a sense be compared to repeated cycles of hypoxia-reoxygenation, the latter study raises hope that empaglifozin could be useful to treat DD in cancer patients. Finally, studies of non-diabetic pigs, exposed to a 2-h balloon occlusion of the proximal left anterior descending coronary artery, showed that empagliflozin could ameliorate diastolic function, histological and molecular remodeling, left ventricle and cardiomyocyte stiffness (Santos-Gallego et al., 2021). While possibly limited in its significance by the experimental manoeuvres utilized to induce acute HF and DD, the latter study unequivocally confirmed that cardioprotective effects of SGLT2i were independent of glycemic control. It goes without saying that SGLT2i have become of paramount importance in cardiovascular medicine (Varzideh, Kansakar, & Santulli, 2021).

Much less is known about SGLT2i relieving DD in cardio-oncologic settings. In limited preclinical *in-vivo* studies empaglifozin prevented doxorubicin-dependent decrease in LVEF as well as deterioration of echocardiographic indices of myocardial plasticity; however, neither protective effect could be duplicated by replacing empaglifozin with a loop diuretic, thus demonstrating that empaglifozine afforded cardioprotection independently of its effects on increasing diuresis and decreasing afterload (Sabatino et al., 2020). As we also said for S/V, the road to further studies of SGLT2i is promisingly paved.

8. Conclusion

In exploring unresolved issues in the field of cancer treatment-related early DD we considered a recurrent leitmotif: little is known about pathophysiology and even less is known about pharmacologic treatment. In addition, we confined our narration to DD as induced by anthracyclines, but many other chemical entities belonging to the new wave of "biologic drugs" will soon confront clinicians with the same problem. Even venerable non-anthracycline drugs, like platinum compounds, can induce early DD in comorbid-free patients (Calabrese et al., 2018). As usual in this setting, evidence that non-anthracycline drugs could harm diastolic function and cause early DD was preceded by reports showing that long-term cancer survivors treated with cisplatin were exposed to an increased risk of grade III-IV DD and ischemic complications (Carver et al., 2007). The pharmacotherapy of cancer-treatment related DD can only improve if a diagnosis is placed as soon as possible and potential drugs are tested in suitable preclinical models.

Finally, there is a need to involve pharmaceutical industry partners early in this research. Companies are intuitively interested in expanding indications of e.g., S/V or SGLT2i, but are reluctant to launch trials that probe the efficacy and safety of these drugs in cancer treatment-related cardiotoxicity. Cancer patients usually represent a small, very marginal subgroup of patients recruited in phase III trials of new CV drugs. Closer interactions between academia and pharmaceutical companies is much needed to accelerate transition of potentially active CV drugs from the general population to the cardio-oncology community.

Conflict of interest statement

The authors have no conflicts of interest to declare.

References

Abbate, A., Arena, R., Abouzaki, N., Van Tassell, B. W., Canada, J., Shah, K., et al. (2015). Heart failure with preserved ejection fraction: Refocusing on diastole. *International Journal of Cardiology*, *179*, 430–440.

Amgalan, D., Garner, T. P., Pekson, R., Jia, X. F., Yanamandala, M., Paulino, V., et al. (2020). A small-molecule allosteric inhibitor of BAX protects against doxorubicin-induced cardiomyopathy. *Nature Cancer*, *1*, 315–328.

Aoki, T., Fukumoto, Y., Sugimura, K., Oikawa, M., Satoh, K., Nakano, M., et al. (2011). Prognostic impact of myocardial interstitial fibrosis in non-ischemic heart failure. -Comparison between preserved and reduced ejection fraction heart failure. *Circulation Journal*, *75*, 2605–2613.

Armenian, S. H., Lacchetti, C., Barac, A., Carver, J., Constine, L. S., Denduluri, N., et al. (2017). Prevention and monitoring of cardiac dysfunction in survivors of adult cancers: American Society of Clinical Oncology clinical practice guideline. *Journal of Clinical Oncology*, *35*, 893–911.

Armstrong, G. T., Joshi, V. M., Ness, K. K., Marwick, T. H., Zhang, N., Srivastava, D., et al. (2015). Comprehensive echocardiographic detection of treatment-related cardiac dysfunction in adult survivors of childhood cancer: Results from the St. Jude Lifetime Cohort Study. *Journal of the American College of Cardiology*, *65*, 2511–2522.

Armstrong, P. W., Lam, C. S. P., Anstrom, K. J., Ezekowitz, J., Hernandez, A. F., O'Connor, C. M., et al. (2020). Effect of vericiguat vs placebo on quality of life in patients with heart failure and preserved ejection fraction: The vitality-HFpEF randomized clinical trial. *Journal of the American Medical Association*, *324*, 1512–1521.

Azer, J., Hua, R., Krishnaswamy, P. S., & Rose, R. A. (2014). Effects of natriuretic peptides on electrical conduction in the sinoatrial node and atrial myocardium of the heart. *The Journal of Physiology*, *592*, 1025–1045.

Belardinelli, L., Shryock, J. C., & Fraser, H. (2006). Inhibition of the late sodium current as a potential cardioprotective principle: effects of the late sodium current inhibitor ranolazine. *Heart*, *92*, iv6–iv14.

Benjamin, R. S., & Minotti, G. (2021). Doxorubicin-dexrazoxane from day 1 for soft-tissue sarcomas: The road to cardioprotection. *Clinical Cancer Research*, *27*, 3809–3811.

Bers, D. M., Barry, W. H., & Intracellular, D. S. (2003). Na^{+} regulation in cardiac myocytes. *Cardiovascular Research*, *57*, 897–912.

Bielecka-Dabrowa, A., Sakowicz, A., Misztal, M., von Haehling, S., Ahmed, A., Pietrucha, T., et al. (2016). Differences in biochemical and genetic biomarkers in patients with heart failure of various etiologies. *International Journal of Cardiology*, *221*, 1073–1080.

Bishu, K., Hamdani, N., Mohammed, S. F., Kruger, M., Ohtani, T., Ogut, O., et al. (2011). Sildenafil and B-type natriuretic peptide acutely phosphorylate titin and improve diastolic distensibility in vivo. *Circulation*, *124*, 2882–2891.

Borlaug, B. A., & Kass, D. A. (2006). Mechanisms of diastolic dysfunction in heart failure. *Trends in Cardiovascular Medicine*, *16*, 273–279.

Boutagy, N. E., Feher, A., Pfau, D., Liu, Z., Guerrera, N. M., Freeburg, L. A., et al. (2020). Dual angiotensin receptor-neprilysin inhibition with sacubitril/valsartan attenuates systolic dysfunction in experimental doxorubicin-induced cardiotoxicity. *JACC. CardioOncology*, *2*, 774–787.

Braunwald, E. (2008). Biomarkers in heart failure. *The New England Journal of Medicine*, *358*, 2148–2159.

Breccia, M., Pregno, P., Spallarossa, P., Arboscello, E., Ciceri, F., Giorgi, M., et al. (2017). Identification, prevention and management of cardiovascular risk in chronic myeloid leukaemia patients candidate to ponatinib: An expert opinion. *Annals of Hematology*, *96*, 549–558.

Brouwers, F. P., de Boer, R. A., van der Harst, P., Voors, A. A., Gansevoort, R. T., Bakker, S. J., et al. (2013). Incidence and epidemiology of new onset heart failure with preserved vs. reduced ejection fraction in a community-based cohort: 11-year follow-up of PREVEND. *European Heart Journal*, *34*, 1424–1431.

Brown, A. J. M., Gandy, S., McCrimmon, R., Houston, J. G., Struthers, A. D., & Lang, C. C. (2020). A randomized controlled trial of dapagliflozin on left ventricular hypertrophy in people with type two diabetes: The DAPA-LVH trial. *European Heart Journal*, *41*, 3421–3432.

Calabrese, V., Menna, P., Annibali, O., Armento, G., Carpino, A., Cerchiara, E., et al. (2018). Early diastolic dysfunction after cancer chemotherapy: Primary endpoint results of a multicenter cardio-oncology study. *Chemotherapy*, *63*, 55–63.

Camilli, M., Del Buono, G., Crea, F., & Minotti, G. (2020). Acute heart failure twenty-nine years after childhood cancer treatment: Role of anthracyclines and insufficient surveillance. *JACC. Cardiooncology*, *2*, 316–319.

Camilli, M., Lombardi, M., Chiabrando, J. G., Del Buono, M. G., Montone, R. A., Biondi-Zoccai, G., et al. (2021). Efficacy of sodium-glucose cotransporter-2 inhibitors in heart failure patients treated with dual angiotensin receptor blocker-neprilysin inhibitor: an updated meta-analysis. *European Heart Journal Cardiovascular Pharmacotherapy*. https://doi.org/10.1093/ehjcvp/pvab034.

Cao, L., Cai, G., Chang, C., Miao, A. Y., Yu, X. L., Yang, Z. Z., et al. (2015). Diastolic dysfunction occurs early in HER2-positive breast cancer patients treated concurrently with radiation therapy and trastuzumab. *The Oncologist*, *20*, 605–614.

Cappetta, D., De Angelis, A., Ciuffreda, L. P., Coppini, R., Cozzolino, A., Miccichè, A., et al. (2020). Amelioration of diastolic dysfunction by dapagliflozin in a non-diabetic model involves coronary endothelium. *Pharmacological Research*, *157*, 104781. https://doi.org/10.1016/j.phrs.2020.104781.

Cappetta, D., Esposito, G., Coppini, R., Piegari, E., Russo, R., Ciuffreda, L. P., et al. (2017). Effects of ranolazine in a model of doxorubicin-induced left ventricle diastolic dysfunction. *British Journal of Pharmacology*, *174*, 3696–3712.

Carver, J. R., Shapiro, C. L., Ng, A., Jacobs, L., Schwartz, C., Virgo, K. S., et al. (2007). American society of clinical oncology clinical evidence review on the ongoing care of adult cancer survivors: Cardiac and pulmonary late effects. *Journal of Clinical Oncology*, *25*, 3991–4007.

Chan, N. Y., Seyedi, N., Takano, K., & Levi, R. (2012). An unsuspected property of natriuretic peptides: Promotion of calcium-dependent catecholamine release via protein kinase G-mediated phosphodiesterase type 3 inhibition. *Circulation*, *125*, 298–307.

Chen, G. Y., & Nunez, G. (2010). Sterile inflammation: Sensing and reacting to damage. *Nature Reviews. Immunology*, *10*, 826–837.

Cohen, J. B., Geara, A. S., Hogan, J. J., & Townsend, R. R. (2019). Hypertension in cancer patients and survivors. Epidemiology, diagnosis, and management. *JACC. Cardiooncology*, *1*, 239–251.

Collier, P., Watson, C. J., Voon, V., Phelan, D., Jan, A., Mak, G., et al. (2011). Can emerging biomarkers of myocardial remodelling identify asymptomatic hypertensive patients at risk for diastolic dysfunction and diastolic heart failure? *European Journal of Heart Failure*, *13*, 1087–1095.

Coppini, R., Ferrantini, C., Yao, L., Fan, P., Del Lungo, M., Stillitano, F., et al. (2013). Late sodium current inhibition reverses electromechanical dysfunction in human hypertrophic cardiomyopathy. *Circulation*, *127*, 575–584.

Cowie, M. R., & Fisher, M. (2020). SGLT2 inhibitors: Mechanisms of cardiovascular benefit beyond glycaemic control. *Nature Reviews. Cardiology*, *17*, 761–772.

Curigliano, G., Lenihan, D., Fradley, M., Ganatra, S., Barac, A., Blaes, A., et al. (2020). ESMO guidelines committee. Management of cardiac disease in cancer patients throughout oncological treatment: ESMO consensus recommendations. *Annals of Oncology*, *31*, 171–190.

Dai, Z., Aoki, T., Fukumoto, Y., & Shimokawa, H. (2012). Coronary perivascular fibrosis is associated with impairment of coronary blood flow in patients with non-ischemic heart failure. *Journal of Cardiology*, *60*, 416–421.

Emdin, C. A., Callender, T., Cao, J., McMurray, J. J., & Rahimi, K. (2015). Meta-analysis of large-scale randomized trials to determine the effectiveness of inhibition of the renin-angiotensin aldosterone system in heart failure. *The American Journal of Cardiology*, *116*, 155–161.

Ewer, M. S., Carver, J. R., & Minotti, G. (2019). Old and new directions of cardio-oncology. *Seminars in Oncology*, *46*, 395–396.

Ewer, M. S., Suter, T. M., Lenihan, D. J., Niculescu, L., Breazna, A., Demetri, G. D., et al. (2014). Cardiovascular events among 1090 cancer patients treated with sunitinib, interferon, or placebo: A comprehensive adjudicated database analysis demonstrating clinically meaningful reversibility of cardiac events. *European Journal of Cancer*, *50*, 2162–2170.

Finkelman, B. S., Putt, M., Wang, T., Wang, L., Narayan, H., Domchek, S., et al. (2017). Arginine-nitric oxide metabolites and cardiac dysfunction in patients with breast cancer. *Journal of the American College of Cardiology*, *70*, 152–162.

Forte, E., Furtado, M. B., & Rosenthal, N. (2018). The interstitium in cardiac repair: Role of the immune-stromal cell interplay. *Nature Reviews. Cardiology*, *15*, 601–616.

Frisk, M., Le, C., Shen, X., Røe, A. T., Hou, Y., Manfra, O., et al. (2021). Etiology-dependent impairment of diastolic cardiomyocyte calcium homeostasis in heart failure with preserved ejection fraction. *Journal of the American College of Cardiology*, *4*, 405–419.

Gager, G. M., von Lewinski, D., Sourij, H., Jilma, B., Eyileten, C., Filipiak, K., et al. (2021). Effects of SGLT2 inhibitors on ion homeostasis and oxidative stress associated mechanisms in heart failure. *Biomedicine & Pharmacotherapy*, *143*, 112169. https://doi.org/10.1016/j.biopha.2021.112169.

Gibson, T. M., Li, Z., Green, D. M., Armstrong, G. T., Mulrooney, D. A., Srivastava, D. K., et al. (2017). Blood pressure status in adult survivors of childhood cancer: a report from the St. Jude Lifetime Cohort Study. *Cancer Epidemiology, Biomarkers & Prevention*, *26*, 1705–1713.

Greene, S. J., Gheorghiade, M., Borlaug, B. A., Pieske, B., Vaduganathan, M., Burnett, J. C., Jr., et al. (2013). The cGMP signaling pathway as a therapeutic target in heart failure with preserved ejection fraction. *Journal of the American Heart Association*, *2*(6), e000536. https://doi.org/10.1161/JAHA.113.000536.

Guo, A., Zhang, C., Wei, S., Chen, B., & Song, L. S. (2013). Emerging mechanisms of T-tubule remodelling in heart failure. *Cardiovascular Research*, *98*, 204–215.

Hale, S. L., Shryock, J. C., Belardinelli, L., Sweeney, M., & Kloner, R. A. (2008). Late sodium current inhibition as a new cardioprotective approach. *Journal of Molecular and Cellular Cardiology*, *44*, 954–967.

Hayashida, W., van Eyll, C., Rousseau, M. F., & Pouleur, H. (1994). Effects of ranolazine on left ventricular regional diastolic function in patients with ischemic heart disease. *Cardiovascular Drugs and Therapy*, *8*, 741–747.

Herat, L. Y., Magno, A. L., Rudnicka, C., Hricova, J., Carnagarin, R., Ward, N. C., et al. (2020). SGLT2 inhibitor–induced sympathoinhibition. *JACC. Basic to Translational Science*, *2*, 169–179.

Hillock, R. J., Frampton, C. M., Yandle, T. G., Troughton, R. W., Lainchbury, J. G., & Richards, A. M. (2008). B-type natriuretic peptide infusions in acute myocardial infarction. *Heart*, *94*, 617–622.

Howard, E., Steingart, R. M., Armstrong, G. T., Lyon, A. R., Armenian, S. H., Voso, T. M., et al. (2019). Cardiovascular events in cancer survivors. *Seminars in Oncology*, *46*, 426–432.

Jeyaseelan, R., Poizat, C., Baker, R. K., Abdishoo, S., Isterabadi, L. B., Lyons, G. E., et al. (1997). A novel cardiac-restricted target for doxorubicinCARP, a nuclear modulator of gene expression in cardiac progenitor cells and cardiomyocytes. *The Journal of Biological Chemistry*, *272*, 22800–22808.

Jeyaseelan, R., Poizat, C., Wu, H. Y., & Kedes, L. (1997). Molecular mechanisms of doxorubicin-induced cardiomyopathy: Selective suppression of Reiske iron–sulfur protein, ADP/ATP translocase and phosphofructokinase genes is associated with ATP depletion in rat cardiomyocytes. *The Journal of Biological Chemistry*, *272*, 5828–5832.

Jiang, C., Deng, L., Karr, M. A., Wen, Y., Wang, Q., Perimbeti, S., et al. (2021). Chronic comorbid conditions among adult cancer survivors in the United States: Results from the National Health Interview Survey, 2002-2018. *Cancer*. https://doi.org/10.1002/cncr.33981.

Kasner, M., Westermann, D., Lopez, B., Gaub, R., Escher, F., Kuhl, U., et al. (2011). Diastolic tissue Doppler indexes correlate with the degree of collagen expression and cross-linking in heart failure and normal ejection fraction. *Journal of the American College of Cardiology*, *57*, 977–985.

Kass, D. A., Bronzwaer, J. G., & Paulus, W. (2004). What mechanisms underlie diastolic dysfunction in heart failure? *Circulation Research*, *94*, 1533–1542.

Klein, R., Nadouri, D., Osler, E., Johnson, C., Dent, S., & Dwivedi, G. (2019). Diastolic dysfunction can precede systolic dysfunction on MUGA in cancer patients receiving trastuzumab-based therapy. *Nuclear Medicine Communications*, *40*, 22–29.

Kopp, L. M., Womer, R. B., Schwartz, C. L., Ebb, D. H., Franco, V. I., Hall, D., et al. (2019). Effects of dexrazoxane on doxorubicin-related cardiotoxicity and second malignant neoplasms in children with osteosarcoma: A report from the Children's Oncology Group. *Cardiooncology*, *28*(5), 15. https://doi.org/10.1186/s40959-019-0050-9.

Krumholz, H. M., Larson, M., & Levy, D. (1993). Sex differences in cardiac adaptation to isolated systolic hypertension. *The American Journal of Cardiology*, *72*, 310–313.

Ladas, E. J., Jacobson, J. S., Kennedy, D. D., Teel, K., Fleischauer, A., & Kelly, K. M. (2004). Antioxidants and cancer therapy: A systematic review. *Journal of Clinical Oncology*, *22*, 517–528.

Lahiri, S., Roy, A., Baby, S. M., Hoshi, T., Semenza, G. L., & Prabhakar, N. R. (2006). Oxygen sensing in the body. *Progress in Biophysics and Molecular Biology*, *91*, 249–286.

Lan, N. S. R., Yeap, B. B., Fegan, P. G., Green, G., Rankin, J. M., Dwivedi, G., et al. (2021). Empagliflozin and left ventricular diastolic function following an acute coronary syndrome in patients with type 2 diabetes. *The International Journal of Cardiovascular Imaging*, *37*, 517–527.

Lebrecht, D., & Walker, U. A. (2007). Role of mtDNA lesions in anthracycline cardiotoxicity. *Cardiovascular Toxicology*, 7, 108–113.

Lipshultz, S. E., Scully, R., Stevenson, K. E., Franco, V. I., Neuberg, D. S., Colan, S. D., et al. (2014). Hearts too small for body size after doxorubicin for childhood ALL: Grinch syndrome. *Journal of Clinical Oncology*, *32*(suppl), 10021A.

Livi, L., Barletta, G., Martella, F., Saieva, C., Desideri, I., Bacci, C., et al. (2021). Cardioprotective strategy for patients with nonmetastatic breast cancer who are receiving an anthracycline-based chemotherapy. *JAMA Oncology*, 7, 1544–1549.

Lovelock, J. D., Monasky, M. M., Jeong, E. M., Lardin, H. A., Liu, H., Patel, B. G., et al. (2012). Ranolazine improves cardiac diastolic dysfunction through modulation of myofilament calcium sensitivity. *Circulation Research*, *110*, 841–850.

Luu, A. Z., Chowdhury, B., Al-Omran, M., Teoh, H., Hess, D. A., & Verma, S. (2018). Role of endothelium in doxorubicin-induced cardiomyopathy. *JACC. Basic to Translational Science*, *3*, 861–870.

Maier, L. S., Layug, B., Karwatowska-Prokopczuk, E., Belardinelli, L., Lee, S., Sander, J., et al. (2013). RAnoLazIne for the treatment of diastolic heart failure in patients with preserved ejection fraction: The RALI-DHF proof-of-concept study. *JACC. Heart Failure*, *1*, 115–122.

Martín-Garcia, A., López-Fernández, T., Mitroi, C., Chaparro-Muñoz, M., Moliner, P., Agustin, C., et al. (2020). Effectiveness of sacubitril–valsartan in cancer patients with heart failure. *ESC Heart Failure*, *7*, 1–5.

Masson, S., Latini, R., Anand, I. S., Vago, T., Angelici, L., Barlera, S., et al. (2006). Direct comparison of B-type natriuretic peptide (BNP) and amino-terminal proBNP in a large population of patients with chronic and symptomatic heart failure: The Valsartan Heart Failure (Val-HeFT) data. *Clinical Chemistry*, *52*, 1528–1538.

McCormack, J. G., Barr, R. L., Wolff, A. A., & Lopaschuk, G. D. (1996). Ranolazine stimulates glucose oxidation in normoxic, ischemic and reperfused ischemic rat hearts. *Circulation*, *93*, 135–142.

McDonagh, T. A., Metra, M., Adamo, M., Gardner, R. S., Baumbach, A., Böhm, M., et al. (2021). 2021 ESC Guidelines for the diagnosis and treatment of acute and chronic heart failure. *European Heart Journal*, *42*, 3599–3726.

McKie, P. M., Schirger, J. A., Costello-Boerrigter, L. C., Benike, S. L., Harstad, L. K., Bailey, K. R., et al. (2011). Impaired natriuretic and renal endocrine response to acute volume expansion in pre-clinical systolic and diastolic dysfunction. *Journal of the American College of Cardiology*, *58*, 2095–2103.

McMurray, J. J. V., Packer, M., Desai, A. S., Gong, J., Lefkowitz, M. P., & Rizkala, A. R. (2014). Angiotensin-neprilysin inhibition versus enalapril in heart failure. *The New England Journal of Medicine*, *371*, 993–1004.

Mecinaj, A., Gulati, G., Heck, S. L., Holte, E., Fagerland, M. W., Larsen, A. I., et al. (2021). Rationale and design of the PRevention of cArdiac dysfunction during adjuvant breast cancer therapy (PRADA II) trial: A randomized, placebo-controlled, multicenter trial. *Cardiooncology*, 7, 33. https://doi.org/10.1186/s40959-021-00115-w.

Menna, P., Calabrese, V., Armento, G., Annibali, O., Greco, C., Salvatorelli, E., et al. (2018). Pharmacology of cardio-oncology: Chronotropic and lusitropic effects of B-type natriuretic peptide in cancer patients with early diastolic dysfunction induced by anthracycline or nonanthracycline chemotherapy. *The Journal of Pharmacology and Experimental Therapeutics*, *366*, 158–168.

Menna, P., Gonzalez Paz, O., Chello, M., Covino, E., Salvatorelli, E., & Minotti, G. (2012). Anthracycline cardiotoxicity. *Expert Opinion on Drug Safety*, *11*, 21–36.

Menna, P., Salvatorelli, E., & Minotti, G. (2008). Cardiotoxicity of antitumor drugs. *Chemical Research in Toxicology*, *15*, 1179–1189.

Michel, K., Herwig, M., Werner, F., Špiranec Spes, K., Abeßery, M., Schuh, K., et al. (2020). C-type natriuretic peptide moderates titin-based cardiomyocyte stiffness. *JCI Insight*, *5*, e139910. https://doi.org/10.1172/jci.insight.139910.

Mincu, R. I., Lampe, L. F., Mahabadi, A. A., Kimmig, R., Rassaf, T., & Totzeck, M. (2021). Left ventricular diastolic function following anthracycline-based chemotherapy in patients with breast cancer without previous cardiac disease—A meta-analysis. *Journal of Clinical Medicine*, *10*, 3890. https://doi.org/10.3390/jcm10173890.

Minotti, G. (2013). Pharmacology at work for cardio-oncology: Ranolazine to treat early cardiotoxicity induced by antitumor drugs. *The Journal of Pharmacology and Experimental Therapeutics*, *346*, 343–349.

Minotti, G., Menna, P., Calabrese, V., Greco, C., Armento, G., Annibali, O., et al. (2019). Pharmacology of ranolazine versus common cardiovascular drugs in patients with early diastolic dysfunction induced by anthracyclines or nonanthracycline chemotherapeutics: A phase 2b minitrial. *The Journal of Pharmacology and Experimental Therapeutics*, *370*, 197–205.

Minotti, G., Menna, P., Salvatorelli, E., Cairo, G., & Gianni, L. (2004). The anthracyclines: Molecular advances and pharmacological developments in antitumor activity and cardiotoxicity. *Pharmacological Reviews*, *56*, 185–229.

Mohammed, S. F., Hussain, S., Mirzoyev, S. A., Edwards, W. D., Maleszewski, J. J., & Redfield, M. M. (2015). Coronary microvascular rarefaction and myocardial fibrosis in heart failure with preserved ejection fraction. *Circulation*, *131*, 550–559.

Molenaar, P., Savarimuthu, S. M., Sarsero, D., Chen, L., Semmler, A. B., Carle, A., et al. (2007). Adrenaline elicits positive inotropic, lusitropic, and biochemical effects through beta2 -adrenoceptors in human atrial myocardium from nonfailing and failing hearts, consistent with Gs coupling but not with Gi coupling. *Naunyn-Schmiedeberg's Archives of Pharmacology*, *375*, 11–28.

Moltzau, L. R., Aronsen, J. M., Meier, S., Skogestad, J., Ørstavik, Ø., Lothe, G. B., et al. (2014). Different compartmentation of responses to brain natriuretic peptide and C-type natriuretic peptide in failing rat ventricle. *The Journal of Pharmacology and Experimental Therapeutics*, *350*, 681–690.

Morrow, D. A., Scirica, B. M., Sabatine, M. S., de Lemos, J. A., Murphy, S. A., Jarolim, P., et al. (2010). B-type natriuretic peptide and the effect of ranolazine in patients with non-ST-segment elevation acute coronary syndromes: Observations from the MERLIN-TIMI 36 (metabolic efficiency with ranolazine for less ischemia in non-ST elevation acute coronary-thrombolysis in myocardial infarction 36) trial. *Journal of the American College of Cardiology*, *55*, 1189–1196.

Moss, A. J., Zareba, W., Schwarz, K. Q., Rosero, S., McNitt, S., & Robinson, J. L. (2008). Ranolazine shortens repolarization in patients with sustained inward sodium current due to type-3 long-QT syndrome. *Journal of Cardiovascular Electrophysiology*, *19*, 1289–1293.

Nagiub, M., Filippone, D., Durrant, D., Das, A., & Kukreja, R. C. (2017). Long-acting PDE5 inhibitor tadalafil prevents early doxorubicin-induced left ventricle diastolic dysfunction in juvenile mice: Potential role of cytoskeletal proteins. *Canadian Journal of Physiology and Pharmacology*, *95*, 295–304.

Nagy, A. C., Cserép, Z., Tolnay, E., Nagykálnai, T., & Forster, T. (2008). Early diagnosis of chemotherapy-induced cardiomyopathy: A prospective tissue Doppler imaging study. *Pathology Oncology Research*, *14*, 69–77.

Novetsky Friedman, D., Tonorezos, E. S., & Cohen, P. (2019). Diabetes and metabolic syndrome in survivors of childhood cancer. *Hormone Research in Pædiatrics*, *91*, 118–127.

O'Connor, C. M., Starling, R. C., Hernandez, A. F., Armstrong, P. W., Dickstein, K., Hasselblad, V., et al. (2011). Effect of nesiritide in patients with acute decompensated heart failure. *The New England Journal of Medicine*, *365*, 32–43.

Olivotto, I., Camici, P. G., Merlini, P. A., Rapezzi, C., Patten, M., Climent, V., et al. (2018). Efficacy of ranolazine in patients with symptomatic hypertrophic cardiomyopathy: The RESTYLE-HCM randomized, double-blind, placebo-controlled study. *Circulation. Heart Failure*, *11*, e004124. https://doi.org/10.1161/circheartfailure.117.004124.

Olson, R. D., & Mushlin, P. S. (1990). Doxorubicin cardiotoxicity: Analysis of prevailing hypotheses. *The FASEB Journal*, *4*, 3076–3086.

Omland, T., Sabatine, M. S., Jablonski, K. A., Rice, M. M., Hsia, J., & Wergeland, R. (2007). Prognostic value of B-type natriuretic peptides in patients with stable coronary artery disease: The PEACE trial. *Journal of the American College of Cardiology*, *50*, 205–214.

Packer, M., Butler, J., Zannad, F., Filippatos, G., Ferreira, J. P., Pocock, S. J., et al. (2021). Effect of Empagliflozin on worsening heart failure events in patients with heart failure and a preserved ejection fraction: The EMPEROR-preserved trial. *Circulation*, *144*, 1284–1289.

Paulus, W. J., & Tschöpe, C. (2013). A novel paradigm for heart failure with preserved ejection fraction: Comorbidities drive myocardial dysfunction and remodeling through coronary microvascular endothelial inflammation. *Journal of the American College of Cardiology*, *62*, 263–271.

Peng, X., Chen, B., Lim, C. C., & Sawyer, D. B. (2005). The cardiotoxicology of anthracycline chemotherapeutics: Translating molecular mechanism into preventative medicine. *Molecular Interventions*, *5*, 163–171.

Penn, M. S. (2008). The role of leukocyte-generated oxidants in left ventricular remodeling. *The American Journal of Cardiology*, *101*, 30D–33D.

Pieske, B., Maggioni, A. P., Lam, C. S. P., Pieske-Kraigher, E., Filippatos, G., Butler, J., et al. (2017). Vericiguat in patients with worsening chronic heart failure and preserved ejection fraction: Results of the SOluble guanylate Cyclase stimulatoR in heArT failurE patientS with PRESERVED EF (SOCRATES-PRESERVED) study. *European Heart Journal*, *38*, 1119–1127.

Pieske, B., Maier, L. S., Piacentino, V., 3rd, Weisser, J., Hasenfuss, G., & Houser, S. (2002). Rate dependence of $[Na^+]_i$ and contractility in nonfailing and failing human myocardium. *Circulation*, *106*, 447–453.

Pinder, M. C., Duan, Z., Goodwin, J. S., Hortobagyi, G. N., & Giordano, S. H. (2007). Congestive heart failure in older women treated with adjuvant anthracycline chemotherapy for breast cancer. *Journal of Clinical Oncology*, *25*, 3808–3815.

Pollack, A., Kontorovich, A. R., Fuster, V., & Dec, G. W. (2015). Viral myocarditis–diagnosis, treatment options, and current controversies. *Nature Reviews. Cardiology*, *12*, 670–680.

Ponikowski, P., Voors, A. A., Anker, S. D., Bueno, H., Cleland, J. G. F., Coats, A. J. S., et al. (2016). ESC Guidelines for the diagnosis and treatment of acute and chronic heart failure: The Task Force for the diagnosis and treatment of acute and chronic heart failure of the European Society of Cardiology (ESC) developed with the special contribution of the Heart Failure Association (HFA) of the ESC. *European Heart Journal*, *37*, 2129–2200.

Redfield, M. M., Chen, H. H., Borlaug, B. A., Semigran, M. J., Lee, K. L., Lewis, G., et al. (2013). Effect of phosphodiesterase-5 inhibition on exercise capacity and clinical status in heart failure with preserved ejection fraction: A randomized clinical trial. *Journal of the American Medical Association*, *309*, 1268–1277.

Richards, D. A., Aronovitz, M. J., Liu, P., Martin, G. L., Tam, K., Pande, S., et al. (2021). CRD-733, a novel PDE9 (phosphodiesterase 9) inhibitor, reverses pressure overload-induced heart failure. *Circulation. Heart Failure*, *14*, e007300. https://doi.org/10.1161/circheartfailure.120.007300.

Rousseau, M. F., Pouleur, H., Cocco, G., & Wolff, A. A. (2005). Comparative efficacy of ranolazine versus atenolol for chronic angina pectoris. *American Journal of Cardiology*, *95*, 311–316.

Roy, C., Slimani, A., de Meester, C., Amzulescu, M., Pasquet, A., Vancraeynest, D., et al. (2018). Associations and prognostic significance of diffuse myocardial fibrosis by cardiovascular magnetic resonance in heart failure with preserved ejection fraction. *Journal of Cardiovascular Magnetic Resonance*, *20*, 55.

Runte, K. E., Bell, S. P., Selby, D. E., Häußler, T. N., Ashikaga, T., LeWinter, M. M., et al. (2017). Relaxation and the role of calcium in isolated contracting myocardium from patients with hypertensive heart disease and heart failure with preserved ejection fraction. *Circulation. Heart Failure*, *10*, e004311. https://doi.org/10.1161/circheartfailure.117.004311.

Sabatino, J., De Rosa, S., Tammè, L., Iaconetti, C., Sorrentino, S., Polimeni, A., et al. (2020). Empagliflozin prevents doxorubicin-induced myocardial dysfunction. *Cardiovascular Diabetology*, *19*, 66. https://doi.org/10.1186/s12933-020-01040-5.

Saiki, H., Moulay, G., Guenzel, A. J., Liu, W., Decklever, T. D., Classic, K. L., et al. (2017). Experimental cardiac radiation exposure induces ventricular diastolic dysfunction with preserved ejection fraction. *American Journal of Physiology. Heart and Circulatory Physiology*, *313*, H392–H407.

Salvatorelli, E., Menna, P., Cantalupo, E., Chello, M., Covino, E., Wolf, F. I., et al. (2015). The concomitant management of cancer therapy and cardiac therapy. *Biochimica et Biophysica Acta*, *1848*, 2727–2737.

Salvatorelli, E., Menna, P., Chello, M., Covino, E., & Minotti, G. (2017). Modeling human myocardium exposure to doxorubicin defines the risk of heart failure from low-dose doxorubicin. *The Journal of Pharmacology and Experimental Therapeutics*, *362*, 263–270.

Santos-Gallego, C., Requena-Ibanez, J. A., San Antonio, R., Garcia-Ropero, A., Ishikawa, K., Watanabe, S., et al. (2021). Empagliflozin ameliorates diastolic dysfunction and left ventricular fibrosis/stiffness in nondiabetic heart failure: A multimodality study. *JACC. Cardiovascular Imaging*, *14*, 393–407.

Savarese, G., Stolfo, D., Sinagra, G., & Lund, L. H. (2021). Heart failure with mid-range or mildly reduced ejection fraction. *Nature Reviews. Cardiology*, *1*, 17. https://doi.org/10.1038/s41569-021-00605-5.

Schwinger, R. H., Munch, G., Bolck, B., Karczewski, P., Krause, E. G., & Erdmann, E. (1999). Reduced Ca(2+)-sensitivity of SERCA 2a in failing human myocardium due to reduced serin-16 phospholamban phosphorylation. *Journal of Molecular and Cellular Cardiology*, *31*, 479–491.

Shi, J., Abdelwahid, E., & Wei, L. (2011). Apoptosis in anthracycline cardiomyopathy. *Current Pediatric Reviews*, 7, 329–336.

Simmonds, S. J., Cuijpers, I., Heymans, S., & Jones, E. A. V. (2020). Cellular and molecular differences between HFpEF and HFreEF: A step ahead in an improved pathological understanding. *Cell*, *9*, 242. https://doi.org/10.3390/cells9010242.

Singh, A., Steadman, C. D., Khan, J. N., Reggiardo, G., & McCann, G. P. (2016). Effect of late sodium current inhibition on MRI measured diastolic dysfunction in aortic stenosis: A pilot study. *BMC Research Notes*, *9*, 64. https://doi.org/10.1186/s13104-016-1874-0.

Smith, L. A., Cornelius, V. R., Plummer, C. J., Levitt, G., Verrill, M., Canney, P., et al. (2010). Cardiotoxicity of anthracycline agents for the treatment of cancer: systematic review and meta-analysis of randomised controlled trials. *BMC Cancer*, *10*, 337–351.

Sokolove, P. M. (1994). Interactions of adriamycin aglycones with mitochondria may mediate adriamycin cardiotoxicity. *The International Journal of Biochemistry*, *26*, 1341–1350.

Solomon, S. D., McMurray, J. J. V., Anand, I. S., Ge, J., Lam, C. S. P., Maggioni, A. P., et al. (2019). Angiotensin–neprilysin inhibition in heart failure with preserved ejection fraction. *The New England Journal of Medicine*, *381*, 1609–1620.

Solomon, S. D., Zile, M., Pieske, B., Voors, A., Shah, A., & Kraigher-Krainer, E. (2012). Prospective comparison of ARNI with ARB on management of heart failUre with preserved ejection fracTion (PARAMOUNT) investigators. The angiotensin receptor neprilysin inhibitor LCZ696 in heart failure with preserved ejection fraction: A phase 2 double blind randomised controlled trial. *Lancet*, *380*, 1387–1395.

Song, J., Yan, R., Wu, Z., Li, J., Yan, M., Hao, X., et al. (2017). (13)N-Ammonia PET/CT detection of myocardial perfusion abnormalities in beagle dogs after local heart irradiation. *Journal of Nuclear Medicine*, *58*, 605–610.

Springer, J., Azer, J., Hua, R., Robbins, C., Adamczyk, A., McBoyle, S., et al. (2012). The natriuretic peptides BNP and CNP increase heart rate and electrical conduction by stimulating ionic currents in the sinoatrial node and atrial myocardium following activation of guanylyl cyclase-linked natriuretic peptide receptors. *Journal of Molecular and Cellular Cardiology*, *52*, 1122–1134.

Stone, P. H. (2008). Ranolazine: New paradigm for management of myocardial ischemia, myocardial dysfunction, and arrhythmias. *Cardiology Clinics*, *26*, 603–614.

Strongman, H., Gadd, S., Matthews, A., Mansfield, K. E., Stanway, S., Lyon, A. R., et al. (2019). Medium and long-term risks of specific cardiovascular diseases in survivors of 20 adult cancers: A population-based cohort study using multiple linked UK electronic health records databases. *Lancet*, *394*, 1041–1054.

Swain, S. M., Whaley, F. S., & Ewer, M. S. (2003). Congestive heart failure in patients treated with doxorubicin: A retrospective analysis of three trials. *Cancer*, *97*, 2869–2879.

Swain, S. M., Whaley, F. S., Gerber, M. C., Weisberg, S., York, M., Spicer, D., et al. (1997). Cardioprotection with dexrazoxane for doxorubicin-containing therapy in advanced breast cancer. *Journal of Clinical Oncology*, *15*, 1318–1332.

Tebbi, C. K., London, W. B., Friedman, D., Villaluna, D., De Alarcon, P. A., Constine, L. S., et al. (2007). Dexrazoxane-associated risk for acute myeloid leukemia/myelodysplastic syndrome and other secondary malignancies in pediatric Hodgkin's disease. *Journal of Clinical Oncology*, *25*, 493–500.

Thavendiranathan, P., & Nolan, M. T. (2017). An emerging epidemic: Cancer and heart failure. *Clinical Science*, *131*, 113–121.

Thireau, J., Karam, S., Roberge, S., Roussel, J., Aimond, F., Cassan, C., et al. (2014). B-adrenergic blockade combined with subcutaneous B-type natriuretic peptide: A promising approach to reduce ventricular arrhythmia in heart failure? *Heart*, *100*, 833–841.

Uthman, L., Baartscheer, A., Schumacher, C. A., Fiolet, J. W. T., Kuschma, M. C., Hollmann, M. W., et al. (2018). Direct cardiac actions of sodium glucose cotransporter 2 inhibitors target pathogenic mechanisms underlying heart failure in diabetic patients. *Frontiers in Physiology*, *9*, 1575. https://doi.org/10.3389/fphys.2018.01575.

van Heerebeek, L., Hamdani, N., Falcão-Pires, I., Leite-Moreira, A. F., Begieneman, M. P., Bronzwaer, J. G., et al. (2012). Low myocardial protein kinase G activity in heart failure with preserved ejection fraction. *Circulation*, *126*, 830–839.

van Heerebeek, L., & Paulus, W. J. (2016). Understanding heart failure with preserved ejection fraction: Where are we today? *Netherlands Heart Journal*, *24*, 227–236.

Varzideh, F., Kansakar, U., & Santulli, G. (2021). SGLT2 inhibitors in cardiovascular medicine. *European Heart Journal - Cardiovascular Pharmacotherapy*, 7, e67–e68. https://doi.org/10.1093/ehjcvp/pvab039.

Vásquez-Vivar, J., Martasek, P., Hogg, N., Masters, B. S., Pritchard, K. A., Jr., & Kalyanaraman, B. (1997). Endothelial nitric oxide synthase-dependent superoxide generation from adriamycin. *Biochemistry*, *36*, 11293–11297.

Vaughn, D. J., Palmer, S. C., Carver, J. R., Jacobs, L. A., & Mohler, E. R. (2008). Cardiovascular risk in long-term survivors of testicular cancer. *Cancer*, *112*, 1949–1953.

Venkataraman, R., Belardinelli, L., Blackburn, B., Heo, J., & Iskandrian, A. E. (2009). A study of the effects of ranolazine using automated quantitative analysis of serial myocardial perfusion images. *JACC. Cardiovascular Imaging*, *2*, 1301–1309.

Wan, S.-H., McKie, P. M., Slusser, J. P., Burnett, J. C., Jr., Hodge, D. O., & Chen, H. H. (2021). Effects of phosphodiesterase V inhibition alone and in combination with BNP on cardiovascular and renal response to volume load in human preclinical diastolic dysfunction. *Physiological Reports*, *9*, e14974. https://doi.org/10.14814/phy2.14974.

Xia, Y., Chen, Z., Chen, A., Fu, M., Dong, Z., Hu, K., et al. (2017). LCZ696 improves cardiac function via alleviating Drp1-mediated mitochondrial dysfunction in mice with doxorubicin-induced dilated cardiomyopathy. *Journal of Molecular and Cellular Cardiology*, *108*, 138–148.

Yeh, E. T. H., Ewer, M. S., Moslehi, J., Dlugosz-Danecka, M., Banchs, J., Chang, H. M., et al. (2019). Mechanisms and clinical course of cardiovascular toxicity of cancer treatment I. Oncology. *Seminars in Oncology*, *46*, 397–402.

Yuan, Y.-P., Ma, Z.-G., Zhang, X., Xu, S.-C., Zeng, X.-F., Yang, Z., et al. (2018). CTRP3 protected against doxorubicin-induced cardiac dysfunction, inflammation and cell death via activation of Sirt1. *Journal of Molecular and Cellular Cardiology*, *114*, 38–47.

Zaid, M. A., Gathirua-Mwangi, W. G., Fung, C., Monahan, P. O., El-Charif, O., Williams, A. M., et al. (2018). Clinical and genetic risk factors for adverse metabolic outcomes in North American testicular cancer survivors. *Journal of the National Comprehensive Cancer Network*, *16*, 257–265.

Zamorano, J. L., Gottfridsson, C., Asteggiano, R., Atar, D., Badimon, L., et al. (2020). The cancer patient and cardiology. *European Journal of Heart Failure*, *22*, 2290–2309.

Zamorano, J. L., Lancellotti, P., Rodriguez Muñoz, D., Aboyans, V., Asteggiano, R., Galderisi, M., et al. (2016). 2016 ESC Position Paper on cancer treatments and cardiovascular toxicity developed under the auspices of the ESC Committee for Practice Guidelines: The Task Force for cancer treatments and cardiovascular toxicity of the European Society of Cardiology (ESC). *European Heart Journal*, *37*, 2768–2801.

Zile, M. R., & Gaasch, W. H. (1990). Mechanical loads and the isovolumic and filling indices of left ventricular relaxation. *Progress in Cardiovascular Diseases*, *32*, 333–346.

Zile, M. R., Gottdiener, J. S., Hetzel, S. J., McMurray, J. J., Komajda, M., McKelvie, R., et al. (2011). Prevalence and significance of alterations in cardiac structure and function in patients with heart failure and a preserved ejection fraction. *Circulation*, *124*, 2491–2501.

FSC
www.fsc.org
MIX
Papier | Fördert
gute Waldnutzung
FSC® C083411

Kolibri 360 GmbH
Ferdinand-Jühlke-Straße 7
99095 Erfurt, Deutschland
produktsicherheit@kolibri360.de